NEUROUROLOGY AND URODYNAMICS

EDITORS:

Subbarao V. Yalla, M.D.

Associate Professor Of Urology, Harvard Medical School;
Chief, Department of Urology, Veterans Administration
Medical Center, West Roxbury, Massachusetts
Associate Surgeon
Brigham & Women's Hospital
Boston, Massachusetts

Edward J. McGuire, M.D.

Professor of Surgery and Head, Section of Urology,
University of Michigan Medical School, Ann Arbor,
Michigan

Ahmad Elbadawi, M.D.

Professor of Pathology and Urology,
State University of New York—Health Science
Center, Syracuse, New York

Jerry G. Blaivas, M.D.

Associate Professor of Urology, College of Physicians
and Surgeons of Columbia University; Director of
Neurourology, Columbia Presbyterian Medical Center,
New York, New York

NEUROUROLOGY AND URODYNAMICS

Principles and Practice

Macmillan Publishing Company
NEW YORK

Collier Macmillan Canada, Inc.
TORONTO

Collier Macmillan Publishers
LONDON

Printed in the United States of America

Macmillan Publishing Company
866 Third Avenue, New York, New York 10022

Collier Macmillan Canada, Inc.
Collier Macmillan Publishers • London

Library of Congress Cataloging-in-Publication Data

Neurourology and urodynamics.

Includes bibliographies and index.
1. Urodynamics. 2. Urinary organs—Innervation.
3. Urinary organs—Diseases. I. Yalla, Subbarao V.
[DNLM: 1. Neurology. 2. Urination Disorders.
3. Urodynamics. 4. Urologic Diseases. WJ 100 N494]
RC901.9.N48 1988 616.6 87-21998
ISBN 0-02-430870-6

Printing: 1 2 3 4 5 6 7 8 Year: 8 9 0 1 2 3 4 5 6

Foreword

Urodynamics has been fortunate to have working within it a remarkable group of clinical and basic scientists. New instrumentation and new insights have led to convincing descriptions of the physiology of normal and abnormal micturition. Treatment and functional rehabilitation, a rarity in neurology, has blossomed in neurourology as a result of these new areas of understanding as well as the advances in self-catheterization, neuropharmacology, and mechanical aids.

Gathering such a varied and distinguished group together for this volume is in itself an event of note. The solution to their differences of terminology must be here. We welcome this monumental collaboration and hope and trust that it will become the premier reference work in the field.

RUBEN F. GITTES, M.D.
Formerly Elliott C. Cutler Professor of Urological Surgery
Chairman, Harvard Program in Urology (Longwood Area)
Chief of Urology
Brigham & Women's Hospital
Boston

Currently Chairman, Department of Surgery and Urologic Surgeon
Scripps Clinic and Research Foundation,
La Jolla, California

Foreword

When four of the leaders in neurourodynamics determine to publish a book covering every aspect of the field in detail, we can be sure that it will be the standard for years to come.

Look at the titles of the chapters listed in the table of contents. Clearly, the editors have selected the experts in each of the many intriguing, important, and practical subdivisions within the larger field. Each of these authors has done original work in his or her field of expertise and is the acknowledged authority in that field.

This book is not one to be read from cover to cover. Rather, it will be used by most to find answers to specific clinical questions; these same readers will return to it again and again, however, to obtain the scientific background needed to interpret new problems—whether they arise in a patient or the laboratory.

The first section provides the experimental basis for understanding the myoneurophysiology, electrophysiology, and mechanics of the urinary tract; this information then leads to the second section, which is concerned with diagnostic techniques. There follow practical sections on the management of specific disorders using modern techniques, both surgical and nonsurgical.

All areas of agreement and controversy are covered here in a readable style with illustrations that are easily understood, making this volume a valuable partner in the laboratory, the clinic, and the office.

FRANK HINMAN, JR., M.D.
Clinical Professor of Urology
University of California
San Francisco

Preface

The art of practicing urology has come a long way and is now recognized as a surgical specialty with several ever-growing scientific dimensions. One area of such growth is "urodynamics and neurourology." For a number of reasons this area has often been regarded as complex, confusing, and of limited value. Despite this attitude, there has been substantial progress in urodynamic technique and application as a result of collaborative efforts by urologists and others. Disagreement regarding various aspects of urodynamics has accompanied progress and, as expected, has generated debate that has shed light on numerous issues.

Only a decade ago urologists were reluctant to get involved in cystometry and urinary flowmetry, which were considered totally alien to their regular everyday clinical practice. However, because of innumerable technological advances and the continued cooperative efforts of the disciplines of engineering, gynecology, gerontology, psychiatry, anatomy, pathology, pharmacology, neurology, neurosurgery, and of course urology, the subspecialty of urodynamics and neurourology has attracted the clinical urologist and has acquired its own unique identity. Present-day urologists, in consort with clinicians and scientists of other disciplines, are currently engaged actively in the analysis of urinary tract function and dysfunction in scientific and clinically applicable urodynamic and neurourologic terms. It is being done in the privacy of institutional research laboratories and clinical practices; through numerous symposia, workshops, and publications in several journals; and most importantly through incessant dialogues and exchange of information at national and international meetings. The subspecialty of urodynamics and neurourology has certainly gathered momentum, has attracted workers in many clinical and basic science disciplines, and is here to stay. Ideas and hypotheses continuously brought up by the several disciplines involved have been generating healthy and sometimes heated debates in private and public forums. The wide spectrum of involvement by all of the above disciplines has resulted in a symphonic blend of urodynamic and neurourologic information that is continually undergoing refined orchestration.

Recognizing the need to include the viewpoints of the involved disciplines in our book, we the editors have chosen prominent experts in all subdivisions of this field of urodynamics and neurourology. The scope of this compilation is based on our conviction that sound clinical and research practice of urodynamics and neurourology today requires a strong understanding of both the basic science and the clinical issues of this field. All contributors have recognized the intended scope of the book and therefore have made every effort to include the recent and important contributions in their respective areas, acknowledging significant contributions of previous workers. Three sections of the book deal with terminology, techniques of evaluation, the disease states, and the principles of management; such sectional arrangement inevitably has produced some overlap of content. Readers may also identify debatable and controversial views in some chapters; we believe, however, that such views are necessary to progress.

Finally, we express our deep gratitude to all our contributors without whose cooperation this endeavor could not have been completed. To our publishers we are indebted for the opportunity to produce this type of presentation, which we believe will remain for many years the most comprehensive source of reference to the researcher in, and the urologist who is actively engaged in or is planning to start a research program in or a sound practice of neurourology and urodynamics.

Subbarao V. Yalla, M.D.
Edward J. McGuire, M.D.
Ahmad Elbadawi, M.D.
Jerry G. Blaivas, M.D.

Acknowledgments

We wish to express our gratitude to all those who have participated in the completion of our book. Our sincere thanks to all our colleagues who have contributed their expertise so generously despite their demanding daily schedules. We especially thank our secretaries at the Veterans Administration Medical Center, West Roxbury, Massachusetts: Jean Federico during the early planning stages and Kathryn Balsavich during the remaining and important stages of this project. We are grateful to both of them for their patience and time. We also thank Leslie Oliver, R.N. from the Neurourology Laboratory at Columbia University College of Physicians and Surgeons, New York; Mona Gardon and Donna Maslak of the Department of Urology at the University of Ann Arbor, Michigan; and Laurie Brandt of the Department of Pathology, State University of New York Health Science Center, Syracuse, New York.

Finally, we express our deep sense of gratitude to our wives and our children for their patience and understanding during the demands of our profession and for their unselfish emotional support during the entire project.

S.V.Y.
E.J.McG.
A.E.
J.G.B.

Contributors

Abel, Gene G., M.D.
Professor of Psychiatry
Emory University School of Medicine
Atlanta, GA 30322

Barrett, David M., M.D.
Professor of Urology
Mayo Medical School
Consultant, Department of Urology
Mayo Clinic and Mayo Foundation
Rochester, MN 55905

Blaivas, Jerry G., M.D.
Associate Professor of Urology
College of Physicians and Surgeons
of Columbia University
Director of Neurourology
Columbia Presbyterian Medical Center
New York, NY 10032

Blendinger, Doris, Ph.D.
President, Stress Management, Inc.
P.O. Box 521
Whitestone, NY 11357

Bloom, Joseph W., Ph.D.
Assistant Professor of Surgery
McMaster University
Faculty of Health Sciences
Hamilton, Ontario L8N3Z5 Canada

Coolsaet, Bo, M.D., Ph.D.
Professor and Chairman
Department of Urology
Sint Josefziekenhuis
2080 Kapellen
Antwerp, Belgium

Diokno, Ananias C., M.D.
Clinical Professor of Urology
University of Michigan
Chief of Urology
William Beaumont Hospital
Ann Arbor, MI 48109

Dyro, Frances M., M.D.
Director of Electro Diagnostic Lab
Brockton/West Roxbury
Veterans Administration Medical Center
1400 VFW Parkway
West Roxbury, MA 02132

Elbadawi, Ahmad, M.D.
Professor of Pathology and Urology
State University of New York
Health Science Center
Syracuse, NY 13210

Fam Bushra A., M.D.
Acting Chief
Spinal Cord Injury Service
Brockton/West Roxbury
Veterans Administration Medical Center
1400 VFW Parkway
West Roxbury, MA 02132

Furlow, William L., M.D.
Director, The Center for Urological
Treatment and Research
2201 Murphy Avenue, Suite 115
Nashville, TN 37203

Giroux, Janet A., R.N.
Spinal Cord Injury Center
Veterans Administration Medical Center
Stanford University
Palo Alto, CA 94304

Goldwasser, Benad, M.D.
Fellow in Neurourology and Genitourinary
Prosthetics
Mayo Clinic and Mayo Foundation
Rochester, MN 55905

Griffiths, Derek F., Ph.D.
Senior Lecturer, Dept. of Urology
Dept. of Biological and
Medical Physics
Erasamus University Rotterdam

Postbus 1738, 300 Dr. Rotterdam
The Netherlands

Hadley, Roger, M.D.
Assistant Professor of Urology
Loma Linda University
School of Medicine
11370 Anderson, Suite 1100
Loma Linda, CA 92354

Jonas, Udo, M.D.
Professor of Urology
Dept. of Urology
Academic Hospital
Leiden, The Netherlands

Kramer, August, E.J.L., Ph.D.
Dept. of Urology
Academic Hospital
Leiden, The Netherlands

Krane, Robert J., M.D.
Professor and Chairman
Department of Urology
Boston University School of Medicine
Boston, MA 02118

Levin, Robert M., Ph.D.
Research Associate
Professor of Urology
University of Pennsylvania
3010 Ravdin Courtyard Bldg.
Philadelphia, PA 19104

Loughlin, Kevin, M.D.
Assistant Professor of Urology Surgery
Harvard Medical School
Staff Physician in Urology
Brigham & Women's Hospital
75 Francis Street
Boston, MA 02115

McGuire, Edward J., M.D.
Professor of Surgery and
Head, Section of Urology,
University of Michigan Medical School,
Ann Arbor, MI 48109

Malkowicz, S. Bruce, M.D.
Chief Resident in Urology
University of Pennsylvania
3400 Spruce Street
Philadelphia, PA 19194

Perkash, Inder, M.D.
Professor of Surgery
Paralyzed Veterans of America
Professor of Spinal Cord Injury
Stanford University
Chief of Spinal Cord Injury
Veterans Administration Medical Center
Palo Alto, CA 94304

Raz, Shlomo, M.D.
Professor of Urology
University of California
Center for the Health Sciences
Room BU 134F
Los Angeles, CA 90024

Regnier, Claude H., M.Sc.
Product Development Specialist
R.L. Medical Devices Corp.
One Blue Hill Plaza, Suite 815
Pearl River, NY 10965
Formerly,
Eris Medical Technology, Inc.
1308 Springfield Avenue
New Providence, NJ 07974

Resnick, Neil M, M.D.
Gerontologist, Beth Israel Hospital
Brigham & Women's Hospital
75 Francis Street
Boston, MA 02115
Instructor in Medicine
Harvard Medical School
Boston, MA 02115

Sarkarati, Mehdi, M.D.
Assistant Chief, Academic Affairs
Spinal Cord Injury Service
Brockton/West Roxbury
Veterans Administration Medical Center
1400 VFW Parkway
West Roxbury, MA 02132
Instructor in Surgery
Harvard Medical School, Boston, MA 02115

Schmidt, Richard A., M.D.
Associate Professor of Urology
University of California
San Francisco, CA 94143

Siroky, Mike B., M.D.
Associate Professor of Urology
Boston University School of Medicine
Chief of Urology

Veterans Administration Medical Center
Boston, MA 02130

Susset, Jacques G., M.D.
Professor of Urology
Brown University
Chief of Urology
Veterans Administration Medical Center
Providence, RI 02908

Talalla, Andrew, M.D.
Professor of Neurological Surgery
McMaster University
Faculty of Health Sciences
Hamilton, Ontario L8N3Z5, Canada

Tanagho, Emil A., M.D.
Professor and Chairman
The Department of Urology
University of California
San Francisco, CA 94143

Wein, Alan J., M.D.
Professor and Chairman
The Division of Urology
University of Pennsylvania
3400 Spruce Street
Philadelphia, PA 19194

Woodside, Jeffrey R., M.D.
Professor of Urology
University of Texas Medical School at Houston
P.O. Box 20708
Houston, TX 77225

Yalla, Subbarao V., M.D.
Chief of Urology
Brockton/West Roxbury
Veterans Administration Medical Center
1400 VFW Parkway
West Roxbury, MA 02132
Associate Surgeon
Brigham & Women's Hospital
Boston, MA 02115
Associate Professor of Urology
Harvard Medical School
Boston, MA 02115

Zimmern, Philippe E., M.D.
Chief Resident in Urology
University of California
Center for the Health Sciences
Los Angeles, CA 90024

Contents

Section Four *PHARMACOLOGY, REHABILITATION, AND OTHER METHODS OF MANAGEMENT*

NEUROUROLOGY AND URODYNAMICS

Section One
Basic Sciences

Neuromuscular Mechanisms of Micturition

1

AHMAD ELBADAWI, M.D.

The urinary bladder serves the dual function of storage and periodic expulsion of urine. During storage the urinary conduit remains closed by the urethral sphincteric mechanism, to prevent untimely leakage of urine while the bladder becomes progressively distended, and allow occasional withholding of urine when it is distended to capacity. With the onset of voiding, the bladder contracts and the urethral conduit is opened to establish flow of the urinary stream. During the storage and expulsion phases of micturition, the ureterovesical junctions remain competent, thereby preventing vesicoureteral reflux, at least in man.

The perpetual repetition of both phases of micturition consistently, efficiently, and with precision depends on the optimally constructed smooth musculature of the bladder, urethra, and ureterovesical junctions, supplemented by the striated urethral sphincter, as well as a complex central and peripheral neural control of both the smooth and striated muscle systems (*1*). In this chapter, current knowledge of the anatomic, structural, pharmacologic, and physiologic bases of the neuromuscular mechanism of micturition in experimental animals and man are reviewed.

ANATOMIC BASIS

The Muscular Apparatus of Micturition

Current knowledge of the muscular anatomy of the urinary bladder and urethra is derived from many detailed dissection and histotopographic studies, mainly of human organs (*2–10*). From collective analysis of these reports, one can reconstruct a nearly unified concept of the anatomic organization of the mammalian vesicourethral muscularis, particularly in man. As yet, the functional correlates of this concept are not fully established. This can be explained in part by the different degrees of emphasis placed by different authors on the functional importance of certain muscle bundles or bundle arrangements. Moreover, muscle bundles of one region that are in direct anatomic continuity with those of another, e.g., in the bladder body and base, or the base and urethra, may perform physiologically different functions during the same phase of the voiding cycle.

Based on available embryologic, anatomic, neuromorphologic, physiologic, and pharmacologic studies in both experimental animals and man, Elbadawi (*1,11,12*) proposed that the mammalian muscular apparatus of micturition is composed of four functional units, each of which appears to have a specific role in both the storage and expulsion phases of micturition. These uints include three smooth and one striated muscular components, i.e., the bladder body detrusor, lissosphincter, ureterotrigonal muscle, and urethral rhabdosphincter (Fig. 1–1).

Bladder Body Detrusor. The bladder body detrusor (*3,4,9*) is composed of a complex array of interlacing muscle bundles of variable thickness. These bundles extend throughout the bladder wall, continually changing their planes and orientation and

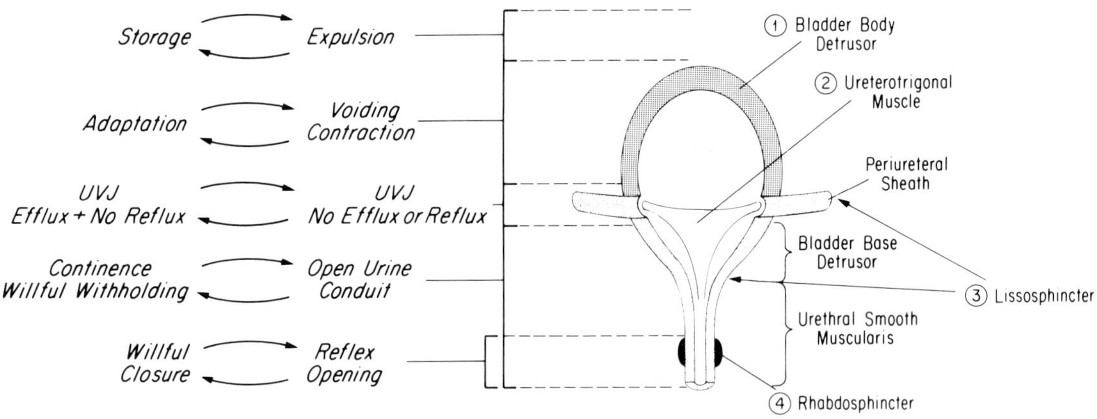

Figure 1–1. The four units of the micturition muscular apparatus (bladder body detrusor, lissosphincter, ureterotrigonal muscle, and rhabdosphincter) and their function in the storage and expulsion phases of micturition.

freely criss-crossing and interlacing with each other, without arrangement as discrete layers. Although Hunter's description (*4*) of the body detrusor implies a constant pattern of bundle decussation and exchange of planes, it is more likely that its bundle organization varies individually. In some experimental animals, particularly the cat, the ventral aspect of the body detrusor is marked by a stout vertical midline bundle that extends from the dome of the bladder almost to its junction with the urethra and is joined by transversely oriented bundles on each side.

Lissosphincter. As proposed by Elbadawi (*11,12*), the lissosphincter comprises the bladder base detrusor, its caudal extensions into the urethra, and its cranial extensions to ensheathe the vesical end of both ureters.

The Bladder Base Component. The concept of functional division of the detrusor into base and body units was introduced on the basis of morphologic patterns of its intrinsic muscular innervation by Elbadawi and Schenk in 1966 (*13*), as a substitute for the traditional units of detrusor and trigone that had prevailed in the earlier literature (*14*). According to this concept, the base is the part of the detrusor, in all walls of the bladder, that lies below the level of entrance of the ureters into its dorsal wall. Although the body and base detrusor are not separated by any identifiable anatomic or histologic boundary, their existence as two units of the muscular apparatus of micturition of different and distinct physiopharmacologic properties has been confirmed in all mammalian species so far studied, including man (*11*). Consequently, the body–base concept has become a key element in all experimental and clinical studies on micturition and its control mechanisms (*15*).

The bladder base region is sizable in man but tends to be short in experimental animals, particularly the rat. The junction of the base and the urethra is well defined in most species, although in some, particularly the rabbit, it is gradual and almost imperceptible.

In the human bladder base, the interlacing detrusor bundles are organized into a ventral and a dorsal group (*2,5,6*). The ventral group includes the following bundles: (a) Two lateral longitudinal bundles that blend together at the level of the bladder neck to form the precervical arc. This arc has a posterior concavity and lies superficial to, but abuts closely against, the detrusor loop (*vide infra*). (b) An outer anterior longitudinal bundle that inserts mainly into the precervical arc. Some fibers of this bundle continue into the retropubic connective tissue to secure a pubic attachment. (c) A slender submucosal plexiform inner anterior longitudinal bundle that extends into the anterior urethral wall as its inner longitudinal fibers.

The dorsal group of base detrusor bundles comprises a heavy posterior and two posterolateral longitudinal bundles. The posterior longitudinal bundle is the most prominent, inserts in part into the deep transverse trigonal muscle (*vide infra*), and is anchored in the midline to the cranial part of the prostate in men or the urethrovaginal septum in women; some lateral fibers of the bundle continue into the external "layer" of the urethral muscularis. The posterolateral longitudinal bundles extend along both sides of the posterior longitudinal bundle, each splitting at the ureteral orifice into a medial and lateral part, called interna and externa by Gil Vernet (*2*). The medial parts of the two sides continue into the deep trigonal muscle, and the lateral parts arch anteriorly to form the detrusor loop, a stout horseshoe-shaped muscular loop with dorsocephalic concavity. The detrusor loop fibers splay out into two bites that lie anteriorly in the base: (a) a distal deeper loop embedded in the urethrovesical junction (described by Gil Vernet (*2*), and (b) a shorter, more cephalic, superficial loop (Heiss's loop) (*10*). These two loops lie, respectively, caudal and cranial to the precervical arc but at a deeper plane in the base wall.

Woodburne (*9*) denied the existence of any annular muscular arrangement surrounding the bladder neck and stated that although arching fibers exist at this level they arch away from the bladder neck. He also described dense elastic tissue in the submucosa and between muscle bundles of the bladder neck to which he attributed continent closure of the vesical outlet and proximal urethra.

Urethral Smooth Muscularis. In most species the prostate is related to the most cranial portion of the male urethra, immediately caudal to the bladder neck. In the male cat, however, the prostate lies very deep in the pelvis, with a few centimeters stretch of preprostatic urethra separating it from the bladder neck.

The following is a simplified version of Young's description (*10*) of the human urethral musculature. Smooth muscle bundles extend from the base detrusor into the entire sphincteric urethra, which includes the "posterior" urethra in men and almost the whole urethra in women. These bundles are arranged in several bundles that are oriented longitudinally (or helically) and circularly.

Urethral Longitudinal Fibers. In men, urethral longitudinal fibers consist of two main groups: (a) the vesicocervical fibers, which extend from the level of the bladder neck to that of the verumontanum; and (b) the prostatourethral fibers, which extend from the latter to the level of the caudal prostate. The two fiber groups are not distinctly separable in the female urethra.

The vesicocervical fibers include inner submucosal and outer longitudinal fibers. The *inner submucosal fibers* consist of three groups, named according to their anatomic positions: (a) the anterior group, arising from the inner longitudinal bundle of the base; (b) two lateral slim bundles, arising from the inner lateral longitudinal base detrusor bundles; and (c) the posterior group, representing the caudal extension of the superficial trigone (*vide infra*) and supplemented by fibers derived from the deep trigonal muscle. All inner submucosal fibers peter out and are partially inserted into the urethral mucosa at the level of the verumontanum. The *outer longitudinal fibers* arise from the posterior longitudinal bundle of the base detrusor and extend (as the vesicoprostatourethral fibers) along the entire length of the male sphincteric urethra. Other similarly oriented fibers of this group lie external (i.e., superficial) to the urethral rhabdosphincter.

The prostatourethral fibers include a single posterior and two anterolateral bundles that arise in the submucosa of the prostatic urethra and end in that of the membranous urethra. The posterior bundle is densely interlaced with elastic fibers and fans out near its termination. The two anterolateral bundles have a common origin at the verumontanum.

Urethral Circular Fibers. The urethral circular fibers have been emphasized by Hutch (*5*) who characterized them as the "heart of the sphincteric urethra." The following groups of urethral circular muscle fibers have been described in the literature. One group—the internal sphincter of Gil Vernet (*2*)—has been demonstrated, particularly in men, immediately below the bladder neck in the form of a ring that is separate and distinct from both the detrusor loop and the deep trigonal muscle. Fibers of this group are sandwiched between the longitudinal vescocervical fibers of the urethral muscularis caudally and the transversely oriented precervical arc of the bladder base cranially. Hutch described the structure commonly known as the capsule of the prostate as the outer circular muscle layer of the prostatic urethra, which he believed to be the involuntary urethral sphincter that maintains constant closure of the urethra (*5*). A well-developed circular muscle layer forms an arc in the anterior wall of the membranous urethra. This muscle embraces the prostatourethral longitudinal fibers and lies internal (deep) to the urethral rhabdosphincter. Another slender submucosal circular muscle ring lies 0.5 cm distal to the inferior margin of the membranous urethra; this muscle probably does not belong to the sphincteric urethral muscularis but might act as a sphincter of ducts of Cowper's glands (*10*).

In women, longitudinal muscle fibers extend along the whole urethra on its anterior and lateral walls and are continuous with the inner plexiform "layer" of the base detrusor. Posteriorly, some external longitudinal fibers also extend from the base detrusor along the entire length of the urethra. When contracting, both groups of muscle fibers participate in shortening of the female urethra, thereby reducing urethral resistance. Although circular muscle fibers are present throughout the entire female urethra, they are prominent only in its middle third (*2*).

Periureteral Sheath Component. In man as well as most experimental animals, cranial extensions of muscle fibers of the bladder base component of the lissosphincter surround all three portions of the distal ureter, i.e., prehiatal (juxtavesical), hiatal (intravesical), and posthiatal ("submucosal"), in the form of two periureteral sheaths: the superficial sheath (including Waldeyer's sheath around the prehiatal segment) and the deep sheath (which derives some of its fibers from the ureteral muscularis) (*16,17*). The two sheaths can be demonstrated grossly by microdissection as well as histologically in sections of the ureterovesical junction. Their component muscle fibers are oriented longitudinally and partially helically around the ureter. The dual periureteral sheath concept has been confirmed anatomically, histologically, and surgically in man (*18,19*).

Ureterotrigonal Muscle. On each side of the human bladder the predominantly longitudinal muscularis of the distal ureters fans out at the ureteral orifices, extending beyond their floor into the suburothelial layer of the trigonal region, to and past the vesicourethral junction (*11*). Muscular extensions from both sides blend to form a thin triangular sheet of thin, compact muscle bundles, the apex of which is at the vesicourethral junction. This sheet has been designated as the superficial trigone (*20*) or simply as the trigonal muscle (*11,21*). Though considered by some (*20*) as a crucial factor in maintaining competence of the ureterovesical junction, this muscle is now believed (*11,21*) to serve no more than as a mechanism of mooring the distal ureter to the bladder. Slim bundles from the apex of the trigonal muscle sheet extend further caudally along the posterior wall of the proximal urethra as far as the verumontanum, to form a part of its inner longitudinal "layer."

The superficial trigonal muscle receives slim reinforcing bundles from lateral and cranial outlying bundles of the bladder base component of the lissosphincter, the underlying deep trigonal part of the lissosphincter, and cranially related bundles of the bladder body detrusor (Elbadawi, unpublished data). This muscle is difficult to dissect separately and is almost inseparably adherent to bladder base urothelium; it exists as the previously described triangular muscular sheet only in man but is represented in the cat, dog, rabbit, and rat by two flimsy suburothelial muscle bundlets that extend between the ureteral orifices and vesicourethral junction, petering out there or extending for variable distances into the cranial part of the urethral muscularis (Elbadawi, unpublished data).

Urethral Rhabdosphincter. Striated muscles related to the urethra include: (a) the urethral rhabdosphincter, which is intimately associated with the prediaphragmatic urethral smooth muscularis of both sexes in man and several animal species (*22*); and (b) the periurethral muscle, which is actually a part of the pelvic diaphragm, lies in a horizontal plane (in man), is separated from the urethral wall by a connective tissue plane, and corresponds to the so-called "external urethral sphincter" (compressor urethrae; muscle sphincter urethrae membranaceae) of classic anatomy textbooks. For many years, anatomy textbooks depicted this external urethral sphincter as the only striated muscle related to the urethra, ignoring the functionally more important rhabdosphincter (*23,24*).

Anatomic descriptions of the human rhabdosphincter are available in both old and recent literature (*25–28*). In women, this muscle forms a complete 1.5 cm long circular ring around the middle third of the urethra, extending cranially as far as the posterior bladder base. In men, the rhabdosphincter has been described as consisting of three parts: (a) a caudal part that forms a complete ring of obliquely oriented fibers around the membranous urethra and is totally integrated in its wall; (b) a middle prostatic part extending longitudinally along the anterior surface of the prostate; and (c) a cranial part, in which the direction of muscle fibers changes from a transverse arcuate orientation around the urethra to an oblique course, and extends from the anterior surface of the prostate cranially, around the bladder neck, and then behind the seminal vesicles to interdigitate with the posterior bundle of the bladder base detrusor.

Proximal extension of the rabdosphincter to the bladder neck region is supported by the constant presence of striated muscle fibers in samples of transurethral resection of the bladder neck, especially its ventral aspect (*29*). Some physiologic studies also support the existence of striated muscle in the bladder neck (*30,31*), which has been observed cystoscopically to contract in response to electrical stimulation of the pudendal nerve (*30*).

In addition to the above-mentioned three parts of the rhabdosphincter, Gil Vernet (*2*) described a more caudal portion that surrounds the proximal bulbous urethra and wraps around both Cowper's glands. He believed that this part is not functionally related to urinary continence but serves a pure genital role by squeezing secretions of Cowper's gland during ejaculation. This most caudal part probably corresponds in women to the urethrovaginal muscle that surrounds the lower one-third of the urethra and the vagina (*2*).

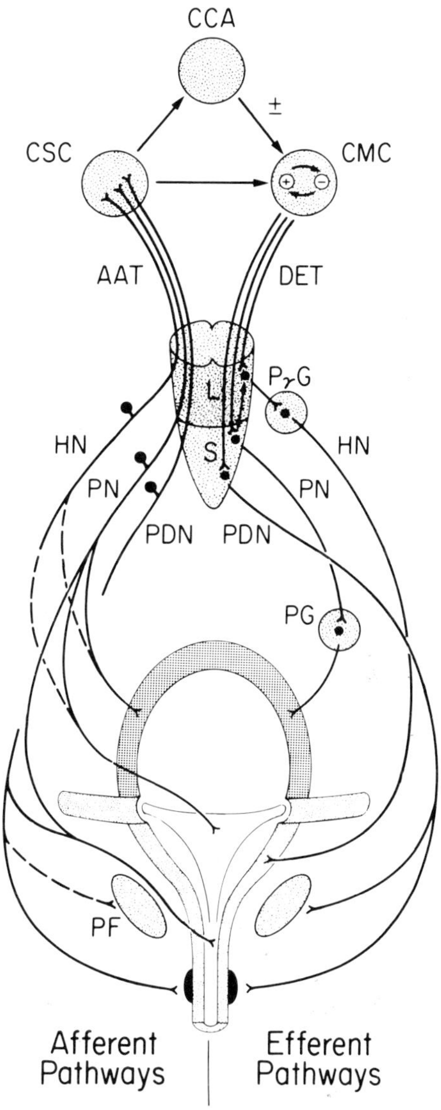

Figure 1–2. Afferent and efferent neural pathways of the micturition muscular apparatus. Dotted area = bladder body detrusor. *Cross-hatched area* = lissosphincter. *Blank area* = ureterotrigonal muscle. *Solid black area* = urethral rhabdosphincter. *PF* = pelvic floor musculature. *PDN* = pudendal nerve. *PN* = pelvic nerve. *HN* = hypogastric nerve. *S* = sacral spinal cord. *L* = lumbar spinal cord. *AAT* = ascending afferent (sensory) tracts in spinal cord. *CSC* = cerebral sensory center (s). *CCA* = cerebral and (cerebellar) control areas of micturition. *CMC* = control medullary centers. *DET* = descending efferent tracts in spinal cord. *PVG* = paravertebral sympathetic ganglion (collateral or ? in sympathetic chain). *PG* = peripheral ganglion (along autonomic nerves or branches of pelvic plexus).

Neural Pathways

Neuraxis. Extensive animal experiments, mainly in the cat, as well as some clinical studies, have led to the identification of several areas in the spinal cord and brain that exercise neural control on the act of micturition (Fig. 1–2). Spinal cord nuclei controlling vesicourethral smooth muscle and the rhabdosphincter are located in the lumbosacral region, their exact locations varying slightly in different species. In man the sympathetic autonomic nucleus is located in the intermediolateral gray matter column of

$T_{10\text{-}12}$ segments, and the parasympathetic autonomic nucleus in the same column of the $S_{2\text{-}4}$ segments (*32–37*).

It is universally accepted that efferent somatomotor innervation of the urethral rhabdosphincter originates in the sacral spinal cord. This has been confirmed by horseradish peroxidase tracing (*38*), whereby the enzyme was localized in the sacral spinal cord following its injection into the urethral rhabdosphincter or pelvic floor muscles. Motoneurons of the urethral rhabdosphincter have now been localized definitively in Onufrowicz's (Onuf's) nucleus (*39*), which lies at the anterior margin of sacral ventral horns and consists of smaller and more spherical neurons than those of the rest of the horns (*39*). The nucleus lies ventral and adjacent to the sacral parasympathetic nucleus; in both cat and rhesus monkey, the former nucleus has been described to lie one segment higher than the latter (*40,41*), which may explain the dissociation represented by involvement of the detrusor with sparing of rhabdosphincter neural control, sometimes observed in myelodysplasia and multiple sclerosis (*32,42,43*). It is also interesting that neurons of Onuf's nucleus resist degeneration in amyotrophic lateral sclerosis, unlike other somatomotor ventral horn neurons (*44*).

It now seems certain that a specific region in the pontine–mesencephalic reticular formation is the main cephalic control center of micturition (*34,35,45,46*). Through descending cephalospinal pyramidal and extrapyramidal pathways, this center exercises facilitatory or inhibitory control on spinal cord nuclei of nicturition (Fig. 1–2). Several other areas in the brain, especially the frontal cerebral cortex, hypothalamus, cerebellum, basal ganglia, and limbic system, have been shown, especially in the cat, to have modulatory, facilitatory, disinhibitory, or inhibitory influence on the pontomesencephalic micturition center. Details of the localization and interconnections of these areas of the brain are available in several reviews (*33–35,37,47*).

Central (Neuraxial) Afferent Pathways. Nerve fibers conveying afferent impulses from the organs of micturition (Fig. 1–2) (*33–35*) represent peripheral axonal projections of dorsal spinal root ganglia corresponding to the same segments as the sympathetic, parasympathetic, and rhabdosphincteric spinal cord nuclei. Central projections of the ganglia enter the spinal cord via the dorsal roots of the corresponding spinal nerves. There is sufficient evidence, however, that a proportion of afferent fibers are contained within the ventral roots in some species, especially the cat (*48*). Upon entering the spinal cord, some afferent fibers establish synaptic relays with neurons of the corresponding spinal nucleus of micturition to close segmental reflex arcs. Other fibers make relays in the dorsal horn of the gray matter of the spinal cord, cross the midline, and ascend in the anterolateral part of the contralateral white matter of the cord via the spinothalamic tract. Still other fibers ascend in the ipsilateral dorsal column of the spinal cord, in the fascicle of Goll and Burdach, making synaptic relays at some more cranially located segment of the cord with secondary sensory neurons, the axons of which cross the midline and ascend in the cord to the brain. It is generally assumed that the thalamus is the main cerebral relay station of afferent fibers conveying impulses from the organs of micturition, with probable postcentral projection to the parietal cerebral cortex.

Peripheral Efferent Pathways to Vesicourethral Smooth Muscle. Peripheral efferent sympathetic and parasympathetic innervation of the vesicourethral smooth muscle, together with the internal genital organs in both sexes, is conveyed, respectively, via the hypogastric nerve (or its equivalent) and the pelvic nerve (nervus erigens; pelvic splanchnic nerve). The exact cord connections, topographic anatomy, and branching pattern of both hypogastric and pelvic nerves vary among species (*11,12,49–56*) and are herein summarized.

Topographic Anatomy of Extrinsic Nerves. Peripheral axonal projections of neurons of the sympathetic spinal nucleus, conveyed by ventral roots of spinal nerves, are connected to the segmentally corresponding ganglia of the lumbar sympathetic chain (*11,12,51,53*). In man, centrifugal fibers of these ganglia join a lumbosacral preaortic plexiform nerve arrangement: the presacral nerve (superior hypogastric plexus), which bifurcates to form the right and left hypogastric nerves. These nerves are represented on each side by an elongate plexus of nerve strands rather than a single nerve trunk. In all animal species, peripheral branches of the lumbar sympathetic ganglia join the inferior mesenteric ganglion, which gives origin to the hypogastric nerves, either as a single trunk that shortly bifurcates (rabbit) or as two separate right and left trunks (other animal species).

Peripheral axonal projections of neurons of the parasympathetic spinal nucleus are conveyed to the bladder and urethra via the ventral roots of sacral spinal nerves and the pelvic nerves. Each pelvic nerve is usually represented by three or four trunks in man, a double trunk in the monkey, or a single trunk in other mammalian species.

At some distance from the urogenital organs, which varies with the species, the hypogastric and pelvic nerves of each side meet, branch repeatedly, and mingle to form the pelvic plexus (plexus of Frankenhäuser; inferior hypogastric plexus in man). The pelvic plexus is represented by a tridimensional network of interconnected nerve strands in the pelvic fascia lateral to the rectum, lower urinary organs, and internal genitalia. In most species, especially man, the plexus is roughly separable grossly as posterior rectal, superior ureterovesical, and inferior vasourethroprostatic (or urethrouterocervical) components. There is sufficient evidence that branches of the pelvic plexus innervate not only the ipsilateral side of the bladder and urethra but to some extent also the contralateral side across midplanes of the organs, especially dorsally (*57*).

Anatomy and Distribution of Peripheral Ganglia. Numerous central and peripheral ganglia intercept the sympathetic and parasympathetic neural pathways to the bladder and urethra (*11,12*). Central ganglia include paravertebral ganglia of the sympathetic chain and the inferior mesenteric ganglion when present, as well as inconstant neuronal cell clusters along the trunk of the pelvic and the termination of the hypogastric nerve (Atta and Elbadawi, unpublished data). Peripheral ganglia lie at or distal to the meeting point of the hypogastric and pelvic nerves, depending on the species. These ganglia lie at a short distance from, adjacent to, and within the bladder and urethra, and include the hypogastric ganglion or its equivalent, pelvic plexus ganglia, and intrinsic preterminal (mural) ganglia within the vesical and urethral walls (*11,21,55,58,59*). Because of their proximity to and intimate association with the vesical and urethral walls, the peripheral ganglia have collectively been designated as the urogenital short neuron system (*11,12,21*). The term "short" neuron emphasizes the analogous topographic distribution of sympathetic and parasympathetic components of the system and distinguishes those of the former from postganglionic sympathetic "long" neurons, the cell bodies of which lie away from the target organs within central sympathetic ganglia (*11,12,55*).

The exact contribution, if any, of central sympathetic ganglia to efferent postganglionic innervation of the bladder and urethra is yet to be determined (*49*). When present, the inferior mesenteric ganglion receives convergent branches from paravertebral lumbar sympathetic ganglia and the celiac plexus, innervates the colon, and gives origin to the hypogastric nerves (*49,55*).

In man, monkey, and dog the hypogastric ganglion is located a short distance from the bladder and urethra at the junction of the hypogastric and pelvic nerves; it supplies all nerve strands that form the ipsilateral pelvic plexus (*5*). In the male rat, the corresponding ganglion is known as the major pelvic ganglion, which is barely visible to the naked eye and lies on the craniodorsal surface of each lateral prostatic lobe (*59*). The same ganglion in the female rat is even smaller and is adherent to the cranial part of the uterine cervix (*59*). The corresponding ganglion in the male guinea pig is composed of two parts: the anterior pelvic ganglion, which lies dorsolateral to the apex of the coagulating gland, and a smaller and less defined posterior pelvic ganglion that lies dorsal to the caudal portion of the gland (*58*).

Pelvic plexus ganglia, associated with branch nerves of the pelvic plexus in all species, are small and visible only under magnification. These ganglia vary in number in different species, being most numerous and widespread in species that lack a well-defined hypogastric or pelvic ganglion, particularly in the cat (Atta and Elbadawi, unpublished data). Pelvic plexus ganglia are freely interconnected by the main strands and side branches of the pelvic plexus.

Clustered as well as individually distributed neuronal cell bodies are constantly associated with the nerves on the surface of and within the bladder and urethra, forming interconnected ganglion complexes, some of which are discernible grossly at both ureterovesical and vesicourethral junctions (*1,11,13,21,22,49,60–62*). Four components of these complexes have been recognized: the vesical, ureterovesical, vesicourethral, and vasourethroprostatic (or urethrocervical) complexes (*21,22*). Of these complexes, the ureterovesical and vesicourethral components seem to be the most prominent in all mammalian species so far studied. The bladder base component of the lissosphincter is supplied largely by the ureterovesical and to some extent the vesicourethral components, whereas the urethral component is innervated cranially by the vesicourethral and caudally by the vasourethroprostatic (or urethrocervical) complexes. In both bladder base and urethral components of the lissosphincter, the mural ganglia are most abundant in the adventitia in association with its large nerves and blood vessels; smaller ganglia and individual neuronal cell bodies exist constantly in the muscular, and sporadically in the suburothelial neuroplexuses of the vesical outlet and urethral conduit (*11,12,21,22,60,61*).

Accessory Efferent Autonomic Pathways. In addition to vesicourethral nerves derived from the pelvic plexus, McCrea and Kimmel (*63*) described an accessory nerve pathway in man derived from the $S_{2\text{-}4}$ pelvic sacral roots and the sympathetic sacral chain. This pathway passes along the vesical blood vessels beneath the endopelvic fascia and enters the bladder at the ureterovesical junction without passing through the pelvic plexus. The authors suggested that this pathway can maintain normal bladder function following interruption of the pelvic plexus during extirpative pelvic surgery. A contribution from the sacral sympathetic chain to the ipsilateral pelvic nerve has also been described (*64,65*).

Efferent Innervation of Urethral Rhabdosphincter. Somatomotor innervation of the rhabdosphincter has traditionally been believed to be conveyed exclusively via the pudendal nerves (Fig. 1–2) (*11,12,35,51*). This has been supported by experiments involving electrical stimulation of the nerves, clinical experience of the beneficial effect of pudendal neurectomy in the treatment of somatic sphincter dyssynergia, and horseradish peroxidase tracing studies (*35, 66–69*). Using gross dissection and histologic study of the adult human and canine as well as fetal human material, some authors could not identify any pudendal nerve-derived innervation of the rhabdosphincter, which they concluded is innervated purely by branches of the pelvic plexus together with the intimately related urethral smooth muscularis (*2,70–73*). In other dissection studies, however, nerve twigs from the pudendal nerve could be traced to the region of the human urethral rhabdosphincter (*63,74*). In a more recent study (*75*), it was concluded that the canine urethral rhabdosphincter receives somatomotor innervation via both pudendal and pelvic nerve, since (a) complete electromyographic silence of the sphincter could be achieved only after combined pudendal and pelvic neurectomy; and (b) positive marking of Onuf's nucleus in the sacral spinal cord was obtained following injection of horseradish peroxidase in either the pudendal or the pelvic nerve. Onuf's nucleus, however, has been shown by the same technique to supply pelvic nerve-conveyed innervation to the feline detrusor (*69*).

It should be noted that authors identifying the pelvic nerves as a partial or the sole source of innervation of the urethral rhabdosphincter have summarily considered or indicated that such autonomic nerve-conveyed innervation is somatomotor in nature (*2,70–73*). This view is not necessarily valid, nor has it been proved by any author; it is possible that any pelvic nerve-conveyed innervation of the rhabdosphincter is in part, or in its entirety, truly autonomic in origin.

Peripheral Afferent Pathways. The afferent (sensory) output of the bladder and urethra originates largely in the region of the vesical outlet and is conveyed by the hypogastric and pelvic nerves, respectively, to the lumbar and sacral segments of the spinal cord (Fig. 1–2) (*51,53,76–79*). Traditionally, the afferent fibers of this output have been considered to be exclusively the peripheral projections of segmental lumbosacral spinal dorsal root ganglia. There is evidence, however, that some afferent fibers from the bladder and/or urethra belong to infraspinal neurons located in peripheral ganglia innervating the organs (Fig. 1–3) and form short circuit infraspinal reflex arcs similar to those pre-

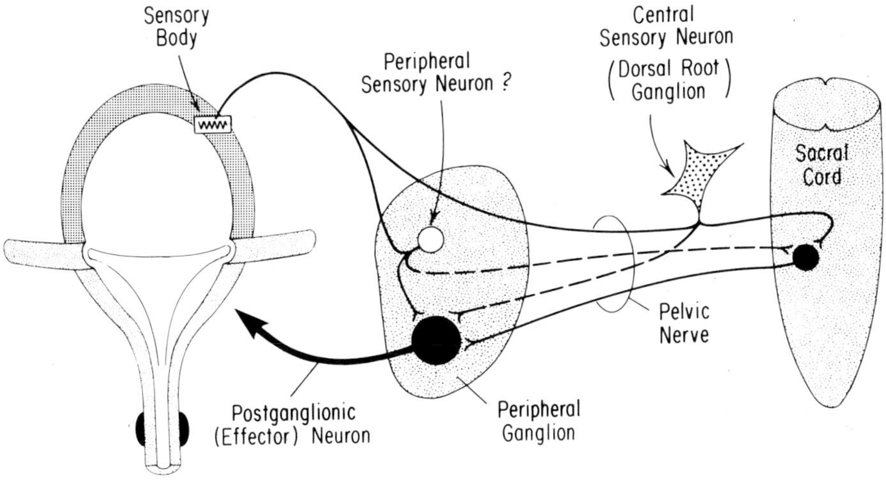

Figure 1–3. Spinal and possible infraspinal (local) afferent neural influence on pastganglionic effector autonomic neurons innervating the muscular apparatus of micturition.

viously described in intestinal and genital ganglia (*80,81*). Along the sympathetic pathway, such local reflex (Fig. 1–4) arcs may be an explanation for the Sowkonin reflex (*82*), and along the parasympathetic pathway they may explain motor detrusor responses obtained by Griffiths (*3*) in the decentralized bladder (Fig. 1–5).

STRUCTURAL BASIS

Muscular Apparatus of Micturition

Detailed descriptions of the structure of the muscular apparatus of micturition are available only in the lissosphincter in both cat and rat (*83*) and in the human body detrusor (*84*).

Ultrastructure of Muscle Cells and Cell Junctions in the Lissosphincter. As in other smooth muscle systems, the muscle cell profiles of the lissosphincter (*83,85*) in both cat and rat are arranged as groups of a variable number of cells and are separated by connective tissue containing collagen, elastic fibers, blood vessels, Schwann cells, and branch nerve bundles. The muscle fascicles are composed predominantly of "dark" cells with a few dispersed "light" cells distinguished, respectively, by the high and low electron density of the sarcoplasm. This different density is believed to be an artifact of specimen fixation *in vitro* (*86,87*).

Muscle cells of the lissosphincter have the characteristic ultrastructural features of smooth muscle elsewhere (*88*). The sarcoplasm is packed with three types of

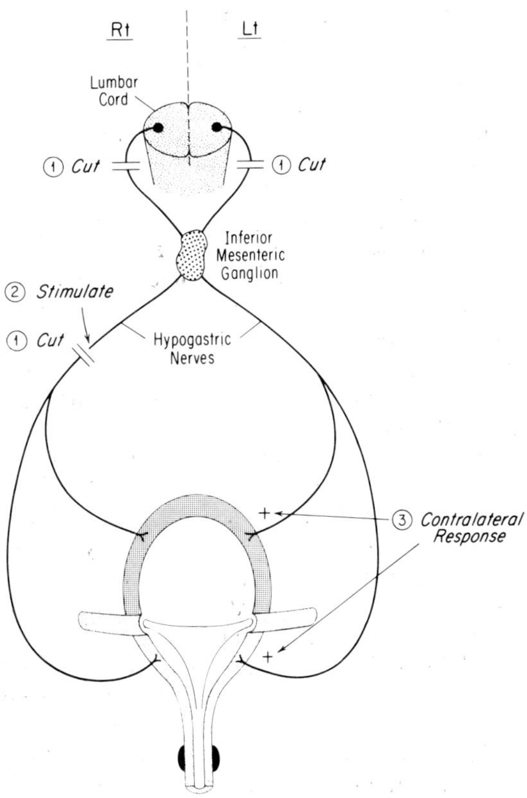

Figure 1–4. Sowkonin's reflex. (From Sowkonin, N.: Innervation der Harnblase. *Pflugers Arch.* 8:600, 1874.)

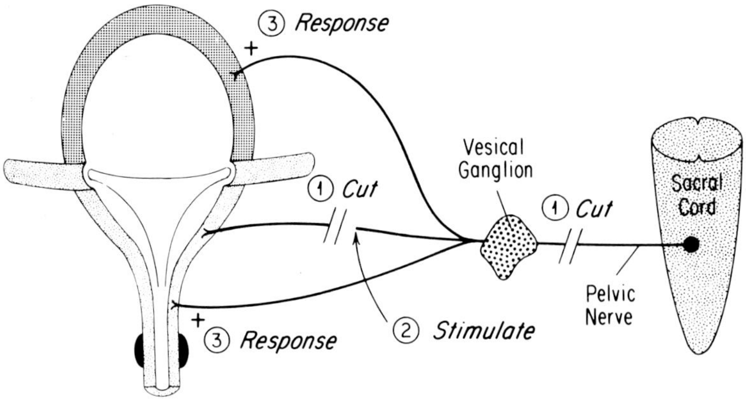

Figure 1–5. "Griffiths' reflex." (From Griffiths, J.: Observations on the urinary bladder and urethra. Part 1. *J. Anat. Physiol.* 25:549, 1895.)

myofilament identified according to their size as thin (7 nm), intermediate (10 nm), and thick (14 to 16 nm) filaments, all of which are regularly arranged as tightly packed bundles. Short electron-dense structures of 30 to 300 nm width, the dense "cigar" bodies, are uniformly distributed throughout the sarcoplasm parallel to myofilaments. Sarcoplasmic reticulum, mitochondria, and the Golgi complex are present usually next to each pole of the nucleus. Flat sacs of smooth sarcoplasmic reticulum are sometimes present beneath the sarcolemma.

The sarcolemma has two related specialized structures that are arranged alternately: the dense bands and caveolae. The dense bands are 200 to 400 nm thick, reinforce the sarcoplasmic side of the sarcolemma, and are penetrated by thin and intermediate myofilaments. Caveolae are flask-shaped in-pocketings of the sarcolemma that have narrow necks and are usually grouped in rows. When their necks are not sectioned, the caveolae appear as small vesicular structures.

The sarcolemma is ensheathed by a ±20 nm thick basal lamina and is separated from it by an electron-lucent space. The basal laminae of contiguous muscle cells are separated by 0.7 to 1.0 μm wide intercellular spaces containing particulate electron-dense material.

Three types of close sarcolemmal contacts are present in the lissosphincter of the cat and rat: adherens, intrusion, and probable nexus-type (gap) junctions. Adherens junctions are the commonest type and occur in two forms. One form resembles the desmosome (macula adherens) with parallel sarcolemmal densities and a 30- to 60-nm separation gap that contains an intermediate central linear density. The other form resembles the zonula adherens (intermediate junction), with similar sarcolemmal densities but a narrower (5–25 nm wide) separation gap that lacks a linear density. The "intrusion" junction is formed by a bulbous muscle cell process that has a characteristic "empty" profile and fits as a "peg in socket" into an invagination in an adjacent muscle cell, with a 5 to 20 nm separation gap. Probable nexus-type contacts are not common in the lissosphincter, occurring mainly at intrusion junctions. At these contacts the sarcolemmas of two contiguous cells appear to be fused at low magnifications, but with higher resolution they are separated by a narrow (2–5 nm) gap—hence the name "gap" junction. No gap junctions have so far been identified in the human body detrusor. (*84*). In addition to their possible function as cellular attachment plaques, the various types of junction, especially the intermediate, and the probable gap junctions are believed to be the medium of myogenic transmission of neural impulses through electrotonic coupling of smooth muscle cells (*89*). Quantitation of the relative frequency distribution and length of muscle cell junctions in the lissosphincter versus the body detrusor is necessary to define the structural basis of differences between the two regions in the myogenic component of neuroeffector transmission.

Functional Structure of Rhabdosphincter. Individual myofibers of the human urethral rhabdosphincter have been reported to be generally smaller than those of the periurethral or other striated muscles (*90*). Muscle spindles have not been identified in either the human or the feline rhabdosphincter (*90–92*).

It is generally accepted that vertebrate striated muscles are composed of one or both of two main myofiber types, i.e., fast and slow fibers, that can be distinguished histologically, histochemically, and ultrastructurally (*93–101*). The fast fiber has: (a) a larger size with uniformly sized and regularly separated fibrils (*fibrillenstruktur*); (b) abundant sarcoplasmic reticulum and glycogen, a modest content of mitochondria, and tubular triads regularly associated with each sarcomere; (c) a thin straight Z-disk as well as a well-defined straight M-line across the center of A-bands; (d) a strongly positive histochemical reactivity to alkaline stable ATPase and phosphorylase but weak reactivity to acid-stable ATPase and oxidative mitochondrial enzymes; and (e) single, acetylcholinesterase-rich, en plaque type motor end-plates. By contrast, the slow fiber: (a) is smaller with irregularly spaced fibrils of variable size (*felderstruktur*); (b) contains relatively little sarcoplasmic reticulum, glycogen particles and tubular triads, but prominent mitochondria that tend to be aligned in rows between every two adjacent sarcomeres; (c) has thick, jagged or zig-zagged Z-disks and absent or poorly defined M-lines; (d) displays strongly positive histochemical reactivity to acid-stable ATPase and oxidative mitochondrial enzymes but is poorly reactive to alkali-stable ATPase and phosphorylase; and (e) is innervated by relatively acetylcholinesterase-poor en grappe type motor end-plates. Some authors have found no significant ultrastructural differences in the pattern of innervation of slow and fast myofibers (*102*). In the cat, the urethralis muscle (*103*), the cranial part of which almost certainly is a part of the rhabdosphincter related to the cranial portion of the postprostatic urethra (Elbadawi and Atta, unpublished data), has been characterized physiologically as a fast muscle and the periurethral muscles (part of the pelvic diaphragm) as slow muscles (*91*). In a combined histochemical and ultrastructural study, what may represent the human urethral rhabdosphincter has been described as consisting exclusively of slow myofibers (*90*). In another study using histochemical stains and volumetric measurements, however, the human rhabdosphincter was reported to consist of equal proportions of slow and fast fibers (*104*). Histochemically, the canine urethral sphincter has been shown to have a 35 percent component of slow and a 65 percent component of fast fibers (*105*).

In a recent study (*92,107*), it has been shown that the feline rhabdosphincter has the same basic ultrastructure as striated muscle elsewhere and, according to available criteria in the literature, is composed of a mixture of fast and slow fibers. The myofiber of the rhabdosphincter is a cylindrical multinucleate cell with most nuclei located beneath the sarcolemma. The sarcolemma is coated by a ± 20 nm thick basal lamina with an intermediate electron-lucent space. The main part of the sarcoplasm is composed of myofilaments arranged as 0.5 to 1.0 μm thick myofibrils. Each myofibril consists of a repetitive series of sarcomeres (the contractile units of striated muscle), with the characteristic arrangement of Z-disks, A- and I-bands, H-zones, and M-lines (*96,108*). Sarcoplasmic reticulum forms a reticular collar around the entire length of each myofibril, and the T-tubule system runs transversely perpendicular to the long axis of the myofiber. At the points of their intersection, these two organelles form specialized structures called sarcoplasmic triads, each of which consists of a central transverse tubule sandwiched between two lateral sacs of sarcoplasmic reticulum that contain osmiophilic material. The triads are most prominent at junctions of the A- and I-bands. Mitochondria, ribosomes, glycogen, and lipid vacuoles are frequently seen in the sarcoplasm between adjacent myofibrils. In some myofibers, the mitochondria are elongated, numerous, and arranged in longitudinal rows running along the entire length of myofibrils (a feature indicated in the literature to be characteristic of slow fibers). Aggregates of spherical and globoid mitochondria are also commonly seen beneath the sarcolemma.

Small fusiform cells abut against myofibers of the feline rhabdosphincter, tightly sandwiched between the sarcolemma and its encoating basal lamina. These cells are identical to the satellite cells of striated muscle (*109,110*); they have single nuclei and scanty cytoplasm that contains some ribosomes and mitochondria but no myofilaments.

Extrinsic Peripheral Neural Pathways

Microstructure of Extrinsic Nerves. Based on the assumption that the pudendal nerves convey somatomotor innervation to the rhabdosphincter as well as the pelvic floor, they should be composed exclusively of myelinated nerve fibers. On the other hand, the main trunks of both hypogastric and pelvic nerves are composed of a mixture of nonmyelinated preganglionic efferent autonomic and myelinated, probably afferent sensory, nerve fibers (*11,49,111,112*). Histochemically, both nerves in animals contain cholinergic as well as adrenergic fibers. The former include all preganglionic sympathetic and parasympathetic autonomic nerves, but the latter by definition are postganglionic sympathetic in origin. The extent of adrenergic fiber contribution to the hypogastric and pelvic nerves varies among species; in the cat it is estimated, respectively, as 40 to 60 percent and 5 to 10 percent (*112*). All major strands of the pelvic plexus in animals are composed of nearly equal populations of cholinergic and adrenergic fibers (*11*). The former includes preganglionic fibers as well as postganglionic parasympathetic fibers originating in ganglia of the urogenital short neuron system (*11,49*). A sympathetic autonomic contribution has been demonstrated not only to the pelvic nerve but also the pudendal nerve in the cat (*64, 65*).

Ultrastructurally, all pelvic plexus nerves in animals are composed of myelinated and nonmyelinated Schwann cell-ensheathed axons (*11,49*). The former are presumably afferent since all efferent autonomic axons are nonmyelinated. Extrinsic nerves in man have not yet been studied histochemically or ultrastructurally in detail.

Microstructure of Peripheral Ganglia. The larger ganglia of the urogenital short neuron system, including pelvic plexus ganglia, consist of intermingled or partially segregated clusters of cholinergic, adrenergic, and small intensely fluorescent (SIF) neurons (*60,61,113,114*). The relative proportion of the three cell types, which can be distinguished both histochemically and ultrastructurally, varies in different species, different animals of the same species, different ganglia, and even between the right and left sides in the same animal. Most small intramural ganglia represent pure clusters of one cell type.

Adrenergic principal neurons in peripheral ganglia, by definition, are postganglionic sympathetic in nature and supply terminal adrenergic innervation to the bladder and urethra. It is almost certain that most cholinergic principal neurons in the ganglia are postganglionic parasympathetic in nature and supply terminal cholinergic innervation to the bladder and urethra. Some, however, may represent a restricted population of postganglionic *sympathetic cholinergic* neurons that modulate secretion of accessory male genital glands, especially the prostate (*49,115*). SIF cells probably play an important role in modulation of the vasomotor function and neurotransmission in the various ganglia. These cells are now accepted as true interneurons, many of which establish efferent synapses with juxtaposed cells of the other two cell types by means of their somas, dendrites, or axonal processes (*116*).

Numerous cholinergic and adrenergic nerve fibers are present within ganglia innervating the vesicourethral muscularis. Many of these fibers are fibers en passage, but some are believed to establish synapses within the ganglia, being intimately associated with some of its neurons. According to traditional dogma, every postganglionic neuron in a peripheral autonomic ganglion has a preganglionic synapse, so that most of the intraganglionic cholinergic synapses must be preganglionic in nature. Morphologic evidence has been provided, however, for the existence in vesical ganglia of both adrenergic and cholinergic postganglionic synapses (*57,62,117*). The existence of adrenergic postganglionic synapses has been confirmed histochemically and ultrastructurally in several species (*12,57*). The adrenergic fibers involved terminate mostly on the preganglionic cholinergic axon that provides the neuron with its preganglionic synapses, rather than on the soma of the neuron (*12,57*). On the other hand, cholinergic postganglionic synapses have been confirmed histochemically and suspected pharmacologically (*12,57*), but remain to be proved ultrastructurally. SIF cells have been shown to receive preganglionic synapses and to establish efferent ("postganglionic") synapses with various neurons in the ganglia (*12*). As mentioned earlier, it is possible that some afferent fibers establish synapses in peripheral vesicourethral ganglia to form infraspinal circuits (*12*). The existence of such synapses, however, needs to be investigated morphologically. Moreover, there is evidence that some neuroterminals within peripheral vesicourethral ganglia contain neuropeptides, especially enkephalin (*118, 118a*).

Intrinsic Efferent Innervation of Vesicourethral Smooth Muscle

Histochemistry. It is now established that the mammalian bladder has dual innervation by cholinergic and adrenergic nerves, with some regional differences in their density and distribution patterns (*13*). These differences were the basis of the concept of dividing the bladder into body and base regions (Fig. 1–6) (*13*). Cholinergic muscular innervation is uniformly rich throughout both body and base detrusor as well as the urethral muscularis of various species (*13,21,22, 113,117,119*). In the rat, however, there is denser cholinergic muscular innervation in the ventral than the dorsal walls of the bladder body, with the reverse pattern in the bladder base, and nearly commensurate intermediate density in the lateral walls of both regions (*120*).

Adrenergic muscular innervation has distinct regional variations in all animal species (Fig. 1–6). In general, this innervation is virtually absent in the bladder dome and is more abundant with greater density and complexity in the proximal urethra than the bladder base, in the base than the body, and in the outer than the inner parts of the walls in any region of the body. The feline base detrusor has commensurate adrenergic innervation in both its ventral and dorsal walls (*13,21,22,113,117*). Adrenergic innervation of the canine bladder base is similar to but less prominent than that in the cat (*83*). In

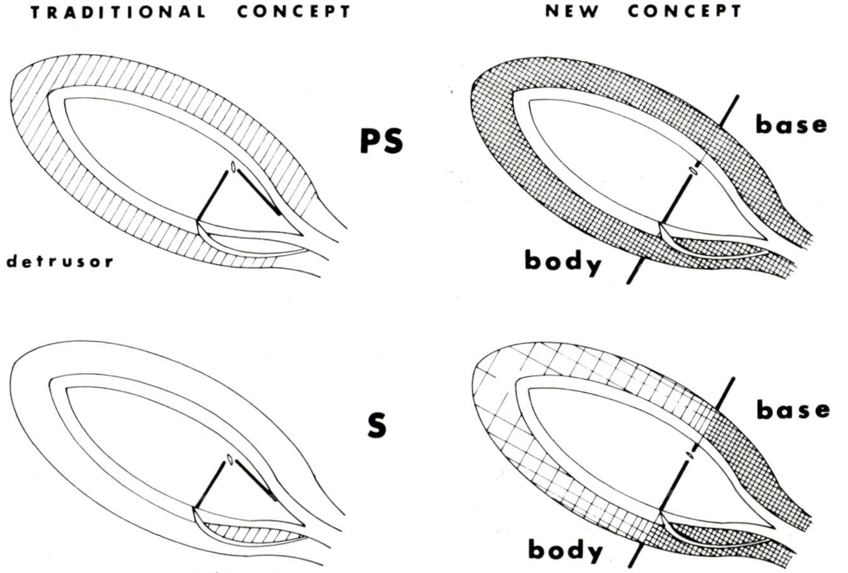

Figure 1–6. Bladder body and base, in contrast to the traditional functional concept, based on the regional density and distribution patterns of intrinsic adrenergic sympathetic and cholinergic parasympathetic nerves in the muscularis.

both rabbit and rat, there is a progressive increase of adrenergic nerve density as the body or base detrusor is followed from the ventral to the dorsal midline at any level (*13,121*). The rat has considerably weaker adrenergic innvervation in the body than other species, except close to its junction with the base (*3,111,122*), and in a peculiar ventral, midline, outer muscle bundle in the body of the male bladder, with adrenergic innervation as dense as that of the dorsal wall of the base (*120*).

In all animal species, the periureteral sheaths have the same distribution pattern and density of both cholinergic and adrenergic nerves as in the bladder base (*11*). The ureterotrigonal muscle, on the other hand, has a distinctly poor innervation that is identical to that of the ureteral muscularis (*11,21*).

Neurohistochemical studies on the human bladder and urethra so far have yielded conflicting observations on the type and relative density of their muscular innervation. These observations have been reviewed in detail elsewhere (*11*). In one study it was reported that there is a uniformly rich cholinergic and sparse adrenergic innervation of the human bladder in both sexes, with sparse cholinergic and adrenergic innervation of the preprostatic urethral muscularis in men and the reverse pattern in women (*123*). No sex differences, however, were observed in either cholinergic or adrenergic muscular innervation in any animal (*11,13,112*) or in other studies on the human detrusor or urethra (*124–128*).

Ultrastructure. So far, the ultrastructure of intrinsic innervation has been described in detail in the bladder base component of the lissosphincter in both cat and rat (83, *129,130*), and in the human body detrusor (*84*).

Nerve trunks in the adventitia of the bladder divide into smaller branch bundles that penetrate its muscularis. Composed of myelinated as well as Schwann cell-ensheathed adrenergic and cholinergic axons, these bundles divide into progressively smaller axon bundles that rapidly lose their myelinated axon component. The smallest axon bundles consist of four to ten adrenergic and/or cholinergic axons, run between and within the muscle fascicles, and end as terminals as each of their component axons innervates one or more muscle cells.

Neuroeffector junctions in the lissosphincter are established by terminals or varicosities of adrenergic and cholinergic axons (Fig. 1–7). Most junctions are of the surface type where the axon is apposed to the surface of the muscle cell, often at a shallow depression. Some axon terminals form invaginated junctions, at which the axon profile occupies a deep groove in, or appears to be totally ensheathed by, the sarcoplasm of the muscle cell. Most junctions are unitary, comprising one axonal and one muscle cell profile. Some are multieffector, with one axon establishing contact with two to four spatially intimate muscle cells. Multiaxonal junctions, formed by two to four adrenergic or cholinergic axon terminals in contact with one muscle cell, are present less frequently. Some muscle cells have neuroeffector junctions formed by one cholinergic and one adrenergic axon: the "diautonomic" junctions (*83*).

It became clear ultrastructurally that the lissosphincter is not innervated on a 1:1 nerve/muscle cell basis, as earlier histochemical studies suggested (*13*). It is doubtful that any part of the vesicourethral muscularis has innervation on such basis (*11,83*). It seems certain that some muscle cells of the lissosphincter have only cholinergic, some only adrenergic, some both cholinergic and adrenergic (diautonomic), and some no neuroeffector junctions of either type (*83*). The neuroeffector junctions in the lissosphincter have 10- to 80- nm gaps and are rarely associated with focal axolemmal or sarcolemmal thickening. The junctions may be close, almost close, or en passage, with a gap width, respectively, of 10 to 25, 25 to 40, and 40 to 80 nm. Since these gaps are as wide as neuroeffector junctions in many other muscle systems, and narrower or much narrower than those in many (e.g., media of blood vessels, teniae coli), it was concluded that all types of neuroeffector junctions described in the lissosphincter mediate neurogenic transmission to its muscle cells (*11,12,83*). Quantitative analysis of the frequency distribution of each type of junction in the lissosphincter versus the body detrusor is essential to consolidate the structural basis of the well documented

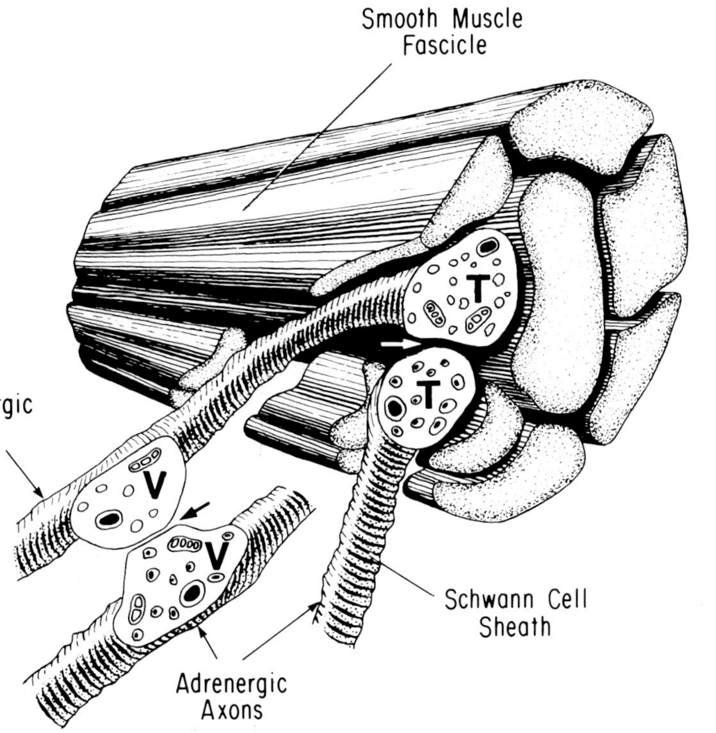

Figure 1–7. Mechanisms of neuromuscular transmission in the lissosphincter. *V* = varicosity of cholinergic and adrenergic axons forming a prejunctional axoaxonal synapse (*arrows*) in the axon bundle. *T*=bare terminals of cholinergic and adrenergic axons forming neuroeffector junctions with muscle cells and an axoaxonal synapse (*arrow*) in the neuroeffector field.

differences in their functional and pharmacologic behavior.

Adrenergic and cholinergic axons of intrinsic muscular neuroplexuses of the lissosphincter run very closely together but are generally separated by the cytoplasm and/or cytomembranes of their ensheathing Schwann cell somas or processes. In an ultrastructural study of the cat and rat bladder base, however, Elbadawi (*129*) discovered direct axolemmal contacts between spatially intimate axons without interposed Schwann cell elements. Such axoaxonal contacts are present in preterminal axon bundles as well as preterminal neuroeffector fields (Fig. 1–7). Most of these contacts are ultrastructurally simple, lacking plasmalemmal specialization as synaptic complexes, and involve two axons that are directly apposed for a 10-nm to 5μm stretch along one or multiple areas, with 15- to 25-nm separation gaps that contain no electron-dense material. Most axoaxonal contacts involve one cholinergic and one adrenergic profile (Fig. 1–7), but a few are formed by two cholinergic, two adrenergic, or one cholinergic, and a probably SIF cell derived profile (*116,129*). Based on an analysis of the available physiopharmacologic literature on peripheral autonomic neurotransmission, Elbadawi (*129*) proposed that the axoaxonal synpases in the lissosphincter are the medium for reciprocal cholinergic/adrenergic interaction of its intrinsic axons peripheral to both spinal cord and ganglia of the pelvic plexus, and are the probable explanation for the prejunctional modulation of neuroeffector transmission in the urethral muscularis (*130*). This has recently been confirmed in the bladder of cat, rabbit, and man (*131*).

Morphologic Basis of Noncholinergic/Nonadrenergic Innervation. *"Purinergic" Nerves?* Despite some pharmacologic observations, the existence of "purinergic" nerves as a distinct and separate nerve entity in the vesicourethral muscularis is questionable for the following reasons (*11*). First, the alleged purinergic transmitter ATP has been known pharmacologically and confirmed ultrastructurally to coexist constantly with the classic neurotransmitters acetylcholine and norepinephrine in the same cholinergic and adrenergic axon terminals, respectively (*132–134*). Second, no nerve population that is separate and distinct from histochemically demonstrable cholinergic and adrenergic nerves has been documented unequivocally in any organ. Third, the ultrastructural axon profile packed with large opaque-core vesicles and (without evidence) claimed to be purinergic (*135,136*), has been identified in the jejunum (in which noncholinergic/nonadrenergic neurotransmission is unequivocal) and the lissosphincter of the cat and rat; but in both organs all such profiles could be traced in serial sections in continuity with ultrastructurally classic cholinergic or adrenergic terminals or varicosities (*83,137*). Fourth, *in vitro* experiments on the guinea pig vas deferens suggest a cotransmitter and not a primary role of ATP in its adrenergic neuroeffector transmission (*138*).

"Peptidergic" Nerves? Immunohistochemical techniques have revealed the presence of neuropeptide-immunoreactive nerves in the lower urinary tract. In the cat and guinea pig, vasoactive intestinal polypeptide (VIP)-immunoreactive nerves have been described in the bladder base, in the trigone, around the ureteral orifices, and at the urethrovesical junction (*139–141*). "VIPergic" muscular nerves have been demonstrated throughout the human bladder, but radioimmunoassay values of the same peptide are higher in the deep trigone than the bladder dome (*142,143*). Since similar nerves are also abundant in the muscularis of the gastroesophageal junction and pylorus (*140*), it has been postulated that the prominent presence of VIPergic nerves is characteristic of sphincteric zones of smooth muscle (*140,144*), and that they probably mediate its noncholinergic/nonadrenergic relaxation (*144,145*).

Substance P-immunoreactive nerves have been demonstrated in the suburothelium and around muscle cells of the proximal urethra of the guinea pig, as well as the human body detrusor (*139,141*). In the human bladder neuropeptide Y-immunoreactive nerves have also been demonstrated in the muscularis of the posterior bladder base in a lesser density than in the body detrusor (*142,143*).

Current morphologic and neurophysiologic data indicate that neuropeptides probably participate as contransmitters or neuromodulators in what is primarily an autonomic adrenergic or cholinergic neuroeffector transmission and do not function as the primary or exclusive vehicle of either (*146–149*). The coexistence of a classic transmitter and one or more neuropeptides in the same neuron has been proved immunohistochemically using special techniques of elusion and restaining, or staining of consecutive sections (*149,150*). Cryostat sections stained immunohistochemically for VIP, photographed, and then rinsed and restained for acetylcholinesterase revealed the presence of both VIP and the enzyme in the same neurons of the exocrine salivary glands of the cat (*151,152*). Avian pancreatic polypeptide and catecholamine synthesizing enzymes coexist in the same neurons of the feline stellate, superior cervical, and celiac ganglia, as shown in histochemically processed consecutive cryostat sections (*149*). Ordinary morphologic and immunocytochemical studies suggest that neuropeptides in peripheral autonomic axons are localized in large dense-core vesicles of the same shapes and sizes as those naturally occurring in small numbers in cholinergic and adrenergic axon terminals and varicosities (*153–155*). The cotransmitter concept of neuropeptide function in autonomic neuroeffector transmission is corroborated by some neurophysiologic studies on innervation of the feline submaxillary salivary gland (*151*), rectum (*156*), and penile vasculature (*157*). The ability of autonomic axons to "switch" functionally from one classic neurotransmitter to another, or from a classic to a putative (especially peptide) neurotransmitter has already been documented during neurigenesis and in association with regenerative/reactive axonal sprouting (*107,158–162*).

Based on the evidence reviewed above, it seems that there is no need to postulate that either "purinergic" or "peptidergic" nerves exist as a separate structural entity in intrinsic innervation of the vesicourethral muscularis, nor perform a function in its neuroeffector transmission in the absence or as a substitute for its classic cholinergic and adrenergic components.

Intrinsic Innervation of Urethral Rhabdosphincter

The urethral rhabdosphincter appears to have a unique somatomotor plus autonomic innervation pattern that so far has been debated. In 1974, Elbadawi and Schenk (*22*) presented histochemical evidence that the male feline rhabdosphincter has triple somatomotor, autonomic cholinergic, and autonomic adrenergic innervation of its myofibers. As in other striated muscles, the somatomotor component was identified as strongly acetylcholinesterase-positive, circumscribed, ovoid motor end-plates on the surface of the myofibers. In addition, and unlike other striated muscles, the male feline rhabdosphincter was found histochemically to have intricate, blood vessel-independent, cholinergic and adrenergic neuroplexuses, the ramifications of which course between and encircle some of its myofibers individually. The presence of direct adrenergic neuroeffector junctions (±40 nm separation gap) with myofibers of the rhabdosphincter has been confirmed in the rat (*85*). Using both light and electron microscopy, some authors denied the presence of any autonomic neuroeffector junctions in the urethra-associated striated muscle cells in the guinea pig, and claimed that all adrenergic axons observed ultrastructurally in relation to these fibers can be traced in serial sections to a neuroeffector relationship with spatially close smooth muscle cells (*163*). Earlier, however, the same authors described intimate histochemical and ultrastructurally en passage contacts between cholinergic axons that have no pre- or postganglionic specilization and subepithelial striated muscle cells in the urethra of the male guinea pig (*164*); it is highly likely that these muscle cells belong to the rhabdosphincter in this species (*11*). Adrenergic innervation of the canine and human "external sphincter" has also been denied in some histochemical and pharmacologic studies (*165,166*); careful analysis of these studies, however, strongly suggests that the structure examined is a part of the periurethral muscle and not the rhabdosphincter itself (*11*).

Ultrastructural studies on the normal and somatically denervated male feline rhabdosphincter (*92,107,158,167,168*) confirm its triple somatomotor/diautonomic innervation pattern as described earlier histochemically (*22*). The normal rhabdosphincter contains interstitial Schwann cell-ensheathed bundles of myelinated, as well as nonmyelinated cholinergic and adrenergic axons; some of these bundles contain only the latter type of axon. Two categories of neuromuscular relationships exist in the normal rhabdosphincter: (a) junctions with classic motor end-plates, and (b) surface axonal junctions without any specialization of the related myofibers.

Junctions with classic motor end-plates have the ultrastructural features of neuromuscular junctions in other striated muscles and are thus considered to be somatomotor in nature (*92*). Myofibers of the male feline rhabdosphincter are innervated by either the en plaque (solitary) or en grappe (clustered) type of end-plates, claimed, respectively, to innervate fast and slow striated myofibers in other muscles (*92,107*). In the male feline rhabdosphincter, however, there is no constant relation between the type of end-plate and the ultrastructural functional type of the related myofiber (*92*).

Because of the absence of sarcolemmal specialization of any kind, all surface nerve–muscle fiber junctions in the male feline rhabdosphincter are considered autonomic in nature (*92*). Such junctions are established by individual axons with the flat, slightly raised, or focally protuberant surface of the myofiber, usually away from its nucleus, and have 50- to 120-nm gaps. The participant axon profile has a Schwann cell sheath only on the side not facing the myofiber. Some myofibers have multiple such junctions. Regardless of the type of axon profile, the surface junctions innervate both slow and fast twitch myofibers as recognized by currently available criteria. No surface junctions exist near a motor end-plate.

The nonspecialized surface junctions with myofibers of the male feline rhabdosphincters are established by cholinergic and adrenergic axon profiles. Some profiles of both axon types contain abundant pleomorphic large dense-core vesicles and on this basis can be considered potentially co-peptidergic (*92*).

Triple innervation of the male feline rhabdosphincter has further been confirmed by studies on the pattern of its innervation following somatic denervation by complete bilateral sacral ventral rhizotomy (*107,158,167,168*). This procedure completely deprives the rhabdosphincter of its somatomotor innervation. Shortly after such denervation the axonal elements of all motor end-plates undergo degeneration and disappear, but the surface junctions persist. Eventually, the end-plates become reinnervated by nonmyelinated autonomic cholinergic and adrenergic (plus possible co-peptidergic elements of both axon types) and the surface junctions appear to be increased in number.

PHYSIOPHARMACOLOGIC BASIS

Neurogenic vesicourethral responses throughout the voiding cycle are determined at the peripheral (infraspinal) level by (*129*): (a) neurotransmission within peripheral vesicourethral ganglia; (b) neuroeffector transmission from postganglionic cholinergic and adrenergic axon terminals and varicosities to vesicourethral smooth muscle cells; and (c) impulse transmission along these postganglionic axons as modified by prejunctional axonal interaction mechanisms. The final muscular response almost certainly involves a myogenic mechanism of electrotonic spread of excitatory neuron influence via muscle cell–cell junctions (Fig. 1–7).

According to traditional neurophysiologic dogma, both cholinergic parasympathetic and adrenergic sympathetic postganglionic (effector-innervating) neurons in peripheral vesicourethral ganglia should be subject primarily to the pharmacologically nicotinic influence of their innervating cholinergic preganglionic synapses. Through the above-described postganglionic and interneuronal synapses, however, the postganglionic neurons are probably subject within the ganglia to several modulatory mechanisms (Fig. 1–8). These mechanisms include (*12,49*): (a) an alpha-adrenergic inhibitory influence that "brakes" transmission in cholinergic and probably autoregulates that in adrenergic postganglionic neurons; (b) a ? postganglionic cholinergic muscarinic excitatory influence that can perpetuate excitatory impulses in postganglionic cholinergic and possibly adrenergic effector neurons; (c) a muscarinic cholinergic-stimulated SIF cell interneuronal circuit that can subsequently inhibit excitatory discharge of postganglionic cholinergic neurons; and (d) neuropeptide-mediated modulatory influence on neurotransmission in postganglionic cholinergic and/or adrenergic intraganglionic neurons. In addition, there is cogent electrophysiologic evidence that postganglionic

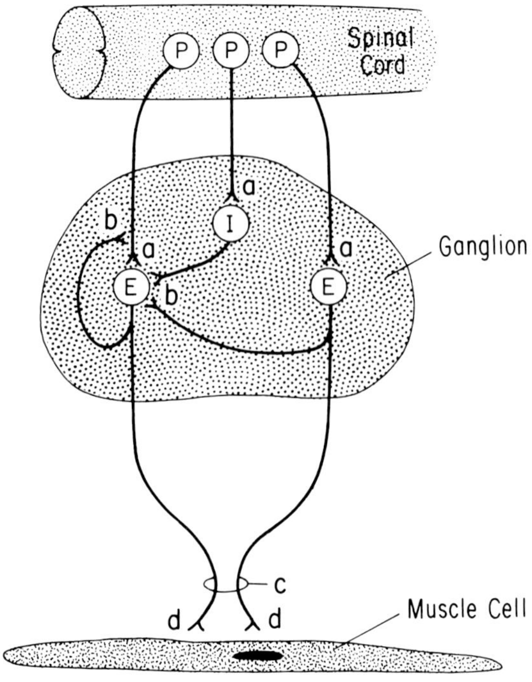

Figure 1–8. Peripheral sympathetic/parasympathetic interactions in vesicourethral muscular function. *P* (left) = preganglionic parasympathetic neuron. *P* (right) = preganglionic sympathetic neuron. *P* (center) = ? preganglionic neuron innervating a SIF cell in peripheral vesicourethral ganglion. *E* (left) = postganglionic effector (muscle-innervating) parasympathetic neuron. *E* (right) = postganglionic effector (muscle-innervating) sympathetic neuron. *I* = inhibitory interneuron (SIF cell). *a* = preganglionic (nicotinic cholinergic) synapse with neurons in peripheral ganglion. *b* = intraganglionic modulatory synapse: excitatory (muscarinic) cholinergic from left E neuron, inhibitory alpha-adrenergic from right E neuron, and inhibitory catecholaminergic from I neuron. *c* = prejunctional axoaxonal synapse between postganglionic adrenergic sympathetic (right) and postganglionic cholinergic (parasympathetic) axonal varicosities and terminals that form individual or conjoint (diautonomic) neuroeffector junctions (*d*) with smooth muscle cells of the bladder and urethra.

parasympathetic neurons innervating the bladder have intrinsic "gating" and "facilitation" properties that, respectively, filter out or potentiate excitatory impulses they receive from the spinal cord.

Available morphologic, physiologic, and pharmacologic observations so far indicate that neuroeffector transmission in the vesicourethral smooth muscle is both neurogenic and myogenic, respectively, through neuroeffector junctions with smooth muscle cells and muscle cell-cell junctions (Fig. 1–6) (*12,83*). Such transmission is elicited through various types of autonomic muscular receptors and is determined by the neuronal output of peripheral vesicourethral ganglia and by prejunctional axonal interaction mechanisms (Fig. 1–7) modulating impulse transmission in postganglionic cholinergic and adrenergic axons innervating muscle cells of the bladder and urethra (*129*).

Since the physiopharmacology of the vesicourethral smooth muscle is reviewed in detail in other chapters in this book, only some pertinent aspects of direct relevance to the discussion of the act of micturition are included in this chapter.

Responses to Electrical Neural Stimulation. Electrical stimulation of efferent parasympathetic pathways to the urinary bladder (sacral ventral roots or pelvic nerve) results in detrusor contraction and voiding in man and experimental animals (*14,67,169–171*). The vesical contraction elicited by this stimulation cannot be blocked completely by atropine, unlike that induced by acetylcholine (*172,173*). This atropine-resistance phenomenon has been recognized since the early years of vesical neurophysiologic studies and has not yet been explained satisfactorily. There is some evidence, however, that it might be related, at least in part, to noncholinergic/nonadrenergic neuroeffector transmission. On the other hand, efferent parasympathetic stimulation has variably been reported to result in an increase (*170,174,175*), a decrease (*176–178*), or no change (*14*) in urethral resistance in various animal species. A noncholinergic/nonadrenergic mechanism of urethral relaxation has been demonstrated *in vivo* in the feline urethra in response to sacral ventral root stimulation and *in vitro* in strips of the human, guinea pig, and rabbit urethra (*179*). The mediator involved in such a mechanism has not yet been identified. Such urethral relaxation, however, is largely blocked by propranolol and was thus thought to be mediated through inhibitory parasympathetic influence on the short adrenergic neurons innervating the urethral musculature (*178*).

The most frequently reported response to hypogastric nerve stimulation in experimental animals is brief detrusor contraction followed by prolonged relaxation that persists for as long as the stimulation lasts (*14,52,67,112,180,181*). The initial contractile response has been characterized either as an alpha-adrenergic (*112,180*) or an atropine-sensitive muscarinic cholinergic (*182*) response, and the subsequent relaxation as a beta-adrenergic response (*112,180–182*). On the other hand, hypogastric nerve stimulation results in an increase in urethral resistance in the cat (*176,178,180*) and dog (*183,184*), an effect that can be blocked by the alpha-adrenergic blockers dihydroergotamine (*177*), phenoxybenzamine (*178,183*) phentolamine, and prazosin (*184*). Hypogastric neurectomy results in a reduction of urethral resistance in both dog and cat (*178,185*). Despite the clearly excitatory effects of sympathetic stimulation on urethral muscular function, some authors have claimed that adrenergic urethral innervation subserves only a sexual function in men, to maintain closure of the bladder neck during ejaculation and thereby prevent "retrograde" flow of semen into the bladder (*123,186,187*). This view is not supported by the fact that the effects of electrical sympathetic stimulation on the urethral muscularis are similar in male and female members of the same species (*176,182*).

Autonomic Receptors and Pharmacologic Responses. Experimental studies on material from man and experimental animals have shown that the anterior part of the bladder base is pharmacologically identical to the deep trigone [trigonal muscle (*11*), posterior base detrusor] but different from the body detrusor (*188,189*). This provided substantial support to the bladder body–base concept proposed originally on purely neuromorphologic grounds by Elbadawi and Schenk (*13*) and led to its current universal acceptance as a key element in the mechanism of micturition (*11,15*).

Muscarinic cholinoceptors are uniformly rich in both body and base detrusor in the cat

(*190,191*), dog (*189*), rabbit (*192,193*), and man (*194,195*), in conformity with the uniformly dense cholinergic muscular innervation of the two regions in these species. The cholinoceptors mediate contraction of the body detrusor to initiate and maintain voiding, as well as its acetylcholine- or cholinomimetic-induced contraction that can be blocked completely by atropine.

Adrenoceptors are also present in both body and base of the bladder in the cat (*126,196*), dog (*188,189,197*), rabbit (*193,198–200*), and man (*194,195,201*), with a selective regional distribution of their subtypes. Alpha-adrenoceptors predominate in the base detrusor and mediate its contraction, whereas beta-adrenoceptors are dominant in the body detrusor and mediate its relaxation (*126,194,202*). This regionally selective distribution of adrenoceptor subtypes in the detrusor has been corroborated by radioligand receptor-binding studies (*203,204*).

Prejunctional Modulation of Neuroeffector Transmission. The bulk of experimental and clinical evidence so far indicates that adrenoceptors of the urethral muscularis, principally of the alpha type, have a crucial role in the mechanism of continence (*18,175,205–212*). This role has been studied well in *in vitro* experiments. Experimental evidence also indicates that cholinoceptors have some role in muscular activity of the urethra, either directly or through its adrenergic innervation (*179,180,196,213, 214*). The results of some of the latter experiments led to the suggestion that the effects of acetylcholine on the circular urethral smooth muscle is mediated by stimulation of norepinephrine release at neuroterminals of the short adrenergic neurons innervating the urethral muscularis, and that its net effect depends on the state of activation of the two adrenoceptor types (*190,196,213*). In another study, however, small doses of acetylcholine increased urethral resistance by a muscarinic atropine-sensitive mechanism (*214*). In yet another study on neuronal release of norepinephrine, it has been shown that adrenergic neuroterminals of the urethral muscularis in both rabbit and man have prejunctional inhibitory alpha$_2$-adrenoceptors and muscarinic cholinoceptors (*179*). Modulatory prejunctional receptors on adrenergic and cholinergic neuroterminals have been demonstrated previously in many organs, especially the vas deferens, and are believed to be a mechanism for interaction of the two subdivisions of the autonomic nervous system at the effector tissue level (*124,131,215–218*). Such interactions have recently been proved to exist in the bladder of cat, rabbit and man (*131*).

Responses to Putative Neurotransmitters. Some purines and neuropeptides appear to modify muscular activity of the bladder and/or urethra. The possible role of ATP in vesical neurotransmission is supported by the demonstration of ATP release on transmural nerve stimulation and the similarity of contractions induced by nerve stimulation to those by ATP in the presence of atropine (*219,220*). ATP contracts strips of the body detrusor, with tachyphylaxis, in man, rabbit, rat, and guinea pig (*221–225*) and has been proposed as the neurotransmitter involved in atropine-resistant detrusor contractions induced by parasympathetic nerve stimulation (*226*). In one study, however, strips of the rabbit bladder base, unlike the body, did not respond *in vitro* to a high concentration of ATP (*193*).

Vasoactive intestinal polypeptide has been reported to lead to reversible and dose-dependent reduction of spontaneous contractions, as well as contractions of strips of the human and porcine vesicourethral muscle in response to cholinomimetics, alpha-adrenergic agonists, and electrical field stimulation (*227,228*). It also has been reported to induce dose-dependent inhibition of baseline tension and carbachol-induced contractions of feline vesicourethral muscle strips (*229*) and to relax strips from both base and body of the rabbit bladder (*230*). The inconsistent effects of VIP on vesicourethral muscle strips reported *in vitro* are probably related to differences in the type of preparation used for study and the species from which it was obtained.

Substance P has an excitatory effect on strips of the guinea pig detrusor and enhances their contractions induced by electrical field stimulation (*231–233*). Prostaglandins (PGs) have also been implicated in vesicourethral muscular function, mainly in relation to the "tone" and spontaneous activity of the detrusor (*232,234,235*). PGE_1

and PGE_2 were reported to relax, and $PGF_{2\alpha}$ to contract strips of the human urethra and detrusor (*236–238*). Since the effects of prostaglandins are resistant to blockade by tetrodotoxin, they do not appear to be related to autonomic neuroeffector transmission (*239*).

Concept of Micturition Reflexes. The concept of micturition reflexes was introduced by Guyon in 1900 (*240*). He described five voiding relfexes, three cephalospinal and two spinal, that elicit bladder contraction in response to vesical distension, urethral urinary flow, or urethral distension by the urine stream. Of these reflexes, a cephalospinal "hind-brain" reflex has both afferent and efferent pathways along the pelvic nerves; a second caphalospinal "hind-brain" reflex has the afferent pathway along the pudendal nerves and the efferent along the pelvic nerves, and the third cephalospinal reflex has both afferent and efferent pathways along the hypogastric nerves. One of the remaining two spinal reflexes, eliciting urethral relaxation, has its afferent and efferent pathways along the pudendal nerves, and the other has its afferent pathway along the pelvic nerves and efferent pathway along the pudendal nerves.

In a series of elaborate neurotomy experiments in the cat, Barrington (1914:1941) described seven reflexes for the initiation and maintenance of voiding, refining and expanding Guyon's pioneering concept (*241–246*). Additional reflexes were introduced in subsequent years to explain these two phases of micturition, as well as its storage and termination phases, by Müller (*247*), Denny-Brown and Robertson (*248*), Garry *et al.* (*249*), Kuru (*35*), Gjone (*250–252*), Pompeius (*253*), Edvardsen (*89,180,254,254a,255*), Ausems (*256*), Sundin *et al.* (*257*), and Mahony *et al.* (*258*).

To my knowledge, 32 micturition reflexes have so far been described, many by multiple authors. The reflexes are triggered by sensory stimuli from the detrusor, vesical mucosa, urethral mucosa, trigone, internal sphincter, "external sphincter," perineal muscles, abdominal muscles, and/or anus; they follow afferent pathways along the pelvic, hypogastric, and/or pudendal nerves to the spinal cord and brain. Some reflexes are spinal (segmental), and others are cephalospinal, involving, respectively, the sacral parasympathetic, lumbar sympathetic, and/or pudendal somatomotor spinal nuclei, or one or more of these nuclei plus pontomesencephalic and/or medullary areas in the brain that are known to control or modulate control of micturition. Efferent impulses resulting from cephalospinal and/or spinal cord influence are transmitted through the pelvic, hypogastric, and/or pudendal nerves to achieve an effector response in the detrusor, trigone, internal sphincter, external sphincter, and/or abdominal and perineal muscles.

Each of the micturition reflexes described has been assigned to function in one of the various phases of micturition, i.e., storage, initiation, maintenance, and termination. Some reflexes have a primary function in one phase and a secondary or potential function in another. Ausems' reflex (*256*) was described primarily for ejaculation, but it can also function as a storage reflex.

Thirteen reflexes serve primarily or secondarily the storage phase of micturition (*35,89,240,248–250,252–254,257,258*). Of these reflexes, nine are spinal, three cephalospinal, and one both spinal and cephalospinal. Afferent stimuli are generated by increased detrusor tension in six reflexes, urethral flow of urine in one, urethral flow plus increased tension in the internal urethral sphincter and trigone in one, and contraction of the perineal muscles in one. These stimuli travel via the pelvic nerves in six reflexes, the pudendal nerves in six, and the hypogastric nerves in one. Of the three cephalospinal reflexes, cephalic control is exercised by inhibitory medullary nuclei in two and the excitatory pontomesencephalic center in one, respectively, on the sacral parasympathetic and pudendal spinal cord nuclei. The peripheral efferent pathway is the pelvic nerves in four reflexes, the pudendal nerves in three, the hypogastric nerves in four, the pelvic plus pudendal nerves in one, and the pelvic plus hypogastric nerves in one. The resultant effector responses achieve relaxation (or reduction of "tone") of the detrusor as well as contraction of the urethral internal and "external" sphincters.

Fourteen reflexes have been advocated primarily or secondarily to explain initiation of voiding (*35,241–248,251,252,254,255,*

258). Of these reflexes, six are spinal and eight are cephalospinal. The afferent sensory stimulus is high detrusor tension in nine reflexes, high internal sphincter tension in one, urethral flow of urine in two, relaxation of the "external" urethral sphincter in one, and relaxation of the pelvic floor plus contraction of abdominal muscles in one. These stimuli travel in the pelvic nerves in nine reflexes, the hypogastric nerves in one, the pudendal nerves in two, and all three nerves in one. Brain influence in the cephalospinal reflexes is exercised through the excitatory medulary region and/or pontine center, resulting in facilitatory and/or disinhibitory impulses to the sacral parasympathetic nuclei as well as inhibitory influence on the pudendal cord nuclei, along descending spinal tracts. The efferent pathway is the pelvic nerve in nine reflexes, the hypogastric nerve in one, the pudendal nerves in one, the pelvic and hypogastric nerve in one, and the pelvic and pudendal nerves in one; the pathway of the remaining reflex (*35*) is uncertain. Efferent stimuli achieve contraction of the detrusor in nine reflexes, contraction of the detrusor and internal sphincter in one, contraction of the detrusor with relaxation of the bladder base and "external" urethral sphincter in one, relaxation of the internal sphincter in one, relaxation of the "external" urethral sphincter in one, and contraction of the detrusor plus contraction of abdominal and relaxation of perineal muscles in one.

Nine reflexes serve the maintenance (continuation) phase of micturition (*35 241–246,251,252,254,255,258*). Seven of these reflexes are cephalospinal, and only two are spinal. Afferent sensory impulses are generated by high tension in the detrusor in five and urine flow through the urethra in four reflexes. The afferent pathway is the pelvic nerve in six reflexes, the pudendal nerve in two, and the pelvic plus hypogastric plus pudendal nerves in one. In the cephalospinal reflexes, excitatory regions in the medulla, pons, and midbrain generate sustained facilitatory and/or disinhibitory influence on the sacral parasympathetic, as well as sustained inhibitory stimuli to the somatomotor pudendal cord nucleus. The efferent pathway is the pelvic nerve in five reflexes, the pelvic and hypogastric nerves in one, the pelvic and pudendal nerves in two, and the pudendal nerves in one. The resultant effector responses are sustained contraction of the detrusor in three reflexes, contraction of the detrusor and internal sphincter in one, contraction of the detrusor plus relaxation of the internal and "external" urethral sphincters in one, sustained contraction of the detrusor plus sustained relaxation of the "external" sphincter in two, and sustained relaxation of the "external" sphincter in two.

Only two primary termination reflexes have been described. The first (*35*) is cephalospinal; its afferent sensory trigger as well as its entire pathway has not been defined clearly, but the resultant effector response is described as relaxation of the detrusor, contraction of the trigone, and contraction of the "external" urethral sphincter. The second termination reflex [12th reflex of Mahony *et al.* (*258*)] is also described as cephalospinal and is triggered by contraction of perineal muscles. The afferent pathway is along the pudendal nerves and the efferent pathway along the pelvic nerves; inhibition of the sacral parasympathetic nuclei with resultant relaxation of the detrusor is achieved through inhibition of excitatory medullary nuclei and excitation of inhibitory medullary nuclei. In addition to the above two reflexes, three spinal primary storage reflexes (*253,257,258*) can be regarded as secondary or potential termination reflexes. Afferent impulses are generated by tension/contraction of perineal muscles in one reflex and anal stimulation in two reflexes; they are conveyed to the spinal cord via the pudendal nerves in two and the hypogastric nerves in one. Detrusor relaxation is elicited by efferent influence via the hypogastric nerves in one reflex and the pelvic nerves in two reflexes.

In addition to the fact that it is almost impossible to commit their details, even partially, to memory, the above reviewed reflexes, whether considered individually or collectively, cannot fully explain any of the phases of micturition or the dynamic transition from one phase to the next. Moreover, (a) some of their designated effector targets have been based on currently obsolete concepts of muscular and neural anatomy, especially in relation to the bladder outlet; (b) they totally ignore competence of the ureterovesical junctions as an integral part of the voiding mechanism in its storage and expulsion phases; (c) they have been based on the assumption that efferent parasympathetic and sympathetic pathways are functionally independent, a premise that has been disproved by evolving concepts of infraspinal direct interaction of the two autonomic divisions at both the ganglionic and prejunctional (effector tissue) levels; and (d) they are not adaptable as pharmacologic models of neuroeffector transmission that clearly indicate the site(s) of action or the target function(s) of each of the drugs that can influence micturition, and thereby can have potential clinical applicability.

"Loops" Concept. Over a number of years, Bradley *et al.* developed the "loops" concept of neural pathways controlling micturition (*34,259*). This concept describes four neural loops (or circuits). Loop I consists of connections between the reticular formation of the brainstem and the frontal cortex. Loop II consists of the ascending afferent tracts in the spinal cord and brainstem, transmitting afferent sensory impulses from the detrusor, as well as descending pathways from the brain to the sacral parasympathetic cord nucleus. Loop III is a spinal reflex arc that comprises afferent sensory axons from the detrusor, their pathway in the sacral spinal cord, the somatomotor pudendal nucleus, and efferent somatomotor axons innervating the "paraurethral striated muscle." Loop IV has a segmental and a neuraxial component; the former comprises pudendal nerve-conveyed afferent and efferent axons innervating the sphincter, and the latter ascending plus descending cephalospinal pathways that control activity of the somatomotor pudendal nucleus in the sacral spinal cord.

Although the "loops" concept has greatly simplified that of micturition reflexes, it has their same shortcomings outlined above. Moreover, (a) it totally ignores function of the lissosphincter in the storage and expulsion phases of micturition to achieve, respectively, continence of urine and establishment of the conduit for urine flow; (b) it totally disregards sympathetic neural pathways as an important, if not a crucial, mechanism of control of vesicourethral storage and voiding functions; and (c) it is not readily or realistically applicable to most forms of clinical neurogenic voiding dysfunction, many of which are due to deficits involving more than one "loop".

Alternative Concept? Current anatomic, morphologic, and physiopharmacologic knowledge indicates that, to be valid and pharmacologically applicable, any proposed neural mechanism of micturition should be based on five main tenets. The mechanism should: (a) be triggered by afferent sensory impulses from all four units of the muscular apparatus of micturition to a variable extent in the various phases of the micturition cycle, but be primarily vesicogenic in all; (b) provide the means for integration and coordination of muscular activity of the four units of the micturition muscular apparatus, including the ureterovesical junctions, during both storage and expulsion phases; (c) be principally diautonomic, i.e., sympathetic and parasympathetic, adrenergic and cholinergic; (d) allow for mutual and reciprocal influence of each autonomic division on the other at the intraganglionic and prejunctional (effector tissue) levels to achieve net effector responses that are determined not only by spinal cord-generated neural stimuli but also the modulatory effect of infraspinal interaction of sympathetic and parasympathetic peripheral postganglionic efferent axons; and (e) recognize the various currently known effector responses of the four units of the micturition muscular apparatus to both parasympathetic and sympathetic efferent neural influence.

Based on the above five tenets, Elbadawi (*260*), proposed the *v*esicogenic *o*rgan-*i*ntegrating *d*iautonomic *e*ffector and *r*eciprocating (VOIDER) reflex as a working hypothesis of the *neural mechanism of micturition. Triggered by sensory output from* various micturition organs, but mainly by *vesicogenic* afferent output, and subject to complex cephalic control, this unitary reflex utilizes *diautonomic* (parasympathetic as well as sympathetic) pathways that elicit multimodal efferent neuroeffector responses. These responses are determined in part by mutually inhibitory infraspinal axonal interaction circuits within vesical ganglia, as well as prejunctionally within the vesicourethral muscularis, and possibly in part by the intraganglionic modulatory influence of SIF cells (and probable co-peptidergic influence) on effector tissue-innervating postganglionic (principal) sympathetic and parasympathetic neurons of vesicourethral ganglia. As an integral part of the above hypothesis, the various pathways and interaction circuits are utilized differently in the various phases of micturition, eliciting different responses in the micturition muscular apparatus. In each phase these responses in any of the four units of the apparatus represent the net result of direct *effector* and indirect *reciprocating* interaction effects of peripheral neural influences, through both of which the neural mechanism of voiding can achieve the continually changing *organ-integrating* function of the muscular apparatus on which consistent performance of normal micturition depends.

Sequential Events of the Micturition Cycle: A Proposal. Based on the above discussion and on current physiopharmacologic knowledge of the mechanism of micturition, Elbadawi (*11,12*) proposed the following sequence of the neural control of micturition (Fig. 1–9). Parts of this proposal are almost certain, but others should be considered as a working hypothesis.

It seems certain that the storage phase of micturition is controlled primarily by sympathetic, and the expulsion phase by parasympathetic vesicourethral innervation. During the storage phase, adrenergic innervation, either directly or via the urogenital short neuron system and/or prejunctional axoaxonal synapses within the vesicourethral muscularis, appears to achieve adaptation of the body detrusor especially in advanced stages of bladder filling, continued continent closure of the lissosphincter, and coordinated competence of both ureterovesical junctions. Opening of the vesical outlet to initiate voiding probably is achieved by relaxation of the vesical outlet by the same parasympathetic discharge that induces micturition contraction of the body detrusor. This relaxation appears to involve a beta-adrenergic mechanism and probably is achieved via parasympathetic/sympathetic interaction circuits within ganglia innervating the bladder and urethra; the axoaxonal synapses that occur frequently in the lissosphincter probably play an even more prominent role in this regard at the prejunctional level. As a working hypothesis, it was proposed (*11,12*) that the urethral relaxation that initiates the voiding stream is replaced by parasympathogenic contraction elicited by the same massive discharge responsible for micturition contraction of the detrusor to sustain a rigidly open vesicourethral outlet, which thereby can withstand the pressure force of the urine stream. Closure of the lissosphincter to terminate voiding remains as the phase of micturition that is most difficult to explain. Elbadawi (*11,12*), however, proposed that this phase is achieved by sympathetic neural discharge when the bladder is completely empty, relaxing the entire vesicourethral muscularis via sympathetic/parasympathetic interaction mechanisms within vesicourethral ganglia or prejunctionally at axoaxonal synapses. Such an influence would restore an adaptable body detrusor, a continent lissosphincter, and a competent but pervious ureterovesical junction in preparation for the next voiding cycle. This proposal is corroborated by data indicating that sympathetic nerve stimulation, whether neurologic or pharmacologic, can interrupt micturition while in progress, and reduce electrical discharges in the pelvic nerves via a mechanism susceptible to alpha-adrenergic blockade (*11*).

The exact role of the rabdosphincter in each phase of micturition still remains to be defined precisely. The concept that the rhabdosphincter is controlled exclusively by the central nervous system through its somatotomotor innervation probably needs revision in view of accumulating data that this structure, at least in some experimental animals, is autonomically innervated by cholinergic and adrenergic axons. Confirmation of such autonomic innervation in man, and its possible role in the function of the rhabdosphincter requires extensive morphologic, physiologic, and pharmacologic investigation. Such studies are necessary, particularly in view of experimental data indicating that the rhabdosphincter, when deprived of its somatomotor innervation, becomes reinnervated purely by autonomic cholinergic and adrenergic axons, with a probable co-peptidergic component in both axon types (*158,168*).

CONCLUDING REMARKS

Since it became known in 1966 that the mammalian urinary bladder has dual cholinergic/adrenergic innervation of its mus-

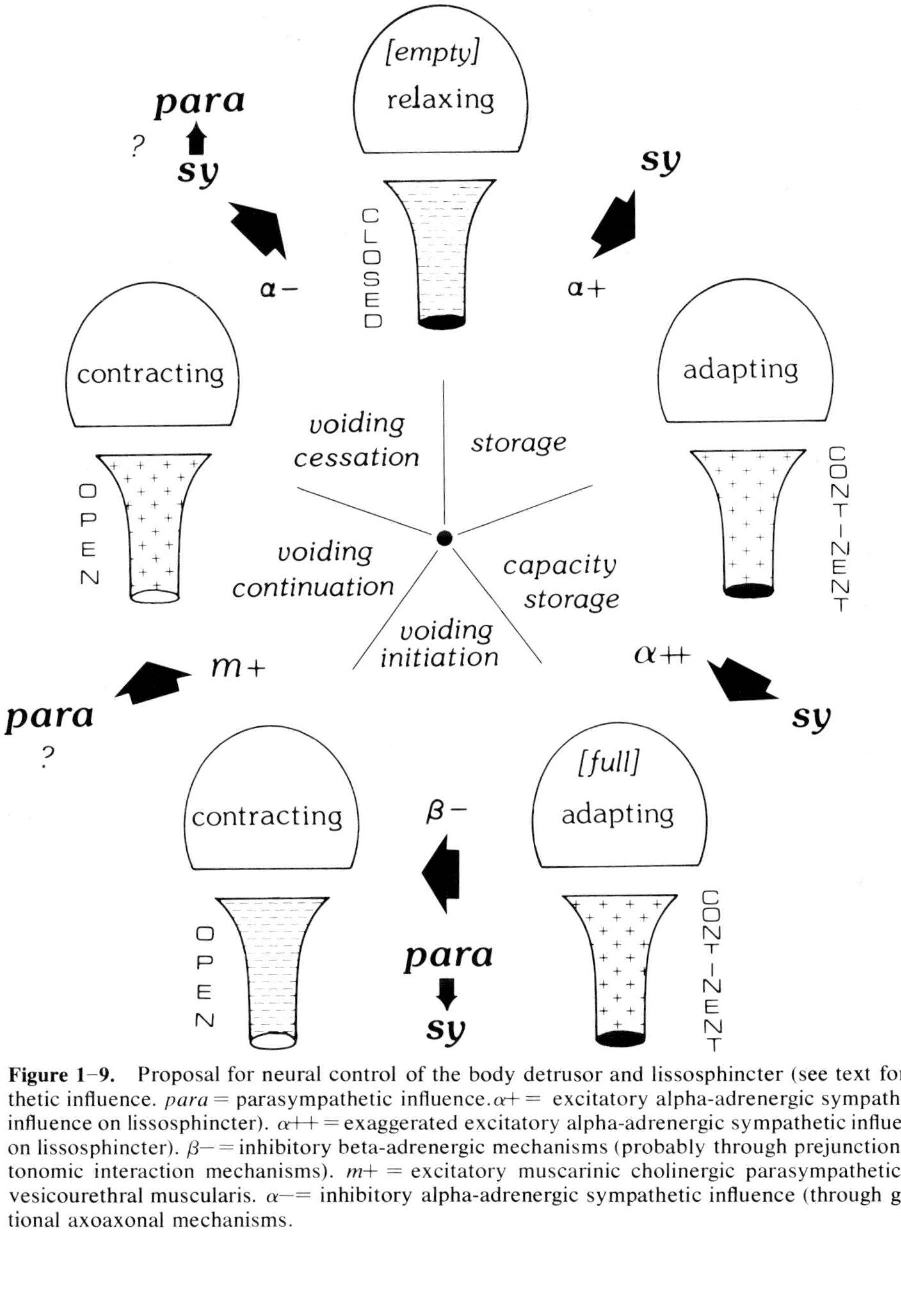

Figure 1–9. Proposal for neural control of the body detrusor and lissosphincter (see text for details). *sy* = sympathetic influence. *para* = parasympathetic influence. *α+* = excitatory alpha-adrenergic sympathetic influence (effector influence on lissosphincter). *α++* = exaggerated excitatory alpha-adrenergic sympathetic influence (effector influence on lissosphincter). *β−* = inhibitory beta-adrenergic mechanisms (probably through prejunctional and ganglionic diautonomic interaction mechanisms). *m+* = excitatory muscarinic cholinergic parasympathetic effector influence on vesicourethral muscularis. *α−* = inhibitory alpha-adrenergic sympathetic influence (through ganglionic and prejunctional axoaxonal mechanisms.

cularis, there has been an avalanche of experimental and clinical data on the physiology and pharmacology of the vesicourethral musculature. These data have invalidated some traditional dogmas, introduced some new concepts, and clarified many issues in regard to the structural and physiopharmacologic basis of micturition. It was inevitable, however, that the depth of the studies that led to these data would raise several new questions that need to be investigated. The most important of such questions is perhaps related to the increasing awareness that the sympathetic and parasympathetic divisions of the autonomic nervous system interact infraspinally (peripherally) at both the ganglionic and prejunctional levels, and that one or more neuropeptides seem to be involved in modulating discharges through these axons, probably by functioning as co-transmitters. It is only through continued intensive investigation in both clinical and experimental models that meaningful answers to such questions can be provided. This is particularly important since data have been accumulating that the intrinsic neuromuscular apparatus of the bladder and urethra may be altered, not only physiologically and pharmacologically but also structurally, in various micturition disorders. Chief among these conditions are acute and chronic vesical distension, persistent urinary tract infection, aging, and neurogenic voiding dysfunctions. Furthermore, experimental studies in the rat indicate that reproductive sex hormones alter the structure and distribution patterns of the cholinergic and adrenergic innervation of the bladder base and probably also the detrusor, so that a hormonal factor may be involved in some micturition disorders involving preferentially one sex, or one age period in either sex (*11,120*). Such influence not only would have an important bearing on our understanding of the pathogenesis of various micturition disorders, but also could be the basis for potentially useful therapeutic modalities, at least in some such disorders.

Acknowledgments

Most morphologic data included in this chapter have been obtained from experimental studies supported by grants AM-28000, NS-17144 and AG-06202 from the USPHS National Institutes of Health.

REFERENCES

1. Elbadawi, A.: Autonomic innervation of the bladder and urethra. *Proc. 16th Cong. Soc. Int. d'Urol.*, Vol. 2, Part 1, Doin, Paris, 1973, pp. 311–316.
2. Gil Vernet, S.: *Morphology and Function of Vesico-prostatourethral Musculature.* Edizioni Canova, Treviso, 1968.
3. Griffiths, J.: Observations on the urinary bladder and urethra. Part 1. *J. Anat. Physiol.* 25:549, 1895.
4. Hunter, DeW. T., Jr.: A new concept of the urinary bladder musculature. *J. Urol.* 71:695–704. 1954.
5. Hutch, J. A.: *Anatomy and Physiology of the Bladder, Trigone and Urethra.* Appleton-Century-Crofts, New York, 1972, pp. 1–180.
6. Lapides, J.: Structure and function of the internal vesical sphincter, *J. Urol.* 80:34–53, 1958.
7. Uhlenhuth, E., Hunter, D. W., Jr., and Loechel, W. F.: *Problems in the Anatomy of the Pelvis.* Lippincott, Philadelphia, 1953, pp. 1–157.
8. Wesson, M. B.: Anatomical, embryological and physiological studies of the trigone and neck of the bladder. *J. Urol.* 4:279–315, 1920.
9. Woodburne, R.T.: Anatomy of the bladder. In Boyarsky, S. (ed.), *The Neurogenic Bladder.* Williams & Wilkins, Baltimore, 1967, pp. 3–17.
10. Young, B. W.: *Lower Urinary Tract Obstruction in Childhood.* Lea & Febiger, Philadelphia, 1972.
11. Elbadawi, A.: Neuromorphologic basis of vesicourethral function. I. Histochemistry, ultrastructure, and function of intrinsic nerves of the bladder and urethra. *Neurourol. Urodyn.* 1:3–50, 1982.
12. Elbadawi, A.: Autonomic muscular innervation of the vesical outlet and its role in micturition. In Hinman, F., Jr. (ed.), *Benign Prostatic Hypertrophy.* Springer-Verlag, New York, 1983, pp. 330–348.
13. Elbadawi, A., and Schenk, E. A.: Dual innervation of the mammalian urinary bladder. A histochemical study of the distribution of cholinergic and adrenergic nerves. *Am. J. Anat.* 119:405–427, 1966.
14. Fagge, C. H.: On the innervation of the urinary passages in dogs. *J. Physiol. (Lond.)* 28:304–315, 1902.
15. Blaivas, J. G.: Why now? *Neurourol. Urodyn.* 1:1–2, 1982 (editorial).
16. Elbadawi, A.: Anatomy and function of the ureteral sheath. *J. Urol.* 107:224–229, 1972.
17. Elbadawi, A., Amaku, E. O., and Frank, I. N.: Trilaminar musculature of the submucosal ureter: anatomy and functional implications. *Urology* 2:409–417, 1973.
18. Koyanagi, T., and Tsuji, I.: Study of ureteral reflux in neurogenic dysfunction of bladder: concept of neurogenic ureter and role of periureteral sheath in genesis of reflux and supersensitive response to autonomic drugs. *J. Urol.* 126:210–217, 1981.
19. Stephens, F. D.: The normal and abnormal ureterovesical hiatus: methods of correction of vesicoureteral reflux and paraureteral diverticula. *J. Contin. Educ. Urol.* Dec. 1978, p. 12.
20. Tanagho, E. A., and Pugh, R. C. B.: The anatomy of the ureterovesical junction. *Br. J. Urol.* 35:151, 1963.
21. Elbadawi, A., and Schenk, E. A.: A new theory of the innervation of bladder musculature. 2. The innervation apparatus of the ureterovesical junction. *J. Urol.* 105:372–374, 1971.
22. Elbadawi, A., and Schenk, E. A.: A new theory of the innervation of bladder musculature. 4. Innervation of the vesicourethral junction and external urethral sphincter. *J. Urol.* 111:613–615, 1974.
23. *Cunningham's Textbook of Anatomy*, 9th ed. W. Wood, New York, 1951.
24. Gray, H.: *Anatomy of the Human Body*, 29th Am. ed. Gross C. M. (ed.) Lea & Febiger, Philadelphia, 1973.
25. Colapinto, V.: The anatomy of the urethral sphincter and the myth of the urogential sandwich. In: *Proceedings 79th Annual Meeting American Urological Association*, Abstr. 244, 1984, p. 132A.
26. Hanes, R. W.: The striped compressor of the prostatic urethra. *Br. J. Urol.* 41:481–493, 1970.
27. Oerlich, T. M.: The urethral sphincter muscle in the male. *Am. J. Anat.* 158:229–264, 1980.

28. Oerlich, T. M.: The striated urogenital sphincter muscle in the female. *Anat. Rec.* 205:223–232, 1982.
29. Bors, E., Comarr, A. E., and Reingold, I. M.: Striated muscle fibers of the bladder neck. *J. Urol.* 72:191–196, 1954.
30. Bors, E.: Effect of electrical pudendal nerve stimulation on the vesical neck; its significance for the function of the cord bladder: preliminary report. *J. Urol.* 67:925–935, 1952.
31. Yalla, S. V., Gabilondo, F. B., Blunt, K. J., Fam, B. A., Castello, A., and Kaufman, J. M.: Functional striated sphincter component at the bladder neck: clinical implications. *J. Urol.* 118:408–411, 1977.
32. Bors, E., and Comarr, A. E.: *Neurological Urology: Physiology of Micturition, its Neurological Disorders and Sequelae.* University Park Press, Baltimore, 1971, pp. 1–454.
33. Buzelin, J. M.: *Urodynamique. Bas Appareil Urinaire.* Masson, Paris, 1984, pp. 3–18.
34. Hald, T., and Bradley, W. E.: *The Urinary Bladder: Neurology and Dynamics.* Williams & Wilkins, Baltimore, 1982, pp. 5–36.
35. Kuru, M.: Nervous control of micturition. *Physiol. Rev.* 45:425–494, 1965.
36. Schmidt, R. A.: Urethral vesical reflexes and their inhibition. In Hinman, F., Jr. (ed.), *Benign Prostatic Hypertrophy.* Springer-Verlag, New York, 1983, pp. 361–372.
37. Wein, A. J., and Raezer, D. M.: Physiology of micturition. In Krane, R. J., and Siroky, M. B. (eds.), *Clinical Neuro-urology.* Little, Brown, Boston, 1979, pp. 35–44.
38. Tanagho, E. A., Schmidt, R. A., and Araujo, C. G.: Urinary striated sphincter: what is its nerve supply? *Urology,* 24:415–417, 1982.
39. Onufrowicz, B.: On the arrangement and function of cell groups of the sacral region of the spinal cord in man. *Arch. Neurol. Psychopathol.* 3:387–412, 1902.
40. Oliver, J. E., Bradley, W. E., and Fletcher, T. J.: Spinal cord distribution of the somatic innervation of the external urethral sphincter in the cat. *J. Neurol. Sci.* 10:11–23, 1970.
41. Rockswold, G. L., Bradley, W. E., and Chou, S. M.: Innervation of the urinary bladder in higher primates. *J. Comp. Neurol.* 193:509–520, 1980.
42. Anderson, J. T., and Bradley, W. E.: Bladder and urethral innervation in multiple sclerosis. *Br. J. Urol.* 48:239–243, 1976.
43. Blaivas, J. G., Bhimani, G., and Labib, K. B.: Vesicourethral dysfunction in multiple sclerosis. *J. Urol.* 122:342–346, 1979.
44. Mannen, T., Iwata, M., Toyokura, Y., and Nagashima, K.: Preservation of certain motor neurons group of the sacral cord in amyotrophic lateral sclerosis: its clinical significance. *J. Neurol. Neurosurg. Psychiatry* 40:255–269, 1977.
45. Blaivas, J. G.: The neurophysiology of micturition: a clinical study of 550 patients. *J. Urol.* 127:958–963, 1982.
46. De Wall, J. G., Griffiths, D. J., Dalm, E., and Holstege, G.: Neurourological investigation of the supraspinal regulation of bladder and urethral function in the cat. In *Proceedings 14th Annual Meeting International Continence Society,* 1984, pp. 235–236.
47. Ruch, T. C.: The urinary bladder: physiology and biophysics. In Ruch, T .C., and Patton, H. D. (eds.). *Circulation, Respiration and Fluid Balance.* Saunders, Philadelphia, 1974, pp. 525–546.
48. Coggeshall, R. E.: Law of separation of function of the spinal roots. *Physiol. Rev.* 60:716–754, 1980.
49. Elbadawi, A., and Goodman, D. C.: Autonomic innervation of accessory male genital glands. In Spring-Mills, E., and Hafez, E. S. E. (eds), *Male Accessory Sex Glands.* Elsevier/North Holland, Amsterdam, 1980, pp. 101–128.
50. Gruber, C. M.: The autonomic innervation of the genitourinary system. *Physiol. Rev.* 13:497–609, 1933.
51. Kuntz, A.: *The Autonomic Nervous System.* Lea & Febiger, Philadelphia, 1945.
52. Kuntz, A., and Saccomanno, G.: Sympathetic innervation of the detrusor muscle. *J. Urol.* 51:535–545, 1944.
53. Mitchell, G. A. G.: *Anatomy of the Autonomic Nervous System.* Livingstone, Edinburgh, 1953, pp. 257–310.
54. Schnitzlein, H. N., Hofman, H. H., Tucker, C. C., and Quigley, M. B.: The pelvic splanchine nerves of the male Rehsus monkey. *J. Comp. Neurol.* 114:659, 1972.
55. Sjöstrand, N. O.: The adrenergic innervation of the vas deferens and the accessory male genital glands. *Acta Physiol. Scand.* [*Suppl.*] 257:1, 1965.
56. Wózniak, W., and Skowrónska, U.: Comparative anatomy of pelvic plexus in cat, dog, rabbit, macaque and man. *Anat. Anz.* 120:457, 1967.
57. Elbadawi, A., Atta, M. A., and Franck, J. I.: Intrinsic neuromuscular defects in the neurogenic bladder. I. Short-term ultrastructural changes in muscular innervation of the decentralized feline bladder base following unilateral sacral ventral rhizotomy. *Neurourol. Urodyn.* 3:93–113, 1984.
58. Costa, M., and Furness, J. B.: Observations on the anatomy and amine histochemistry of the nerves and ganglia which supply the pelvic viscera and on the associated chromaffin tissue in the guinea-pig. *Z. Anat. Entwickl.-Gesch.* 140:85, 1973.
59. Langworthy, O. R.: Innervation of the pelvic organs of the rat. *Invest. Urol.* 2:491, 1965.
60. Elbadawi, A., and Schenk, E. A.: The peripheral adrenergic innervation apparatus. I. Intraganglionic and extraganglionic adrenergic ganglion cells. *Z. Zellforsch.* 87:218–225, 1968.
61. Elbadawi, A., and Schenk, E. A.: Intra- and extraganglionic peripheral cholinergic neurons in urogential organs of the cat. *Z. Zellforsch.* 103:26–33, 1970.
62. Elbadawi, A., and Schenk, E. A.: Parasympathetic and sympathetic postganglionic synapses in ureterovesical autonomic pathways. *Z. Zellforsch.* 146:147–156, 1973.
63. McCrea, L. E., and Kimmel, D. L.: The importance of nerve supply of the urinary bladder in surgery of the rectosigmoid. *J. Int. Coll. Surg.* 17:651–657, 1952.
64. Downie, J. W., Champion, J. A., and Nance, D. W.: A quantitative analysis of the afferent and extrinsic efferent innervation of specific regions of the bladder and urethra in the cat. *Brain Res. Bull.* 12:735–740, 1984.
65. Kuo, D. C., Hisamitsu, T., and de Groat, W. C.: The sympathetic projection from sacral paraver-

tebral ganglia to the pelvic nerve and to postganglionic nerves on the surface of the urinary bladder and large intestine of the cat. *J. Comp. Neurol.* 226:76–86, 1984.
66. Bors, E., and Comarr, A. E.: Effect of pudendal neurectomy operations on the neurogenic bladder. *J. Urol.* 72:666, 1954.
67. Langworthy, O. R., Kolb, L. C., and Lewis, L. G.: *Physiology of Micturition, Experimental and Clinical Studies with Suggestions as to Diagnosis and Treatment.* Williams & Wilkins, Baltimore, 1940, pp 1–211.
68. Tasker, J. H.: Pudendal neurectomy. *Br. J. Urol.* 33:397–398, 1961.
69. Yamamoto, T., Satomi, H., Ise, H., Takamata, H., and Takahashi, K.: Sacral spinal innervation of the rectal and vesical smooth muscles and the sphincteric striated muscles demonstrated by the horseradish peroxidase method. *Neurosci. Lett.* 7:41–47, 1978.
70. Gil Vernet, S.: L'innérvation somatique et vegétative des organes génitourinaires. *Acta Urol. Belg.* 32:265–293, 1964.
71. Gil Vernet, S.: Maladie du col vésical ou prostatisme sans hypertrophie de la prostate. *Urol. Int.* 18:216–226, 1964.
72. Winkler, G.: Contribucion al estudeo de la innervacion de las visceras pelvianas. *Arch. Esp. Urol.* 20:259–279, 1967.
73. Winkler, G.: L'innérvation des viscères pelviens chez le mouton: participation du nerf honteux interne. *Arch. Anat.* 40:85–89, 1967.
74. Tuchschmid, D., Lahläidi, A., and von Niederhäusern, W. Y.: Contribution a l'étude de l'innérvation de sphincter strié de l'urètre. *Helv. Chir. Acta* 40:525–529.
75. Morita, T., Nishizawa, O., Noto, H., and Tsuchida, S.: Pelvic nerve innervation of the external sphincter of the urehtra as suggested by urodynamic and horseradish peroxidase studies. *J. Urol.* 131:591–595, 1984.
76. Stach, W., Fanghänel, J., and Schultz, E. Afferente terminal-organe in der Wand der Harnblase ver scheidner laboratoriumstiere und ihre Topographie. *J. Neurovisc. Rel.* 31:26, 1970.
77. Uemura, E., Fletcher, T. F., and Bradley, W. E.: Distribution of lumbar afferent axons in muscle coat of cat urinary bladder. *Am. J. Anat.* 139:389–398, 1974.
78. Uemura, E., Fletcher, T. F., and Bradley, W. E.: Distribution of lumbar and sacral afferent axons in submucosa of cat urinary bladder. *Anat. Rec.* 183:579–588, 1975.
79. Uemura, E., Fletcher, T. F., Dirks, V. A., and Bradley, W. E.: Distribution of sacral afferent axons in cat urinary bladder. *Am. J. Anat.* 136:305–314, 1973.
80. Purinton, T., Fletcher, T., and Bradley, W.: Sensory perikarya in autonomic ganglia. *Nature [New Biol.]* 231:63–64, 1971.
81. Ungvary, G., and Léranth, C.: Termination in the prevertebral abdominal sympathetic ganglia of axons arising from the local (terminal) vegetative plexus of visceral organs: peripheral reflex arcs. *Z. Zellforsch.* 110:185–191, 1970.
82. Sowkonin, N.: Innervation der Harnblase. *Pflugers Arch.* 8:600, 1874.
83. Elbadawi, A.: Ultrastucture of vesicourethral innervation. I. Neuroeffector and cell junctions in the male internal sphincter. *J. Urol.* 128:180–188, 1982.
84. Daniel, E. E., Cowan, W., and Daniel, V. P.: Structural bases for neural and myogenic control of human detrusor muscle. *Can. J. Physiol. Pharmacol.* 61:1247–1272, 1983.
85. Watanabe, H., and Yamamoto, T. Y.: Autonomic innervation of the muscles in the wall of the bladder and proximal urethra of male rats. *J. Anat.* 128:873–886, 1979.
86. Ganote, E., and Moses, H. L.: Light and dark cells as artifacts of tissue fixation. *Lab, Invest.* 18:740–745, 1968.
87. Garfield, R. W., and Daniel, E. E.: Light and dark smooth muscle cells in estrogen-stimulated rat myometrium. *Can. J. Physiol. Pharmacol.* 54:822, 1976.
88. Gabella, G.: Structure of smooth muscles. In Bülbring, E., Brading, A. F., Jones, A. W., and Tomita, T. (eds.), *Smooth Muscle: An Assessment of Current Knowledge.* University of Texas Press, Austin, 1981, pp. 1–46.
89. Burnstock, G., and Iwayama, T.: Fine structural identification of autonomic nerves and their relation to smooth muscle. *Prog. Brain Res.* 34:389–404, 1971.
90. Gosling, J. A., and Dixon, J. S.: Light and electron microscopic observations on the human external urethral sphincter. *J. Anat.* 129:216, 1979.
91. Bowen, J. M., Timm, G. W., and Bradley, W. E.: Some contractile and electrophysiologic properties of the periurethral striated muscle of the cat. *Invest. Urol.* 13:327–330, 1976.
92. Elbadawi, A., and Atta, M. A.: Ultrastructure of vesicourethral innervation. IV. Evidence for somatomotor plus autonomic innervation of the male feline rhabdosphincter. *Neurourol. Urodyn.* 4:23–36, 1985.
93. Gillespie, C. A., Simpson, D. R., and Edgerton, V. R.: High glycogen content of red as opposed to white skeletal muscle fibers of guinea pigs. *J. Histchem. Cytochem.* 18:552–558, 1970.
94. Hess, A.: The structure of vertebrate slow and twitch muscle fibers. *Invest. Ophthalmol.* 6:217–228, 1967.
95. Hess, A.: Vertebrate slow muscle fibers. *Pharmacol. Rev.* 50:40–62, 1970.
96. Lentz, T. L.: *Cell Fine Structure. An Atlas of Drawings of Whole-Cell Structure.* Saunders, Philadelphia, 1971, pp. 84–102.
97. Mitko, L., and Kilarski, W.: Correlation between nerve terminal size and muscle fiber diameter in urodela extrinsic eye muscle. *Z. Mikrosk.-Anat. Forsch.* 89:1015–1029, 1975.
98. Murata, F., and Ogata, T.: The ultrastructure of neuromuscular junctions of human red, white and intermediate striated muscle fibers. *Tohoku J. Exp. Med.* 99:289–301, 1969.
99. Padykula, H.A., and Gauthier, G. F.: The ultrastructure of the neuromuscular junctions of mammalian red, white and intermediate skeletal muscle fibers. *J. Cell Biol.* 46:27–41, 1970.
100. Peter, J. B., Barnard, R. J., Edgerton, V. R., Gillespie, C. A., and Stempel, K. E.: Metabolic profiles of three fiber types of skeletal muscle in

guinea pigs and rabbits. *Biochemistry* 11:2627–2633, 1972.
101. Schiaffino, S., Hanzlikova, V., and Pierobon, S.: Relations between structure and function in rat skeletal muscle fibers. *J. Cell Biol.* 47:107–119, 1970.
102. Santa, T., and Engel, A. G.: Histometric analysis of neuromuscular junction ultrastructure in rat red, white and intermediate muscle fibers. In Desmedt, J. E. (ed.), *New Developments in Electromyography and Clinical Neurophysiology*, Vol. 1. Karger, Basel, 1973, pp. 202–221.
103. Martin, W. D., Fletcher, T. F., and Bradley, W. E.: Innervation of feline perineal musculature. *Anat. Rec.* 180:15–29, 1974.
104. Schroder, H. D., and Reske-Nielsen, E.: Fiber types in the striated urethral and anal sphincters. *Acta Neuropathol. (Berl.)* 60:278–282, 1983.
105. Bazeed, M.A., Thüroff, J. W., Schmidt, R. A., and Tanagho, E. A.: Histochemical study of urethral striated musculature in the dog. *J. Urol.* 128:406–410.
106. Elbadawi, A.: Le support anatomique des voies urinaires. In Buzelin, J. M., Richard F., and Susset, J. G. (eds.): *Physiologie et Pathologie Functionelle des Voies Urinaires.* Vigot Publishing Co., Paris, 1987. In press.
107. Atta, M. A.: Vesicourethral Neuromuscular Defects in Lower-Motor Neurogenic Voiding Dysfunction. An Experimental Study in the Cat. M.D. (Ph.D.) Thesis, Alexandria University, Alexandria, Egypt, 1985, pp. 1–402.
108. Mastaglia, F. L., and Walton, J.: *Skeletal Muscle Pathology*. Churchill Livingstone, Edinburgh, 1982, pp. 1–87.
109. Mauro, A.: Satellite cell of skeletal muscle fibers. *J. Biophys. Biochem. Cytol.* 9:493–495, 1961.
110. Muir, A. R.: The structure and distribution of satellite cells. In Mauro, A., Shafiq, S. A., and Milhorat, A. T. (eds.), *Regeneration of Striated Muscle and Myogenesis. International Congress Series* 218. Excerpta Medica, Amsterdam, 1970, pp. 91–100.
111. Elmér, M.: Autonomic Innervation of the Rat Urinary Bladder. Thesis, University of Lund, Lund, Sweden, 1975, pp. 1–31.
112. Sundin, T., Dahlström, A.: The sympathetic innervation of the urinary bladder and urethra in the normal state and after parasympathetic denervation at the spinal root level: an experimental study in cats. *Scand. J. Urol. Nephrol.* 7:131–149, 1973.
113. Elbadawi, A., and Schenk, E. A.: A new theory of the innervation of bladder musculature. 1. Morphology of the intrinsic vesical innervation apparatus. *J. Urol.* 99:585–587, 1968.
114. Owman, C., and Sjöstrand, N. O.: Short adrenergic neurons and catecholamine-containing cells in vas deferens and accessory male genital glands of different mammals. *Z. Zellforsch.* 66:300, 1965.
115. Smith, E. R.: The canine prostate and its secretion. *Adv. Sex Horm. Res.* 1:167, 1975.
116. Elbadawi, A.: Ultrastructure of vesicourethral innervation. III. Axoaxonal synapses between postganglionic cholinergic axons and probably SIF-cell derived processes in feline lissosphincter. *J. Urol.* 133:524–528, 1985.
117. Elbadawi, A., and Schenk, E. A.: A new theory of the innervation of urinary bladder musculature. III. Postganglionic synapses in ureterovesicourethral autonomic pathways. *J. Urol.* 105:372–374, 1971.
118. deGroat, W. C., Booth, A. M., Hisamitsu, T., and Kawatani, M.: The role of enkephalins in the neural control of bladder capacity. In *Proceedings 6th Annual Urodynamics Society Symposium*, 1984, p. 29.
118a. de Groat, W. C., and Kawatani, M.: Neural control of the urinary bladder: possible relationship between peptidergic inhibitory mechanisms and detrusor instability. *Neurourol. Urodyn.* 4:285–300, 1985.
119. Elbadawi, A.: Bladder innervation. *Urology* 2:331–332, 1973 (editorial).
120. El-Sadr, A.: Modulation of Bladder Base Innervation by Reproductive Hormones: A New Concept of the Neural Control of Vesical Outlet Function. Thesis, Alexandria University, Alexandria, Egypt, 1982, pp. 1–311.
121. Slack, B. E., Downie, J. W., and Elbadawi, A.: Paradoxical resistance to adrenolytic agents of field-stimulated bladder base of rabbit. *J. Pharmacol. Exp. Ther.* 220:216–222, 1982.
122. Alm, P., and Elmér, M.: Adrenergic and cholinergic innervation of the rat urinary bladder. *Acta Physiol. Scand.* 94:36–45, 1975.
123. Gosling, J. A., Dixon, J. S., and Lendon, R. G.: The autonomic innervation of the human male and female bladder neck and proximal urethra. *J. Urol.* 118:302–305, 1977.
124. Elbadawi, A.: Comparative anatomy in animals. In Torrens, M. J., and Morrison, J. M. (eds.): *The Neurophysiology of Micturition*. Springer Verlag, London, 1987. In press.
125. Alm, P.: Cholinergic innervation of the human urethra and urinary bladder: a histochemical study and review of methodology. *Acta Pharmacol. Toxicol. (Copenh.)* 43:56–62, 1978.
126. Ek, A., Alm, P., Andersson, K-E., and Persson, C. G. A.: Adrenergic and cholinergic nerves of the human urethra and urinary bladder: a histochemical study. *Acta Physiol. Scand.* 99:345–352, 1977.
127. Kluck, P.: The autonomic innervation of the human urinary bladder, bladder neck and urethra: histochemical study. *Anat. Rec.* 198:439–448, 1980.
128. Nordling, J., and Christensen, B.: Human sympathetic bladder innervation. *Urol. Int.* 33:359–365, 1978.
129. Elbadawi, A.: Ultrastructure of vesicourethral innervation. II. Postganglionic axoaxonal synapses in intrinsic innervation of the vesicourethral lissosphincter: a new structural and functional concept in micturition. *J. Urol.* 131:781–790, 1984.
130. Mattiasson, A., Andersson, K-E., and Sjögren, C.: Adrenoceptors and cholinoceptors controlling noradrenaline release from adrenergic nerves in the urethra of rabbit and man. *J. Urol.* 131:1190–1195, 1984.
131. Mattiasson, A., Andersson, K.-E., Elbadawi, A., Morgan, E., and Sjögren, C.: Interaction between adrenergic and cholinergic nerve terminals in the urinary bladder of rabbit, cat and man. *J. Urol.* 137:1017–1019, 1987.

132. Iijima, T.: Occurrence of uranaffin-positive synaptic vesicles in both adrenergic and non-adrenergic nerves of the rat anococcygeus muscle. *Cell Tissue Res.* 220:427–433, 1981.
133. Nathanson, J. A.: Cyclic nucleotides and nervous system function. *Physiol. Rev.* 57:157–256, 1977.
134. Richards, J. G., and da Prada, M.: Uranaffin reaction: a new cytochemical technique for the localization of adenine nucleotide in organs storing biogenic amines. *J. Histochem. Cytochem.* 25:1322–1336, 1977.
135. Burnstock, G.: Purinergic nerves. *Pharmacol. Rev.* 24:509, 1972.
136. Burnstock, G., and Iwayama, T.: Fine structural identification of autonomic nerves and their relation to smooth muscle. *Prog. Brain Res.* 34:389–404, 1971.
137. Daniel, E. E., Taylor, G. S., Daniel, V. P., and Holman, M. E.: Can nonadrenergic inhibitory varicostities be identified ultrastructurally? *Can. J. physiol. Pharmacol.* 55:243–250, 1977.
138. Sneddon, P., and Westfall, D. P.: Pharmacological evidence that adenosine triphosphate and noradrenaline are co-transmitters in the guinea pig vas deferens. *J. Physiol. (Lond.)* 347:561–580.
139. Alm, P., Alumets, J., Hakanson, R., and Sundler, F.: Peptidergic nerves in the genitourinary tract. *Neuroscience* 2:751–754, 1977.
140. Alumets, J., Fahrenkrug, R., de Muckadell, S., Sundler, F., and Uddman, R.: A rich VIP nerve supply is characteristic of sphincters. *Nature* 280:155–156, 1980.
141. Hökfelt, T., Schulzberg, M., Elde, P., Nilsson, G., Terenius, L., Simonds, S., and Goldstein, M.: Peptidergic neurons in peripheral tissues including the urinary tract: immunohistochemical studies. *Acta Pharmacol. Toxicol. (Copendh.)* 43:79–89, 1978.
142. Gu, J., Blank, M. A., Huang, W. M., Islam, K. N., McGregoir, G. P., Christofiedes, N., Allen, J. M., Bloom, S. R., and Polak, J. M.: Peptide-containing nerves in human urinary bladder, *Urology* 24:353–357, 1984.
143. Islam, K. N., Gu, J., Blank, H. A., Bloom, S. R., Polak, J. M., and Shuttleworth, K. E. D.: Peptide-containing nerves in human urinary bladder. In *Proceedings 79th Annual Meeting, American Urological Association,* Abstract 359, 1984, pp. 193A.
144. Goyal, R. K., Rathan, S., and Said, S. I.:VIP as a possible neurotransmitter of non-cholinergic non-adrenergic inhibitory neurons. *Nature* 288:378–382, 1980.
145. Matsuzaki, Y., Hamasuki, Y., and Said, S. I.: A possible transmitter of noradrenergic relaxation of guinea pig airways. *Science* 210:1252–1253, 1980.
146. Cuello, A. C.: *Co-Transmission,* Macmillan, London, 1982, pp. 1–259.
147. Lundberg, J. M., Hökfelt, T.: Coexistence of peptides and classical neurotransmitters. *Trends Neurosci.* 6:325–333, 1983.
148. Lundberg, J. M., Hedlund, B., Anggard, A., Fahrenkrug, J., Hökfelt, T., Tatemoto, T., and Bartfai, T.: In Bloom, S. R., Polak, J. M., and Lindenlaub, E. (eds), *Systemic Role of Regulatory Peptides.* 1982, pp. 145–168.
149. Lundberg, J. M., Terenius, L., Hökfelt, T., Martling, C.R., Tatemoto, T., Mutt, V., Polak, J., Bloom, S., and Goldstein, M.: Neuropeptide-Y (NPY)-like immunoactivity in peripheral noradrenergic neurons and effects of NPY on sympathetic fibres. *Acta Physiol. Scand.* 116:477–480, 1982.
150. Tramu, G., Pillez, A., and Leonardelli, J.: An efficient method of antibody elution for successive or simultaneous location of two antigens by immunocytochemistry. *J. Histochem. Cytochem.* 26:322–324, 1978.
151. Lundberg, J. M.: Evidence for coexistence of vasoactive intestinal polypeptide (VIP) and acetylcholine in neurons of cat exocrine glands: morphological, biochemical and functional studies. *Acta Physiol. Scand.* [Suppl.] 496:1–57, 1981.
152. Lundberg, J. M., Hökfelt, T., Schultzberg, M., Uvaus-Wallensten, K., Kohler, C., and Said, S. I.: Occurrence of vasoactive intestinal polypeptide-like immunoreactivity in certain cholinergic neurons in the cat: evidence from combined immunohistochemistry and acetylcholinesterase. *Neuroscience* 4:1539–1559, 1979.
153. Chan-Palay, V., Jonsson, G., and Palay, S. L.: Serotonin and substance P coexist in neurons of the rat central nervous system. *Z. Zellforsch.* 135:287–314, 1978.
154. Larsson, L-I.: Ultrastructural localization of a new peptide (VIP). *Histochemistry* 54:170–176, 1977.
155. Pickel, V., Reis, D., and Leeman, S.: Ultrastructural localization of substance P in neurons of the rat spinal cord. *Brain Res.* 122:504–540, 1977.
156. Andersson, P-O., Bloom, S. R., Edwards, A. V., Jarhult, J., and Mellander, S.: Neural vasodilatation control in the rectum of the cat and its possible mediation by vasoactive intestinal polypeptide. *J. Physiol. (Lond.)* 344:49–67, 1983.
157. Andersson, P-O., Bloom, S. R., and, B. L., and Mellander, S.: Hemodynamics of nerve induced penile erection in the dog: possible mediation by vasoactive intestinal polypeptide. *J. Physiol. (Lond.)* 350:209–224, 1984.
158. Atta, M. A., and Elbadawi, A.: The denervated rhabdosphincter loses somatomotor cholinergic and acquires adrenergic/probably co-peptidergic innervation. In *Proceedings 14th Annual Meeting International Continence Society,* 1984, pp. 261–262.
159. Atta, M. A., Franck, J. I., and Elbadawi, A.: Intrinsic neuromuscular defects in the neurogenic bladder. II. Long-term innervation of the unilaterally decentralized feline bladder base by regenerated cholinergic, increased adrenergic and emergent probable "peptidergic" nerves. *Neurourol. Urodyn.* 3:185–200, 1984.
160. Ceccarelli, B., Clementi, F., and Mantegazza, P.: Adrenergic reinnervation of smooth muscle of nictitating membrane by preganglionic sympathetic fibers. *Arch. Int. Pharmacodyn. Thér.* 196:293–295, 1972.
161. Jan, Y. N., and Jan, L. Y.: Coexistence and corelease of cholinergic and peptidergic transmitters in frog sympathetic ganglia. *Fed. Proc.* 42:2929-2933, 1983.
162. Landis, S. C.: Development of cholinergic sympathetic neurons: evidence for transmitter plasticity in vivo. *Fed. Proc.* 42:1633–1638, 1983.
163. Dixon, J. S., and Gosling, J. A.: Light and electron

microscopic observations on the adrenergic nerves and striated muscle cells of the guinea-pig urethra. *Am. J. Anat.* 149:121–126, 1977.

164. Dixon, J. S., and Gosling, J. A.: The morphology and innervation of the subepithelial "striated" muscle cells in the male guinea-pig urethra. *Cell Tissue Res.* 174:281–288, 1976.
165. Rossier, A. B., Fam. B. A., Lee, I. Y., and Sarkarati, M.: Neuropharmacological urodynamic evaluation of the smooth and striated components of the external urethral sphincter in neurogenic bladder. In *Proceedings 76th Annual Meeting American. Urological Association*, abstract 568, 1981, p. 233.
166. Wein, A. J., Benson, G. S., and Jacobowitz, D.: Lack of evidence for adrenergic innervation of the external urethral sphincter. *J. Urol.* 121:324–326, 1979.
167. Atta, M. A., and Elbadawi, A.: Intrinsic neuromuscular defects in the neurogenic bladder. IV. Loss of somatomotor and preservation of autonomic innervation of the male feline rhabdosphincter following bilateral sacral ventral rhizotomy. *Neurourol. Urodyn.*, 4:219–229, 1985.
168. Elbadawi, A., and Atta, M.A.: Intrinsic neuromuscular effects in the neurogenic bladder. V. Autonomic re-innervation of the male feline rhabdosphincter following somatic denervation by bilateral sacral ventral rhizotomy. *Neurourol. Uro*dyn. 5:65–85, 1985.
169. Brindley, G. S.: Control of the bladder and urethral sphincters by the surgically implanted electrical stimulators. In Chisolm, G. D., and Williams, D. I. (eds.), *Scientific Foundations of Urology*. Year Book, Chicago, 1982, pp 464–470.
170. Creed, K. E., and Tulloch, A. G. C.: The effect of pelvic nerve stimulation and some drugs on the urethra and bladder of the dog. *Br. J. Urol.* 50:398–405, 1978.
171. Susset, J. G., Boctor, S. N., Rossini, F., Robinovitch, H., and MacKinnon, K. J.: Implantable electronic vesical stimulator: review of literature and report of a successful case. *Can. Med. Assoc. J.* 95:1128–1131, 1966.
172. Ambache, N., and Zar, M. A.: Non-cholinergic transmission by postganglionic motor neurones in the mammalian bladder. *J. Physiol. (Lond.)* 210:761–783, 1970.
173. Taira, N.: The autonomic pharmacology of the bladder. *Annu. Rev. Pharmacol.* 12:197–208, 1972.
174. Graber, P., and Tanagho, E. A.: Urethral responses to autonomic nerve stimulation. *Urology* 6:52–58, 1975.
175. Kiruluta, H. G., Downie, J. W., and Awad, S. A.: The continence mechanism: the effect of bladder filling on the urethra. *Invest. Urol.* 18:460–465, 1981.
176. Elliott, T. R.: The innervation of the bladder and urethra. *J. Physiol. (Lond.)* 35:367–445, 1906-1907.
177. Girado, J. M., and Campbell, J. B.: The innervation of the urethra of the female cat. *Exp. Neurol.* 1:44–64, 1959.
178. McGuire, E. J., and Herlihy, E.: Bladder and urethral responses to isolated motor root stimulation. *Invest. Urol.* 16:219–223, 1978.
179. Mattiasson, A.: On the Peripheral Nervous Control of the Lower Urinary Tract. Thesis, University of Lund, Lund, Sweden, Part VI, 1984, pp. 117–127.
180. Edvardsen, P.: Nervous control of urinary bladder in cats. IV. Effects of autonomic blocking agents on response to peripheral nerve stimulation. *Acta Physiol. Scand.* 72:234–247, 1968.
181. Sigg, E. B., and Sigg, T. D.: Sympathetic stimulation and blockage of the urinary bladder in the cat. *Int. J. Neuropharmacol.* 3:241–252, 1964.
182. De Sy, W., Lacroix, E., and Leusen, I.: An analysis of the urinary bladder response to hypogastric nerve stimulation in the cat. *Invest. Urol.* 11:508–516, 1974.
183. Awad, S. A., and Downie, J. W.: The effect of adrenergic drugs and hypogastric nerve stimulation on the canine urethra: a radiologic and urethral pressure study. *Invest. Urol.* 13:298–301, 1976.
184. Andersson, K-E., Ek, A., Hedlund, H., and Mattiasson, A.: Effects of prazosin on isolated human urethra and in patients with lower motor neuron lesions. *Invest. Urol.* 19:39–42, 1981.
185. Cumes, D., Govan, D. E., and Mensah-Dwumah, M.: The effect of sympathectomy on the urethral pressure profile in the experimental animal. *Invest. Urol.* 16:281–283, 1979.
186. Bruschini, H., Schmidt, R. A., and Tanagho, E. A.: The male genitourinary sphincter mechanism in the dog. *Invest. Urol.* 15:284–287, 1978.
187. Gallizia, P.: The smooth sphincter of the vesical neck; a genital organ. *Urol. Int.* 27:341–354, 1972.
188. Raezer, D. M., Benson, G. S., Wein, A. J., and Duckett, J. W., Jr.: The functional approach to the management of the pediatric neurogenic bladder: a clinical study. *J. Urol.* 117:649–653, 1977.
189. Rohner, T. J., Raezer, D. M., Wein, A. J., and Schoenberg, H. W.: Contractile responses of dog bladder neck muscle to adrenergic drugs. *J. Urol.* 105:657–661, 1971.
190. Nergårdh, A.: Autonomic receptor function in the lower urinary tract, a survey of recent experimental results. *J. Urol.* 113:180–185, 1975.
191. Nergårdh, A., and Boréus, L. O.: The functional role of cholinergic receptors in the outlet region of the urinary bladder: an in vitro study of the cat. *Acta Pharmacol. Toxicol. (Copenh.)* 32:467–490, 1973.
192. Downie, J. W., and Dean, D. M.: The contribution of cholinergic postganglionic neurotransmission to contraction of rabbit detrusor. *J. Pharmacol. Exp. Ther.* 203:417–425, 1977.
193. Levin, R. M., Shofer, F. S., and Wein, W. J.: Cholinergic, adrenergic and purinergic responses of sequential strips of rabbit urinary bladder. *J. Pharmacol. Exp. Ther.* 212:536–540, 1980.
194. Benson, G. S., Wein, W. J., Raezer, D. M., and Corriere, J. N., Jr.: Adrenergic and cholinergic stimulation and blockade of the human bladder base. *J. Urol.* 116:174–175, 1976.
195. Ek, A., Alm, P., Andersson, K-E., and Persson, C. G. A.: Adrenoceptors and cholinoceptor mediated responses of the isolated human urethra. *Scand. J. Urol. Nephrol.* 11:97–102, 1977.
196. Nergårdh, A.: The functional role of adrenergic receptors in the outlet region of the urinary bladder: an in vitro and in vivo study in the cat. *Scand. J. Urol. Nephrol.* 8:100–107, 1974.

197. Raz, S., Zeigler, M., and Caine, M.: Isometric studies on canine urethral musculature. *Invest. Urol.* 9:443–446, 1972.
198. Downie, J. W., Dean, D. M., Carro-Ciampi, G., and Awad, S. A.: A difference in sensitivity to alpha-adrenergic agonists exhibited by detrusor and bladder neck of the rabbit. *Can. J. Physiol. Pharmacol.* 53:525–530, 1975.
199. Edvardsen, P., and Setekleiv, J.: Distribution of the adrenergic receptors in the urinary bladder of cats, rabbits and guinea pigs. *Acta Pharmacol. Toxicol. (Copenh.)* 26:437–445, 1968.
200. Salimi, M., Setekleiv, J., and Skobba, T. J.: The sensitivity of adrenergic excitatory and inhibitory receptors in the smooth muscle of rabbit urinary bladder. *Acta. Pharmacol. Toxicol. (Copenh.)* 27:213–224, 1969.
201. Awad, S. A., Bruce, A. W., Carro-Ciampi, G., Downie, J. W., Lin, M., and Marks, G. S.: Distribution of alpha and beta adrenoreceptors in the human urinary bladder. *Br. J. Pharmacol.* 50:525–529, 1974.
202. Van Buren, G. A., and Anderson, G. F.: Comparison of the urinary bladder base and detrusor to cholinergic and histaminergic receptor activation in the rabbit. *Pharmacology* 18:136–142, 1979.
203. Levin, R. M., and Wein, A. J.: Quantitative analysis of alpha and beta adrenergic receptor densities in the lower urinary tract of the dog and rabbit. *Invest. Urol.* 17:75–77, 1979.
204. Levin, R. M., and Wein, A. J.: Distribution and function of adrenergic receptors in the urinary bladder of the rabbit. *Mol. Pharmacol.* 16:441–448, 1979.
205. Creed, K. E.: The role of the hypogastric nerve in the bladder and urethral activity of the dog. *Br. J. Pharmacol.* 65:357, 1979.
206. Donker, P. J., Invanovici, F., and Noach, E. L.: Analysis of the urethral pressure profile by means of electromyography and the administration of drugs. *Br. J. Urol.* 44:180–193, 1972.
207. Koyanagi, T.: Further observations on the denervation supersensitivity of the urethra in patients with chronic neurogenic bladders. *J. Urol.* 122:348–351, 1979.
208. Koyanagi, T.: Studies on the sphincteric system located distally in the urethra: external urethral sphincter revisited. *J. Urol.* 124:400–406, 1980.
209. Koyanagi, T., and Tsuji, I.: The mechanism of continence after prostatectomy. *Urol. Int.* 32:353–367, 1977.
210. Koyanagi, T., Arikado, K., Takamatsu, T., and Tsuji, I.: Relevance of sympathetic dyssynergia in the region of external urethral sphincter: possible mechanism of voiding dysfunction in the absence of (somatic) sphincter dyssynergia. *J. Urol.* 127:277–282, 1982.
211. Murray, K., Stone, A. R., Bunni, N., Chawla, J., and Stephenson, T. P.: An assessment of the effect of alpha-adrenergic blockade on sphincteric function in spinal injury patients and its clinical significance. In *Proceedings 79th Annual Meeting American Urological Association,* Abstract 245, 1984, p. 165A.
212. Raz, S., and Caine, M.: Adrenergic receptors in the female canine urethra. *Invest. Urol.* 9:319–323, 1972.
213. Nergårdh, A.: The interaction between adrenergic and cholinergic receptor functions in the outlet region of the urinary bladder. *Scand. J. Urol. Nephrol.* 8:108–113, 1974.
214. Persson, C. G. A., and Andersson, K-E.: Adrenoceptor and cholinoceptor mediated effects in the isolated urethra of the cat and guinea pig. *Clin. Exp. Pharmacol. Physiol.* 3:415–431, 1976.
215. Westfall, T. C.: Local regulation of adrenergic neurotransmission. *Physiol. Rev.* 57:657–728, 1977.
216. Langer, S. Z.: Presynaptic receptors and their role in the regulation of transmitter release. *Br. J. Pharmacol.* 60:481–497, 1977.
217. Langer, S. Z.: Presynaptic regulation of the release of catecholamines. *Pharmacol. Rev.* 32:337–362, 1981.
218. Stjarne, L., and Brindin, J.: $Beta_2$-adrenoreceptors facilitating noradrenaline secretion from the human vasoconstrictor nerves. *Acta Physiol. Scand.* 97:88–93, 1976.
219. Burnstock, G., Cocks, T., Crowe, R., and Kasakov, L.: Purinergic innervation of the guinea pig urinary bladder. *Br. J. Pharmacol.* 63:125–138, 1978.
220. Burnstock, G., Cocks, T., Kasakov, L., and Wong, H. K.: Direct evidence for ATP-release from non-adrenergic non-cholinergic ("purinergic") nerves in the guinea-pig taenia coli and bladder. *Eur. J. Pharmacol.* 49:145–149, 1978.
221. Andersson, K-E., Husted, S., and Sjögren, C.: Contribution of prostaglandin to the adenosine-induced contractions of rabbit urinary bladder. *Br. J. Pharmacol.* 70:443–452, 1980.
222. Brown, C., Burnstock, G., and Cocks, T.: Effect of adenosine 5-triphosphate and B-Y-methylene ATP on the rat urinary bladder. *Br. J. Pharmacol.* 65:97–102, 1979.
223. Sjögren, S., and Andersson, K.-E.: Inhibition of the ATP-induced contraction in the guinea-pig urinary bladder in vitro and in vivo. *Acta Pharmacol. Toxicol. (Copenh.)* 44:221, 1979
224. Downie, J. W., and Larsson, C.: Prostaglandin involvement in contractions in rabbit detrusor by field stimulation and by adenosine 5-triphosphate. *Can. J. Physiol. Pharmacol.* 59:253–260, 1981.
225. Husted, S., Sjögren, S., and Andersson, K.-E.: Direct effects of adenosine and adenine nucleotides on isolated human urinary bladder and their influence on electrically induced contractions. *J. Urol.* 130:392–398, 1983.
226. Burnstock, G., Dumsday, B., and Smythe, A.: Atropine-resistant excitation of the urinary bladder: the possibility of transmission via nerves releasing purine nucleotide. *Br. J. Pharmacol.* 44:451–461, 1972.
227. Kinder, R. B., Restorick, J., and Mundy, A. R.: Inhibition of the responses to nerve mediated stimuli and of spontaneous activity of the human detrusor in vitro by vasoactive intestinal polypeptide. In *Proceedings 14th Annual Meeting International Continence Society,* 1984, pp. 231–232.
228. Klarskov, P., Gerstenberg, T., and Hald, T.: Vasoactive intestinal polypeptide influence on lower urinary tract smooth muscle from human and pig. *J. Urol.* 131:1000–1004, 1984.
229. Larsen, J. J., Ottesen, B., Fahrenkrug, J., and Fahrenkrug, L.: Vasoactive intestinal polypeptide

in the male genitourinary tract. *Invest. Urol.* 19:211–213, 1981.

230. Levin, R. M., and Wein, A. J.: Effect of vasoactive intestinal polypeptide on the contractility of the rabbit urinary bladder. *Urol. Res.* 9:217–218, 1981.
231. Erspamer, G. F., Negri, G., and Piccinelli, D.: The use of preparations of urinary bladder smooth muscle for bioassay of and discrimination between polypeptides. *Naunyn. Schmiedebergs Arch. Pharmacol.* 279:61–82, 1973.
232. Husted, S., Sjögren, C., and Andersson, K-E.: Substance P and somatostatin and excitatory neurotransmission in rabbit urinary bladder. *Arch. Int. Pharmacodyn. Ther.* 252:72–85, 1981.
233. Johns, A.: The effect of indomethacin and substance P on the guinea pig urinary bladder. *Life Sci.* 29:1803–1809, 1981.
234. Abdel-Rahman, M., Coulombe, A., and Elhilali, M.M.: Detrusor dynamics. I. Effect of prostaglandin F_2 on tension-length relationship. *Invest. Urol.* 18:278–280, 1981.
235. Abdel-Rahman, M., Coulombe, A. M., and Elhilali, M. M.: Detrusor dynamics. II. Effects of prostaglandins and their synthesis inhibitor on stress-relaxation time course. *Invest. Urol.* 18:281–284, 1981.
236. Andersson, K.-E., and Forman, A.: Effects of prostaglandins on the smooth muscle of the urinary tract. *Acta Pharmacol. Toxicol. (Copenh.)* 43:90–95, 1978.
237. Bultitude, M. I., Hills, N. A., and Shuttleworth, K. E. D.: Clinical and experimental studies on the action of prostaglandins and their synthesis inhibitors on detrusor muscle in vitro and in vivo. *Br. J. Urol.* 48:631–637, 1976.
238. Persson, C. G. A.: Inhibitory effect at the bladder urethral junction. *Acta Physiol. Scand.* 97: 139–141, 1976.
239. Andersson, K.-E., Ek, A., and Persson, C. G. A.: Effect of prostaglandins on the isolated human bladder and urethra. *Acta Physiol. Scand.* 100:165–171, 1977.
240. Guyon, J. F.: Role de nerf erécteur sacré dans la miction normale. *C. R. Soc. Biol.* 52:712–713, 1900.
241. Barrington, F. J. F.: The nervous mechanism of micturition. *Q. J. Exp. Physiol.* 8:33–71, 1915.
242. Barrington, F. J. F.: The relation of the hind-brain to micturition. *Brain* 44:23–53, 1921.
243. Barrington, F. J. F.: The effect of lesion of the hind- and mid-brain on micturition in the cat. *Q. J. Exp. Physiol.* 15:81–102, 1925.
244. Barrington, F. J. F.: The component reflexes of micturition in the cat. Parts I and II. *Brain* 54:177–188, 1931.
245. Barrington, F. J. F.: The localization of pathways subserving micturition in the spinal cord of the cat. *Brain* 6:126–136, 1933.
246. Barrington, F. J. F.: The component reflexes of micturition in the cat. Part III. *Brain* 64:239–243, 1941.
247. Müller, L. R.: Die Blaseninnervation. *Dtsch. Arch. Klin. Med.* 101:81–106, 1918.
248. Denny-Brown, D., and Robertson, E. G.: On the physiology of micturition. *Brain* 56:149–190, 1933.
249. Garry, R. C., Roberts, T. D. M., and Todd, J. K.: Reflexes involving the external urethral sphincter in the cat. *J. Physiol. (Lond.)* 149:653–665, 1959.
250. Gjone, R.: Peripheral autonomic influence on the motility of the urinary bladder in the cat. II. "Tone." *Acta Physiol. Scand.* 66:72–80, 1966.
251. Gjone, R.: Peripheral autonomic influence on the motility of the urinary bladder in the cat. III. Micturition. *Acta Physiol. Scand.* 66:81–90, 1966.
252. Gjone, R.: A dual peripheral and supraspinal autonomic influence on the urinary bladder: a survey of previous and new concepts based on experimental results. *J. Oslo City Hosp.* 15:173–182, 1965.
253. Pompeius, R.: Detrusor Inhibition Induced from Anal Region in Man. Thesis, Elanders Boktryckeri AB, Kungsbacka, Sweden, 1966.
254. Edvardsen, P.: Nervous control of the urinary bladder in the cat. *Acta Neurol. Scand.* 43:543–563, 1967.
254a. Edvardsen, P.: Nervous control of urinary bladder in cats. I. The collecting phase. *Acta Physiol. Scand.* 72:157–171, 1968.
255. Edvardsen, P.: Nervous control of the urinary bladder in cats. II. The expulsion phase. *Acta Physiol. Scand.* 72:172–182, 1968.
256. Ausems, M. M.: Pätienten Met Chronische Blaasklachten. *Overg. Neederl. Tigesch.* 115:1808–1811, 1971.
257. Sundin, T., Carlsson, C-A., and Kock, N. G.: Detrusor inhibition induced from mechanical stimulation of the anal region and from electrical stimulation of pudendal nerve afferents. *Invest. Urol.* 11:374–378, 1974.
258. Mahony, D. T., Laferte, R. O., and Blais, D. J.: Integral storage and voiding reflexes: neurophysiologic concept of continence and micturition *Urology* 9:95–106, 1977.
259. Bradley, W. E., Timm, G. W., and Scott, F. B.: Cystometry. II. Central nervous system organization of detrusor reflex. *Urology*, 5:578–580, 1975.
260. Elbadawi, A.: The Voider reflex: a new unitary concept of the infraspinal reflex control of micturition. In *Proceedings 79th Meeting American Urological Association* 1984, p. 284A.

2

Upper Urinary Tract Function

BO COOLSAET, M.D., Ph.D.

NORMAL FUNCTION

The function of the upper urinary tract is to transport urine from the renal papillae via the renal calices, renal pelvis, and ureter to the bladder (*1*). The function of the calices and pelvis is twofold: They function as a reservoir where urine from the papillae is collected, and they act as an active conduit for urine to the ureter.

Reservoir function is made possible by maintaining low intrapelvic baseline pressure, which permits continuous outflow of urine from the collecting tubules. Under normal conditions intracapillary pressure in the glomeruli is approximately 105 cm H_2O, which greatly exceeds pressures of 17 cm H_2O in the proximal tubules and 34 cm H_2O colloidosmotic pressure (*2*). In addition, effective filtration pressure easily overcomes mean baseline pelvic pressures of 6 to 7 cm H_2O.

The renal pelvic capacity is 4 to 8 ml, but in "disease" capacities of several hundred milliliters are encountered. Even under these conditions low baseline pressures are maintained owing to the geometry of the system, active relaxation of the densely woven network of smooth muscle fibers, and passive viscoelastic relaxation of the wall. This viscoelastic relaxation makes possible changes of the unstretched length of the wall tissue. These phenomena have been investigated extensively on smooth muscle of the bladder wall (*3,4*) and the ureter (*5*).

The upper urinary tract is an adaptive system. Dimensions and active and passive characteristics alter in order to meet the functioning requirements resulting from physiologic changes. These changes are caused by changes in diuresis and bladder filling. Diuretic input changes from one individual to another and from one measurement to another depending on the degree of hydration. Normally, urine flow varies from 0.5 to 1.0 ml per minute per ureter, whereas maximum urine flow seldom exceeds 7.0 ml per minute per ureter. Pressure in the normal upper tract is mainly related, however, to detrusor pressures. These pressures apparently are of greater influence than the diuretic input.

Conduit function is influenced by several mechanisms, some of which are still not completely understood.

The muscle coat of the renal calices and pelvis is composed of two morphologically and histochemically (*6*) distinct types of smooth muscle cell (Fig. 2–1). The outer-layer muscle cell type is identical to the ureteral smooth muscle coat; but a distinct inner layer of the minor and major calices and the pelvis consists of atypical smooth muscle cells. These atypical cells are devoid of the enzyme product cholinesterase, in contrast to the outer muscle layer, which demonstrates nonspecific cholinesterase. It is not known what role is played by this atypical muscle cell layer.

Muscle cells in the wall of the upper urinary tract are considered to be "latent" pacemaker cells. Previously it has been thought that pacemaker activity originates in the upper part of the ureter. There is now experimental evidence to show that under normal conditions activity is dominated by pace-

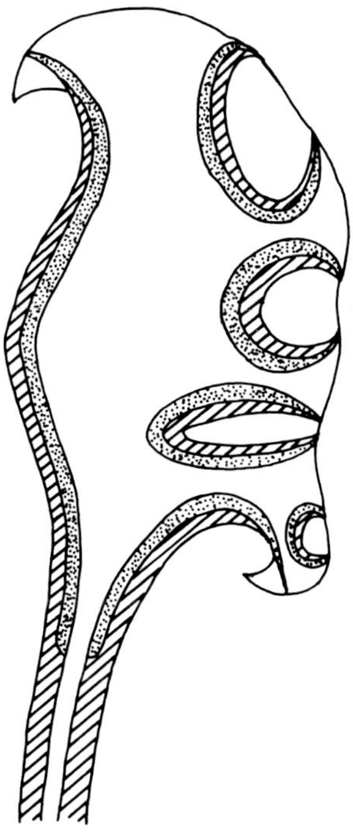

Figure 2–1. According to Gosling, the muscle coat of the renal calices and pelvis is composed of two morphologically and histochemically distinct types of smooth muscle cells. (From Gosling, J.A., *et al.: Slide Atlas of Urinary Tract Anatomy.* Gower Medical Publishing, London, 1982.)

maker cell activity arising at the sites where the minor calices are attached to the renal parenchyma. Each minor calix possesses these cells. Minor calices are linked by similar cells. There is a frequency gradient in the spontaneous activity of the upper tract musculature (Fig. 2–2). The highest spontaneous frequency is generated at the site of the minor calices; frequency decreases down the renal pelvis and ureter (*7,8*). Muscle cells with slower spontaneous activity are dominated by higher-frequency cells. The cells that generate the highest frequency at the minor calix site hence act as a primary pacemaker. All minor calices are able to generate a contraction. This contraction is propagated to other calices that are functionally coupled. This coupling system is not completely understood.

Contractions of the walls of the minor calices are normally coapting and act therefore as a pumping mechanism by which urine outflow from collecting tubules is facilitated and protected against intrapelvic pressure increases, unless dilatation disrupts this important defense mechanism. These contractions occur 10 to 12 times per minute. Because the autonomic nerve system is represented only sparsely in the upper tract (*5*) activity is propagated directly from one muscle cell to another by way of close contacts.

Contractions at the calix site induce a coordinated pelvic contraction three to four times per minute, to a maximum of six per minute. These pelvic contractions progress on to the pelvoureteric region (Fig. 2–3). Notwithstanding previous opinions, there is no sphincter at this region. Not all pelvic

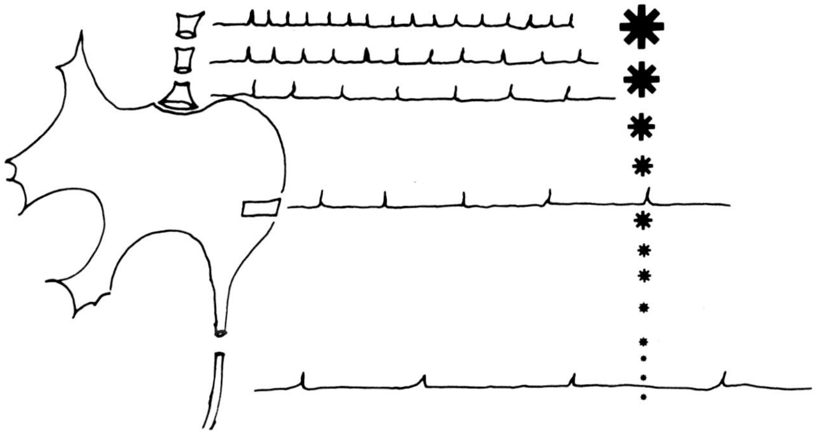

Figure 2–2. Frequency gradient in the spontaneous activity of the upper tract smooth musculature. The highest spontaneous frequency is generated at the minor calices site and decreases down the renal pelvis and ureter.

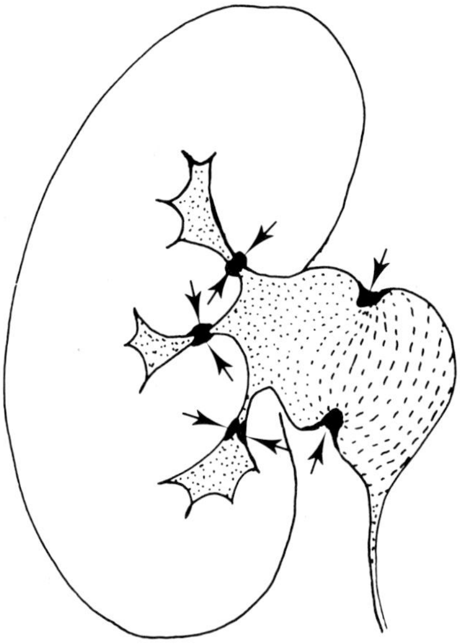

Figure 2–3. Contractions at the calyx site are coapting and act as a pumping mechanism. They induce pelvic contractions that progress onto the pelvoureteric region.

contractions are transmitted to the ureter. Depending on diuresis and hence on intrapelvic volume, pressure, or pelvic wall tension, and probably other factors, boluses are launched down the ureter. At a normal urinary flow rate, approximately one of three pelvic contractions is transmitted distally. This 3:1 ratio increases to a 1:1 ratio at higher rates of diuresis. Pelvic pressure changes during each filling cycle. It increases from approximately 2 cm H_2O to 15 cm H_2O at bolus launching. After launching, the pelvic pressure drops to its baseline value, and the cycle of filling and building up pressure and launching restarts.

These contraction waves are propagated from smooth muscle cell to smooth muscle cell by means of intercellular junctions. The spread of action potentials is possible in many directions. Direction is normally dictated by the frequency gradient, however, which shows the highest frequency at the minor calices site. Ureteral peristalsis is apparently initiated by propagating action potentials from the renal pelvis combined with distension of the ureter by urine. The mechanism of bolus launching is not completely understood. It appears to consist in a rather complicated regulating mechanism that is determined by action potentials and wall stress factors. It seems most likely that disturbance of this regulating mechanism is the cause of functional obstruction in this area, resulting in so-called hydronephrosis. The uncoordinated pelvic contractions result in a hypertrophic muscle coat (Fig. 2–4), and propagation to the ureter and bolus launching are impaired. Indeed, a true organic stenosis is absent, in most of the investigated pyeloureteral junction.

The ureter has a transporting function. It is in a nearly continuous state of change and motion. The peristaltic contraction coapts the ureteral wall completely and moves with a constant velocity of 3 to 4 cm/s distally toward the bladder. Bolus dimensions vary with diuresis, ureteral and periureteral factors, and bladder changes (*9*). During normal diuresis the peristaltic impulse moves at constant velocity, and the contracting ring prevents intraureteric reflux of urine (Fig. 2–5). The velocity of the leading edge of the bolus, however, changes along the ureter depending on mechanical factors, e.g., the geometry of the ureter, probably changes in wall properties, and extraureteral structures. Therefore, the width and the length of the bolus are not uniform on its way from the renal pelvis to the bladder. Viscoelastic properties of the ureteral wall itself do not appear to show systematic changes. They are probably of minor importance. The precise causes of the

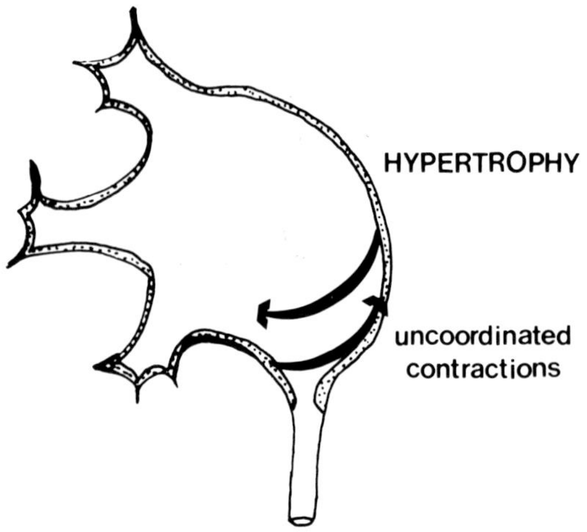

Figure 2–4. It is likely that widening of the renal pelvis is caused by uncoordinated pelvic contractions that result in impaired bolus launching.

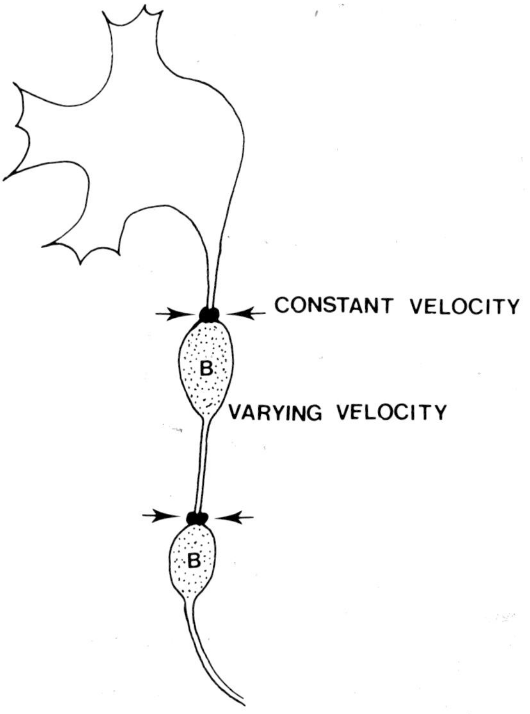

Figure 2–5. Ureteral contraction ring moves toward the bladder at a constant velocity. The velocity of the leading edge of the bolus (*B*) changes along the ureter.

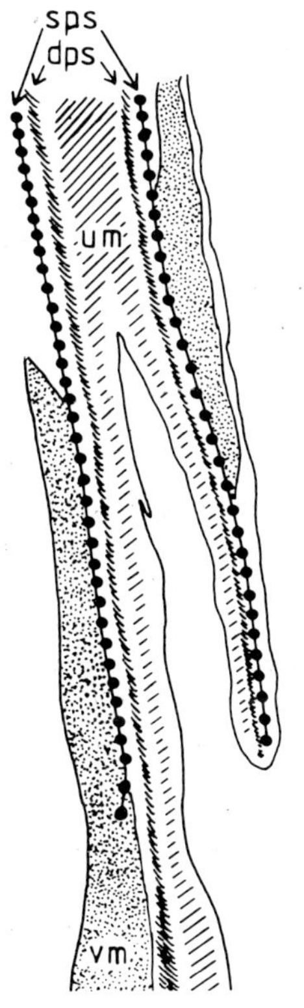

Figure 2–6. Ureterovesical junction according to Elbadawi. *sps* = superficial periureteral sheath. *dps* = deep periureteral sheath. *um* = ureteral muscle. *vm* = vesical muscle.

changes at the leading edge of the bolus are still not completely understood.

At the distal end of the ureter the urine bolus passes through the ureterovesical junction (Fig. 2–6). The intramural course is approximately 1.5 cm (*10*). This ureterovesical junction acts as a one-way valve in preventing regurgitation of urine from the bladder lumen into the ureter. Resistance to antegrade flow from the ureter through the ureterovesical junction toward the bladder and prevention of vesicoureteral reflux are influenced by a complex mechanism consisting of morphological and functional factors (Fig. 2–7), including passive and active characteristics, forces in the bladder wall surrounding the distal ureteral segment, detrusor pressure, prevesical ureteral activity, and coaptation of the ureteral wall.

There are both *passive and active characteristics of the ureteral wall.* The intramural part of the distal ureter is not a passive, inert structure. Indeed, peristaltic activity superimposes high-pressure peaks on slow-pressure waves originating from an encircling de-

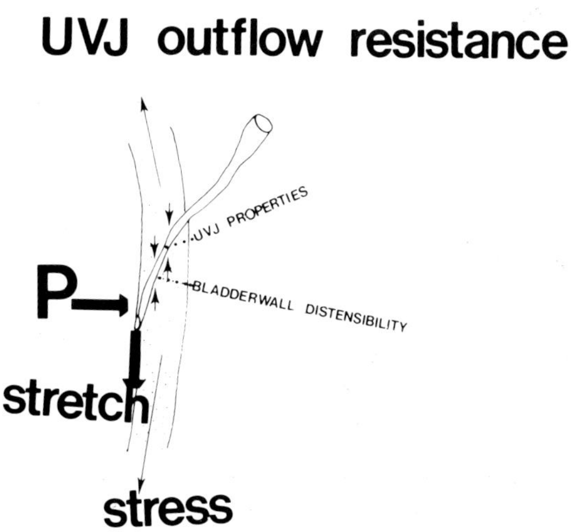

Figure 2–7. Resistance to antegrade flow toward the bladder and prevention of reflux are influenced by a complex mechanism consisting in detrusor pressure (*P*), bladder wall stretch, bladder wall stress, distensibility of the surrounding bladder wall for bolus passage, and properties of the ureterovesical junction itself.

trusor muscle coat (*11*). Baseline resistance pressure to antegrade flow at the ureterovesical junction exceeds the detrusor pressure by 5 cm H_2O (Fig. 2–8).

Forces in the bladder wall surrounding the distal ureteral segment. Bolus passage through the ureterovesical junction is influenced by the morphologic characteristics of the surrounding bladder wall tissue. Supple surrounding tissue exerts minimal resistance to dilatation of the intramural ureter by bolus passage. One of the major controversies, however, concerns the impact of bladder wall tension or bladder wall stress. It is well known that bladder wall stress increases with increasing bladder volume, as can be easily understood by Laplace's equation (Fig. 2–9). The pressure, on the other hand, remains nearly constant, owing to geometric and merely viscoelastic properties.

Some experiments have clearly shown that antegrade resistance to flow in the pig and the human is related to detrusor pressure and to forces originating from active bladder wall contraction (*12*). Bladder wall stress, on the other hand, appears to be of less importance. In other experiments (*13*), more influence has been attributed to bladder wall stress. Because the radius of a hole within a tissue increases with increasing tension or stress in that tissue, the compression of a tube within that hole decreases with increasing stress. Hence, it is expected that the resistance to flow through that tube will decrease when passive stress in surrounding tissue increases. On the other hand, a contraction of that tissue compresses the tube and hence increases resistance. It appears that increased stretch of the ureterovesical junction caused by bladder filling considerably influences resistance to antegrade flow and is of major importance in preventing vesicoureteral reflux. Hence bladder wall stress appears to influence ureterovesical junction dynamics only indirectly, by stretching it.

In contrast, *Detrusor pressure* directly affects the ureterovesical junction. Increased detrusor pressure due to filling of the bladder or involuntary or voiding contractions results in a nearly parallel increase of resistance to flow at the ureterovesical junction (Fig. 2–10). Detrusor pressure is transmitted

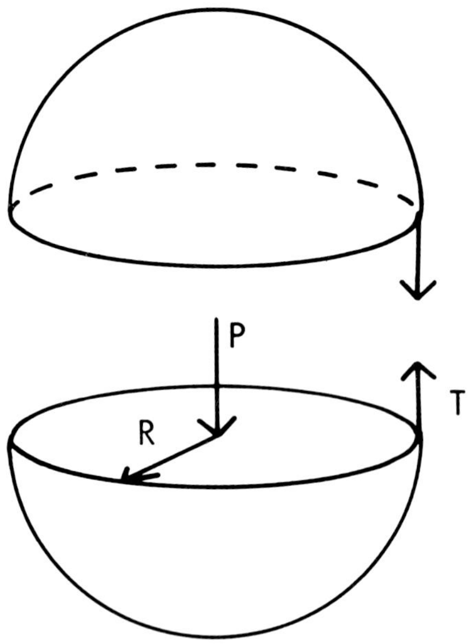

Figure 2–9. Representation of Laplace's formula. The halves of a sphere are forced apart by a force ($P \cdot \Pi R^2$) and held together by a force ($T \cdot 2\ \Pi R$). Hence $S = P \cdot R/2d$, where S is stress in N/m^2, P is pressure, R is radius, and d is wall thickness.

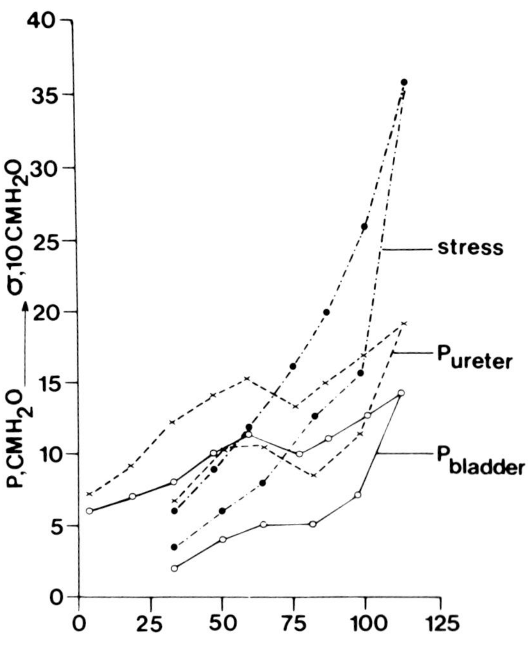

Figure 2–8. Baseline resistance to antegrade flow pressure (P_{ureter}) at the ureterovesical junction exceeds bladder pressure ($P_{bladder}$) with 5 cm H_2O. It is independent of the calculated stress in the bladder wall.

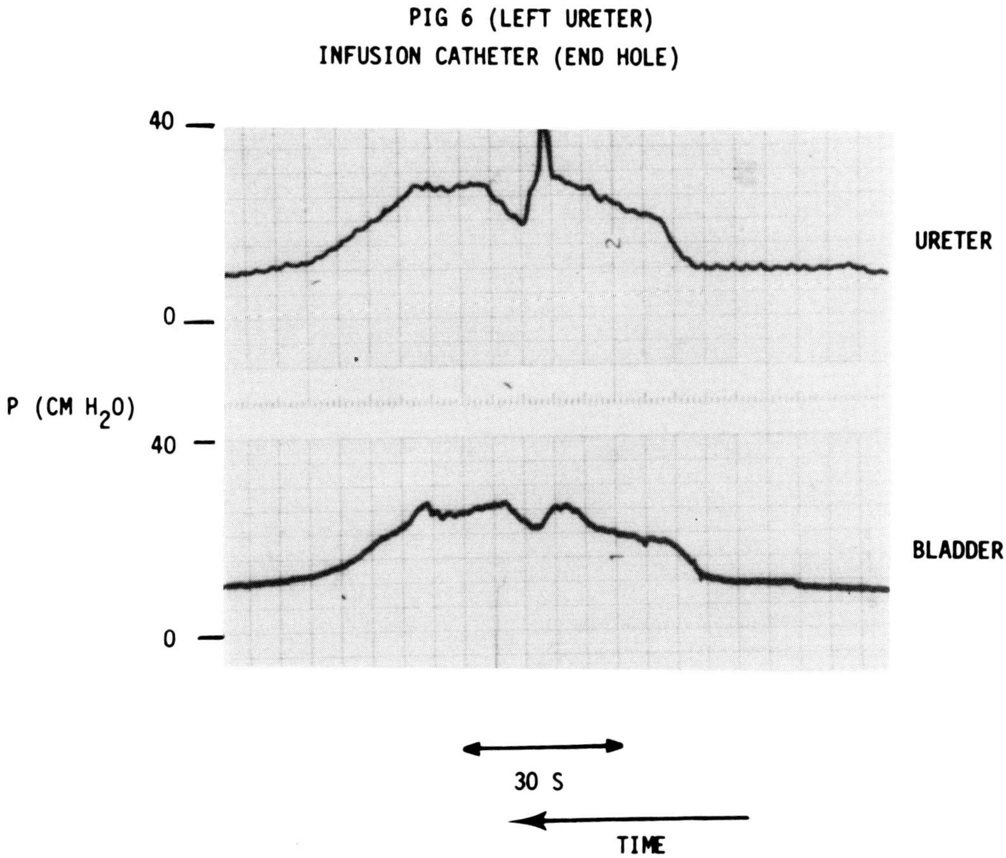

Figure 2–10. Measurement of resistance to flow pressure in the ureter during an unstable detrusor contraction. Pressure in the ureter increases with the increase of detrusor pressure. An additional pressure peak is observed in the ureter that is caused by ureteral wall contraction.

to the submucosal part of the ureter and has a direct effect on the outflow of urine at the ureteral orifice.

Prevesical ureteral activity, pressure generation in the ureter, and coaptation of the ureteral wall prevent urine from regurgitating. The impact of these mechanisms might change during bladder filling, and hence the degree of stretch of the bladder wall and trigone by which the length and course of the intramural ureter changes.

PHYSIOLOGIC ADAPTIVE MECHANISMS

Diuresis

Alterations of upper tract dynamics depend on, among other factors, the requirement to transport varying amounts of urine (*14*). Reduced urine excretion leads to a decreased frequency of activity, and increased urine production enhances activity and the force that is developed by the contraction waves. Therefore an increased diuretic load enhances a combination of physiologic adaptive mechanisms. Indeed, smooth muscle behavior depends on, among other factors, the amount of stretch and the rate at which the stretch is applied. Moreover, in the upper urinary tract stretch of the wall influences the frequency of peristaltic activity and the force generated by the induced contractions.

Frequency. With increasing urine flow, the propagation of action potentials from the renal pelvis to the ureter increases so that each pelvic contraction is transmitted to the proximal ureter (Fig. 2–11). In humans this increase in frequency is limited, generally increasing to twice normal or, at the maximum, three times normal frequency.

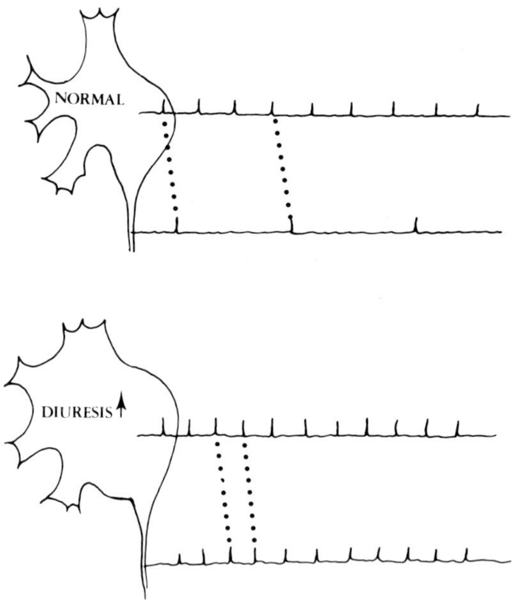

Figure 2–11. Increased diuresis causes increased pelvic contractions and increased contraction transmission to the proximal ureter.

Force. The force that is developed increases to a maximum at an optimum level of steady-state passive force, as has been demonstrated on detrusor muscle strips (*15*). The pressure measured in the lumen results from the force generated in the wall but also depends on the diameter of the system. Indeed, according to Laplace's equation

$$P = \frac{T \cdot d}{R}$$

the intraluminal pressure increase is inversely influenced by dilatation of the system.

Although at high diuresis the renal pelvis is distended with several milliliters of urine, its diameter seldom increases more than 25 percent in the normal human (*16*). All these factors result in a gradual increase of intrapelvic pressure with increasing flow. Pressure reaches its upper limit of approximately 25 cm H_2O at 4 to 7 ml/minute depending on the species. From that level, pressure increases only slightly with increasing flow rate. At low diuresis, pelvic pressure fluctuates between 2 and 10 cm H_2O, and during osmotic diuresis the pressure averages 10 to 15 cm H_2O. It increases to an average of 25 cm H_2O during extreme diuresis when a continuous stream occurs. The main change that occurs with increasing diuresis is an increase of the urine bolus. Although peristaltic wave propagation velocity remains unchanged, each peristaltic wave expels a larger volume of urine. Hence boluses become longer, and their diameter increases. Several phases can be arbitrarily distinguished (Fig. 2–12):

During normal diuresis, boluses are isolated from each other. One of every three pelvic contractions is propagated to the ureter. The ureteral wall coapts at the contracting ring; and the ring at the rear end moves with a constant velocity of 3.0 to 5.0 cm/s.

With increasing flow, bolus length increases and pelvic contractions more frequently propagate ureteral peristaltic contraction. The leading edge of the bolus approximates the contraction ring of the preceding bolus. The ureter is nearly completely filled, divided by still coapting contraction waves; pressure in the bolus increases owing to increased resistance at the leading edge, where it touches the preceding contraction ring.

At still higher flow rates, distension of the ureter increases. Contraction frequency does not increase further. Pressure in the bolus exceeds the contraction pressure of

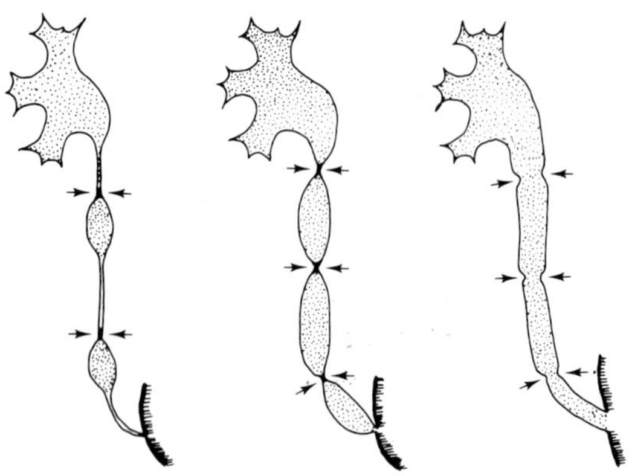

Figure 2–12. Several phases can be distinguished depending on diuresis. **A.** During normal diuresis boluses are isolated from each other by coapted ureteral wall. **B.** With increasing flow rates the bolus length increases; the leading edge of the bolus approximates the contraction ring of the preceding bolus. **C.** At still higher flow rates, distension of the ureter increases and exceeds the pressure in the contraction ring; the ureter becomes an open tube.

the ring; and contraction pressure is no longer sufficient to coapt the ureteral wall. The ureter then is completely open, and transport is no longer effected by active peristaltic activity; contractions still occur and can be observed as impressions, but they do not contribute to transport.

Transport is effected by peristaltic activity up to flow rates of approximately 5 ml/minute per ureter. At higher rates the ureter becomes the shape of an open tube, connecting the renal pelvis and the bladder. Resistance to flow at the ureterovesical junction is then determined almost entirely by the detrusor pressure, the pressure in the renal pelvis depends on the detrusor pressure via the fluid-filled open tube connection, and vesicoureteral reflux is prevented only by the mechanical downstream forces of the urine flow.

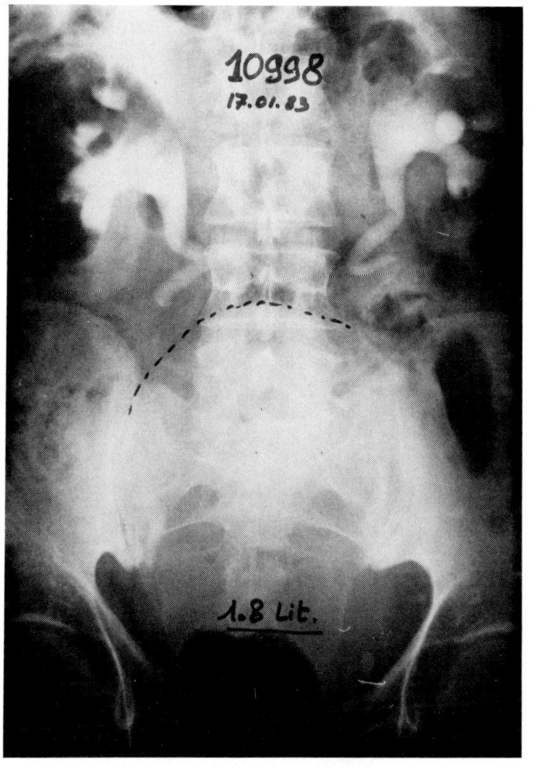

Figure 2–13. Intravenous urography with upper tract dilatation in a highly compliant bladder.

Bladder Filling

Bladder filling causes alterations in upper tract activity that are similar to those observed in chronic outflow obstruction. This increased resistance to antegrade flow is effected by an increase of detrusor pressure during filling and by mechanical stretching of the intramural ureteral segment among other things; it is influenced by an increase of bladder wall stress (*17*).

The individual action force of these factors depends on the intravesical volume and the amount of stretch of the vesical wall. Stretch of the wall not only increases resistance of the intramural ureter but changes its course through it. By changing the direction of the ureter in the wall, the relative impact of pressure and wall stress also changes. Large bladder wall stretch, which occurs at high intravesical volume, might cause increased ureterovesical outflow resistance, whereas detrusor pressure remains low in some high compliant bladders (Fig. 2–13). With increasing bladder filling, changes occur similar to those observed during high diuresis (Fig. 2–12). At low intravesical volume, outflow from the ureter toward the bladder is free. Bolus information, launching, and transportation are unimpeded.

As filling of the bladder proceeds slowly, detrusor pressure increases little, whereas stress in the bladder wall increases more steeply. Resistance increases mostly by the stretch of the ureterovesical junction. The upper tract adapts to these changing requirements by increasing peristaltic activity. Frequency and baseline pressure increase in order to maintain an antegrade urine flow toward the bladder. With increasing resistance, however, changes occur similar to those observed during high diuresis. The ureter becomes more dilated, and boluses approach the contraction ring of the preceding boluses. Bolus pressure increases and exceeds the contraction ring pressure. The contraction rings no longer coapt, and the ureter becomes an open tube, as can be seen on intravenous urography when the bladder is full. Ureteral efflux toward the bladder ceases when the detrusor pressure exceeds approximately 45 cm H_2O. This phase occurs during normal micturition. The intravesical volume that stops ureteral outflow varies from one individual to the next. This suppression of ureterovesical efflux of urine is more or less maintained when micturition is actively postponed, and evacuation of urine by the nephron becomes impossible.

REFERENCES

1. Kiil, F.: *The Function of the Ureter and Renal Pelvis*. Saunders, Philadelphia, 1957.
2. Kinn, A. Ch.: Urodynamics and Renal Function in Hydronephrosis. Thesis, Stockholm 1982.
3. Coolsaet, B. L. R. A., van Duyl, W. A., van Mastrigt, R., and van der Zwart, A.: Viscoelastic properties of the bladder wall. *Urol. Int.* 30:16, 1975.
4. Van Mastrigt, R., Coolsaet, B. L. R. A., van Duyl, W. A.: Passive properties of the urinary bladder in the collection phase. *Med. Biol. Eng. Comput.* 16:471, 1978.
5. Weiss, R., Bassett, A. L., and Hoffman, B. F.: Dynamic length-tension curves of cat ureter. *Am. J. Physiol.* 222:388, 1971.
6. Gosling, J.A., and Dixon, J.S.: Species variation in the location of upper urinary tract pacemaker cells. *Invest. Urol.* 11:418, 1974.
7. Constantinou, C. E.: Renal pelvic pacemaker control of ureteral peristaltic rate. *Am. J. Physiol.* 226:1413, 1974.
8. Golenhofen, K., and Hannappel, J.: Normal spontaneous activity of the pyelo-ureteral system in the guinea pig. *Pflugers Arch.* 341:257, 1973.
9. Durben, G., and Gerlach, R.: The velocity of urine bolus under different conditions. In *Proceedings I.S.D.U. Meeting*, Antwerp, 1979.
10. Elbadawi, A.: Anatomy and function of the ureteral sheath. *J. Urol.* 102:224, 1972.
11. Blok, C., van Venrooij, G. E. P. M., and Coolsaet, B. L. R. A.: Dynamics of the ureterovesical junction. In *Workshop on Upper Urinary Tract Urodynamics*, Springer-Verlag, Heidelberg, 1985.
12. Coolsaet, B. L. R. A., van Venrooij, G. E. P. M., and Blok, C.: Detrusor pressure versus wall stress in relation to ureterovesical resistance. *Neurourol. Urodyn.* 1:105, 1982.
13. Tanagho, E. A., Meyers, F. H., and Smith, D. R.: The trigone: anatomical and physiological considerations. 1. In relation to the ureterovesical junction. *J. Urol.*, 100:623, 1968.
14. Briggs, M. E., Constantinou, C. E. and Govan, D. E.: Dynamics of the upper urinary tract: the relationship of urine flow rate and rate of ureteral peristalsis, *Invest. Urol.* 10:56, 1972.
15. Griffiths, D. J., van Mastrigt, R., van Duyl, W. A., and Coolsaet, B. L. R. A.: Active mechanical properties of the smooth muscle of the urinary bladder. *Med. Biol. Eng. Comput.* 17:281, 1979.
16. Whitfield, H. N., Britton, K. E., Hendry, W. F., and Wickham, J. E. A.: Furosemide intravenous urography in the diagnosis of pelviureteric junction obstruction. *Br. J. Urol.* 51:445, 1979.
17. Coolsaet, B. L. R. A., Griffiths, D. J., van Mastrigt, R., and van Duyl, W. A.: Urodynamic investigation of the wide ureter. *J. Urol.* 124:666, 1980.

Electrophysiology of the Lower Urinary Tract

3

FRANCES M. DYRO, M.D.

Electromyography is a method of measuring electrical activity of muscle fibers and, in turn, of studying the nerve and muscle components of the motor unit. The first electrical measurements in the sphincters were made by Beck (*1*), who recorded from the anal sphincter. Early studies on the urethral sphincter were carried out by Petersen and Franksson (*2*). Since that time electromyography of the sphincters and pelvic floor musculature has become an important part of urodynamic studies.

THE MOTOR UNIT AND ITS PATHOPHYSIOLOGY

The motor unit is composed of an anterior horn cell, its axon, Schwann cells elaborating myelin around the axon, and muscle fibers innervated by it (Fig. 3–1). The anterior horn cell is an alpha motor neuron giving rise to myelinated fibers of 6 to 20 μm diameter. These fibers branch distally and innervate a varying number of muscle fibers, ranging from three fibers per axon in the extraocular

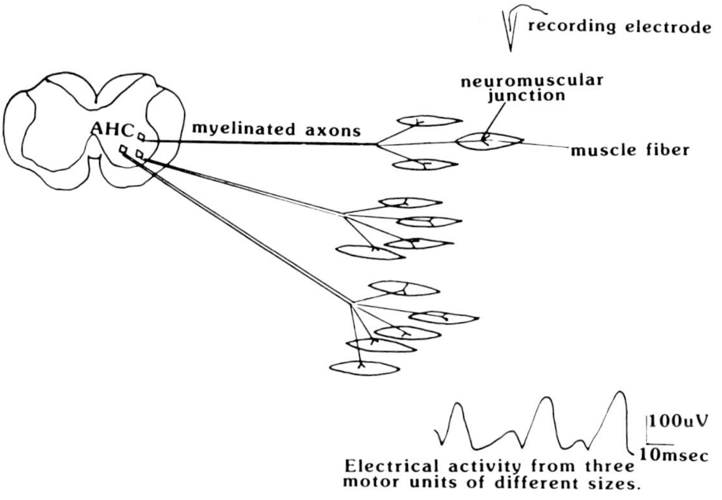

Figure 3–1. Motor unit and electrical response in the normal state. AHC = anterior horn cells in the ventral horn of the spinal cord. This is rather a simplistic representation of the motor unit and its components. The reader is advised to refer to Chapter 1 for further details related to the neurophysiology, the ultrastructure of the neuromuscular apparatus, and more updated literature.

muscles to several hundred in large limb muscles. The anterior horn cell bodies supplying the sphincters are at the sacral cord level in the nucleus of Onufrowicz (Onuf's nucleus).

The myoneural junction is a composite structure with a presynaptic portion belonging to the nerve and a postsynaptic portion belonging to the muscle. The presynaptic region contains a large number of mitochondria and particles called synaptic vesicles that are storage areas for acetylcholine. The postsynaptic region or endplate is characterized by gutters or troughs that are actually infoldings of muscle membrane.

Disorders of the motor unit result if any part of the motor unit malfunctions. The anterior horn cell may be damaged by trauma to the anterior horn of the spinal cord or by ischemia. Degenerative disorders such as amyotrophic lateral sclerosis result in the loss of anterior horn cells but spare Onuf's nucleus. Viral infection, most notably poliomyelitis, may produce acute and delayed loss of cells. Loss of the anterior horn cell results in wallerian degeneration of the axon and its branches.

Myelin or the Schwann cells may be affected without loss of the axons. However, because myelin is necessary for saltatory conduction, segmental loss of myelin results in slowing of nerve conduction that may be rather marked (one-eighth of normal). The peripheral nerve may be damaged by local trauma. If conduction is temporarily blocked at one point but the axon is intact, it is referred to as *neurapraxia* (Fig. 3–2). This condition most commonly results from a pressure palsy. There is usually good return of function, the time required for recovery being related to the duration of compression. Conduction below the level of the block remains normal. If there is a conduction block and the axon distal to the injury begins to degenerate, it is called *axonotmesis*. Recovery can occur with the axon regenerating at the rate of 1 to 3 mm/day through sheaths of remaining connective tissue. Complete loss of neural function as a result of complete anatomic loss of continuity is called *neurotmesis*. After complete transection of a nerve, wallerian degeneration takes place. For up to 3 to 4 days, stimulation of the nerve distal to the injury can produce a response.

Segmental loss of myelin or overall increase in the length of the nodes of Ranvier or even intramyelinic edema may occur after exposure to some toxic chemicals. In the extreme case, the axon remains intact but nerve conduction is completely blocked. Axonal degeneration with secondary involvement of myelin is usually the result of metabolic derangement of the whole axon. Systemic metabolic disorders are causative, although the exact mechanisms and the rapid reversal in uremic neuropathy after transplant are not understood.

The muscle fibers in adults are 60 to 80 μm in diameter. There are multiple subsarcolemmal nuclei. After fixation in formalin and staining with hematoxylin and eosin, the fibers are pink. When fresh muscle samples are quick-frozen then stained for ATPase activity, it becomes apparent that some fibers are high in ATPase activity at pH 9.4. Called type II fibers, it is these fibers that respond with fast twitch, but they fatigue rapidly. They are supplied by large motor neurons and are the last to respond to a stimulus and the first to fatigue. These fibers are typified by the "white meat" in the breast of the chicken, enabling it to fly short distances to escape danger. The fibers that

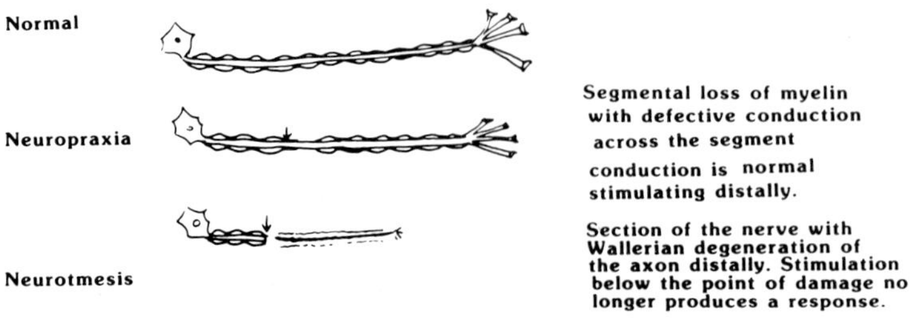

Figure 3–2. Types of conduction block.

are low in ATPase fire slowly and rhythmically for long periods. These type I fibers are smaller, are innervated by smaller axons, and are rich in oxidative enzymes. The fibers provide a baseline level of contraction. The axons supplying them have a low threshold and conduct at slower rates than those of type II fibers. These fibers are typified by the "dark meat" of the chicken leg (a rough approximation). There is evidence for a subdivision of type II into IIA and IIB, with the IIA fibers being fatigue-resistant (*3*).

The composition of human muscle is one-third type I and two-thirds type II. If the axon supplying a number of fibers is lost either through anterior horn cell loss or peripheral nerve damage, remaining axons send sprouts to reinnervate the orphaned muscle fibers. This action results in grouping of fiber types because the adopted muscle fibers take on the properties of the other fibers in the same motor unit. The most striking example of the phenomenon occurs in amyotrophic lateral sclerosis where a whole muscle may be innervated by a few remaining anterior horn cells giving rise to a few motor unit potentials of extremely high amplitude (the result of summation of electrical activity of many fibers in each motor unit) (Fig. 3–3).

Some of the myopathies are characterized by abnormalities of certain fiber types. In myotonic dystrophy there is typically type I atrophy. In some cases there is predominance of certain fiber types at birth. In the muscular dystrophies fibers from motor units die and become necrotic. There is usually a decrease in the size of the action potential with fewer fibers firing. There is relative sparing of muscle fibers in the sphincters, extraocular muscles, and the iris. Curiously, these muscles all have persistent tonic activity.

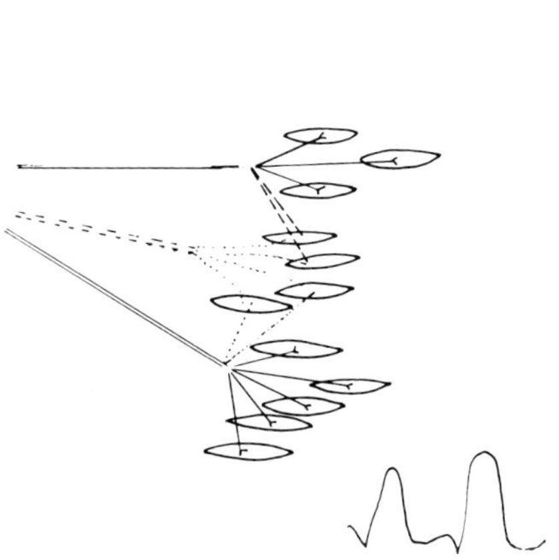

Figure 3–3. Loss of axons resulting in reinnervation and "giant units."

ELECTROMYOGRAPHY

The electrical activity generated by activation of a motor unit can be measured in a variety of ways. Each method used looks at a potential difference between the electrically active muscle and a neutral point on the body surface.

Surface electrodes are used by many groups. These electrodes may be applied to the skin of the perineum or perianal regions (*4,5*). Electrodes have been mounted on urethral catheters (*6*) on an anal plug (*7*). Kiesswetter has used electrodes mounted on vaginal tampons to record from the external sphincter (*8*). Although this type of electrode is painless and easy to use, the recording obtained may be difficult to interpret. Surface electrodes provide a record of total net activity of the muscles in the vicinity. Groups using surface electrodes process the recordings through electronic integrators or pulse counters and record the activity on a strip chart recording along with the cystometrogram. In addition to contraction of the periurethral striated muscles, the surface electrodes also pick up activity generated by contraction of abdominal and hip girdle muscles (especially the iliopsoas and glutei). If electromyographic activity is being monitored only on a graphic recording with a slow chart speed, it is impossible to distinguish the source of the activity. Another drawback of surface electrodes is difficulty in maintaining good contact. Electrodes mounted on catheters suffer from electrical discontinuities, e.g., when the patient is voiding around the catheter.

Intramuscular recording yields more specific information. The technique was first described by Petersen and Franksson, who used flexible wires introduced through long hypodermic needles (*2*). Most investigators now use commercially available electrodes of either monopolar or concentric type.

Types of Electrodes

Wire electrodes. Wire electrodes are composed of Teflon-coated, stainless steel wire that is sanded with an emory board to bare the tip for 3 mm. A length of wire is then threaded through a 26- or 27-gauge needle. The tip of the wire is bent back sharply prior to insertion into the needle. After the needle and wire are inserted, the needle is pulled back while the wire fishhooks itself into place. Care must be taken not to damage the coating, as such damage gives artifactual and spurious recordings.

Monopolar Electrodes. Monopolar electrodes are Teflon-coated wire electrodes of about 30 gauge. They do not require an introducer. Several companies manufacture these electrodes including Cavan Company, which makes a disposable electrode (available through the Electrode Store, Yucca Valley, CA 92284). Monopolar electrodes are used with surface electrodes, which act as ground and reference electrodes. Monopolar electrodes are well tolerated, sturdy, and inexpensive. They have a recording area of 500 μm.

Concentric (Coaxial, Bipolar) Needle Electrodes. Concentric needle electrodes are available through Teca Medelec and Disa (Philips). They consist of an active wire center and a concentric needle shaft. Their outer diameter is 0.45 mm with a core pickup area of 0.07 mm (125 × 580 μm). These electrodes are thicker than monopolar electrodes (20–26 gauge) but do not require a surface reference electrode. The beveled tip can be sharpened. They are more stable electrically. The Disa electrode uses a cable attachment that sometimes disconnects and may be difficult to reconnect after a patient is prepped and draped.

All electrodes mentioned are available in 25, 37, 50, 75 mm lengths. The 75-mm electrode is used in men, and the 25-mm electrode is suitable for women and for anal sphincter recording (Fig. 3–4).

Single Fiber Electrodes. Single fiber electrodes are fine concentric electrodes with a modified recording area. There have been a

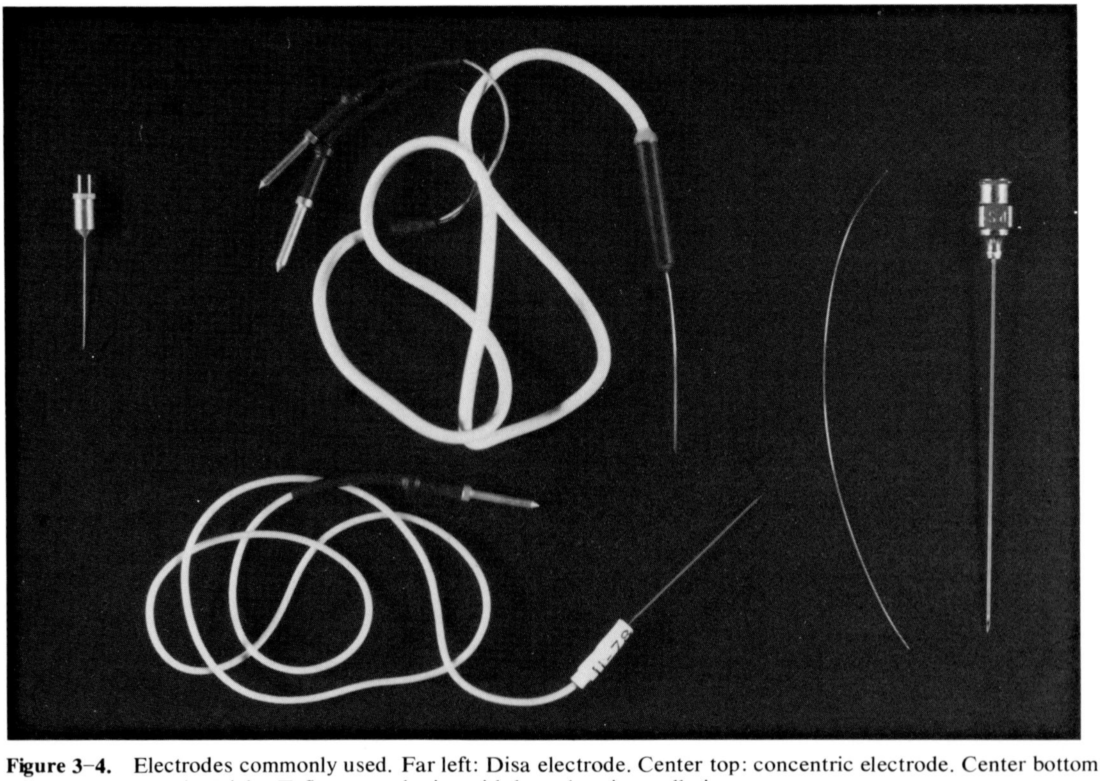

Figure 3–4. Electrodes commonly used. Far left: Disa electrode. Center top: concentric electrode. Center bottom: monopolar electrode. Right: Teflon-coated wire with hypodermic needle inserter.

few reports of their use for counting firing frequency of motor unit fibers.

Electromyography Equipment

There are several companies now manufacturing electromyographic (EMG) equipment. The essential features are an oscilloscope with wide frequency response (30–10,000 Hz) to allow visualization of individual motor units and possible abnormal spontaneous activity, an audio signal so that EMG activity can be monitored audibly while other measurements are being made, and a fast moving chart device. Most equipment uses graphic recorders or photography. Monitoring EMG activity only on a strip chart recorder can make baseline shifts and 60-cycle interference resemble muscle activity. A stimulator that triggers the oscilloscope sweep and that can be varied in terms of pulse duration, amplitude, and frequency is necessary for performing reflex studies. These instruments are commercially available. No special modifications are necessary. Stimulation may be carried out by applying a bipolar stimulator to the skin, stimulating a nerve using an intramuscular electrode, or using ring electrodes.

Performance of Sphincter EMG

The patient is placed on his back with hips flexed and externally rotated or in dorsal lithotomy position. The perianal or periurethral tissue may be made analgesic with ethyl chloride spray or lidocaine ointment. The needle is inserted in the anal sphincter at the mucocutaneous junction, monitoring the sound on the electromyograph (Figs. 3–5 to 3–7). The external urethral sphincter is found in women by inserting the needle just lateral to the urethral meatus to a depth of 15 mm. In the male patient the needle is inserted in the perineum at midline about 1.5 to 2.0 cm anterior to the anus. A gloved finger in the rectum monitors the position of the prostate while the electrode is being directed toward its apex. Final localization is made by monitoring motor unit activity electromyographically (listening to the frequency or "sharpness" of motor unit potentials sampled) and by examining the needle position fluoroscopically. If the needle is recording motor unit activity but appears to be superficial to the periurethral striated muscle, the muscle being sampled is most likely to be the bulbocavernosus muscle. Electrode insertion may also be made through the urethra using cystoscopic monitoring.

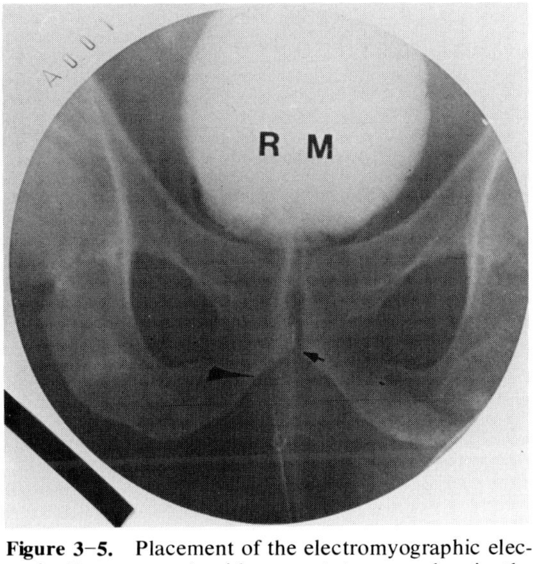

Figure 3–5. Placement of the electromyographic electrode (*large arrow*) with respect to a marker in the urethral catheter (*small arrow*).

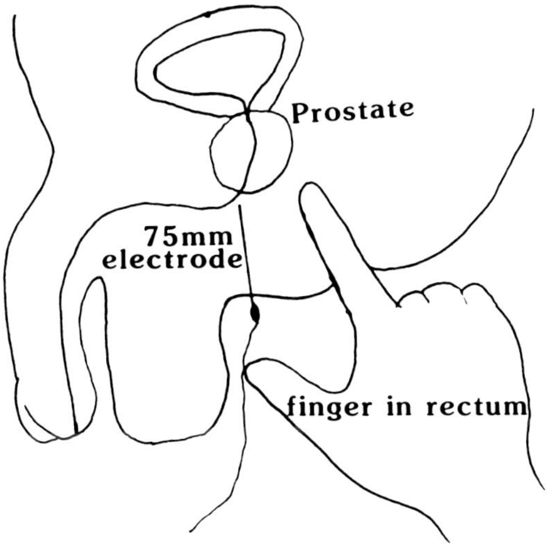

Figure 3–6. Surface anatomy and placement of electrode in male patients.

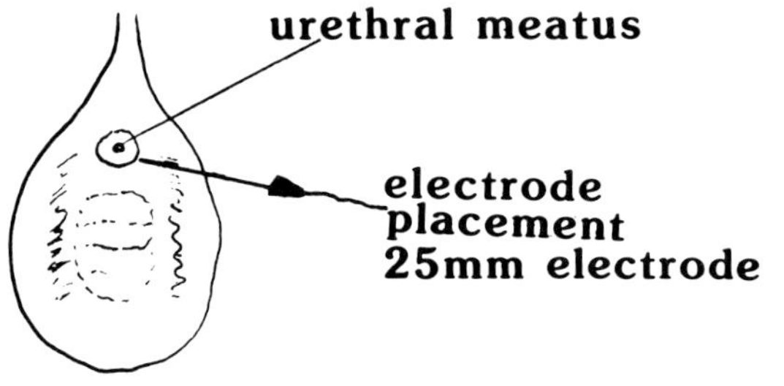

Figure 3–7. Placement of electrode in female patients.

Interpretation of E.M.G.

At rest there is continuous baseline activity consisting of motor unit potentials of 100 to 500 μV firing at rates of one to four per second (Fig. 3–8). Amplitude varies with the age of the patient, being lower in infants and increasing with maturation (*9,10*). This baseline activity is generated by slow twitch fibers and is least when the bladder is empty, increasing with bladder filling (*11,12*) in normal subjects. Silencing occurs only with voiding or defecation. If the muscle is silent at rest, it is probably not the sphincter (*13*). Each motor unit potential recorded represents the electrical activity generated by action potentials of muscle fibers within that unit. The signal derived is a triphasic wave with an initial positive deflection (*14*).

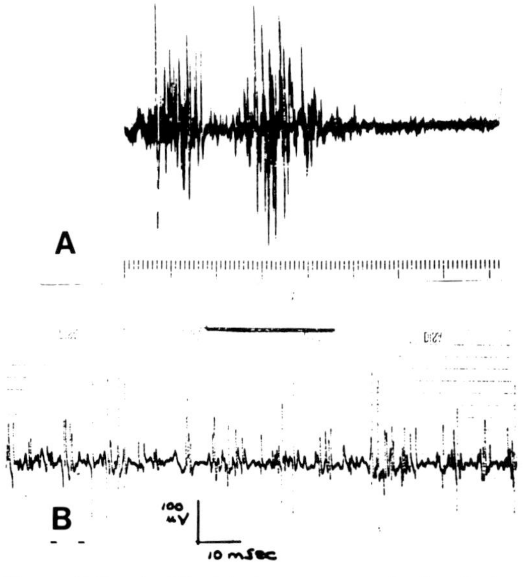

Figure 3–8. **A.** Electrical measurement of voluntary contraction and relaxation of the external urethral sphincter (EUS) at slow sweep speed. **B.** Motor unit potentials in EUS at a faster sweep to show motor unit morphology.

If the electrode is inserted near a neuromuscular junction, spontaneous miniature end-plate potentials produced by random release of packets of acetylcholine may be recorded as monophasic negative waves of less than 100 μV and 1 to 3 ms duration. This situation produces a "seashell" noise on the speaker. End-plate spikes are short-duration discharges distinguished from fibrillation potentials by their initial negative phase. When this pattern is recorded the needle is moved slightly because recording in this area is uncomfortable for the patient.

Motor unit potentials recorded at one point within muscle vary in amplitude, appearance, and firing pattern. If the patient is asked to voluntarily contract a muscle, additional motor units are recruited, as those firing tonically increase their rate of discharge.

Each muscle has a characteristic pattern of recruitment. The ratio of the rate of firing of individual motor units to the number firing is the *recruitment ratio*. In normal muscle it averages less than 5.

The appearance of the motor units is affected by the type of electrode being used and the frequency range of the amplifiers. It is recommended that one type of electrode be used consistently. The amplitude and form of a motor unit also varies with the placement of the needle within the muscle. There is less variation in a small muscle, e.g., the striated sphincter. The amplitude of individual motor unit potentials is a function of the innervation ratio, i.e., the number of axons per motor unit territory. The sphincters, facial muscles, and extraocular muscles normally contain few units in the 2 to 3 mV range. Children do not achieve an adult pattern until about 70 weeks (*15*).

Insertional activity is assessed as the needle electrode is passed through the muscle. Note is made of whether insertional activity is increased, indicating membrane instability, or decreased, indicating loss of muscle cells (passage of the needle sometimes gives an indication of the presence of fibrosis).

Spontaneous activity is that occurring with the muscle at rest. In addition to the neuromuscular junction end-plate noise, spontaneous activity includes fibrillations, positive waves, fasciculations, and myotonia or com-

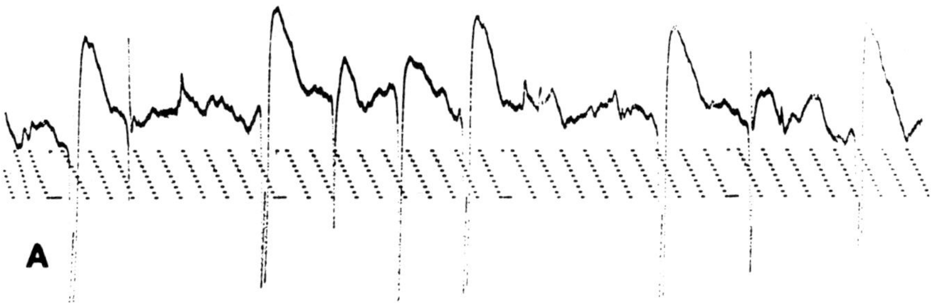

Figure 3–9. Positive waves.

plex repetitive discharges (Figs. 3–9 to 3–11).

Fibrillation potentials are action potentials of single muscle fibers. If they are recorded extracellularly, they appear as 20- to 200-μV potentials that resemble tiny motor unit potentials. There is an initial positive phase. The positive sharp wave is of longer duration and is characterized by a 20- to 200-mV positive deflection followed by a long-duration negative phase. This pattern indicates a muscle fiber potential recorded from a damaged part of the muscle fiber. It has the same significance as the fibrillation potential, i.e., loss of innervation of a fiber for any reason or damage to a muscle fiber (as with primary muscle disease). These potentials appear 10 days to 2 weeks after denervation. Prolonged runs of positive waves and fibrillations may be seen with myotonic dystrophy, glycogen storage diseases, myositis or muscle trauma. Complex repetitive discharges are the action potentials of groups of muscle fibers firing synchronously and rapidly (Fig. 3–11). Single-fiber recording suggests that they represent ephaptic activation of groups of adjacent muscle fibers. These discharges are of abrupt onset and also stop abruptly. They have been described in women with incontinence (*16*), in enuretic girls (*17*), and in a number of other neuropathic and myopathic conditions.

Fasciculation potentials are randomly discharging groups of muscle fibers. They may be seen in fatigued skeletal muscles and are most commonly associated with anterior horn cell disease. They are infrequent in sphincter muscles probably because of the low innervation ratio and the relative sparing of Onuf's nucleus by motor neuron disease.

Motor unit potentials in the striated sphincters and muscles of the pelvic floor range from 100 μV to 3 mV with a mean of 500 μV. Most motor units are triphasic, but in the sphincters 10 to 15 percent may be polyphasic

The amplitude and duration of the motor unit depend on the number of muscle fibers making up the unit and their distribution within the muscle. As denervation and reinnervation take place, motor unit potentials become longer in duration and higher in amplitude. This change is a result of increased fiber density or an increase in the number of fibers supplied by a single motor neuron. In the sphincters these long-duration units may be seen with reinnervation follow-

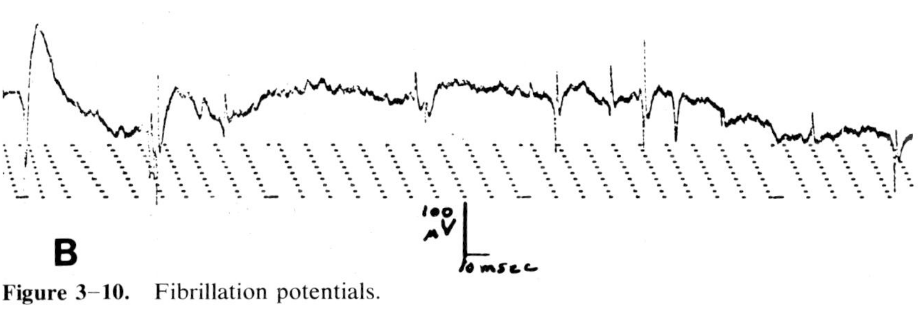

Figure 3–10. Fibrillation potentials.

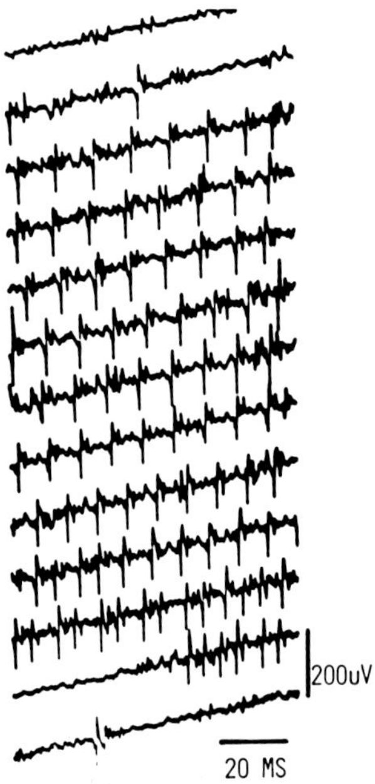

Figure 3–11. Complex repetitive discharges from the external urethral sphincter. The discharge begins and ends abruptly.

ing injury to pudendal nerves or lower sacral roots, or with dysraphisms.

The Onuf's nucleus is a group of motor neurons in the second sacral anterior horn thought to be a center innervating the perineal muscles (*18, 19*). Medial cell groups in the third sacral segment are not spared.

The pelvic floor is generally considered to derive its nerve supply from the pudendal nerve and from a direct branch of S_3 and S_4 roots. The pudendal nerve arises from the anterior primary rami of second, third, and fourth sacral nerves (*20*). The direct branch from $S_{3\text{-}4}$ also carries sensory fibers from the posterior urethra and anal canal (*21–24*).

Polyphasic potentials have five or more phases, i.e., "an area of a potential on either side of the baseline" (*14*). A *complex potential* has multiple reversals of direction without baseline crossings. These potentials have the same significance and are seen in myopathies and neuropathies. The underlying physiology is the firing of fibers within a motor unit at great variability instead of near synchrony. Polyphasia in sphincters most often signifies neuropathy. There is relative sparing of motor units in the sphincters with muscular dystrophies.

An *interference pattern* is that pattern of firing generated by voluntary contraction. It is reduced when motor units are decreased in number or when central mechanisms governing recruitment are affected.

SMOOTH MUSCLE ELECTROPHYSIOLOGY

Contractile properties of smooth muscle are similar to those of striated muscle, but the velocity of shortening and rate of actomysin adenosine triphosphatase activity are much slower in smooth muscle resulting in slower relaxation. The maximum force is comparable but requires less myosin. It appears to be due to a more compliant cross-bridge in smooth muscle and slower transitions between several cross-bridge states (*25*).

The smooth muscle of the bladder is composed of muscle fibers of the detrusor and the trigone. The detrusor is a mesh of smooth muscle bundles organized in layers. The smooth muscle cells may form "tight junctions" representing low-resistance extrasynaptic pathways of excitation (electrical rather than pharmacologic). Smooth muscle cells are smaller than skeletal muscle cells. They may be 2 to 5 μm in diameter and 50 to 200 μm in length. No cross-striations are visible because the contractile mechanism of actin and myosin filaments are oriented longitudinally without clear periodicity. Transmitter substances, (particularly adrenergic agents such as norepinephrine), cholinergic agents, and unknown transmitters activate the individual muscle cells, producing contraction. Bülbring showed that distension and stretch in smooth muscle fibers lowers the transmembrane potential (*26*). Such partial depolarization renders the cells hyperexcitable. These *in vitro* studies were performed using strain gauges to measure slow potentials and microelectrodes to measure intracellular units. There is a nonneural component of bladder tonus attributable to the elastic properties of smooth muscle and collagen.

Contraction in smooth muscle occurs more slowly (about one-fifth as fast as skeletal muscle) and has a longer refractory period

(*27*). Transmembrane potential is about −60 mV, in contrast to −80 to −85 mV in skeletal muscle.

Stimulation of a smooth muscle fiber by a transmitter may produce a spike that is sodium- and potassium-dependent as in skeletal muscle. Calcium ions may be involved in excitation-contraction coupling. There is a spontaneous slow wave potential seen on prolonged recording of smooth muscle (gut, ureter). If the threshold potential (−35 mV) is exceeded, a spike occurs; it may be elicited by stretch (*28,29*). Attempts to measure detrusor electrical activity *in vivo* have been controversial. Early measurements were made by Franksson and Petersen (*30*). Corey *et al.* attempted recording with sterling silver ball electrodes passed through a urethral sound and held against the bladder wall (*28*). They recorded 500-700-μV waveforms of low frequency (two to three per minute) from empty bladder (*31–33*). High-frequency low-amplitude potentials found by Doyle *et al.* (*31*) and Jones *et al.* (*32*) (5–35 mV, up to 170 Hz) using monopolar needle electrodes either transvaginally or transurethrally appear to be independent of rectus abdominus activity. Others who have studied smooth muscle include Abdel-Rahman *et al.* (*34*), Bradley *et al.* (*7*), Burnstock and Prosser (*35*), and Craggs and Stephenson (*36*).

It must be remembered that electrical activity recorded with extracellular electrodes is a summation of synchronous potentials generated and conducted by smooth muscle cells. Studies at the intracellular level are scarce. *In vitro* measurements using glass micropipettes have confirmed a resting potential of −50 mV. Other types of recording have involved inserting hook-shaped needle electrodes (Grass Co., EZ subdermal needles) through the serosa using bipolar concentric needle electrodes or suction electrodes. Takaiwa *et al.* have used a special urethral catheter with two carbon fiber electrodes to carry out detrusor EMG (*37*). They found activity in the 100 ms range with amplitudes of up to 0.2 mV. Pelvic nerve stimulation has been reported to produce 10- to 40-Hz activity in itself. Smooth muscle EMG *in vitro* is fraught with difficulties, errors, and artifacts. A totally satisfactory method of measurement has yet to be developed.

REFLEX ACTIVATION MANEUVERS

A number of maneuvers elicit changes in the baseline activity of muscles of the pelvic floor or striated sphincter mechanism. Pressing on the bladder suprapubically (Credé maneuver), increased intraabdominal pressure (Valsalva maneuver or cough), and stimulation of perianal or perineal skin evoke reflex increases in sphincter activity. Manual stimulation of the glans or clitoris produces an increase in sphincter activity referred to as the bulbocavernosus reflex. This reflex is retained in lesions above the sacral segments (Fig. 3–12) (*38–42*).

Bladder filling also causes a reflex increase in motor unit activity. Initiation of a voluntary detrusor contraction is preceded by total electrical silencing (relaxation) of even the tonic activity in the periurethral striated muscle. Silencing may precede detrusor contraction by as much as 20 to 30 seconds and lasts during detrusor contraction; it is followed by a burst of activity possibly serving to express urine remaining in the urethra. If the patient strains to initiate voiding, there is a burst of sphincter activity. Occasional patients have trained themselves to silence the sphincter while increasing intraabdominal pressure. Other patients have paradoxical silencing of sphincter activity with bulbocavernosus stimulation.

Kawakami has reported that stretching the anal sphincter reduces external urethral sphincter activity (*43*). Bradley and Teague

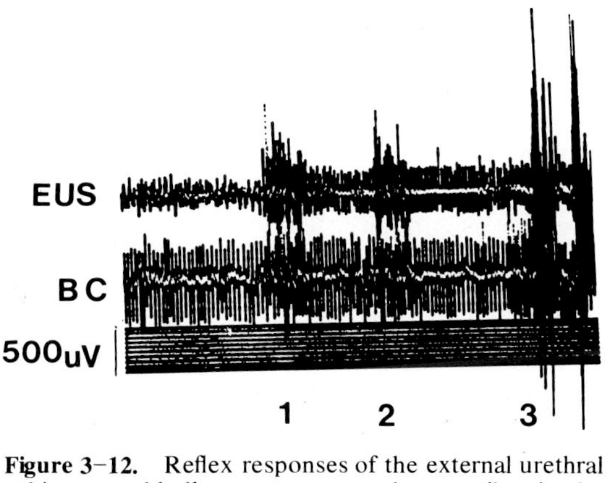

Figure 3–12. Reflex responses of the external urethral sphincter and bulbocavernous muscle to tactile stimulation of the glans (*1*), credé maneuver (*2*), and cough (*3*).

studied decerebrated cats and showed interaction at the sacral spinal cord level of the detrusor and the external urethral and anal sphincters (*44*). This reflex contraction of detrusor evoking depression of tonic sphincter activity was thought to occur via synaptic inhibition of alpha and gamma motor neuron pathways.

EVOKED RESPONSE MEASUREMENT

Evoked response measurements combine the techniques of electroencephalography and conduction velocity measurements. The brain responds to a variety of stimuli with a discrete response that is usually lost in recordings of ongoing cortical activity. It is possible to extract this response using computer averaging techniques. It is also possible to record similar signals along the course of the spinal cord. This technique is invaluable for monitoring cord function in patients with spinal cord injury.

There has been interest in measuring conduction in the central nervous system after stimulation of the lower urinary tract. Gerstenberg *et al.* stimulated the urethra (*45*). Badr *et al.* (*46,47*) stimulated patients with a square wave pulse of 0.5 ms, 20 to 25 mA (at sensory threshold but below pain threshold), at 1 to 2 Hz using wire electrodes inserted cystoscopically into the bladder wall just above the trigone. Because the signal obtained was of low amplitude, as many as 1000 responses were averaged. Recording at the vertex of the skull produced maximum responses. Subsequently they used monopolar suction electrodes with a diphasic stimulus. Their hypothesis was that the signal thereby obtained represented solely autonomic afferents, whereas monopolar stimulation may be recruiting pudendal afferents as well.

The suction electrode consists of an ethylene disposable catheter with a stainless steel suction cap at the distal part and a valve at the proximal part allowing suction to be applied by syringe. The response obtained was a complex signal with an initial positive deflection. Mean peak latencies were N 45 (negative), P_{60} (positive), N 80, and P_{100} ms.

Haldeman *et al.* stimulated the dorsal nerve of the penis or the clitoris and measured averaged responses over the spinal cord and over the sensory cortex (*48*). Subsequently, Kaplan (*49,50*) and Imabayashi *et al.* (*51*) studied the response in a number of abnormal conditions finding latencies to the major peaks to be prolonged in neuropathy, myelopathy, and spinal cord injury. This technique promises to be useful for assessing the integrity of central pathways.

BULBOCAVERNOSUS REFLEX

The presence of a bulbocavernosus reflex depends on the integrity of the pudendal nerves and the sacral segments of the spinal cord. In humans the reflex is affected by sacral cord injury, demyelinating disease, developmental abnormalities, diseases of the sacral roots, and peripheral neuropathy. Various attempts have been made to quantitate the reflex arc measurement.

Rushworth was one of the first investigators to observe an EMG response in the bulbocavernosus muscle on electrical stimulation of the pudendal nerve (*42*). Subsequently, several other groups using needle electrodes in the bulbocavernosus muscle or surface electrodes on the perineum have found a response with an average latency of 35 ms. A response at 50 to 80 ms has been recorded from the anal sphincter by Bradley and Teague (*44*). Bradley *et al.* (*7*) also stimulated the bladder using electrodes mounted on catheters. A standardized technique has been developed to measure reflex responses from the external urethral sphincter. Others have made similar measurements (*52–56*).

Stimulation of the pudendal nerve can be carried out using ring electrodes around the penis in men or with a bipolar stimulator placed on the clitoris in women (Fig. 3–13). In children there is a technical problem because the stimulating electrode is so close to the recording electrodes that a large stimulus artifact is seen (*57*). The stimulus is usually an electrical square wave pulse 0.05 to 1.00 ms in duration and 0 to 300 V in amplitude. Sensory threshold in normal adults is 60 to 80 V. Stimulating in this way one can record with needle electrodes in the external urethral sphincter (or bulbocavernosus or anal sphincter) a complex EMG response with clear-cut components. The first component (R_1) occurs with a latency of 20

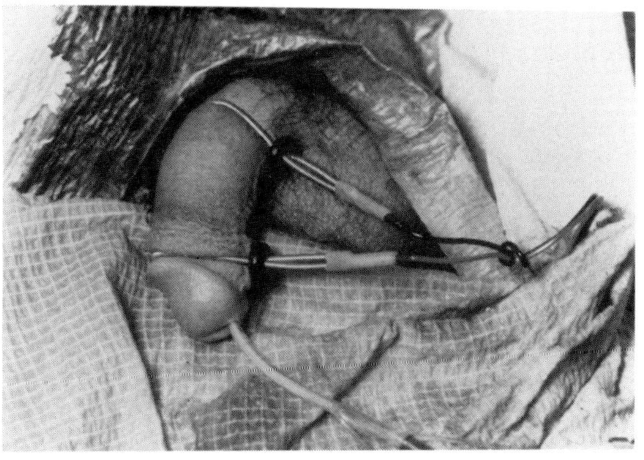

Figure 3–13. Ring electrodes placed around the penis for electrical sacral reflex arc stimulation.

to 45 ms and a duration of 10 to 30 ms. This component appears with the lowest threshold and decreases in latency as the stimulating voltage increases. A second component (R_2) may occur at 50 to 120 ms with higher stimulating voltage. The second component also decreases in latency with higher voltage or with repeated stimulation (Fig. 3–14). Some observers distinguish a third component (R_3) at 112 to 140 ms.

The first component is thought to represent an oligo- or monosynaptic response at one sacral level. The second component may be polysynaptic and involve several spinal levels (Fig. 3–15). The third component may represent the response of higher centers. A stretch reflex may be measured by placing a Fogarty balloon catheter at the external urethral sphincter and filling it rapidly. Hallett *et al.* have found that this stimulus produces a response similar to that seen with electrical stimulation (*57*). It is different from anal sphincter, which relaxes when stretched.

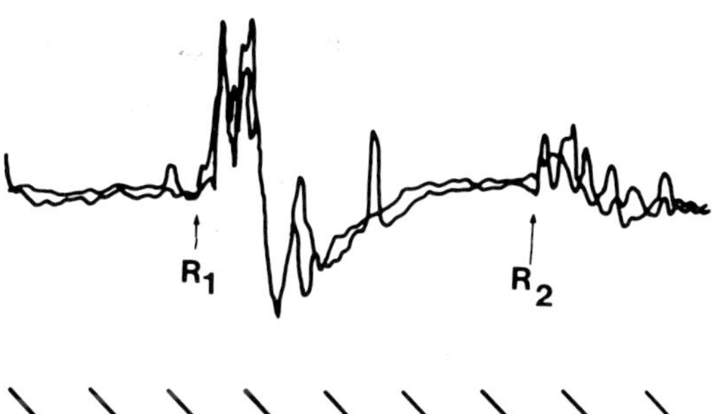

Figure 3–14. Flexor reflex responses R_1 and R_2 occurring at 26 m/s (R_1) and 66 m/s (R_2).

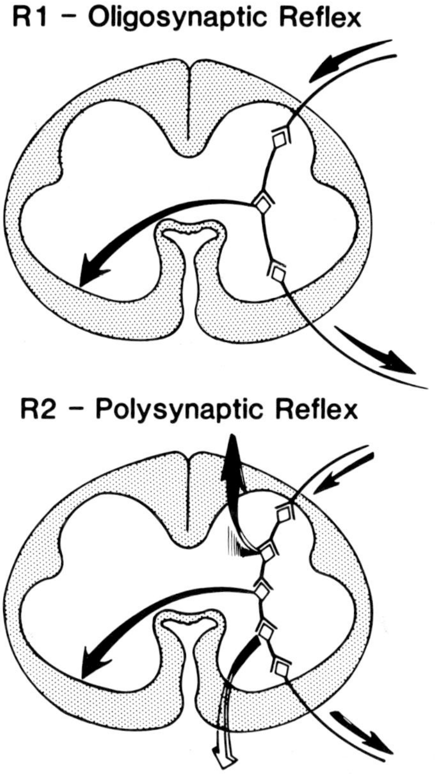

Figure 3–15. Postulated pathways for R_1 and R_2 components of the flexor reflex. (Courtesy of Dr. Stuart Bauer.)

In patients with upper motor neuron lesions stimulation of the posterior tibial nerve can produce contraction of the external urethral sphincter. These reflexes are generally acknowledged to be flexor reflexes because they are reliably reproduced by a given stimulus and have two components. The fibers stimulated in the penis are probably A alpha fibers. Bladder afferents belong to A delta and C fibers. High baseline activity may obscure a response. There may also be voluntary suppression of the response in the same way that contraction of skeletal muscle may have a depressive influence owing to effects of afferents from the muscle in the reflex loop.

CONDUCTION VELOCITIES

Attempts have been made to measure conduction velocities in sensory and motor nerves. Chantraine has determined motor conduction velocities in the internal pudendal nerve (*13*). It is possible to stimulate sacral roots with a needle electrode; Chantraine used needle electrodes to stimulate the pudendal nerve at two points. The placement of the electrode was determined by the locations of the lesser sciatic notch, the iliae crest, the greater trochanter and the ischial tuberosity.

ANAL SPHINCTER RECORDING

Anal sphincter recording may be useful for evaluating patients with fecal incontinence, evaluating children with imperforate anus prior to surgical correction, and as an alternate to urethral sphincter EMG (*58*). Anal sphincter EMG has been used to evaluate neurologic deficits of the sacral segments of the cord, particularly lower motor neuron involvement of S_2–S_4.

This technique is used with caution because of some difference in the root supply and peripheral innervation of the two sphincters (*23*). The characteristics of the two sphincters differ in that the anal sphincter may be silent. Amplitudes and phases of motor units are comparable.

Changes seen with fecal incontinence, especially in diabetics with fecal incontinence and autonomic neuropathy, are similar to those seen in skeletal muscle with neuropathy, the mean motor unit duration being 6.9 ms in control patients and 9.3 ms in those with neuropathy (*58*). Single fiber recordings show increased fiber density (*22*).

Schiller *et al.* found lower anal sphincter pressures in diabetic patients, indicating abnormal internal anal sphincter function probably due to defects in the autonomic innervation of the smooth muscle or external anal sphincter (*59*).

In 1891 Rossolimo described a reflex contraction of the anal sphincter when the anal mucosa or perianal skin is stimulated. Experiments in dogs enabled him to localize the reflex to the sacral cord (*60*).

Pedersen *et al.* studied reflex response of electrical perianal stimulation while obtaining EMG records from the external anal sphincter (*61*). A response was obtained with an average minimum latency of 50 ms when stimulation was with 1-ms pulses separated by 1 ms in five pulse trains. Upon stimulation of the posterior tibial nerve behind the medial malleolus, a reflex reaction of the anal sphincter could be recorded.

More recently, studies have been reported on the nature of cerebral responses evoked by the stimulation of vesico-urethral junction and dorsal nerve of the penis (*62,63*). Also, attempts have been made by Dyro and Yalla to study the refractoriness of the striated urethral sphincter during voiding (*64*).

It is hoped that as our techniques for investigating the interaction between the detrusor and sphincters become more sophisticated, new light will be shed on the normal process of micturition. This step in turn, may enable us to intervene electrophysiologically in pathologic detrusor or sphincter function.

REFERENCES

1. Beck, A.: Elecktromyographische Unter Suchungen am Sphincter ani. *Arch Physiol.* 224:278–292, 1930.
2. Petersen, I., and Franksson, C.: Electromyographic investigation of disturbances in the striated muscle of the urethral sphincter. *Br. J. Urol.* 27:154–161, 1955.
3. Brandstater, M., and Lambert, E. H.: Motor unit anatomy. In Desmedt, J. E. (ed.), *EMG and Clinical Neurophysiology,* Vol. 1. Karger, Basel, 1973, pp. 14–22.
4. Maizels, M., and Firlit, C. F.: Pediatric urodynamics: a clinical comparison of surface versus needle pelvic floor/external sphincter electromyography. *J. Urol.* 125:518, 1980.
5. Barrett, D. M.: Disposable (infant) surface electrocardiogram electrodes in urodynamics: a simultaneous comparative study of electrodes. *J. Urol.* 124:663, 1980.
6. Nordling, J., Meyhoff, H. H., Walter, S., and Andersen, J. T.: Urethral electromyography using a new ring electrode. *J. Urol.* 120:571, 1978.
7. Bradley, W. E., Timm, G. W., Rockswold, G. L., and Scott, F. B.: Detrusor and urethral electromyelography. *J. Urol.* 114:891–894, 1975.
8. Kiesswetter, H.: EMG-pattern of pelvic floor muscles with surface electrodes. *Urol. Int.* 31:60–69, 1976.
9. Buchthal, F., Guld, C., and Rosenfalck, P.: Action potential parameters in normal human muscles and their dependence on physical variables. *Acta Physiol. Scand.* 32:200–219, 1954.
10. Buchthal, F., Pinelli, P., and Rosenfalck, P.: Action potential parameters in normal human muscle and their physiological determinants. *Acta Physiol. Scand.* 32:219–229, 1954.

11. Jesel, M., Isch-Treussard, C., and Isch, F.: Electromyography of striated muscle of anal and urethral sphincters. In: Desmedt, J. E. (ed.). *New Developments in Electromyography and Clinical Neurophysiology*, Vol. 2. Karger, Basel, 1973, pp. 406–420.
12. Mai, J., and Pedersen, E.: Central effect of bladder filling and voiding. *J. Neurol. Neurosurg. Psychiatry* 39:171–177, 1976.
13. Chantraine, A.: EMG examination of the anal and urethral sphincters. In: Desmedt, J.E. (ed.), *New Developments in Electromyography and Clinical Neurophysiology*, Vol. 2. Karger, Basel, 1973, pp 421–432.
14. Daube, J.: *Needle Examination in Clinical Electromyography*, AAEE minimonograph No. 11, 1-29, 1979.
15. Waylonis, G. W., and Aseff, J. N.: Anal sphincter electromyography in the first two years of life. *Arch. Phys. Med. Rehabil.* 54:525, 1973.
16. Butler, W. J.: Pseudomyotonia of the periurethral sphincter in women with urinary incontinence. *J. Urol.* 122:838–840, 1979.
17. Dyro, F. M., Bauer, S., Hallett, M., and Khoshbin, S.: Complex repetitive discharges in external urethral sphincters of children. *Neurourol. Urodyn.* 2:39–44, 1983.
18. Onuf (Onufrowicz), B.: Notes on the arrangement and function of thecell groups in the sacral region of the spinal cord. *J. Nerv. Ment. Dis.* 26:498–504, 1899.
19. Iwata, M., and Hirano, A.: Sparing of the Onufrowicz nucleus in sacral anterior horn lesions. *Ann. Neurol.* 4:245–249, 1978.
20. Wunderlick, M., and Swash, M.: The overlapping innervation of the two sides of the external anal sphincter by the pudendal nerves. *J. Neurol. Sci.* 59:97–109, 1983.
21. Henry, M. M., and Swash, M.: Assessment of pelvic floor disorders and incontinence by electrophysiological recording of the anal reflex. *Lancet* 2:1290–1291, 1978.
22. Neill, M. E., and Swash, M.: Increased motor unit fibre density in the external anal sphincter muscle in ano-rectal incontinence: a single fibre EMG study. *J. Neurol. Neurosurg. Psychiatry* 43:343–347, 1980.
23. Percy, J. P., Swash, M., Neill, M. E., and Parks, A. G.: Electrophysiological study of motor nerve supply of pelvic floor. *Lancet* Jan. 3:16–17, 1981.
24. Swash, M.: Early and late components in the human anal reflex. *J. Neurol. Neurosurg. Psychiatry* 45:767–769, 1982.
25. Ursilo, R. C.: Electrical activity of the isolated nerve-urinary bladder strip preparation of the rabbit. *Am. J. Physiol.* 408:412, 1961.
26. Bülbring, E.: Correlation between membrane potential spike discharge and tension in smooth muscle. *J. Physiol. (Lond.)* 128:200, 1955.
27. Warshaw, D. H., and Fay, F. S.: Tension transients in single isolated smooth muscle cells. *Science* 219:1438–1441, 1983.
28. Corey, E. L., Boyce, W. H., Vest, S. A., and French, C. R.: Electropotential changes in human urinary bladder: a method of measurement. *J. Appl. Physiol.* 3:631–638, 1951.
29. Boyce, W. H.: Bladder electromyography, a new approach to the diagnosis of urinary bladder dysfunction. *J. Urol.* 67:650–671, 1952.
30. Franksson, C., and Petersen, I.: Electromyographic recordings from the normal human urinary bladder, internal urethral sphincter and ureter. *Acta physiol. Scand.* [*Suppl.*] 106:150–156, 1953.
31. Doyle, P. T., Hill, D. W., and Stanton, S. F.: Electromyography of detrusor muscle. *J. Urol.* 114: 298, 1975.
32. Jones, W. G., LaJoie, W. J., and Cosgrove, M. D.: Electromyography in pathological bladder. *Urology* 4:186, 1974.
33. LaJoie, W. J., Cosgrove, M. D., and Jones, W. G.: Electromyographic evaluation of human detrusor muscle activity in relation to abdominal muscle activity. *Arch. Phys. Med. Rehabil.* 57:382, 1976.
34. Abdel-Rahman, M., Coulombe, A., Abdel-Hakim, A., Galeano, C., and Elhilali, M.: Vesicourethral electromyography: facts or artefacts. *Br. J. Urol.* 54:381–386, 1982.
35. Burnstock, G., Prosser, C. L.: Conduction in smooth muscles; comparative electrical properties. *Am. J. Physiol.* 199:553–559, 1960.
36. Craggs, M. D., and Stephenson, J. D.: The real bladder electromyogram. *Br. J. Urol.* 48:443–451, 1976.
37. Takaiwa, M., Shiraiwa, Y., Katahira, K., and Tsukahara, S.: A new urinary bladder electromyogram technique. *Urol. Int.* 38:1–4, 1983.
38. DiBenedetto, M., and Yalla, S. V.: Electrodiagnosis of striated urethral sphincter dysfunction. *J. Urol.* 122:361–365, 1979.
39. Dick, H. C., Bradley, W. E., Scott, F. B., and Timm, G. W.: Pudendal sexual reflexes. *Electrophysiol. Invest. Urol.* 3:376, 1974.
40. Pedersen, H., Harving, H., Klemar, B., and Torring, J.: Human anal reflexes. *J. Neurol. Neurosurg. Psychiatry* 41:813–818, 1978.
41. Pierce, J. M., Boberge, J. T., and Newmann, M. M.: Electromyographic demonstration of bulbocavernosus reflex. *J. Urol.* 83:319, 1960.
42. Rushworth, G.: Diagnostic value of the electromyographic study of reflex activity in man. *Electroencephalogr. Clin. Neurophysiol.* 25(Suppl.): 65–73, 1967.
43. Kawakami, M.: Electromyographic investigation of the human external sphincter muscle of anus. *Jpn. J. Physiol.* 4:196, 1954.
44. Bradley, W. E., and Teague, C. T.: Electrophysiology of pelvic and pudendal nerves in the cat. *Exp. Neurol.* 35:378 1972.
45. Gerstenberg, T., Hald, T., and Meyhoff, H. H.: Urinary cerebral evoked potentials mediated through urethral sensory nerves—a preliminary report. *Prog. Clin. Biol. Res.* 78:141, 1981.
46. Badr, G. G., Carlsson, C-A., Fall, M., Friberg, S., Lindstrom, L., and Ohlsson, B.: Cortical evoked potentials following stimulation of the urinary bladder in man. *Electroencephalogr. Clin. Neurophysiol.* 54:494–498, 1982.
47. Badr, G. G., Fall, M., Carlsson, C-A., Lindstrom, L., Friberg, S., and Ohlsson, B.: Cortical evoked potentials obtained after stimulation of the lower urinary tract. *J. Urol.* 131:306–309, 1984.
48. Haldeman, S., Bradley, W. E., Bhatia, N. N., and Johnson, B. K.: Pudendal evoked responses. *Arch. Neurol.* 39:280, 1982.

49. Kaplan, P. E.: Somatosensory evoked responses obtained after stimulation of the pelvic and pudendal nerves. *Electromyogr. Clin. Neurophysiol.* 23:99–102, 1983.
50. Kaplan, P. E.: A somatosensory evoked response obtained after stimulation of the contralateral pudendal nerve. II. With diabetic neuropathy and benign prostatic hypertrophy. *Electromyogr. Clin. Neurophysiol.* 22:517–519, 1982.
51. Imabayashi, K., Ohnuma, T., and Nishimura, Y.: Evoked potential recording in the central nervous system after electrostimulation of the lower urinary tract. In: *Proceedings UDS*, New Orleans, 1984.
52. Jolesz, F. A., Cheng-Tao, X., Ruenzel, P. W., and Henneman, E.: Flexor reflex control of the external sphincter of the urethra in paraplegia. *Science* 216:1243–1245, 1982.
53. Siroky, M. B., Sax, D. S., and Krane, R. J.: Sacral signal tracing: the electrophysiology of the bulbocavernosus reflex. *J. Urol.* 122:661–664, 1979.
54. Vereecken, R. L., DeMeirsman, J., Puers, B., and Van Mulders, J.: Electrophysiological exploration of the sacral conus. *J. Neurol.* 227:135–144, 1982.
55. Vodusek, D. B., Janko, M., and Lokar, J.: Direct and reflex responses in perineal muscles on electrical stimulation. *J. Neurol. Neurosurg. Psychiatry* 46:67–71, 1983.
56. Yalla, S. V., DiBenedetto, M., Blunt, K. J., Sethi, J. M., and Fam, B. A.: Urethral striated sphincter responses to electrobulbocavernosus stimulation. *J. Urol.* 119:406–409, 1978.
57. Hallett, M., Bauer, S., Khoshbin, S., and Dyro, F.: Reflexes of the external urethral sphincter in children. *Arch. Neurol.* 41:942–945, 1984.
58. Bartolo, D. C. C., Jarratt, J. A., and Read, N. W.: The use of conventional electromyography to assess external sphincter neuropathy in man. *J. Neurol. Neurosurg. Psychiatry* 46:1115–1118, 1983.
59. Schiller, L. R., Santa Ana, C. A., Schmulen, A. C., Hendler, R. S., Harford, W. V., and Fordtran, J. S.: Pathogenesis of fecal incontinence in diabetes mellitus. *N. Engl. J. Med.* 307:1666–1671, 1982.
60. Rossolimo, G.: Der Analreflex, seine Physiologie und Pathologie. *Neurol. Centralbl.* 10:257–259, 1891.
61. Pedersen, E., Klemar, B., Schroder, H. D., and Torring, J.: Anal sphincter responses after perianal electrical stimulation. *J. Neurol. Neurosurg. Psychiatry* 45:770–773, 1982.
62. Sarica, Y., and Karacan, I.: Cerebral responses evoked by stimulation of the vesicourethral junction in normal subjects. *EEG Clin Neurophysiol.* 65:440–446, 1986.
63. Opsomer, R. J., Guerit, J. M., Wese, F. X., and Van Cangh, P. J.: Pudendal cortical somatosensory evoked potentials. *J. Urology*, 135:1216–1218, 1986.
64. Dyro, F. M., and Yalla, S. V.: Refractoriness of urethral striated sphincter during voiding: studies with afferent pudendal reflex arc stimulation in male subjects. *J. Urol.* 135:732–736, 1986.

Editorial comment: The readers may find some of the neurophysiological and related aspects of the bladder and its outlet mentioned in this chapter rather simplistic and controversial. For more details on the neuromuscular physiology and for updated experimental work, the readers are advised to refer to Chapter 1 by Dr. Elbadawi.

Editors

4

Applied Electronics

CLAUDE H. REGNIER, M.Sc.

The measurement of urodynamic variables is made possible by converting a nonelectrical physiological signal, e.g., flow or pressure, into a form that can be read and interpreted easily, e.g., a strip chart or screen display. In order to achieve such measurements, various steps are required to convert the physiologic signal into an electric form that can be displayed with sufficient magnitude. Whether the variables are measured from the lower urinary tract or any other part of the body, those steps are conceptually the same; the source of the signals is always a living tissue. Biomedical instrumentation thus provides the tools by which the measurement of physiologic variables and parameters can be achieved. Any medical instrument uses transducers, signal-processing devices, and displays to convert information about living systems to a form that can be perceived easily.

Although some forms of biomedical instrumentation (including those that monitor urodynamics) are unique to the field of medicine, many are adaptations of widely used physical measurements. A thermistor, for example, changes its electrical resistance with temperature, regardless of whether the temperature is that of an engine or airflow generated through the displacement of urine. The principles are the same. Another example is the strain gauge, which is commonly used to measure stress in structural components. It operates on the principle that electrical resistance is changed by the stretching of a wire or a piece of semiconductor material. Because pressure can be translated into strain by various means, intravesical pressure can be measured by an adaptation of this device. The major difference between this system of medical instrumentation and conventional instrumentation systems is thus the source of the signals.

This chapter outlines the basic principles used in the measurement of urodynamic variables. The man–instrument system is presented as a basic concept of instrumentation that depicts the various functional components involved in the measurement. Each component of the system is then described and applied to urodynamics, particularly the principles for measuring pressure, flow rate, and electromyographic (EMG) potentials. Emphasis is placed on the current role of microcomputers in providing the capability to perform on-line measurements by converting signals to digital values directly from the transducers. Finally, basic notions about electrical safety in urodynamics are discussed.

BASIC CONCEPTS USED IN INSTRUMENTATION

Definition of an Instrumentation System

An instrumentation system can be defined as the set of instrument and equipment utilized in the measurement of one or more characteristics or phenomena, plus the presentation of information obtained from those measurements in a form that can be read and interpreted (*1,2*). In general, the basic objectives of such a system fall into one of the following categories: information gathering, diagnosis, evaluation, monitoring, and control. The general field of biomedical instrumentation involves, to some extent, all of the preceding objectives. The man–instrument system can be defined as an overall instrumentation system that includes both the human subject and the instrumentation required for the various measurements in this particular subject. The function of medical instrumentation in this system is to provide the clinician and researcher with various tools for obtaining reliable and meaningful measurements from humans. Several factors, however, are associated with the difficulty of obtaining valid measurements: (a) safety considerations; (b) the environment of the hospital in which these measurements are to be performed; (c) the medical personnel usually involved in the measurement; and (d) ethical and legal considerations. Because of the major interaction between the instrument system and the patient being measured, it is essential that the person on whom measurements are made be considered an integral part of the instrumentation system.

Components of the Man–Instrument System

The man–instrument system is shown in Figure 4–1; the primary flow of information is from left to right. The basic components of this system are essentially the same as in any instrumentation system.

Measurand. The measurand denotes the physical quantity, property, or condition that the system measures. The accessibility of the measurand is important because it may be internal or external on the body surface. Urodynamic parameters are common measurands in clinical urodynamics; for example, intra-urethral or vesical pressures are internal and flow measurement is obviously external.

Transducer. The transducer is defined here as a device capable of converting one form of energy or signal to another. Each transducer is used to produce an electrical signal that is an analog of the phenomenon being measured, regardless of which physiologic parameter it addresses. The transducer should interface with the living system with minimal interference. In urodynamics, urine flow rate, urethral and bladder pressures, and sphincter EMG potentials are common phenomena recorded with different types of transducer; their output is always an electric signal. Two or more transducers may be used simultaneously to obtain relative variations between phenonmena. A complete micturition study (bladder and rectal pressures, urine flow rate, and anal sphincter EMG during voiding) would require, for instance, four types of transducer used in parallel. Surface and needle electrodes, strain gauges, flowmeters, thermistors, accelerometers, and microphones are examples of transducers.

Signal Conditioning Equipment. Signal conditioning equipment amplifies, modifies, or in any other way changes the electric output of the transducer; it is also used to combine or relate the output of two or more transducers. Although the output signal is

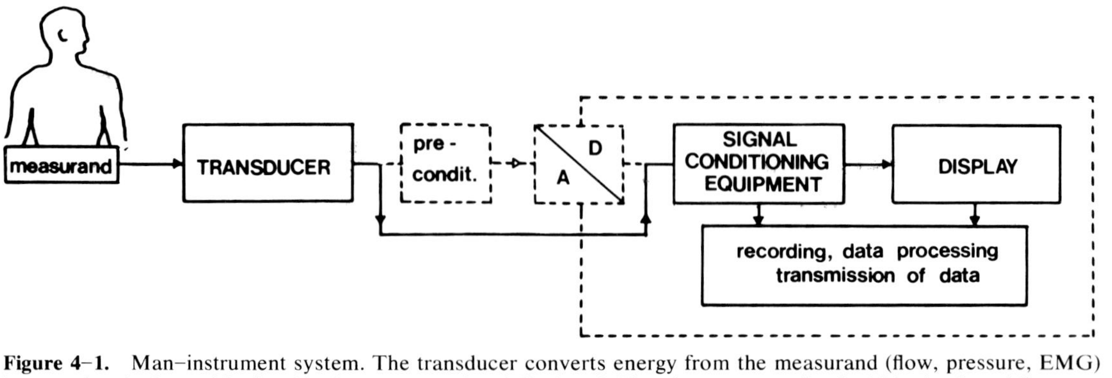

Figure 4–1. Man–instrument system. The transducer converts energy from the measurand (flow, pressure, EMG) into an electric form; this signal is then processed and displayed. The elements contained within the dotted lines can be computerized; in such cases the signal is preconditioned and converted from analog to digital before being processed by the computer. (Modified from Cromwell, L., *et al.: Biomedical Instrumentation and Measurements*. Prentice-Hall, Englewood Cliffs, N.J., 1973.)

often greatly modified with respect to the input, both input and output remain electric signals. It is usally at this stage that the signal is amplified, filtered (to reduce some artifacts), or matched to the impedance of the transducer. Signal conditioning equipment may also compensate for undesirable transducer characteristics or average repetitive signals to reduce noise. In essence, then, the purpose of the signal conditioning equipment is to prepare signals suitable for operating the display or recording equipment that follows.

Display Equipment Display equipment converts the electric output of the signal conditioning equipment to a form that can convey the information obtained by the measurement in a meaningful way. In urodynamics the most common types of display are visual (e.g., a digital reading of a pressure manometer) or audible (e.g., the sound produced on a speaker by EMG potentials.

Recording, Processing, and Transmission of Data. Data recording, processing, and transmission are necessary to store the measured information for possible later use or to transmit it from one location to another. Graph paper is commonly used in urodynamics, but computer control can be employed when automatic storage or processing of data is required; in the latter case, an on-line analog-to-digital converter may be part of the instrumentation system. The current development of microcomputers has made it possible to achieve all signal processing, e.g., amplifying or filtering, within the computer. The dotted line on Figure 4–1 shows how the components of the man–instrument system can be integrated into a single computerized unit.

Measurement Constraints

The various urodynamic parameters measured from the human body are seldom deterministic; the measured quantities vary with time, even when all controllable factors are fixed. There is an inherent variability, e.g., anatomic variations, which require large tolerance on the measurements. The typical urodynamic parameter measurement and frequency ranges are listed in Table 4–1. We can see from this table that the pressures encountered in urodynamics are quasistatic, or low-frequency signals, whereas EMG potentials have a higher frequency range. EMG signals can also vary from 20 to 4000 μV (4 mV), which is a ratio of 200 from the smallest possible EMG signal to the largest possible EMG signal. Care must be taken to determine that the complete instrumentation system, including the input device, can reproduce the full dynamic range without introducing distortion or nonlinearity. The characteristics of instrument performance are usually based on the frequency of such signals.

Fortunately, most urodynamic parameters are readily accessible for measurement. The problem remains, however, that many other variables within the human body are not accessible for measurement and might intercorrelate with the investigation. Measurement of bladder "tone" from a compliance curve is a striking example where the neuroactive element interferes with pressure

Table 4–1. Typical Urodynamic Parameter Measurement and Frequency Ranges*

PARAMETER	PRINCIPAL MEASUREMENT RANGE	PRINCIPAL FREQUENCY RANGE (Hz)
Bladder pressure	1–100 cm H_2O	10
Urethral pressure	1–100 cm H_2O	20
Abdominal pressure	1–100 cm H_2O	10
Urinary flow rate	1–50 ml/s	5
Electromyography	0.2–4.0 mV	10,000

*Pressures encountered in urodynamics are relatively low frequency signals, whereas EMG signals have a higher frequency range. The characteristics of instrument performance are usually based on the frequency of such signals.

readings; intravesical pressure results from the sum of two components, active and passive. Urodynamic variables, like most variables that can be measured from the human body, should therefore be considered as stochastic processes, i.e., time variables related to other variables in a nondeterministic way. They must be represented by some kind of statistical or probabilistic distribution. In other words, urodynamic measurements taken under a fixed set of conditions at one time are not necessarily the same as similar measurements made under the same conditions at another time; statistical methods must be employed in order to estimate relations among variables.

Urodynamic measurements are affected in some way by the presence of the measuring transducer, e.g., uroflowmetry. Susset (*3*) showed that peak flow rate has a tendancy to be below normal in the first ten voidings obtained within a week (Fig. 4–2); it stabilizes later on and is interpreted as a partial psychological inhibition. Some individuals who would otherwise have a normal flow rate show inhibited readings whenever they are in the physician's office. It is a fear response on the part of the patient involving the autonomic nervous system. The effect of the presence of the measuring device should be minimal in urodynamic instrument design.

The operation of instruments imposes additional constraints; equipment must be reliable, simple to operate, and capable of withstanding physical abuse and exposure to corrosive chemicals. The safety of patients and medical personnel must also be considered in all phases of design and testing of instruments.

GENERAL CHARACTERISTICS OF INSTRUMENTS

In order to compare commercially available urodynamic instruments (and evaluate new instrument design), quantitative criteria for the performance of such instruments are needed. Such criteria must clearly specify how well the instrument measures the desired input and how much the output depends on interfering and modifying inputs. Although many factors affect the performance of these instruments, some of the gener-

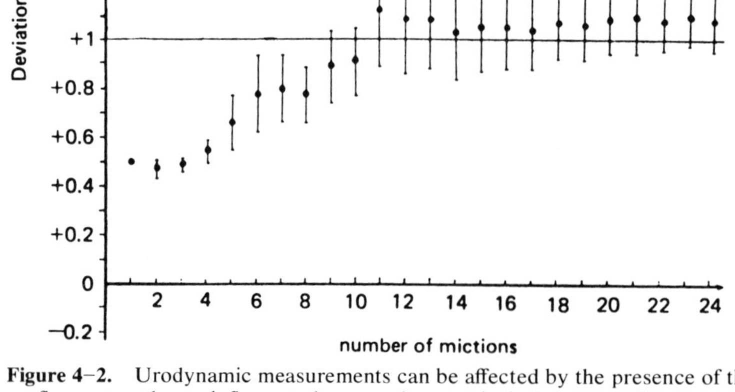

Figure 4–2. Urodynamic measurements can be affected by the presence of the measuring transducer. In the case of uroflowmetry, the peak flow rate has a tendency to be below normal in the first ten voidings as a result of a partial psychological inhibition. These values represent the average for five individuals. (From Hinman, F., Jr. [ed.]: *Benign Prostatic Hypertrophy*. Springer-Verlag, New York, 1983.)

al requirements can be characterized into signal, environment, medical, and economic factors. The type of transducer selected usually stipulates as well the signal conditioning equipment, so that urodynamic and biomedical instrument specifications at large include more than just deciding what type of transducer to use. For each urodynamic piece of equipment, in particular, the technical specifications should be given by the manufacturers and designers.

The terms used have been listed by Olson (*1*) and are summarized below to facilitate evaluation of the completeness of such specifications. For convenience, the list is subdivided into the following categories: input and transducer specifications, signal-processing specifications, output specifications, and errors and reliability

Input and Transducer Characteristics

Input Ranges. The input ranges define the maximum ranges of allowed input quantities that are applicable for various conditions. In other words, the measuring instrument has a scale on which the reading of the measurement appears; each scale has a lower and an upper value, and the difference between the two defines the range. Pressure recording instruments usually have more than one scale, and each scale has a different range. For instance, a scale of ±20 cm H_2O per division (one division = 1 cm on the graph paper = 5 cm full scale) has a range of ±100 cm H_2O. It is always desirable to choose the scale that is mid-range for the measurement. Pressure, flow rate, and EMG signals are the most common input quantities used in urodynamics. The input range for pressure transducers is usually 250 cm H_2O. The maximum operating range is the largest input that does not damage the instrument; it is commonly 1000 cm H_2O for pressure transducers.

Frequency Response. The frequency response denotes the response of the measuring instrument with time. How fast can the instrument respond to a change of the parameter being measured? Ideally, the urologist uses an instrument that responds rapidly enough to include the most rapid change in such parameter; that is, the instrument must be capable of adequately responding to the highest frequency that can occur. The instruments are generally designed to respond not only to the average value of the signal but also the highest Fourier harmonic of the signal. Most commercially available instruments used in urodynamics have a frequency response that goes much beyond the typical ranges expressed in Table 4–1. Frequency ranges for pressure manometers depend on the type of transducer being used; it is usually 100 Hz for standard external transducers and 5 kHz for tip transducers. Such instruments are therefore largely suitable for recording bladder, rectal, or urethral pressures, which have a frequency in the order of 10 to 20 Hz. A time constant is often used as a measure of frequency response for a given system; it is defined as the time required for this system to register 63 percent of its final reading when subjected to a step change in input. A large time constant thus corresponds to a low-frequency response.

Sensitivity. The sensitivity of an instrument can be defined as (a) the amount of signal required to produce a unit of deflection or (b) the amount of deflection per unit of signal, i.e., the overall instrument output per unit input. For example, an EMG amplifier can have a sensitivity of 20 or 100 μV per division (one division = 1 cm on graph paper = 5 cm full scale). Range and sensitivity are interrelated; the greater the range, the less sensitive is an instrument per unit of deflection.

Input Impedance. The input impedance measures the degree to which instruments disturb the quantity being measured, as biomedical transducers and instruments usually convert nonelectric quantities into voltage or current. The generalized input impedance is defined as the ratio of the effort input variable (voltage, flow, pressure) to the flow input variable (current, velocity, flow). It depends on the rate at which energy is being transferred across the tissue–transducer interface. The time rate of such energy transfer should be minimized, and therefore the generalized input impedance should be as large as possible in order to minimize the flow variable, as biologic source impedances are usually unknown, variable, and difficult to measure and control. The best measurement of voltage at the surface of the skin requires, for example, that the EMG signal be transferred to the amplifier without attenuation, distortion, or drift. It is best accomplished when the impedance across the skin–electrode interface, called the source impedance, is as low as possible, and the input impedance of the amplifier is high, at least 100 or 1000 times the source impedance. When the amplifier input impedance/source impedance ratio is high, little power is transferred from the skin to the amplifier. This situation implies that a minimum of current per unit area flows through the skin electrode and then to the amplifier input.

Transient Response Time. The transient response time gives the degree of damping that results from a step input. For example, it measures the time necessary for a flowmeter to give a steady-state response when a rapid and constant change in volume is applied. Transient analysis is also commonly used to evaluate the frequency response of a manometer–catheter system because such systems respond to some rapid change in pressure.

Input Common Mode Rejection Ratio. The common mode rejection ratio (CMRR) is a quantity used to measure the departure from the ideal characteristics of differential amplifiers. As is discussed in more detail below, a differential amplifier results if both of its inputs are free to sense active potentials, in contrast to single-ended amplifiers where the voltage reference level is provided by some ground point. In other words, a signal common to both inputs of a differential amplifier does not affect the output. Differential amplifiers are in practice not ideal in their rejection of common mode signals. Their rejection is limited to a factor of 10,000:1 or 1,000,000:1 with respect to the amplitude of the differential voltage (*4*). The quality of a differential amplifier or CMRR is then defined as

CMRR = (amplification of the differential voltage)/(amplification of the common-mode voltage)

If, for example, an EMG amplifier has a gain of 1000 for differential input voltages, and common-mode signals are at the same time attenuated by a factor of 100, the CMRR is 100,000. Thus a common-mode signal of 1 V appears at the output of the amplifier with an amplitude of 10 mV. At the same time, the EMG of 1 mV is amplified to 1 V, which means that the level of the common-mode signal is 1 percent of the EMG amplitude, a reasonable value. If the common-mode signal was 10 V in the example mentioned above, the signal would have been 10 percent, which is not permissible. It is thus of great advantage to make the common-mode voltage in the first place as small as possible. It can be done by proper grounding of the patient.

Signal-Processing Specifications

Compensation. Compensation is necessary when undesirable transducer characteristics enhance a nonlinear output response (see below for linearily).

Zero Suppression. Zero suppression denotes an adjustment to compensate for various sources of drift (see below for sources of drift).

Filtering. Filtering defines electronic restrictions on the processor frequency response. It is used in urodynamics mostly for EMG recording when certain frequencies are undesirable (e.g., 60 Hz). It is possible to use different filter types in order to eliminate a certain range of frequencies from the measurement, e.g., low frequencies up to 6 or 7 Hz. However, difficulties may arise when the undesirable frequency is contained within the frequency range of the signal. Filters are usually specified for EMG amplifiers in terms of a cutoff frequency.

Interfacing. Interfacing denotes digital interfacing capability. It is necessary if computer control is part of the instrumentation system.

Output Specifications

Output Quantity. Output quantity is usually a voltage or current that drives a display device that may be a part of the instrument. For instance, the output voltage of a mictiograph can be 5 V maximum corresponding to 10, 25, or 50 ml/s depending on the range in use.

Output Range. The output range defines the range of linear output and the level of output saturation. It corresponds to the maximum output quantity that is allowable for a particular instrument.

Output Impedance. Output impedance denotes the generalized output effort variable divided by the output flow variable. The output impedance should be minimized as the flow variable in this case should be as large as possible.

Writing Speed. Writing speed is important to measure the frequency response of the display device. It is particularly important in transient analysis. It usually ranges from 0.5 to 20.0 mm/s. It has only relative importance if the data can be stored within a computer, as such data can be called back for further anaylsis.

Errors and Reliability

Accuracy. The accuracy of a single measured quantity is the true value minus the measured value, and the difference is divided by the true value. Accuracy is a measure of the total error without regard to the type or source of the error; it can be expressed as percent of reading, percent of full scale, $\pm$ number of digits per digital readouts, $\pm$ one-half the smallest analog scale division, or the sum of these. The accuracy usually varies over the normal range of the quantity measured. For example, the accuracy of a multirange urine flowmeter decreases as the full scale of the quantity decreases; i.e., the flowmeter is less accurate at 10 ml/s than at 50 ml/s. It is thus important that the accuracy of an instrument be expressed in terms of both percent of reading and percent of full scale.

Precision. The precision of a measurement expresses the number of distinguishable alternatives from which a given result is selected. For instance, a manometer that displays 23.24 cm H_20 is more precise than one displaying 23.2 cm H_20. High precision measurements, however, do not imply high accuracy, as the latter varies with range and variable biologic input as defined above.

Resolution. Resolution denotes the smallest incremental quantity that can be measured with certainty. It expresses the degree to which nearly equal values can be differentiated and depends on the variable being measured. For instance, resolution for urine flow rate is commonly 0.1 ml/s and 1 second for the voiding time.

Reproducibility. Reproducibility is defined by the ability of an instrument to give the same output for an input applied over a period of time. It does not imply accuracy.

Statistical Control. Statistical control means that random variations in measured quantities, resulting from all factors that influence the measurement, are tolerable. Random variations encountered in EMG recording can be a difficult problem, as the measurand and the instrument may introduce statistical variations that make the output nonreproducible.

Static Sensitivity. A static calibration curve is performed by holding all inputs (desired, interfering, or modifying) except one. As one input is varied incrementally over the normal operating range, the static sensitivity of an instrument can be defined as the ratio of the incremental output quantity to the incremental input quantity. Static sensitivity may be constant only for a limited range of input, as shown in Figure 4–3, and thus depends on the output range of the instruments.

Zero Drift. Zero drift occurs when all output values increase or decrease by the same absolute amount, but the slope of the static sensitivity curve shown in Figure 4–3 remains unchanged. Several factors can cause such a drift, manufacturing misalignment, variations in ambient temperature, hysteresis, vibrations, and shock. Fast changes due to motion of the patient, for instance, cause zero drift to appear at the out-

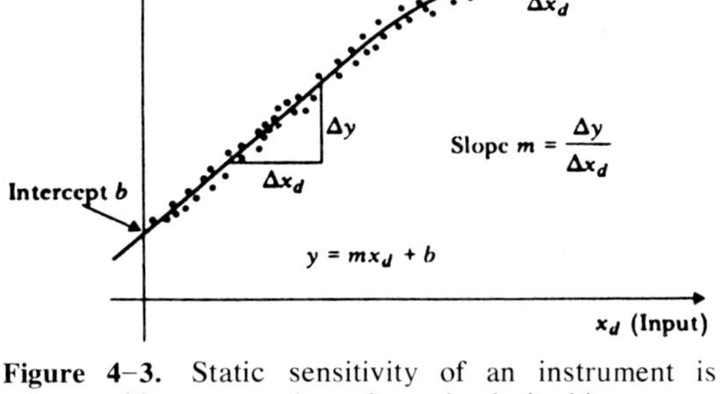

Figure 4–3. Static sensitivity of an instrument is expressed by a curve that relates the desired input x_d to the output y. Static sensitivity may be constant for only a limited range of inputs. (From Doebelin, E. O. (ed.): *Measurement Systems: Application and Design*. McGraw-Hill, New York, 1975.)

put in pressure measurements. Zero drift for standard pressure manometers is usually 0.2 cm H_20 per degree centigrade for temperature and 0.2 cm H_20 per 24 hours for long term stability. A drift of less than 0.1 percent per degree centigrade is usually desirable.

Sensitivity Drift. Sensitivity drift results when the slope of the static sensitivity curve changes (either increases or decreases) after an interfering input. Such drift causes an error that is proportional to the magnitude of the input. Manufacturing tolerances, power supply variations, nonlinearities, and changes in ambient temperature and pressure can cause such a drift. Figure 4–4 shows a static sensitivity curve affected by both zero and sensitivity drifts. In practice, the sensitivity drift is often referred to as a drift in the "gain" of the system.

Linearity. Linearity exists for an instrument when the calibration curve is a straight line. In practice, no instrument has a perfect linear response, so a measure of deviation from linearity is needed. It should be noted also that high accuracy does not necessarily imply linearity. Nonlinearity defines a deviation from linear operation; for instance, hysteresis results when some of the energy applied to the instruments for an increasing input is not recovered when the input decreases. All instruments have some degree of hysteresis because the second law of thermodynamics prohibits perfect reversibility. The input–output characteristics are therefore different for increasing input and decreasing input. All instruments also exhibit saturation if the input magnitudes are too large; it is another common type of nonlinearity. For example, in Figure 4–3 the characterisitic is linear for input up to some level, but the slope of the curve decreases and becomes zero for large inputs. Such transition may be smooth or abrupt depending on the type of nonlinearity.

Noise. Noise is defined as maximum peak-to-peak electric (or nonelectric) noise referred to the input. Operational amplifiers have transistor input junctions, which generate both noise–voltage and noise–current sources. The amplitude of the noise varies with frequency; for instance, at low frequencies a large amount of noise is present, whereas at higher frequencies the noise is lower. Noise can be generated through various sources of interference, e.g., electric or mechanical. It is therefore advisable to increase the frequency of the signal when noise is present in order to differentiate more easily the noise from the recorded signal.

Signal/Noise Ratio. The signal/noise ratio denotes the ratio of the value of the signal to that of the noise, expressed in decibels. It is an important parameter in EMG recording because it represents the degree to which the signal is faithfully reproduced. Such ratio depends on the signal frequency and the noise bandwidth.

Stability. The stability of an instrument characterizes the drift of its output as a function of time, temperature, humidity, acceler-

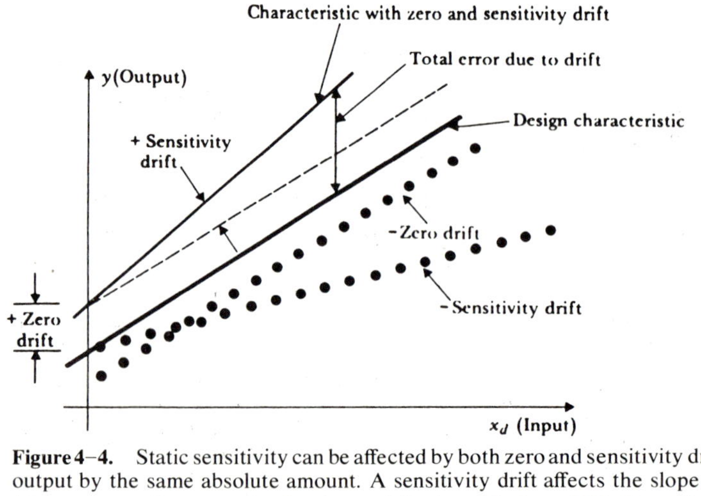

Figure 4–4. Static sensitivity can be affected by both zero and sensitivity drifts. A zero drift increases (or decreases) the output by the same absolute amount. A sensitivity drift affects the slope of the curve. (From Doebelin, E. O. (ed.): *Measurement Systems: Application and Design*. McGraw-Hill, New York, 1975.)

ation, and vibration. In other words, it denotes the warm-up time.

BASIC ELECTRONIC TERMINOLOGY

Many electronic terms are used to describe the basic operations of biomedical instruments. In order to gain proper understanding of the instrumentation it is necessary to be somewhat familiar with the terminology and language used in the various descriptions (*5*). It is essential to know the material discussed in this section in order to form conventional points of reference for study of the instrumentation itself.

Voltage

Voltage is a term used to describe a condition of potential difference. It is simply the force that activates the flow of current in a circuit. There are two basic types of voltage: Direct current (DC) voltage is often supplied by batteries, whereas alternating current (AC) voltage is that obtained from electric outlets. A volt (V) is the basic unit of measurement of potential difference. Most of the electronic instrumentation under discussion is initially powered by 120 or 240 V of alternating current. In all electronic circuits voltage is measured at two points: the positive pole and the negative pole. Both of these poles must be connected to the circuit under power or to the measurement device in order to establish a flow of current. When both poles of a source of voltage are connected to an electronic circuit, current begins to flow from the negative pole to the positive pole. In DC voltage circuits the polarity remains constant. The positive pole is always positive, and the negative pole likewise remains the same. However, AC circuits maintain a continual reversal of polarity. The rate of change or alternation in AC circuits is described in Hertz (Hz) or cycles per second (cps), which are equivalent terms. Common household current reverses at a rate of 60 Hz, which means that the polarity of the voltage reverses itself 60 times per second. The human body can also be thought of as the chemical generator of electric voltage and currents.

Amperage

Just as the volt is the basic unit of potential difference, the ampere is the basic unit of current. We can describe current as the flow of electrons through a specific circuit. A single ampere is the equivalent of the movement of approximately six trillion electrons past a specific point in the circuit. In practical measurement, however, the number of electrons is almost never stipulated by counts but is always expressed in amperes. Like voltage, the flow of electrons is always in one direction in DC circuits, whereas in AC circuits the current flow reverses itself at the established frequency rate. Measuring instruments that are intended to provide voltage or current indications are called, respectively, voltmeter and ammeter.

Conductance and Conductor

The amount of current that flows in a conductor, i.e., a device that provides a path of current flow, as a result of the applied voltage is a function of the number of electrons in each of its atoms that is free to drift or move in the conductor; the current is also a function of a variety of other factors, e.g., the temperature of the conductor. The property of the conductor that describes its ability to conduct quantitatively is referred to as its conductance. Electric wiring is a prime example of a conductor, as it allows electrons to pass freely through its copper or sometimes aluminum material. There is no material that provides a completely perfect path for electron flow. Even the finest conductor provides some resistance to this flow. Conductance is measured in Siemens but the mho is the basic unit of conductivity. It is the reverse term of ohm, which is utilized for resistance.

Resistance and Resistor

It is usually more practical to use a term that means the reciprocal of conductance; this term is resistance. Resistance can be thought of as opposition to the flow of current. The resistance of a conductor to the flow of current is a function of the length of the conductor, its cross-sectional area, and the nature of the conductor itself. The unit of resistance is the ohm, named after George Simon Ohm, the physicist who first described it. In most electronic circuits resistance takes the form of a lamped constant called a resistor. It usually consists of a small device that provides a specific resistance to the flow of the current when placed in the circuit. When a material has a higher ohms rating than the mho value, it is usually called a resistor. When the reverse is true, it is usually called a conductor. Although the average human body conducts electricity, it is more a resistor than a conductor; its average resistance approximates 50,000 ohms. A device that measures resistance is called an ohmmeter. Ohm's law expresses the constant relation existing between current (I), voltage (V) and resistance (R): $V = (R) \times (I)$.

Power

When current passes through an electric resistance, power is generated. This power may take the form of a sound, visual effects, mechanical processes, heat, etc. The amount of power utilized in electronic circuits is expressed in watts. As previously described, a resistor impedes the flow of current. When such impedance occurs, a heating effect takes place, and a certain portion of circuit power is disposed of through resistor heat, which is dissipated into the surrounding air. There is a maximum amount of heat that a device or instrument can safely distribute in a heat exchange with the surrounding air. Whenever there is a flow of current, there is always a power factor (P); this factor is directly dependent on current and voltage within the circuit. It is expressed by: $P = (V) \times (I)$. One watt represents the power utilized in a circuit of 1 volt and 1 ampere.

Capacitance and Capacitor

The movement of electrons and the accumulation charge on a conductor causes it to exhibit capacitance, which may be defined as the ratio of the charge to the potential difference or voltage between two points on the conductor. The capacitor is able to store energy when charged. In other words, when current is fed through a capacitor, electric power is stored within this device to perform various electronic functions. The basic unit of capacitance is the farad, named after Michael Faraday. However, the farad is such a large unit that only microfarad and picofarad are commonly used as rating terms for capacitors in various medical instrumentation circuits.

Inductance and Inductor

Inductance is a phenomenon that occurs when the magnetic field generated by a solenoid (a coiled wire) tends to decelerate the electrons traveling the wire. A solenoid has an inductance that is expressed in henrys, named after Joseph Henry. Such device offers considerable opposition to alternating current with a frequency rate that falls within the range of the coil. It therefore generates a voltage or electromotive force opposite to the one driving the current.

Semiconductor Devices

Most biomedical instrumentation of modern design makes 100 percent use of semicondutor devices, which have replaced the older vacuum tube. Semiconductor devices contain no moving parts, and they are not subject to damage through vibration or moderate shocks. Semiconductors are made from crystalline materials (normally silicone or germanium) that are chemically treated and then combined. This material is then mounted in a small plastic or metal case with protruding lids for electronic connections. Semicondutor devices include many components that perform a myriad of electronic functions. The major devices are the transistor, the diode, and the integrated circuit.

Transistor. Transistors have the ability to amplify or increase electric power; this action is called power amplification and is often rated in terms of multiplication. For example, a component with an amplification factor of 10 can produce an output equivalent to ten times the input. Transistors have voltage, power, and frequency ratings that are specified by manufacturer operation sheets supplied with each unit. There are three leads protruding from a transistor that are connected to the collector, emitter, and base of the component, the three basic sections.

Diode. Diodes have the characteristic of passing currents freely in one direction while blocking or highly opposing the flow in the opposite direction. Diodes can pass only direct currents. Therefore when an alternating current is applied to a diode, only one-half cycle of the AC wave is conducted; the other half is completely dropped. It means that a diode converts alternating current to direct current, and this trait is used for rectification purposes—the changing of AC to DC—in power supplies. Therefore an AC input is changed at the diode output to a wave that is no longer of a changing polarity.

Integrated Circuit. An integrated circuit is a semiconductor device that contains many of the components already discussed on a tiny piece of semiconductor material. Transistors, diodes, resistors, and their associated connections are chemically produced from the basic silicone crystal material. The integrated circuit is a complete, functional circuit with no discrete or moving parts. The integrated circuit crystalline chip is housed in a small plastic or metal container with many leads brought to the exterior for connection to the various internal circuit points. Because each integrated circuit is a complete circuit, different uses and ratings apply for the many thousands of units. Thus biomedical instruments that would otherwise have required several rooms of electronic circuitry can now be made small enough to be carried easily. The stability and reliability of operation have been increased a hundredfold by these devices because of their compact, solid-state construction.

Schematic Diagrams

Electronic circuits can appear extremely complicated, but it should be remembered that almost every complex electronic circuit is composed of a multitude of simple circuits. Each of these less complicated circuits is connected to another, resulting in a pyramid of circuits and components. It is convenient to draw, pictorially, the mulititude of components that make up a complex electronic circuit. Schematic diagrams, then, provide an easy means of accurately displaying the electronic workings and components of any electronic circuit. Each part of the circuit is represented by a symbol that can be easily drawn. Figure 4–5 shows a modified "flashlight" circuit that is nearly equivalent to the portable flashlight used in the home.

The battery is indicated with its schematic representation, as are the lightbulb and switch. The lines connecting these symbols to each other represent wires in the actual circuits. The battery symbol has a plus (+) and a minus (−) on either side to indicate polarity. Table 4–2 represents a chart of schematic representations that are often used.

Block Diagrams

A block diagram serves a more useful purpose than the schematic diagram. It does not usually show individual components but, rather, the major circuit sections. In a typical block diagram, the blocks may have thousands of electronic components, but it is simply represented by one type of diagram. A block diagram is useful in determining where problems lie within a piece of instrumentation. It gives a starting point from which to work when determining the exact cause of inoperation. Once a particular circuit area is found to be questionable, the technician refers to the schematic diagram for this portion of the circuit for a more comprehensive search of the problem. A block diagram is

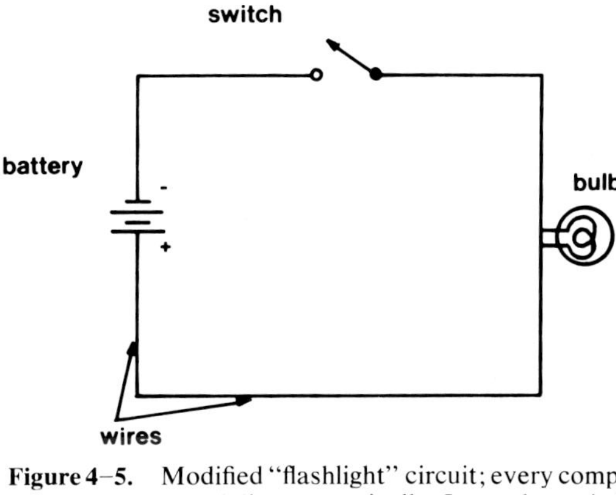

Figure 4–5. Modified "flashlight" circuit; every component is represented diagrammatically. In urodynamic instruments, electronic circuits are represented by a multitude of simple circuits connected one to another, resulting in a pyramid of circuits and components.

Table 4–2. Schematic Representation of Commonly Used Electronic Symbols
Electronic circuits found in urodynamic instruments are drawn pictorially by a multitude of simply circuits made up of those symbols.

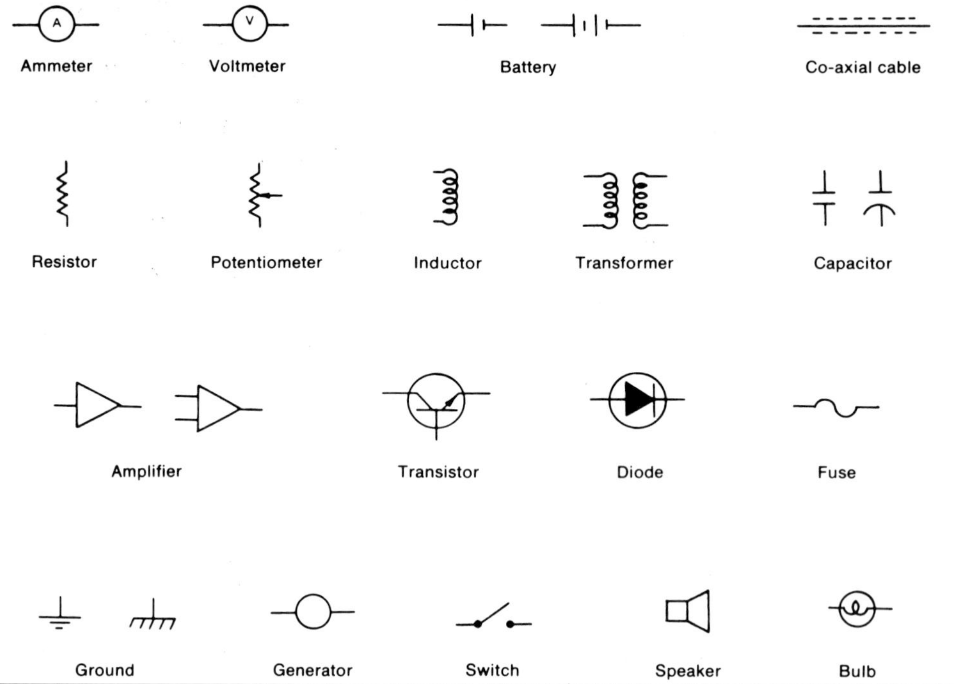

also known as a functional diagram, rather than the intricate electronics it contains.

AMPLIFIERS AND SIGNAL CONDITIONING

Most of the bioelectric signals encountered in urodynamics are small and require amplification. Amplifiers are used in a general sense for interfacing with transducers that measure the given variable; in addition to simple amplification, the amplifier may also modify the signal to produce frequency filtering or nonlinear effects. Some of the general principles used in signal processing are presented and discussed in this section in relation to urodynamics; however, for a more detailed description, we refer the reader to the literature (*4,6–13*).

Basic Principles of Amplifiers

Transducers are used for converting the activity of nonelectric sources (ionic current, flow, pressure) into electric signals, which results in a wide range of voltages. One thing that all these electric voltages have in common is that their amplitudes are rather small, being of the order of 1 μV up to 10 mV. These values are normally too small to register on chart recorders or displays. It is therefore necessary to increase these small voltages to higher values, of the order of volts; electronic amplifiers have thus been developed. An electronic amplifier amplifies input voltages in a certain frequency band to higher output voltages. For example, a 1-mV EMG voltage picked up by two electrodes and connected to an amplifier with an amplification factor (often called a gain) of 1000 appears at the output of the amplifier as a voltage of 1V. In addition, this 1-V voltage source may be able to deliver enough current to drive, for instance, the pen motor of a paper recorder. It is not possible to draw this current directly from the original voltage source; thus in addition to amplifying the input voltage, an amplifier increases the power of the source. An amplifier is represented schematically by means of a triangle with input and output leads (Fig. 4–6). The letter A is used to represent the internal gain, which may be fixed or adjusted manually by means of a potentiometer. This front panel may be designated "gain," "amplitude," or "sensitivity."

In order to discuss amplifiers, it is first necessary to make a point clear concerning the measurement of voltage at the input leads. Voltage is always measured relative to some reference potential, and amplifiers amplify a voltage relative to some reference. In this sense, all amplifiers can be thought of as having two inputs: the signal to be amplified and the reference level. Many amplifiers are "single-ended," and the voltage reference level is provided by some ground point. This ground is at a constant potential, is free of noise, and is usually associated with the power supply ground of the system. The ground is normally carried through to the source voltage, and both the source voltage and the amplifier then operate relative to the same ground.

Some amplifiers invert the data signal during the process of amplification. The plus or minus signs are used to indicate whether the amplifier is noninverting or inverting, and the convention is followed of not showing the reference ground point.

Amplifiers can be built that do not require the use of one of the inputs as a stable ground reference. A "differential" amplifier results if both inputs are free to sense active potentials and are connected in an inverting and a noninverting arrangement. The rejection of common-mode signals is one of the main reasons for using the differential amplifier in bioelectric measurements; it is widely used in clinical urodynamics to record EMG potentials. In theory, a common-mode input voltage is eliminated from the output; in practice, however, it is not the case. The gain of the amplifier has to be such that no distortion in the output can occur. If there is a large gain, the output signal may show flat parts because of the signal level exceeding the voltage limit of the amplifier in use.

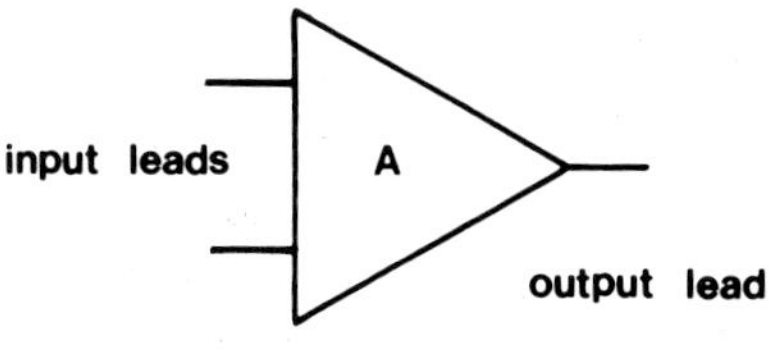

Figure 4–6. Schematic representation of an amplifier. A single-ended amplifier results if one of the input leads is a ground point. A differential amplifier results if both input leads are free to sense active potential. A = gain of the amplifier.

Basic Characteristics of Amplifiers

An important characteristic of an amplifier is the band of frequencies it passes. Every electronic system has a limited frequency band, often set to fixed values of low and high cut off frequencies or externally adjustable by means of built-in filters. Using an amplifier with an inadequate frequency characteristic results in distortion of the amplified signal.

In addition to passive components such as resistors, capacitors, and inductors, an amplifier always contains one or more active components that do the job of amplification. The active component in early amplifiers was the electronic valve or vacuum tube, resembling an ordinary light bulb but with some additional plates and grids inside, and consequently more internal connections. Although the invention of the electronic valve made it possible to build electronic amplifiers for the first time, today they are rarely found inside urodynamic instruments.

The function of a transistor is similar to that of the valve, but its appearance is quite different. The transistor is a solid-state device that has the advantages that it is small and lightweight, and does not consume much energy. The input voltage going through a transistor is transformed into an output voltage with a higher amplitude; that is, the input voltage is multiplied by a certain gain factor "A." Amplifier stages can be connected in series, increasing the total gain to any required value. The transistors and resistors necessary for an amplifier with a certain gain can be directly constructed in one piece of silicone with the proper connections to each other already built in. This configuration results in a complete amplifier with, for instance, a gain of 10,000; it is called an integrated circuit. The technology of manufacturing integrated circuits is the most important development of recent years, especially with respect to biomedical instrumentation.

Signal Conditioning

Signal conditioning usually denotes electronic processing of the amplified signal that can achieve one or several of the following tasks: filtering, integration, differentiation, analog-to-digital conversion.

Signal Filtering. Filtering is one of the important parameters to consider when designing or specifying an amplifier. A signal that is passed through signal conditioning electronics may undergo many time changes in amplitude and phase. Moreover, even with their input shorted, amplifiers produce electric noise that arises from resistors and from the operation of active circuit elements. This noise is random and can have varying spectral compositions. Amplifier noise can also appear as baseline displacements and large-amplitude transient events. Filters are employed to extract or eliminate some particular part of the signal. This separation is performed on the basis of the frequency ranges of the desired and undesired signals. For example, the input signal to a filter may be composed of the bioelectric signal of interest and a noise signal that has a different frequency composition. The purpose of filtering the combined signal is to remove the noise. If the filter were ideal, the noise would be completely eliminated in the output. Without adequate filtering, a recorded signal may be difficult to interpret; Figure 4–7 shows a pressure signal recorded in the absence of, and with excessive, filtering. Appropriate filtering must be used to faithfully reproduce the desired signal.

Low-pass filters are useful for attenuating high-frequency noise, whereas high-pass filters are used for amplifying small AC voltages. A series combination of the low-pass filter and the high-pass filter results in a band-pass filter, which amplifies frequencies over a desired range and attenuates higher and lower frequencies. The recording of vesical or urethral pressures usually requires an amplifier with a DC frequency range of 15 to 20 Hz, whereas for EMG measurements the frequency range can go up to several kilohertz (see Table 4–1 for urodynamic parameter ranges).

The problem with most amplifying systems is the presence of voltages other than the voltage of interest; such "artifacts" are often amplified and may seriously disturb the recording. This effect can be caused by capacitive coupling between the amplifier input leads and any conducting materials in the vicinity. If one of these materials, e.g., a wire, has an alternating voltage with respect to the input lead of the amplifier, this voltage is also measured. Urodynamics laboratories usually contain electric power lines from the main supply, and thus most measuring devices are affected by the capacitive coupling with the mains. One remedy for this interference is to use coaxial cables shielded by a flexible woven coating of conducting material connected to earth, which results by no voltage pickup by the input of the amplifier (Fig. 4–8).

Differential amplifiers have been devel-

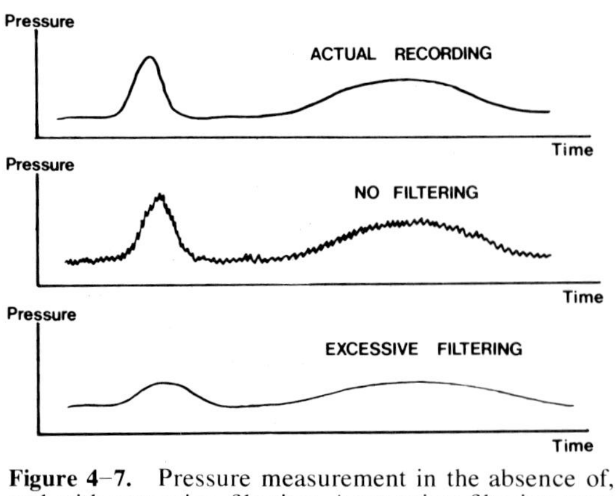

Figure 4–7. Pressure measurement in the absence of, and with excessive, filtering. Appropriate filtering must be used to faithfully reproduce the desired signal; it is part of "signal conditioning."

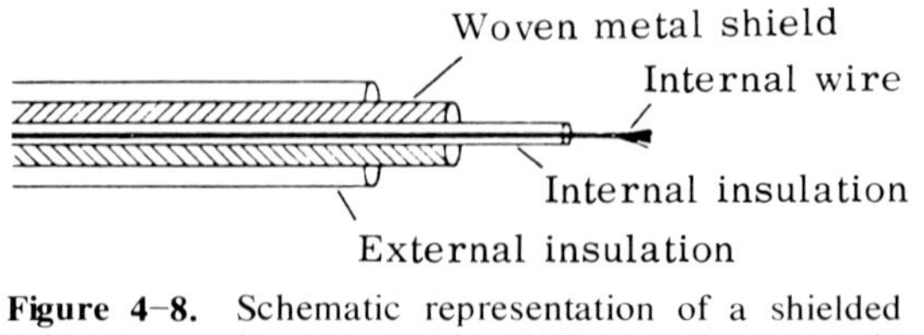

Figure 4–8. Schematic representation of a shielded cable. Such cables are used in EMG recordings to avoid voltage pickup by the input of the amplifier. (From Bergveld, P.: Electronic amplifiers. In Bergveld, P. [ed.]: *Electromedical Instrumentation: A Guide for Medical Personnel.* Cambridge University Press, Cambridge, 1980.

oped for amplifying only differential, not common-mode, signals. There is no difference in the amplitude of the voltage between two points of the body due to capacitive coupling with the mains.

Signal Integration. Integration is generally used to calculate the area under a given curve; for instance, the integration of a urine flow curve (versus time) represents the total voided volume. In a similar way, the integration of external vesical power (pressure × flow) divided by the voiding time represents the work done for one voiding cycle. Integration can be performed through electronic circuitry. Applications in urodynamics are various; integration is used in uroflowmeters when flow rate is directly recorded and voided volume is being displayed. It is also used in EMG measurements to provide an "integrated EMG."

Signal Differentiation. Differentiation can be defined as the rate of change of a given signal as a function of time; it is the reverse function of integration. Such function is used frequently to calculate urinary flow rate when the volume or mass of urine is being recorded by the transducer; after differentiation the signal represents the volumetric or mass flow rate as a function of time.

Analog-to-Digital Conversion. Most urodynamic data are in the form of analog signals, so analog-to-digital conversion is required if the data are to be stored or analyzed by means of a computer. An analog-to-digital converter (ADC) quantifies the given signal (curve) into a series of discrete digital numbers; theoretically, the sampling frequency must be at least twice the highest frequency of the recorded signal in order to obtain an accurate representation. Figure 4–9 shows a cystometrogram digitally converted; the computer assigns on a time scale a series of digital numbers that are stored and can be retrieved for subsequent analysis.

Conventional approaches have been to convert the analog data from a recorded signal into a digital form via ADC circuitry. Current trends are integrating these two functions into one system. The following section discusses how microcomputers can intrinsically achieve an analog/digital (A/D) conversion during signal processing.

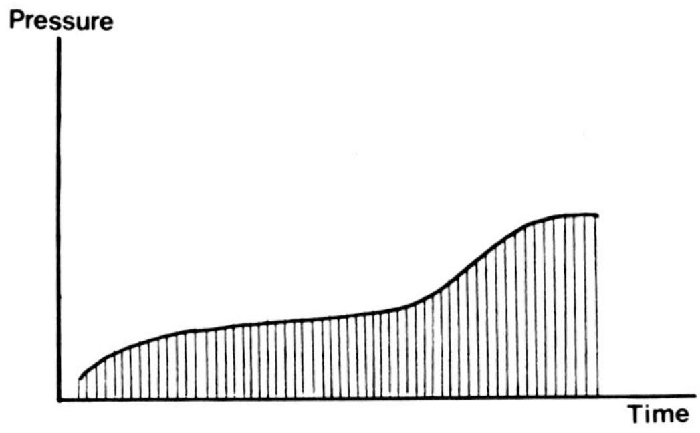

Figure 4–9. Analog-to-digital conversion. The analog values of the pressure recording are converted to a series of digital values and stored in the computer. Such data can then be retrieved for subsequent analysis. The rate of sampling usually equals twice the highest frequency of the recorded signal.

Use of Microcomputers in Signal Processing

Signal amplifying and conditioning has been handled traditionally by using relatively simple analog electronic circuits. Such functions, however, can be enhanced through the use of microcomputers. The use of microcomputer as a "process controller" results in fewer integrated-circuit packages, as well as the capability for self-calibration and detection of errors: this reduced complexity enhances the reliability of the instrument. At present, several attempts have been made to "computerize" urodynamic studies (*14–21*) and proved to enhance more completeness and efficiency in urodynamic studies. One study (*17*) reported extremely accurate recording of urodynamic events, with a higher-frequency response than existing units. However, most authors have used the computer in series to the conventional urodynamic equipment, resulting in two sets of data. Regnier recently reviewed such past applications and discusses the overall impact of microcomputers in the field of urodynamics (Regnier, C. H.: Current and future applications of computers in urodynamics. *Neurourol. Urodyn.* 5:343–371, 1986). Three generations of computerized systems are described below; they depict the existing trend of today's urodynamic systems toward computerized urodynamic signal processing. Three generations of computerized systems are described below; they depict the existing trend of today's urodynamic systems toward computerized urodynamic signal processing.

First Generation Systems. In early computerized systems one approach required the use of an instrumentation tape recorder. For instance, the analog signal (e.g., a flow curve) can be converted through frequency modulation and recorded on magnetic tape; subsequently the tape is replayed and the information digitized (A/D conversion) and then fed into the computer for analysis. Rollema (*22*) processed a large number of data obtained from uroflowmetry curves in men based on this approach. It is clear here that the computer is mostly used for processing the collected data and not for collecting it. One other approach consisted in reading a strip chart and digitizing the analog data for subsequent analysis.

Second Generation Systems. Direct online processing of the urodynamic recording was achieved in the second-generation systems. The A/D conversion was done from the amplified analog signal, which permits storage of the urodynamic curve in real time. Kramer and Jonas (*23*) described a system they developed based on this approach. Jacobs *et al.* (*17*) described a similar system. This generation of signal processing requires the use of a separate computer to be hooked in series to the conventional urodynamic equipment; this results into two sets of data, i.e., analog and digital, and two sets of controls, i.e., urodynamic and computer.

Third Generation Systems. In the third generation systems the urodynamic signal is processed in a digital form; the microcomputer contains all the necessary hardware to measure, digitize, process, record, and store all test data, which eliminates the conventional signal-amplifying and conditioning units. Figure 4–10 illustrates this approach.

Microcomputerized urodiagnostic systems that control processing of the urodynamic data are now commercially available. The electric impulses from the various transducers are directly converted to digital bits of information that are then processed by the microcomputer ("process controller"). In other words, all signals are sent through a custom data acquisition board that is plugged into the microcomputer. This connection allows extremely accurate recordings, as the data can be sampled at a rate exceeding the frequency response of pen recorders. Because control of the hardware comes from the computer, sensitivity settings and calibration procedures are also automated.

The various components of the man–instrument system still clearly exist. The implication is, however, that the microcomputer is an integral part of the system, com-

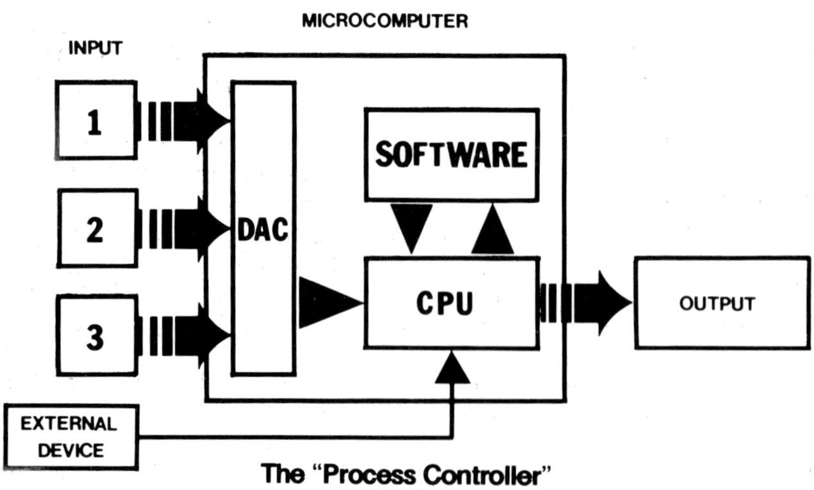

Figure 4–10. Block diagram of a microcomputerized urodiagnostic system. The signals from the transducers are sent to a data acquisition board installed within the computer. The digital bits of information are then processed by the control center, all controls being run from the software. The microcomputer here is an integral part of the system, which gives at the same time all the features that a computer can do. (From Regnier, C, H.: *Neurourol. Urodyn.* 5:343–371, 1986.)

bining all the steps of signal processing under one control.

Summary

In summary, amplifiers are used to increase small voltages (resulting from the transducers) into larger ones. In order to reproduce the amplified signal as faithfully as possible and derive additional parameters, signal conditioning is necessary; filtering, integration, differentiation, and A/D conversion are examples of signal conditioning. This goal is usually achieved with conventional electronic units; however, microcomputers offer more advanced capabilities by processing the signal through data acquisition boards that are contained within the computer itself.

MEASUREMENT OF PRESSURE

The measurement of bladder and urethral pressures is a fundamental tool in clinical urodynamics, essential in the understanding and assessment of urinary tract function. Bladder pressure, for instance, is routinely measured by means of catheters in urodynamic units. It is generally necessary to use techniques capable of measuring time-varying pressures despite the low-frequency nature of pressures encountered in urodynamics. Fluid manometers, used for measuring constant pressures, are too slow to respond adequately to rapid pressure variations because of the large fluid inertia. In addition, rapid pressure changes would cause the fluid to oscillate, precluding accurate measurement. One must then resort to pressure transducers especially designed to handle high-frequency phenomena. Physiologic pressures are generally more difficult to measure than pressures in a physical experiment. Their reproducibility with time is sometimes not good, and several artifacts due to patient motion or probe displacement with respect to the patient can alter the signal corresponding to the particular event to be recorded. Figure 4–11 shows two cystometrograms recorded successively in a dog.

The variability from one subject to another is even greater. Therefore it is not surprising that the measurement of physiologic pressures has presented a challenge to the instrument designer, especially in the areas of mechanical and electronic miniaturization and signal processing. Significant progress has been made in the domain of microprobes.

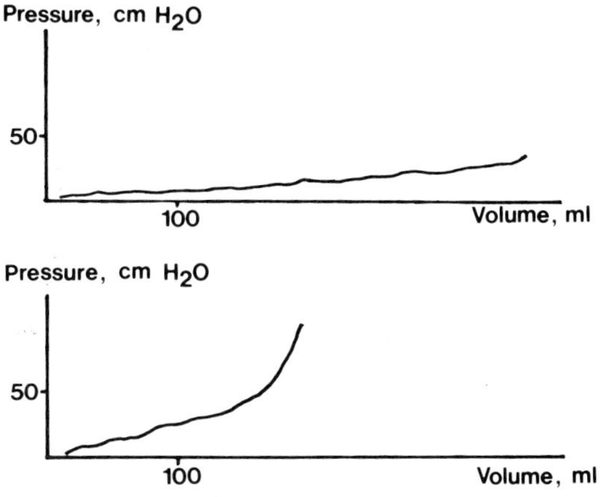

Figure 4–11. Variability of a cystometrogram with time. The measurements were taken successively on a dog. The variability from one subject to another is even greater.

Traditionally, pressure units used in medicine and physiology have been different from those used in physics, which has led to a lack of uniformity in the systems reported in the urodynamic literature; it was thus recommended in 1975 by the International Continence Society Committee on standardization of terminology (*24*) that all results be given in international system (SI) units. It is particularly important in order to avoid confusion when other parameters that are a function of pressure are computed. The basic unit of pressure in the SI system is centimeters of water.

This section outlines the fundamental basis of pressure transducers in relation to urodynamics. For a more complete description, we refer the reader to the literature (*2,25–30*).

Basic Mechanisms and Principles of Pressure Transducers

Resistive Transducers. *Potentiometers.* The simplest device for measuring displacement is the linear or rotational potentiometer. Examples of both are shown in Figure 4–12. The point at which dis-

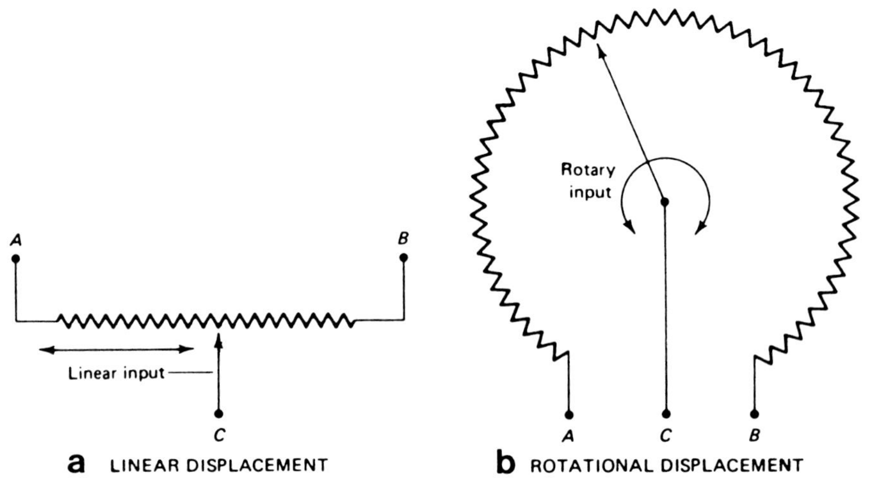

Figure 4–12. Two types of potentiometric device for measuring displacement: linear (a) and rotational (b). Pressure can be measured by coupling the displacement to a mechanical diaphragm. The resistance elements may be excited by either *dc* or *ac* voltages. (From Cromwell, L., *et al.: Biomedical Instrumentation and Measurements.* Prentice-Hall, Englewood Cliffs, N.J. 1973.)

placement is to be measured is simply attached to a sliding contact that can move along a path of linear electric resistance. A voltage between the wiper at either end of the resistor making up the potentiometer varies with the position of the wiper.

This principle has been used for one of the oldest resistive types of pressure transducer. However, the major difficulty with this type of transducer remains the amount of friction of the wiper on the wire or resistor. A true displacement transducer should not require any force to move the contact. Transducers utilizing solid-state materials have now replaced the older transducer. A device with moving parts is indeed more prone to stress and mechanical failure than a device that is electronic and nonmovable in nature.

Strain Gauges. A strain gauge is a length of conductive material, e.g., a fine wire, or a piece of semiconductor material that is stressed or compressed in proportion to displacement. When stretched, the wire or other device elongates and at the same time is reduced in its cross-sectional area, thereby increasing its electric resistance. Similarly, when the gauge is compressed, the resistance is lowered. This principle can be applied to measure the bending or the displacement of a diaphragm. Most transducers used in urodynamic measurements are of this type, e.g., the Statham P231D. The sensitivity of a strain gauge is determined by a gauge factor, whereas the percentage of resistance changes per unit change in length. The average gauge factor for metals is about 2, whereas the gauge factor for silicone (semiconductor material) is about 120. To increase sensitivity, several lengths of wire are usually stretched or compressed simultaneously and connected in series. Wire strain gauges are of two basic types: bonded and unbonded. In the bonded strain gauge, the wire is bonded to a thin piece of plastic or paper that is cemented to the material to which the stress is applied, as shown in Figure 4–13.

In the unbonded strain gauge, the wires of the strain gauge are wound under tension between isolating posts. Figure 4–14 shows a typical unbonded strain-gauge pressure transducer. Here four unbonded gauges are attached to two otherwise isolated members, called the armature and the frame. A diaphragm is directly coupled by the armature to the unbonded strain-gauge system. Mechanical stops are provided to prevent an overload from breaking the wires. Without applied force, the wires are stretched with the armature centered in the frame. As force is applied (by pressure), tension on two of the gauges is increased, and tension on the two other gauges is decreased.

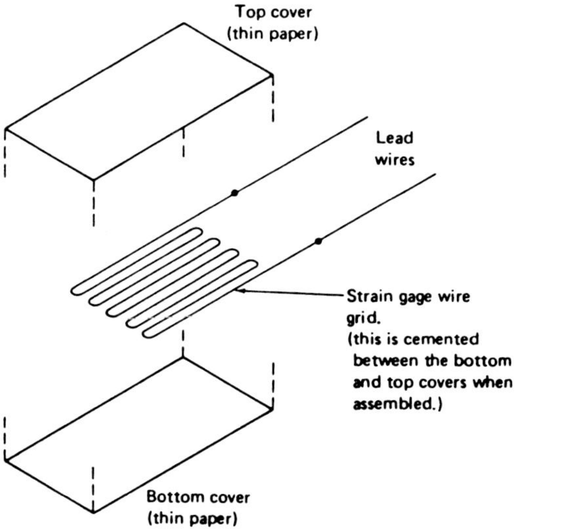

Figure 4–13. Typical bonded strain-gauge configuration. This principle can be used to measure pressure, force, or displacement. When the gauge is compressed, the resistance is lowered. Changes in resistance are detected by electronic circuitry. (From Cromwell, L., *et al.*: *Biomedical Instrumentation and Measurements*. Prentice-Hall, Englewood Cliffs, N.J., 1973.)

Both bonded and unbonded strain gauges are found in many other forms of transducers designed for biomedical applications. Depending on the nature of the device to which the gauge is bonded, any strain gauge transducer may actually be designed to measure displacement, force, pressure, or acceleration. The difference between a transducer designed to measure displacement and one designed to measure force or pressure is merely the amount and ease with which the supporting structure bends. With silicone strain gauges, much smaller transducers can be used to obtain force and displacement measurements. The higher sensitivity also permits stiffer gauges with higher-frequency responses, up to 2000 Hz with semiconductor strain gauges. Because semiconductor strain-gauge bridges are often temperature-sensitive, however, they must be calibrated initially as well as periodically.

Inductance Transducers. In a self-inductance transducer the diaphragm is coupled to a coil, and its displacement is detected from variations in coil inductance obtained by moving the coil over a fixed core. Although such transducers have some mechanical limitations, (e.g., they are usually linear over a limited range of displacement), they do have a few practical applications. Figure 4–15 shows an arrangement wherein a metal core is moved into and out of the center of a coil to vary the inductance as the core is displaced.

An inductive transducer has an advantage in not being affected by the DC electric properties of its environment. However, it may be affected by external magnetic fields because of the proximity of magnetic materials. Inductance transducers can be miniaturized, and a catheter tip inductance transducer was first designed by Wetterer (*31*). That these devices have low power requirements and produce large variations in inductance makes them attractive as well for radiotelemetry applications. Mutual induc-

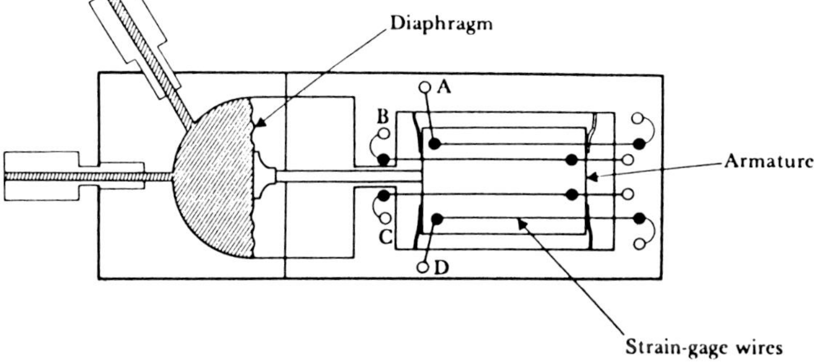

Figure 4–14. Typical unbonded strain-gauge pressure transducer. Displacement of the diaphragm is transmitted to a system composed of a moving armature and an unbonded strain gauge. With increasing pressure, the strain on gauge pair B and C is increased, whereas that on gauge pair A and D is decreased. The reasons these systems are used so frequently is that they have stability and sensitivity. (From Webster, J. G. [ed.]: *Medical Instrumentation: Application and Design*. Houghton Mifflin, Boston, 1978.)

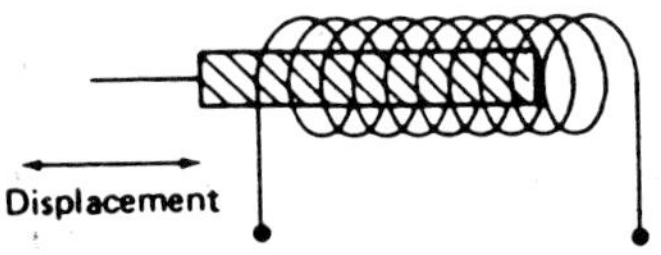

Figure 4–15. Self-inductance transducer. Pressure is measured by coupling the coil to a diaphragm; displacement of the coil is detected from variations in coil inductance obtained by moving the coil over a fixed core. (From Cromwell, L., *et al.*: *Biomedical Instrumentation and Measurements*. Prentice-Hall, Englewood Cliffs, N.J. 1973.)

tance transducers employ two coils whose variation in mutual magnetic coupling is used to measure displacement. Van Citter (*32*) provided a good description of applications of mutual inductance transformers in measuring changes in diameter of internal organs (kidney, major blood vessels, and left ventricle). The induced voltage in this case is a function of the geometry of the coils.

Differential transformers are also based on the principle of inductance. A transformer is a component in which two or more continuous loops of wire are wrapped around a ferrous core, forming the primary coil. Elsewhere on the magnetic core, another coil of one or more continuous loops of insulated wire is wrapped around the core. This second coil is referred to as the secondary coil. The linear variable differential transformer (LVDT) is based on this principle and is widely used in physiologic research and clinical medicine to measure pressure as well as displacement and force. A diagram of such device is shown in Figure 4–16. The transformer has a movable core that is attached to the point at which displacement is to be measured. Its output is the difference between the voltages induced in the two secondaries, which is proportional to the amount of displacement of the cores, and in a polarity corresponding to the direction in which the core is moved. The movable core is attached to the pressure-sensing diaphragm.

A differential transformer is able to measure extremely small variations in displacement (and therefore pressure), even as small as 0.000001 inch. One problem with this type of transducer, however, is that it is not linear for large amounts of displacement.

Capacitance Transducers. The principle of capacitance transducers is to measure the change in electric capacitance between the displaced diaphragm and a plate. If one plate of a capacitor is connected to a point at which displacement or movement is to be measured and the other plate is fixed as a reference, any change in the relative position of two plates is reflected as a change in the capacity. Figure 4–17 shows a diaphragm of a capacitance displacement transducer; changes in capacitance may detect pressure by coupling one of the plates to a diaphragm.

A variation of this technique consists in inserting the moving plate between two fixed plates forming two capacitors so that motion of the plate increases one capacity while decreasing the other. Such systems have the advantage of providing accurate measurements of displacement.

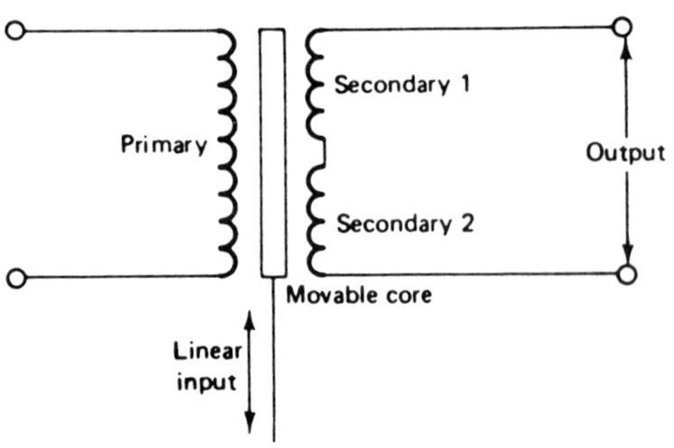

Figure 4–16. Linear variable differential transformer. Displacement is measured through a movable core. Pressure can be measured on this prinicple with a much higher sensititvity than that for strain gauges; it requires, however, more complex signal-processing instrumentation. (From Cromwell, L., *et al.*: *Biomedical Instrumentation and Measurements*. Prentice-Hall, Englewood Cliffs, N.J., 1973.)

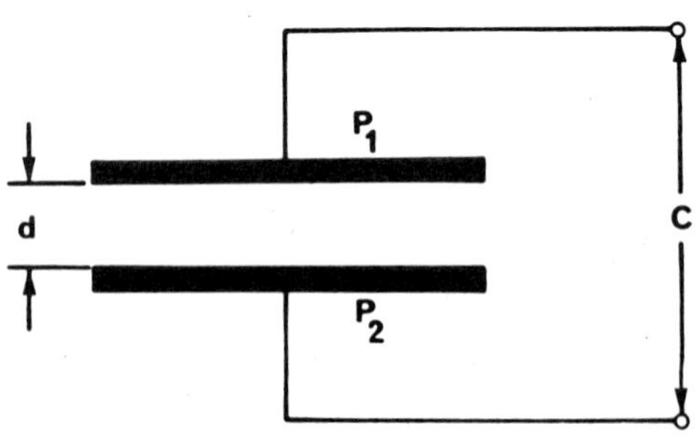

Figure 4–17. Capacitance displacement transducer. Capacitance changes as *d* is changed; capacitance also varies as the area of the moving plate directly over the fixed plate is changed. A pressure transducer results if one of the plates is coupled to a diaphragm. (From Yanof, H.M.: *Biomedical Electronics*, 2nd ed. Davis, Philadelphia, 1972.

Piezoelectric Transducers. The piezoelectric effect is the capacity of certain substances to produce an electric charge proportional to the amount of deformation when they are physically deformed. The piezoelectric effect is found naturally in Rochelle salt, quartz, ammonium, and dihydrogen phosphate and can be introduced by treatment into barium titantate. When contacts are applied to the face of the piezoelectric material, an electric signal is obtained. The piezoelectric element is therefore equivalent to a voltage generator, delivering a voltage proportional to the applied force, collected in series with a capacitor. Transducers utilizing the principle of the piezoelectric effect are called piezoelectric transducers. They are used to measure physiologic displacement (and therefore pressure) as well as heart sounds (*33*). The principle of operation is that when an isometric crystal lattice is distorted a charge reorientation takes place, causing relative displacement of negative and positive charges. The displaced internal charges induce surface charges of opposite polarity on opposite sides of the crystal. Surface charge can be determined by measuring the difference in voltage between electrodes attached to the surface. The total induced charge is therefore directly proportional to the applied force. Figure 4–18 demonstrates a piezoelectric transducer.

Dynamic Requirements of Pressure Transducers in Liquid-Filled Systems

It is important to understand the dynamic properties of a pressure-measurement system in order to preserve the best dynamic accuracy of the measured pressure. A liquid-filled catheter transducer is a hydraulic system that can be represented by some sort of parameter models. Figure 4–19 shows the physical model of a catheter–transducer system; an increase in pressure at the input of the catheter causes a flow of liquid to the right from the catheter tip, through the catheter, and into the transducer. This liquid shift causes a deflection of the transducer diaphragm, which is sensed by an electromechanical system. The response of such a system depends largely on the characteristics of the liquid catheter.

Response of a Rigid Catheter–Transducer System. The problem of a rigid catheter–transducer system was investigated by Hansen (*34*) and developed by McDonald (*35*). The fluid motion in the catheter (manometer line) is coupled to the displacement and bending of the diaphragm in the transducer. In turn, this bending can be converted to an electric signal by a strain gauge mounted on the diaphragm. The diaphragm opposes a restoring force to any change in pressure, and this restoring force induces oscillations. If the catheter is perfectly rigid, the system has a natural frequency. Such frequency depends on the radius and length of the catheter, the fluid inertia, and the compliance of the diaphragm. For a given transducer, damping can be increased by decreasing the catheter diameter and increasing the length. The behavior of such a system as a function of damping is best illustrated by its response to a step change in pressure (Fig. 4–20). If there is no damping, the system oscillates forever at the natural frequency. If the damping is large, the diaphragm reaches its equilibrium position exponentially without oscillations.

This simple analysis rests on the assumption of parabolic velocity profiles in the catheter to compute the damping. This assumption is invalid if the flow is unsteady, as it certainly is when it oscillates. A more exact analysis was carried out by Lambossy (*36*), but the improvement in the prediction is marginal.

Transducer Connected to an Elastic Catheter. In the preceding analysis the compliance of the catheter was neglected in comparison with the diaphragm compliance. We now consider the opposite situation where the catheter is elastic and the diaphragm compliance is negligible. In such a system

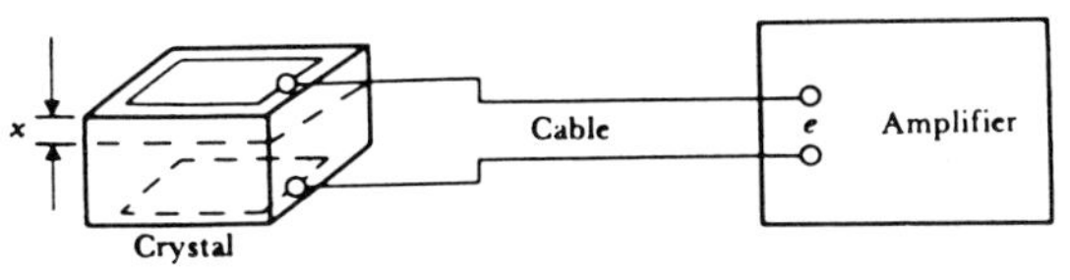

Figure 4–18. Piezoelectric transducer. When the crystal is physically deformed, it produces an electric charge proportional to the amount of deformation. This principle is used to measure any kind of vibration pattern, e.g., pressure and heart sounds. (From Doebelin, E.: *Measurement Systems; Application and Design*. McGraw-Hill, New York 1975.)

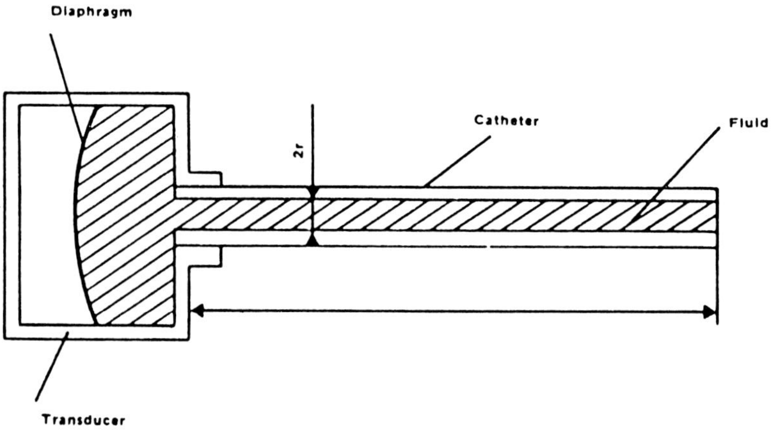

Figure 4–19. Catheter coupled to a diaphragm-type pressure transducer. The response of such a system depends largely on the characteristics of the liquid catheter. (Reprinted with permission from Feinberg, B., and Fleming, D.: *CRC Handbook of Engineering in Medicine and Biology*. Copyright 1978, CRC Press, Inc., Boca Raton, FL.)

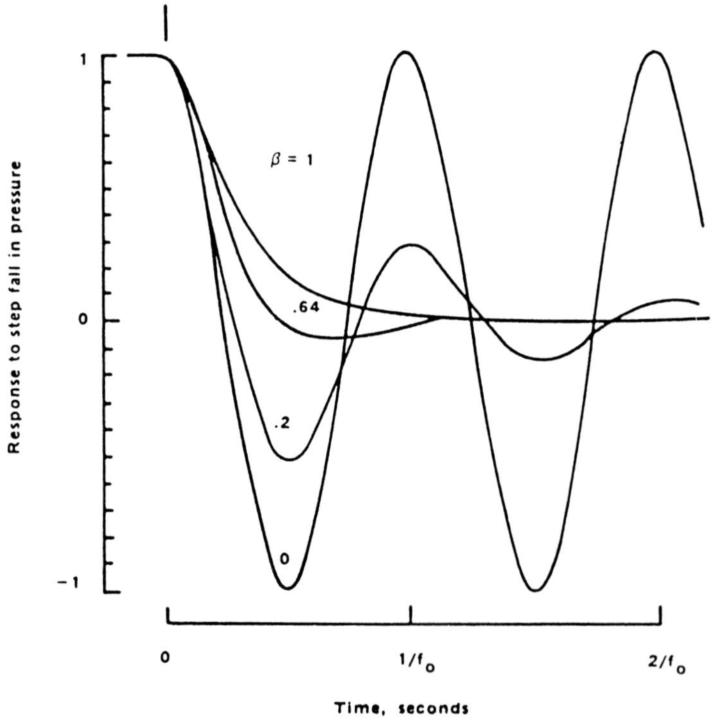

Figure 4–20. Response of a rigid catheter–transducer system to a step fall in pressure for four values of the damping factor β. fo = the natural oscillating frequency and depends on the characteristics of the catheter as well as the compliance of the diaphragm. The damping factor can be decreased by increasing the catheter diameter and decreasing its length. If β is more than 1, the diaphragm reaches its equilibrium position exponentially without oscillation. (From Gabe, I. T.: Pressure measurement in experimental physiology. In Bergel, D.H. [ed.]: *Cardiovascular Fluid Dynamics*. Vol. 1. Academic Press, London 1972.)

waves propagate in the catheter wall with a certain speed depending on the compliance and cross-sectional area of the catheter as well as the fluid inertia. For a short catheter, there is a high resonant frequency. Damping is again due to fluid viscosity and wall viscoelasticity. Figure 4–21 shows the transient response of a transducer connected to various lengths of tubing; it clearly demonstrates the influence of catheter length on the damping factor. When elastic tubing is used it is therefore indicated to choose tubing of short length and large diameter.

Determination of Frequency Response of Pressure Transducers. The dynamic response of a catheter–transducer system must be tested if accurate recordings of bladder and urethral pressures are desired. There are two basic methods for determining the response characteristics. One involves measuring the transient step response for the system by applying a sudden pressure change to the transducer (e.g., by occluding the infusion side whole) and recording the resultant damped oscillations of the system. Such test has been described by Peura (*37*). The transient response of the transducer is in the form of a damped exponential, and the observer can calculate from such curves the damping ratio as well as the undamped natural frequency.

The other technique consists in applying a pulsatile pressure wave of variable frequency and amplitude, usually sinusoidal.

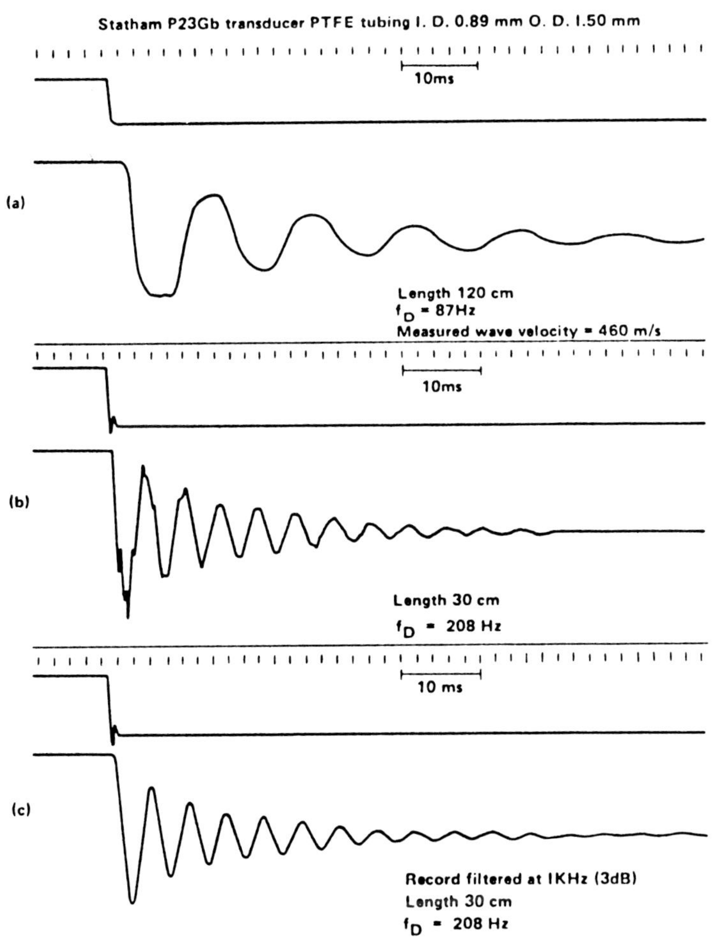

Figure 4–21. Response of an elastic catheter–transducer system to a step fall in pressure for different catheter lengths. The shorter the catheter, the higher is the resonant frequency; the damping is due to fluid viscosity and wall viscoelasticity. (From Gabe, I. T.: Pressure measurement in experimental physiology. In Bergel, D.H. [ed.]: *Cardiovascular fluid Dynamics*, Vol. 1. Academic Press, London, 1972.)

Such a test requires specialized equipment (e.g., a pressure–generator test system) but can be built from commercially available units (*38,39*). This technique is useful for determining more directly the amplitude and phase of the output as a function of frequency. In urodynamics such dynamic characteristics are essential for urethral pressure profile recordings and depend on the catheter withdrawal speed. One must ensure that for a given withdrawal speed any sudden change in pressure is recorded rapidly enough. Brown *et al.* (*40*) established a minimal acceptable speed response to 200 cm $H_2 0$/s.

Factors Affecting Pressure Measurement Accuracy. *Presence of Air Bubbles.* The presence of air bubbles in the manometric system makes the system more compliant and thus tends to increase the damping and cause potential distortion problems. Using the above described techniques, Shapiro and Krovetz (*41*) found that even minute air bubbles increased the compliance of the catheter–manometer system and drastically decreased the damped natural frequency. The same authors demonstrated that by using a PE-190 catheter of 10 to 100 cm lengths the damped natural frequency decreased by approximately 50 to 60 percent for an unboiled-water case, compared to a boiled-water case.

Frequency–Response Limitations. Water and saline are not perfect liquids as they have a finite volume modulus of elasticity. Therefore a theoretical upper limit in high-frequency response exists for a water-filled transducer–catheter system. The solution to that problem has been solved by Peura (*37*), who established the limit to 700 Hz for a 50 mm long needle (20 gauge) directly connected to the transducer.

Effect of Catheter Material. Shapiro and Krovetz (*41*) found that because Teflon is slightly stiffer than polyethylene it has a slightly higher frequency response at any given length. Silastic, on the other hand, has increased compliance and caused a marked decrease in frequency response.

Effect of Connectors. The same authors (*41*) suggested that the fewest possible number of connectors be used and that all connectors be tight-fitting and have a water seal. They concluded that the connector serves as a simple series hydraulic damper that decreases the frequency response.

Direct Measurement of Pressure

Liquid-Filled Catheter Connected to External Transducers. The liquid-filled catheter connected to external transducers comprises one of the most frequently used techniques because the transducer, which is external to the body, does not need to be miniaturized and is less expensive and much more rugged than the miniaturized catheter-tip transducers. The pressure sensor is available in various pressure ranges and is connected to the measuring site by a saline-filled catheter inserted in the bladder and urethra. The frequency response of this technique is limited by the natural oscillating frequency of the fluid column. The main factors deteriorating the frequency response of pressure-measuring systems are the use of non rigid connecting tubes and the presence of air bubbles. Each increases the volume displacement of the transducer and the damping. In addition, nonrigid tubes may add another resonant frequency, which can produce signal distortion. A balance must therefore be struck between the length and diameter of connecting tubes and the volume displacement of the transducer in order to optimize the damping. To obtain good results, it is important to (a) carefully flush all air bubbles in this system, (b) use stiff catheters of the shortest possible length and large enough diameters to have high resonant frequencies, and (c) mount the transducer at approximately the same height as the measurement site to avoid hydrostatic effects (symphysis pubis).

It should also be remembered that a pressure is always measured with respect to some reference level. Such a level should be the atmospheric pressure.

Catheter-Tip Transducers. The inconvenience of interposing a liquid column between the measuring site and the transducer has led to the development of miniaturized transducers that are mounted at the tip of a catheter. Filtering and amplifying remain external to the patient, but signal transmission along the catheter is electric and not through a liquid column. The use of tip transducers has become somewhat controversial because of the artifact induced by the patient's movements and zero reference drift (*42,43*). For instance, tip transducers used during filling of the bladder are subject to increasing hydrostatic pressure caused by a building mass of liquid proportional to the volume infused. However, this system offers the best frequency response.

Fiber optic Transducers. The fiber optic pressure transducer consists of a bifurcated fiberoptic bundle with a pressure-sensitive membrane at the common end. One leg of the bundle is connected to a light source and transmits light to the reflecting backside of the membrane. As membrane is deflected by pressure, a varying amount of light is reflected back into the fibers in the other leg of the bundle, which leads to a photodetector. The pressure acting on the membrane thus affects the amount of reflected light and the electric signal from the photodetector (*44*). This time-saving technique has been developed for intravesical, intraurethral, and rectal pressure recordings, and has been used on several patients with various urologic problems (*45*). The potential frequency response of such a transducer is about 25 kHz, with excellent linearity, hysteresis, and baseline drift.

Measurement of Pressure in a Flowing Fluid

Urethral pressure profilometry during voiding requires the measurement of pressure in a flowing fluid. Static and dynamic pressures can be measured in such tests with a manometer connected through small pressure taps drilled in a tube wall. If the orifice edge is dented or rounded, it may produce a stagnation point, and the pressure measured will be intermediate between static pressure (P) and total pressure (P_0) (sometimes called stagnation pressure), which according to Bernouilli's equation is the sum of static and dynamic pressures:

$$P_0 = P + \tfrac{1}{2}\rho V^2$$

where V denotes fluid velocity, $\frac{1}{2}\rho V^2$ is dynamic pressure, and ρ is density. When measuring urethral pressure during voiding by means of a catheter, the pressure taps must be on the catheter side in order to register static pressure. If the tap is at the catheter end and facing the flow, the catheter registers the total pressure. If the catheter hole is at the rear of the catheter with respect to the flow (by pulling in the direction of flow), there is a small separation region around the end, and the pressure there can be less than the static pressure, depending on the catheter/vessel area ratio and on the Reynolds number. This difference between the measured pressure and the static pressure is of the order of dynamic pressure.

MEASUREMENT OF URINARY FLOW

There are numerous ways of recording urine flow rate as a function of time. Historically, Rehfish has been reported to be the first to record voided volume by using an air displacement method (*46*). Literature on the subject offers rather complete surveys of the various existing methodologies (*3,22,47–50*). Here we summarize only the most important techniques used and discuss their underlying principles.

Basic Mechanisms of Flow Transducers

Air Displacement. Air displaced by the urine flow cools a hot wire that is maintained at constant temperature. The amount of current needed to keep this temperature constant is directly proportional to the urine flow. Flowmeters based on this principle have proved to have excellent longevity (*3*), the major reason being that the device does not contain any movable parts, which reduces the chance of mechanical failure. Such instruments are lightweight and portable, and can be used with men in a standing position as well as with women in a sitting position. Cooling of the hot wire is based on the characteristics of self-heated thermistors; thermistors are thermally sensitive resistors whose primary function is to exhibit a change in electric resistance with a change of temperature. They are passive electronic semiconductors whose electric resistance varies with temperature and lies between that of conductors and insulators. An important characteristic of thermistors is their extreme sensitivity to relatively minute temperature changes. Thermistors are characterized by large temperature coefficients and a nonlinear resistance–temperature relation. Proper electronic circuitry provides a linear response in the desired range of flows encountered in a clinical situation. Figure 4–22 shows a typical resistance ratio versus temperature characteristics for a self-heated thermistor.

Rotating Disk. The rotating disk consists of a disk rotating at constant speed that is slowed by the urinary flow directly projected on it. The better the flow, the more the disk rotation is depressed. The amount of electric power required to maintain the rotational speed of the disk is proportional to the mass flow rate. The risk of mechanical failure is usually increased with this type of instrument because it contains movable parts.

Such devices consist of a mechanical unit and an electronic unit. Microprocessors can be used to provide automatic calculation of parameters and take into account the frictional problems of the rotating disk.

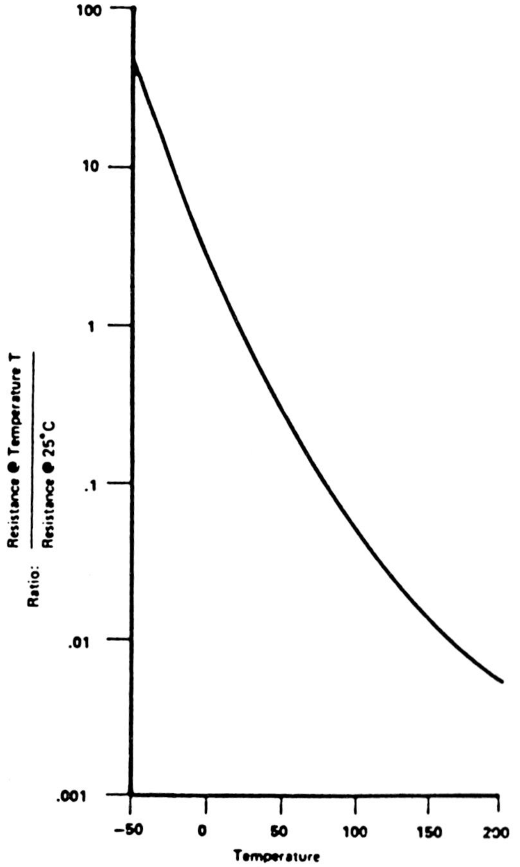

Figure 4–22. Typical resistance ratio versus temperature characteristics. If the temperature varies as a result of a change in ambient conditions, the resistance of the thermistor predictably changes as a function of its temperature. This principle is used for some types of urinary flowmeter; the urine flow displaces air, which in turn cools a self-heated thermistor.

Weight Principle. The weight principle is as follows: For a fluid of constant density the weight is proportional to the volume; flow rate is then obtained by mathematic differentiation. "Load cell" flowmeters are based on this principle. Signal differentiation is needed to convert the volume of urine (versus time) into a flow rate signal.

Other Techniques. There are other techniques that can be used to record urine flow rate, e.g., volumetric, electromagnetic, spectrometric, or momentum flux methods. Each of these techniques has been described extensively. There are also potential new methodologies that may be more sensitive to small-scale changes (*51*).

Methods for Testing the Accuracy of Uroflowmeters

Despite the increasing emphasis placed on the measurement of urine flow rate, few studies have addressed the need to develop techniques for testing the accuracy of uroflowmeters. The reliability and accuracy of the clinical measurements is usually taken for granted, which results in a lack of routine checking and calibration of the flowmeters.

Techniques. The first technique is obvious; it consists in comparing the recording of a constant flow to a known flow increment. Flow is recorded repeatedly at various flow rates. A second technique uses a source of flow that is interrupted in rapid sequences. This method, which measures the delay of recording on the curve, reflects the responsiveness of the apparatus. However, urinary flow is essentially variable, increasing to a maximum and decreasing thereafter. An apparatus that feeds the uroflowmeter with water at a flow rate that varies along such a pattern was developed by Susset (*3*). The principle of such device is a prism that sinks at constant speed in a basin of water (Fig. 4–23). Because of the shape of the prism the water is displaced at increasing speed, which

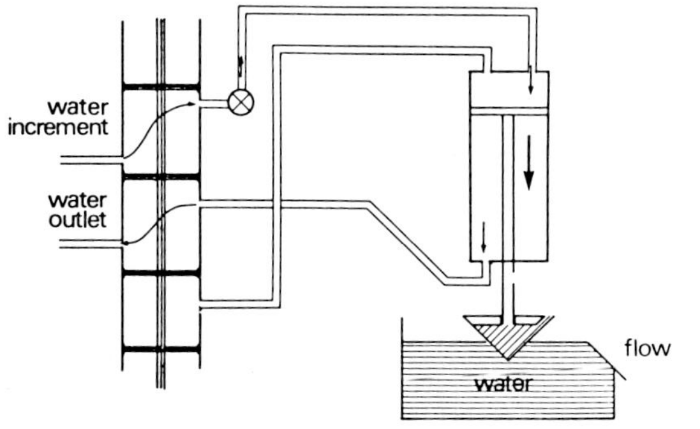

Figure 4–23. Device used for testing urine flowmeters. Because of the prismatic shape of the mobile, water is displaced at increasing speed and feeds the flowmeter to be tested directly. This principle simulates an increasing-decreasing pattern of flow.

varies at a constant rate. The water displaced directly feeds the flowmeter to be tested. The prism is moved by a piston that moves according to the action of constant water pressure (city water). A pressure regulator is placed between the source of the water and the piston, allowing the speed of the piston to increase or decrease. The water displaced by the prism goes over a razor-sharp edge of fiberglass placed in an absolutely horizontal position in order to provide a regular flow. Reversing the direction of the pressure valve allows the piston to return at its original position.

Three types of uroflowmeter based on different principles were tested according to the three techniques mentioned (*52*). The flowmeter based on air displacement showed an excellent response at both constant flow and constant flow variations; the response to interrupted flow was satisfactory, showing little delay in recording. The device based on the rotating disk principle showed good to excellent accuracy at repeated constant flow determinations as well as at constant flow variations. Response to interrupted flow was only satisfactory, showing slight damping expressed by a delay in recording. A limiting factor was represented by some variations in recording due to the site of impact of the urinary jet. The flowmeter based on the weight principle showed fair to good responsiveness to constant flow and to constant flow variations. It did not respond to interrupted flow at a rapid rate because of the built-in inertia of the device. The study concluded that accuracy in urinary flow recording was necessary in order to establish the limits of normal and to prepare proper curve analyses.

Rollema (*22*) extensively studied uroflowmetry in men; the accuracy of the flowmeter used was assessed by testing a series of constant flow rates at different target points of the stream. The study provided an excellent review of the various factors involved in the overall accuracy of the recording. It was concluded that in practical use the accuracy of the flow rate measurement can be assessed by comparing the volume in the measuring container with that computed from the flow rate signal. In this way it was found that the error rarely exceeded 2 ml/s, though momentarily a wag artifact could cause much larger aberrations. Only when the stream hit the edge of the grid did an appreciably larger error occur. The same author also developed a microprocessor-controlled analysis and interpretation of uroflow curves in relation to urinary outflow impairment (*53–55*).

Griffiths *et al.* (*56*) described a simple device for testing urine flowmeters. The device is made from readily available components, is portable, is easy to use, and does not require special care in setting up. The flow rate is accurate to within 0.5 ml/s. The study reported that the nursing staff were able to do regular calibration checks on the urine flowmeters and that some flowmeter deficiencies could be exposed. Using such a tester, examples of artifactual peak flow rates were recorded. Other techniques have also been proposed for routine calibration of uroflowmeters (*57–59*).

Criteria for Accuracy. In uroflowmetry (and pressure) recordings accuracy of the measurement is an essential criterion, although it can be misleading. The most common parameters used to describe accuracy are the percentage of reading error and the percentage of full-scale error. The former is relative to the measured value, whereas the latter is relative to the maximum full-scale value. This statement implies that a full-scale error is generally smaller than a reading error, as it is divided by a larger number; it also implies that a reading error decreases proportionally to an increasing measured value. At full scale both errors are the same. Most manufacturers unfortunately do not clearly specify the error that is being used, which can be confusing. For example, a flowmeter with a 50 ml/s full scale has a cited accuracy of ± 5 percent; if the accuracy is a full-scale error, the maximum absolute error is 2.5 ml/s; the problem is that 2.5 ml/s corresponds to a 25 percent reading error for a measured flow of 10 ml/s. Ideally, both accuracy errors are cited.

It is recommended that calibration tests be performed routinely; they can be done by recording a series of known constant flow rates and plotting the measured value (from the flowmeter) versus the injected flow rate (from a constant-infusion pump, for instance). For each flow rate the accuracy can then be assessed in terms of the percent of reading error and the percent of full-scale error; adjustment can be made to compensate for any gain or zero drifts observed from the calibration curves.

MEASUREMENT OF BIOELECTRIC SIGNALS

Bioelectric signals are recorded routinely in urodynamics, particularly at the levels of the anal and urethral sphincters. These signals are an essential tool in overall patient assessment. Such signals are the electric manifestation of neuromuscular activation associated with a contracting muscle; it is an exceedingly complicated signal that is partly affected by the characteristics of the instrumentation used to detect and observe it. This section describes the basic principles that apply to the recording of an EMG. The reader is also referred to the literature for a more complete and technical insight (*60–68*).

Origin of Biopotentials

Skeletal muscle is organized functionally on the basis of motor units. The motor unit is the smallest unit that may be activated by a volitional effort, in which case all constituent muscle fibers are activated synchronously (*60*). The component fibers of the motor unit extend lengthwise in loose bundles along the muscle. In cross-section, however, the fibers of a given motor unit are interspersed with fibers of other motor units. Thus the component muscle fibers of the single motor unit (SMU) constitute a distributed, unit bioelectric source located in a volume conductor consisting of all other muscle fibers, both active and inactive. The evoked extracellular field potential from the active fibers of an SMU has a triphasic form of brief duration (3–15ms) and an amplitude of 20 to 2000 μV depending on the size of the motor unit. The frequency of discharge usually varies from 10 to 100 per second. In order to measure and record potentials at sphincteric levels, it is necessary to provide some interface between the body and the electronic measuring apparatus. This interface function is carried out by biopotential electrodes. An electrode therefore carries out the transducing function because current is carried in the body by ions, whereas it is carried by electrons in the electrode and its lead wire (Fig. 4–24). The electrode serves as a transducer to change an ionic current into an electronic current.

The disadvantages of recording the EMG with the convenient surface electrode is that it can be used only with superficial muscles and it is sensitive to electric activity over a wide area. Various types of monopolar, bipolar, and multipolar insertion-type electrodes are commonly used for EMG recording from deep muscles and SMUs. This type of electrode generally records local activity from small regions within the muscle in which it is inserted.

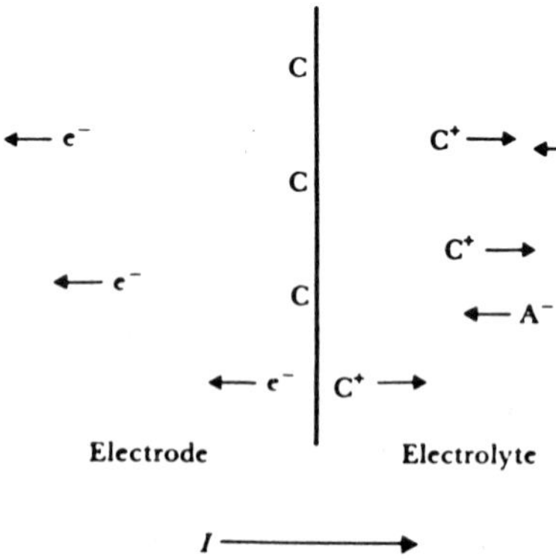

Figure 4–24. Electrode–electrolyte interface with current crossing from left to right. The electrode consists of metallic atoms (*C*); the electrolyte is an aqueous solution containing cations of the electrode metal (C^+) and anions (A^-). (From Webster, J.G. [ed.]: *Medical Instrumentation and Design*. Houghton Mifflin, Boston, 1978.)

Basic Principles for Measuring Biopotentials

Electrode—Electrolyte Interface. An electrolyte is defined as a nonmetallic electric conductor in which current is carried by the movement of ions (*61*). Electrolytes are present in the body and form an interface with electrodes to carry out a transducing function. Such interface is necessary to provide the biopotential electrode with the capability of conducting current. A net current that crosses the interface, passing from the electrode to the electrolyte, consists of: (a) electrons moving in a direction opposite to that of the current in the electrode; (b) cations moving in the same direction as the current; and (c) anions moving in a direction opposite to that of the current in the electrolyte. What actually occur are chemical reactions at the interface. Those reactions are often reversible and reach a state of equilibrium. The electrode is usually made up of atoms of the same material as the cations, so that the chemical reactions at the interface are reversible. Two types of electrode are theoretically possible regarding what happens to the electrode when a current passes between it and the electrolyte. Polarizable electrodes are those in which no actual charge crosses the interface when a current is applied; the current at the interface is a displacement current. Nonpolarizable electrodes are those in which current passes freely across the interface. Such characteristics are important features when choosing the electrodes.

Electrode—Skin Interface and Motion Artifact. When biopotentials are recorded from the surface of the skin, an additional interface must be considered—the interface between the electrode–electrolyte and the skin—in order to understand the behavior of electrodes. When coupling an electrode to the skin, we usually use an electrolyte paste containing Cl^- as principle anion to maintain good contact. The skin consists of three principle layers: the epidermis (outermost layer), the dermis, and the subcutaneous layer. The interface between an electrode and the skin through the agency of electrolyte paste imply a series resistance of the paste. The epidermal layer is also found to have an electric impedance. The outer surface of the epidermis, on the other hand, consists of dead material, the stratum corneum, which has electric characteristics different from those of live tissue. The effect of this stratum corneum is usually reduced by removing part of it, i.e., by vigorous rubbing with alcohol. When two electrodes are in electrolyte and one moves while the other remains stationary, a potential difference appears between the two electrodes during this movement. This potential is known as motion artifact and can be a serious cause of interference during the measurement of biopotentials.

Types of Electrode

Metal Plate Electrodes. The metal plate electrode is one of the most frequently used forms of a metallic conductor in contact with the skin and uses an electrolyte paste to establish and maintain contact. Stainless steel, platinum, or gold-plated disks are usually used to minimize the chance that the electrode will enter into chemical reactions with perspiration or the paste. Such "solid" electrodes have the disadvantage not to conform to a change in body surface topography, which can result in additional motion artifact.

Floating Electrodes. Floating electrodes avoid or diminish the source of motion artifact previously described. The principal feature of the electrode is that the actual electrode element (or metal disk) is recessed in a cavity so that it does not come in contact with the skin itself (Fig. 4–25). Instead, the element is surrounded by electrolyte paste in the cavity. Because the cavity does not move with respect to the metal disk, it does not produce any mechanical movement of the double layer of charge. In practice, the electrode is filled with electrolyte paste and then attached to the skin surface by means of a double-sided adhesive tape ring.

Flexible Electrodes. Flexible electrodes conform to a change in body surface topography. They can be made of a mesh woven from fine silver wire attached to a lead wire and substituted for the gauze sponge portion of a small plastic bandage (Fig. 4–26). They are often used for infants because they do not cause severe skin ulceration at pressure points.

Dry Electrodes. It is possible with dry electrodes to record surface biopotentials by a direct contact to the skin without an inter-

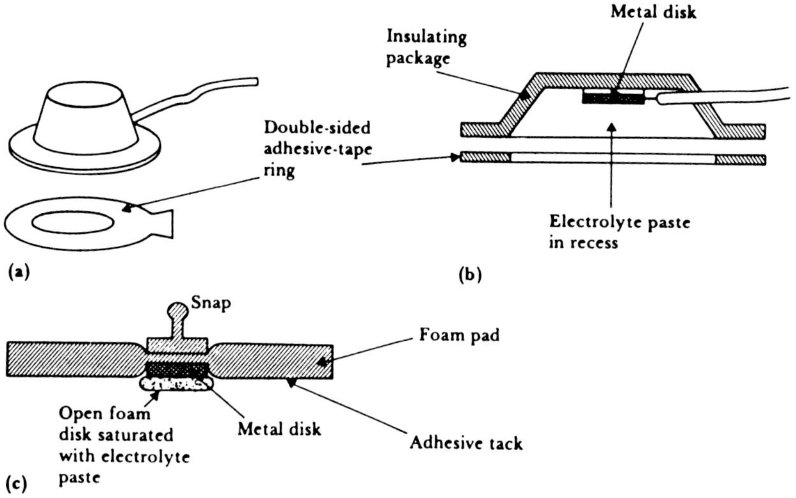

Figure 4–25. Examples of floating metal body-surface electrodes. **a.** Recessed electrode with top-hat structure. **b.** Cross-sectional view of electrode in **a. c.** Cross-sectional view of a disposable foam-pad electrode; the recess in this electrode is formed from an open foam disk, saturated with electrolyte paste, placed over the metal electrode. (From Webster, J. G. [ed.]: *Medical Instrumentation: Application and Design*. Houghton Mufflin, Boston, 1978.)

mediate layer of electrolyte paste. The significant feature of these electrodes is a self-contained, high-input impedance. However, many artifacts are associated with this method: low-frequency response, changing voltage, and electric interference (static electricity or pickup voltages).

Internal Needle Electrodes. Internal needle electrodes do not have to contend with the electrolyte–skin interface and its associated limitations. The electrode coupling behaves entirely like the electrode –electrolyte interface as no electrolyte paste is required to maintain its interface. There are many types of internal electrode (Fig. 4–27).

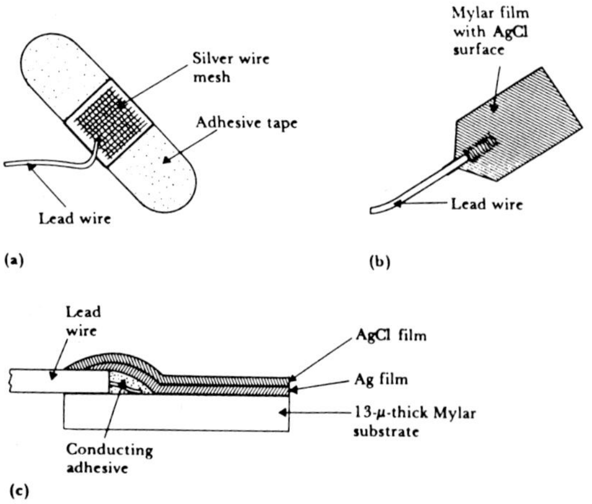

Figure 4–26. Flexible body-surface electrodes. **a.** Silverwire mesh electrode on an adhesive-tape bandage. **b.** Flexible thin-film neonatal electrode. **c.** Cross-sectional view of the thin-film electrode in **b.** (From Webster, J. G. [ed.]: *Medical Instrumentation: Application and Design*. Houghton Mifflin, Boston, 1978.)

The basic needle electrode consists of a solid needle (usually made of stainless steel) with a sharp point. A lead wire is attached to the other end of the needle, and the joint is encapsulated in a plastic hub to protect it. Multiple electrodes containing two wires placed within the lumen of the needle can also be formed and connected differentially; such electrodes are sensitive to electric activity only in the immediate vicinity of the electrode tip.

Electrodes for Electric Stimulation of Tissue. Electrodes designed to electrically stimulate tissue differ in that current of the order of many amperes crosses the electrode–electrolyte interface. Constant voltage stimulation is usually used in urodynamics for sacral evoked response studies. The choice of materials for stimulating electrodes must take into consideration chemical reactions occurring at the electrode–electrolyte interface. Thus the best stimulating electrodes are made from metals such as stainless steel, as they undergo minimal chemical

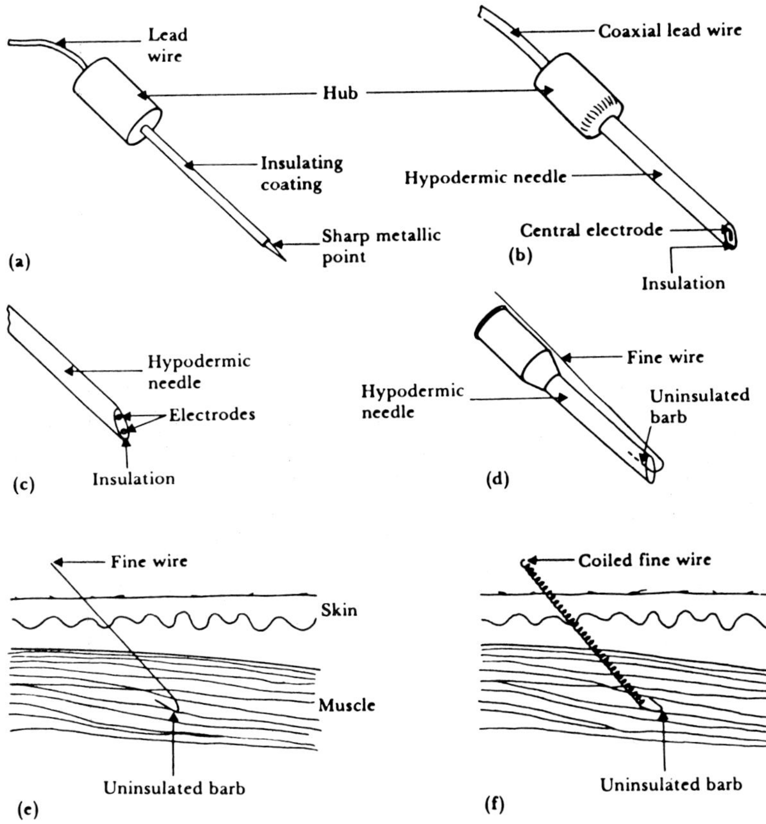

Figure 4–27. Needle and wire electrodes for transdermal measurement of biopotentionals. They are commonly used in urodynamics for sacral evoked response studies. **a.** Insulated needle electrode. **b.** Coaxial needle electrode. **c.** Bipolar coaxial electrode. **d.** Fine-wire electrode connected to hypodermic needle, before being inserted. **e.** Cross-sectional view of skin and muscle, showing fine-wire electrode in place. **f.** Cross-sectional view of skin and muscle, showing the coiled fine-wire electrode in place. (From Webster, J.G. [ed.]: *Medical Instrumentation: Application and Design*, Houghton Mifflin, Boston, 1978.)

reactions. The polarization of these electrodes, however, is large.

Practical Hints for Using Electrodes

Any part of the electrode that may be exposed to the electrolyte should be of the same material. For example, a third material, e.g., solder, should not be used to connect the electrode to its lead wire unless it is certain that it will not be in contact with the electrolyte. Electromechanical reactions can easily be set up between two materials and result in additional polarization or even corrosion of one of the metals. Electrodes placed on the skin surface have a tendency to become wet and come off. However, the problem need not arise if the electrodes are well designed. The lead wire to the surface electrode should be extremely flexible, yet strong. The insulation of the lead wire and the electrode can also present problems. Some of the insulating materials can absorb water and therefore become more conductive. If the lead wire is made of a material different from that of the electrode, the problem just described can result and enhance an important electric noise. It is therefore important to consider and understand the insulating material used for choosing a good electrode. Finally, proper isolation and grounding of instrumentation and the patient is essential to minimize the artifacts that occur during EMG recording.

DISPLAY AND TRANSMISSION OF DATA

After processing, the data finally interface with the instrument operator in the form of a chart, a screen display, a digital readout, or some other device. In conventional urodynamics the data are usually recorded directly on a paper chart using a pen or thermal recorder. In more advanced computerized systems, the digital data are plotted on an output device and can be retrieved for subsequent analysis. This section briefly describes some basic principles of paper chart recorders and discusses the present implication of microcomputers in the display and transmission of urodynamic data.

Basic Principles of Paper Chart Recorders

A measured signal generally consists of a voltage that must be displayed in order that it may be interpreted for diagnosis; the signal can be made audible by means of an amplifier and a loudspeaker, but mostly it is presented in a visible form. In principle, this step can be accomplished in two ways: by means of an analog representation or a digital representation of the amplitude of the signal. With an analog indication, the voltage is usually represented by the meter needle, which moves along a calibrated scale. It is, however, easier to read displayed data from a long distance when digital techniques are used. Here the amplitude of a signal is directly given in digits by means of illuminated figures, as in a pocket calculator.

There are various ways to record the signal on a chart recorder (*26,69*). The basic components of paper chart recorders are generally the same; they contain an electromechanical device that converts the electric input signal to a mechanical movement and a writing mechanism that produces a hard copy of the mechanical movement. Different principles can be applied to make such recordings: ink pen, thermal pen, ink jet, and/or light beam. The major differences among those techniques remain their frequency response and their cost. Ink or thermal pen recorders are usually limited to 50-Hz signals, whereas ink jet recorders have a higher frequency response (up to 700 Hz); the latter, however, are more expensive.

Paper chart recorders are commonly used in urodynamic units; the recorded data, however, cannot be retrieved or rescaled subsequently. It should be pointed out also that frequency response is directly limited by the writing speed of the paper; if the paper is not moving fast enough, high-frequency signals cannot be recognized.

Use of Microcomputers in the Display and Transmission of Data

Microcomputerized urodynamic systems can record and save all measurements obtained during a given investigation; all measurements are displayed graphically on a monitor screen and simultaneously recorded by a graphics printer. In such systems the display is independent from the rate at which the signal has been sampled; i.e., the signal can be sampled at a rate different from that of the printer, as all of the data can be stored. This method offers a particular advantage for EMG recordings because a strip chart is usually limited by the frequency response of the pen recorder. By sampling an EMG signal at a high rate and storing the signal in the computer, the same signal can then be fully replotted. Moreover, specific portions of the signal can be "windowed" and expanded on a full screen for further anaylsis. Storage of the data thus provides the capability to recall the information at any time for subsequent analysis; this method can be used for generating a graphic summary of the urodynamic investigation because the data can be compressed, expanded, rescaled, or edited. The user can archive selected curves, as opposed to several feet of chart paper. Such data can also be transmitted to a distant remote terminal; for example, the signal can be modulated by a modem through a telephone line and demodulated by a modem at the remote location. An entire urodynamic investigation or patient history can thus be transferred to another location for a second opinion or simply on a referral basis. Although telephone lines represent the most practical approach to date, there are more powerful ways of data transmission, e.g., radio or cable systems.

SAFETY CONSIDERATIONS

The safety aspects of any electronic equipment used in a patient environment should be considered; urodynamic instruments should therefore comply with the standards that have been established by various commissions. This section outlines some basic safety considerations, and the reader is referred to the literature for more detailed information (*69–72*).

General Considerations

Under most circumstances intact dry skin limits the flow of current through the body to safe levels. Furthermore, the application of current to the body surface usually results in distribution of that current in such a way that only a small fraction of it may pass through the myocardium. However, urodynamic procedures sometimes defeat these natural safeguards. Endoscopy can, for instance, introduce current into the body through low resistance mucous membranes rather than skin; moreover, the anesthetized patient does not react to painful sensations or withdraw from a current source. There are numerous hazardous sources of current. Direct contact with a live conductor is an obvious one. Any line-powered electric device may also be a source of current if there is a connection between the power source and metal case or some other accessible conductive part of the device. This connection can be by means of a direct short circuit, conduction of current through relatively conductive substances such as dirt or biologic fluids, indirect coupling through capacitive or inductive effects, or incorrect connections: inproperly wired electric outlets, probes plugged into the wrong jacks in a device, etc. Whether such a source is hazardous depends on the magnitude of the current available, the intimacy of an individual's contact with the source and the ground, and the individual's physical condition. Most electrically hazardous situations require simultaneous contact with a source of current and a ground pathway. The term "ground" here refers to any return path to the source of the current, regardless of whether it is connected to the earth. For current to flow, it must leave the source, pass through objects that are capable of conducting electricity, and return to the source. Such a system is called a circuit. In many circuits the ground is earth, but it need not be. For a physiologic effect to occur, the body must become part of an electric circuit; i.e., current must enter the body at one point and leave at some other point.

Potential Electric Hazards in Urodynamics

Exposure of the body to currents of varying amplitude occurs in some urodynamic procedures. The best example is sacral evoked response studies; in this test currents that may go up to 90 mA are applied to the penile skin or the clitoris. However, those currents have an extremely short pulse duration, usually not exceeding 0.5 ms, and are applied at low frequencies. It should nevertheless be remembered that three general effects can occur when electric current flows through biologic tissue: (a) resistive heating of tissue; (b) electric stimulation of excitable tissue (nerve and muscle); and (c) electrochemical burns (for direct current). Figure 4–28 summarizes the approximate range of currents that produce each effect in a 70-kg man for 1- to 3-second exposure to 60-Hz current applied to the hands. A shock hazard also exists in any patient's electric environment between the two conductors supplying either a 240- or a 120-V appliance. Because the neutral wire on a 120-V circuit is connected to ground, a connection between the hot conductor and any grounded object poses a shock hazard.

Preventive Maintenance of Urodynamic Equipment

The purpose of preventive maintenance is to ensure that: (a) the equipment is operating properly; (b) the equipment and all accessories, cables, and power cords are safe; and (c) the equipment is mechanically in good condition with no missing parts or loose switches or knobs. Many organizations are continually developing and revising codes, standards, and regulations that affect health care facilities. However, clear and widely accepted codes and standards for electric safety have not yet emerged.

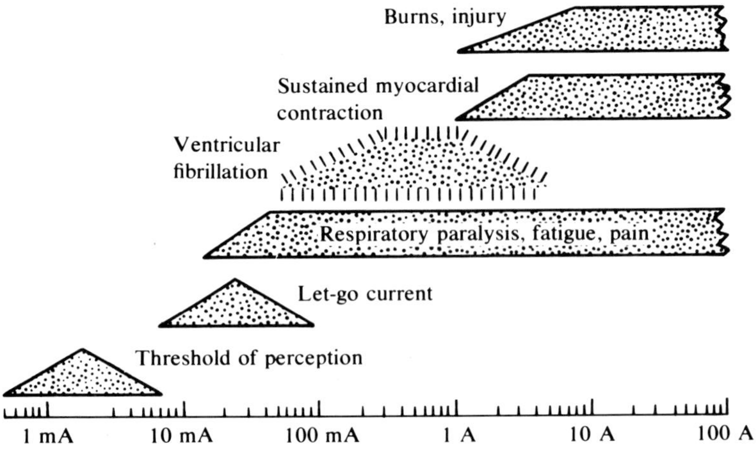

Figure 4–28. Physiologic effects of electricity. Threshold or estimated mean values are given for each effect in a 70-kg man for 1- to 3-second exposures to 60-Hz current applied to copper wires grasped by the hands. (From Webster F. G. [ed.]: *Medical Instrumentation: Application and Design*, Houghton Mifflin, Boston, 1978.)

Periodic testing and inspection of all AC receptacles and grounded surfaces are essential, as ground faults sometimes develop. For example, if a power plug is constantly pulled, the wire connecting the instrument to the grounding-pin third wire might break. Such a faulty ground connection on an electric bed would allow AC voltage to exist on the bed frame as a result of capacitive coupling between the bed frame and the primary wiring in the bed. Ground-fault alarms and interrupters are devices that sense these abnormal conditions and either cut the power or give an alarm. When these protective devices are not available, routine checks with a low-resistance ohmmeter should be made to detect either a ground fault or a resistance between the instrument case and the power-cord ground pin. Every patient should also be completely isolated and insulated from all grounded objects and all sources of electric current. Even if an isolated power system is used, low-resistance grounds that can carry currents of up to circuit-breaker ratings are clearly essential for the patient's protection. Hospital-grade receptacles, plugs, and heavy-duty low-leakage power cords should be used.

SUMMARY

The fundamental principles of biomedical instrumentation that are applicable to the field of urodynamics are presented in this chapter. The man–instrument system has been used as a conceptual approach to describe the steps involved in the measurement of urodynamic variables; it includes the conversion of a physiologic phenomenon into an electric signal that can be processed and displayed. This conversion is achieved on the basis of existing principles that are known and used in other fields of medicine as well as for physical measurements. General characteristics of biomedical instruments have been outlined to assist the urologist in his understanding and choice of urodynamic equipment, and the basic mechanisms for measuring pressure, flow, and electromyographic potentials have been described using specific examples.

The potential of microcomputers in urodynamics has also been presented as an efficient and powerful way of recording and processing data. It is viewed as the current trend toward the future generation of urodynamic systems. It is important to realize, however, that microcomputers do not change the various components of the man–instrument system; the signal is simply amplified, processed, and displayed through the computer itself, in contrast to the practice of using separate units to achieve the same functions.

REFERENCES

1. Olson, W. H.: Basic concepts of instrumentation. In Webster, J. G. (ed.), *Medical Instrumentation; Application and Design*. Houghton Mifflin, Boston, 1978, pp. 1–42.
2. Cromwell, L., Weibell, F. J., Pfeiffer, E. A., and Usselman, L. B.: *Biomedical Instrumentation and Measurements*. Prentice-Hall, Englewood Cliffs, N.J., 1973, pp. 10–24.
3. Susset, J. Development of nomograms for application of uroflowmetry. In Hinman, F. (ed.), *Benign Prostatic Hypertrophy*. Springer-Verlag, New York. 1983, pp. 528–538.
4. Bergveld, P.: Electronic amplifiers. In Bergveld, P., (ed.), *Electromedical Instrumentation: A Guide for Medical Personnel*. Cambridge University Press, Cambridge, 1980, pp. 69–78.
5. Traister, R. J.: Electronic terminology, In Traister, R. J. (ed.), *Principles of Biomedical Instrumentation and Monitoring*. Reston Publishing, Reston, VA, 1981, pp. 51–85.
6. Dymond, A. M.: Instrumentation for bioelectric measurements. In Feinberg, B. N., and Fleming, D. G., (eds.), *CRC Handbook of Engineering in Medicine and Biology. Section B, Instruments and Measurements*. Vol. I. CRC Press, Boca Raton, 1978, pp. 14–24.
7. Webster, J. G.: Amplifiers and signal processing. In Webster, J. G. (ed.), *Medical Instrumentation: Application and Design*. Houghton Mifflin, Boston, 1978, pp. 103–137.
8. Yanof, H. M.: *Biomedical Electronics*, 2nd ed. Davis, Philadelphia, 1972.
9. DuBory, J.: Common biomedical circuits. In Horesta, G. J., and Manning, A. V., (eds.), *Introduction to Biomedical Electronics*. McGraw-Hill, New York, 1978, pp. 249–252.
10. Thomas, H. E.: *Handbook of Biomedical Instrumentation and Measurement*. Reston Publishing, Reston, VA, 1974.
11. Stout, D. F., and Kaufman, M.: *Handbook of Operational Amplifier Circuit Design*. McGraw-Hill, New York, 1976.
12. Wait, J. V., Huelsman, L. P., and Korn, G. A.: *Introduction to Operational Amplifier Theory and Applications*. McGraw-Hill, New York, 1975.
13. DuBory, J.: Converting physiological changes into electric signals. In Horesta, G. J., and Manning, A. V. (eds.), *Introduction to Biomedical Electronics. A Guide for Medical Personnel*. McGraw-Hill, New York, 1978, pp. 64–103.
14. Abrams, P., Lewis, P., Murray, K., and MacLachlan, D.: A computerized system for the acquisition, analysis and storage of urodynamic data. In *Proceedings 79th AUA Meeting*, New Orleans, 1984, abstract 249.
15. Kramer, A., and Jonas, U.: Computer urodynamics—evaluation of practicability of on-line computing in the urodynamics laboratory. In: *Proceedings 79th AUA Meeting*, New Orleans, 1984, abstract 250.
16. Roskar, E., Suhel, P., Kralj, B., and Roskar, A.: Microcomputer controlled urodynamic diagnostic system. In *Proceedings 1st Joint Meeting ICS*–UDS, Los Angeles, 1980, pp. 166–173.
17. Jacobs, S., Sebern M., Donnell, R., and Lawson, R.: Computer-assisted urodynamics. *J. Urol.* 132:716–717,1984.
18. Van Mastrigt, R.: Using a minicomputer in urodynamics. In: *Proceedings XIIth ICS Meeting*, Leiden, 1982, pp. 167–168.
19. Van Mastrigt, R., Thon, H., and de Giessen, H.: Analog data collection via a telephone line: a microprocessor-based remote-controlled data-acquisition system. *Med. Biol. Eng. Comput.* 21-2:229–231, 1983.
20. Van Mastrigt, R.: A computer program for on-line measurement, storage, analysis and retrieval of urodynamic data. *Computer Programs In Biomedicine*. 1984.
21. Schäfer, W., Hannapel, J., Gerlach, R., and Lutzeyer, W.: Computer analysis of urodynamic data in BPH. In *Proceedings 79th AUA Meeting*, New Orleans, 1984, abstract 251.
22. Rollema, H.: *Uroflowmetry in Males. Reference Values and Clinical Application in Benign Prostatic Hypertrophy*. Thesis Kooyker International Booksellers, Leiden, 1981.
23. Kramer, E. J., and Jonas, U.: The use of computers in urodynamic investigations. In Yalla, S. (ed.), *The Principles and Practice of Urodynamics and Neurourology*. Macmillan, New York, 1987.
24. International Continence Society Committee on Standardization of Terminology (Chairman: T. Hald): *The Standardization of Terminology of Lower Urinary Tract Function*. Glasgow, United Kingdom, 1984.
25. Peura, R. A., and Webster, J. G.: Basic transducers and principles. In Webster, J. G., (ed.), *Medical Instrumentation; Application and Design*. Houghton Mifflin, Boston, 1978, pp. 49–98.
26. Abrams, P., Feneley, R., and Torrens, M.: *Urodynamics (Clinical Practice in Urology)*. Springer-Verlag, New York, 1983, pp. 28–96.
27. Jaffrin, M. Y: Pressure, flow, and volume measurements in blood. In Feinberg, B. N., Fleming, D. G., (eds.), *CRC Handbook of Engineering in Medicine and Biology. Section B, Instruments and Measurements*. Vol. I, CRC Press, Boca Raton, 1978, pp. 165–177.
28. Gabe, I. T.: Pressure measurement in experimental physiology. In Bergel, D. H. (ed.), *Cardiovascular Fluid Dynamics*. Vol. 1. Academic Press, London, 1972.
29. Traister, R. J.: Medical transducers and electrodes. In Traister, R. J. (ed.), *Principles of Biomedical Instrumentation and Monitoring*, Reston Publishing, Reston, VA, 1981, pp. 87–108.

30. Geddes, L. A.: *The Direct and Indirect Measurement of Blood Pressure.* Year Book, Chicago, 1970.
31. Wetterer, E.: Eine neue manometrishe Sonde mit electrishe Transmission. *Z. Biol.* 101:332–350, 1943.
32. Van Citter, R. L.: Mutual inductance transducer. *Methods Med. Res.* 11:26–30.
33. Geddes, L. A., and Baker, L. E: Piezoelectric transducers, In Geddes, L. A., and Baker L. E. (eds.), *Principles of Applied Biomedical Instrumentation.* Wiley, New York, 1975, pp. 127–136.
34. Hansen, A. T.: Pressure measurement in the human organism. *Acta Physiol. Scand.* [*Suppl. 68*] 19:1–227, 1949.
35. McDonald, D. A.: *Blood Flow in Arteries.* Edward Arnold, London, 1960.
36. Lambossy, P.: Manometres a l'observation des variations de la pression sanguine. *Helv. Physiol. Acta* 10:138–160, 1952.
37. Peura, R. A.: Blood pressure and sound. In Webster, J. G. (ed.), *Medical Instrumentation; Application and Design.* Houghton Mifflin, Boston, 1978, pp. 273–326.
38. King, G.: An experimental station for teaching cardiovascular manometry. *Med. Res. Eng.* 11:26–28, 1972.
39. Stegall, H. F.: A simple inexpensive sinusoidal pressure generator. *J. Appl. Physiol.* 22:591–592, 1967.
40. Brown, M., Sutherst, J., and Shawer, M.: A standard specification for the speed of response of urethral pressure measuring apparatus. *Clin. Phys. Physiol. Meas.* 1:255, 1980.
41. Shapiro, G. G., and Krovetz, L. J.: Damped and undamped frequency responses of underdamped catheter manometer systems. *Am. Heart J.* 80:226–236, 1970.
42. Schäfer, W., Gerlach, R., and Hannapel, J.: Microtip versus standard transducers: what do they really measure? In *Proceedings 12th ICS Meeting,* Leiden, 1982, pp. 53–55.
43. Anderson, R. S., Shepherd, A. M., and Feneley, R. C. L.: Microtransducer urethral profile methodology: variations caused by transducer orientation. *J. Urol.* 130:727–728, 1983.
44. Hansen, T. E., and Munkhaugen, A. M.: Fiber-optic sensors for medical and electrotechnical applications using bifurcated fiber bundles. In *Conference on Lasers and Electro-Optics (CLEO),* Washington, DC, 1981, paper F14.
45. Kvarstein, B., Aase, O., Hansen, T. E., and Dobloug, P.: A new method with fiberoptic transducers used for simultaneous recording of intravesical and urethral pressure during physiological filling and voiding phases. *J. Urol.* 130:504–506, 1983.
46. Rehfish, E.: Ueber der mechanisms des harnblasen verschlusses und der harnentleerung. *Virchows Arch.* [*Pathol. Anat.*] 150:111–151, 1897.
47. Siroky, M. B., and Krane, R. J.: Hydrodynamic significance of flow rate determination. In Hinman, F. (ed.), *Benign Prostatic Hypertrophy.* Springer-Verlag, New York, 1983, pp. 507–522.
48. Layton, T. N., and Drach, G. W.: Urinary flow rates; measurement and adjustment. In Hinman, F. (ed.), *Benign Prostatic Hypertrophy.* Springer-Verlag, New York, 1983, pp. 523–527.
49. Zinner, N. R., Sterling, A. M., and Ritter, R. C.: The urinary drop spectrometer in diagnosis. In Hinman, F. (ed.), *Benign Prostatic Hypertrophy.* Springer-Verlag, New York, 1983, pp. 553–558.
50. Blaivas, J. G.: A critical appraisal of specific diagnostic techniques. In Krane, R. J., and Siroky, M. B. (eds.), *Clinical Neuro-Urology.* Little, Brown Boston, 1979, pp. 77–80.
51. Donker, P. J., Zinner, N. R., and Sterling, A. M.: Future prospects for urodynamics study in clinical evaluation of benign prostatic hypertrophy. In Hinman, F. (ed.), *Benign Prostatic Hypertrophy.* Springer-Verlag, New York, 1983, pp. 642–648.
52. Susset, J., Picker, P., Kretz, M., and Jorset, R.: Critical evaluation of uroflowmeters and analysis of normal curves. *J. Urol.* 109:874–878, 1973.
53. Rollema, H.: Microprocessor controlled interpretation of urinary flow patterns. Presented at the *2nd Joint Meeting ICS-UDS,* Aachen, 1983.
54. Rollema, H.: New variables for automatic analysis and interpretation of uroflow curves; reference values and evaluation in benign prostatic hypertrophy. In *Proceedings 79th AUA Meeting,* New Orleans, 1984.
55. Rollema, H.: Microprocessor-controlled analysis and interpretation of uroflow curves; the value of estimated bladder contraction velocity in the detection of urinary outflow impairment. Presented to the *Dutch Urological Society,* Amsterdam, 1984.
56. Griffiths, C. J., Murray, A., and Ramsden, P. D.: A simple uroflowmeter tester. *Br. J. Urol.* 55:21–24, 1983.
57. Ryall, R. L., and Marshall, V. R.: An office method for calibrating a uroflowmeter. *J. Urol.* 127:482–483, 1982.
58. Von Garrelts, B., and Strandell, P.: Apparatus for calibration of a uroflowmeter. *Scand. J. Urol. Nephrol.* 6:29–31, 1972.
59. Rowan, D., McKenzie, S., McNee, G., and Glen, E. S.: A technical and clinical evaluation of the Disa uroflowmeter. *Br. J. Urol.* 49:285–291, 1977.
60. Clark, J. W.: The origin of biopotentials. In Webster, J. G. (ed.), *Medical Instrumentation; Application and Design.* Houghton Mifflin, Boston, 1978, pp. 143–184.
61. Neuman, M. R.: Biopotential electrodes. In Webster, J. G. (ed.), *Medical Instrumentation; Application and Design.* Houghton Mifflin, Boston, 1978, pp. 215–267.
62. Miller, H. A., and Harrison, D. C.: *Biomedical Electrode Technology.* Academic Press, New York, 1974.
63. Tam, H. W., and Webster, J. G.: Minimizing electrode motion artefact by skin abrasion. *IEEE Trans. Biomed. Eng.,* BME-24:134–139, 1977.
64. Webster, J. G.: Interference and motion artifact in biopotentials. In *IEEE 1977 Region 6 Conference Record,* 1977, pp. 53–64.
65. DuBory, J.: Interference and instability. In Horesta, G. J. and Manning, A. V. (eds.), *Introduction to Biomedical Electronics. A Guide for Medical Personnel.* McGraw-Hill, New York, 1978, pp. 105–143.
66. De Luca, C. J.: Physiology and mathematics of myoelectric signals. *IEEE Trans. Biomed. Eng.* BME-26: 313–325, 1979.

67. Stulen, F. B., and De Luca, C. J.: Frequency parameters of the myoelectric signal as a measure of muscle conduction velocity. *IEEE Trans. Biomed. Eng.* BME-28: 515–523, 1981.
68. Blaivas, J. G.: Sphincter electromyography. *J. Neurourol. Urodyn.* 2:269–288, 1983.
69. Olson, W. H.: Electrical safety. In Webster, J. G. (ed.), *Medical Instrumentation; Application and Design.* Houghton Mifflin, Boston, 1978, pp. 667–700.
70. DuBory, J.: Patient safety. In Horesta, G. J., and Manning, A. V. (eds.), *Introduction to Biomedical Electronics.* McGraw-Hill, New York, 1978, pp. 36–63.
71. Bergveld, P.: Electrical safety. In Bergveld, P. (ed.), *Electromedical Instrumentation. A Guide for Medical Personnel.* Cambridge University Press, Cambridge, 1980, pp. 115–127.
72. International Electrotechnical Commission: Safety of medical electrical equipment. Part 1. General requirements. *IEC*, 601-1, Geneva, 1977.

Mechanics of Micturition

5

DEREK F. GRIFFITHS, Ph.D.

Micturition is a mechanical process that is under neuromuscular control. The mechanical aspects therefore form only a substrate on which the control system acts. Much commonly encountered pathology is associated with a defect in the control system; the types of purely mechanical defect that can give rise to pathologic micturition are relatively few in number. In principle therefore the subject of this chapter is a simple topic.

Micturition results from an interplay between the expulsive action of the bladder and the impedance offered to that action by the urethra. To simplify the discussion we first consider these two aspects separately (Fig. 5–1).

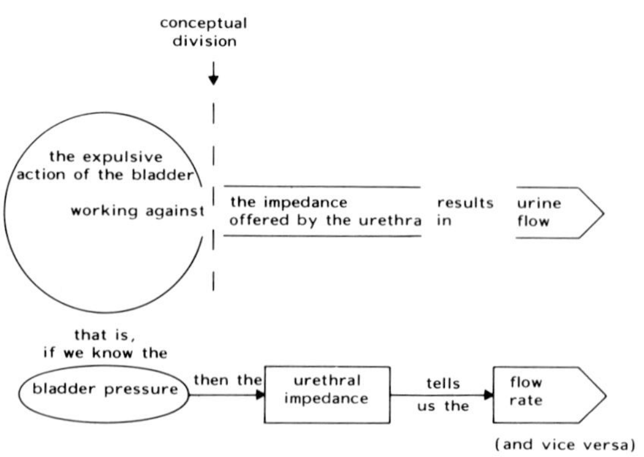

Figure 5–1. Meaning of urethral impedance.

EXPULSIVE ACTION OF THE BLADDER

At the simplest level the expulsive action is represented by the pressure of the urine in the bladder, the intravesical pressure (p_{ves}). Commonly the intravesical pressure is higher during micturition than at rest as a consequence of the expulsive effort. The intravesical pressure can be raised in two ways: extrinsically or intrinsically. It is therefore convenient to divide it into two components:

$$p_{ves} = p_{abd} + p_{det}$$

The intrinsic component (p_{det}) represents the contribution to p_{ves} from forces in the detrusor itself; it is called the detrusor pressure. The extrinsic component p_{abd} represents the contribution from the surrounding structures, grouped together under the term abdominal pressure. It can be increased by abdominal straining. In urodynamic practice p_{ves} is measured directly; p_{abd} is estimated indirectly, e.g., by measuring the pressure in the rectum; and an estimate of p_{det} is obtained by subtracting p_{abd} from p_{ves}.

Although hydrodynamically the contributions p_{abd} and p_{det} may appear to be equally significant, physiologically they are not comparable for the following reasons:

1. Normal micturition is accomplished principally by an active contraction of the detrusor, resulting in an increased value of p_{det}; abdominal straining is of relatively smaller significance.
2. In the absence of an active detrusor contraction (e.g., because of pathology), abdominal straining alone is inefficient in

emptying the bladder; in fact, voiding in this way may not even be possible.

3. When voiding occurs as a result of an active detrusor contraction, superimposed abdominal straining is usually relatively inefficient in increasing the flow rate (*1*).

Nevertheless, if the detrusor contraction is inadequate to empty the bladder, as in urethral obstruction or underactive detrusor function, abdominal straining may be employed to assist emptying. The relative inefficiency of abdominal straining is discussed again under Distensible Tube Approach, below.

Physiologically, then, the expulsive action of the bladder is reflected primarily in the intrinsic contribution to the intravesical pressure, the detrusor pressure (p_{det}). In principle, p_{det} can result from passive (viscoelastic) forces in the bladder wall, from active contraction of the detrusor or from that mysterious entity known as muscle tone. During physiologic micturition the most important of these actions is the active contraction. Because the active contraction is controlled by the parasympathetic innervation of the detrusor, the detrusor pressure at any given moment obviously depends on (a) the intrinsic strength of that particular detrusor muscle and (b) the level of neural stimulation at that moment. Measurements indicate that it depends also on (c) the volume of urine in the bladder and (d) the rate of flow of urine out of the bladder (*2*) (Fig. 5–2).

Therefore when we attempt to assess or compare the strength of detrusor contractions, the temptation to look only at the detrusor pressure must be resisted. A detrusor pressure of 50 cm H_2O, for example, can represent in one case a strong and in another a weak detrusor contraction, depending on the flow rate and the volume in the bladder.

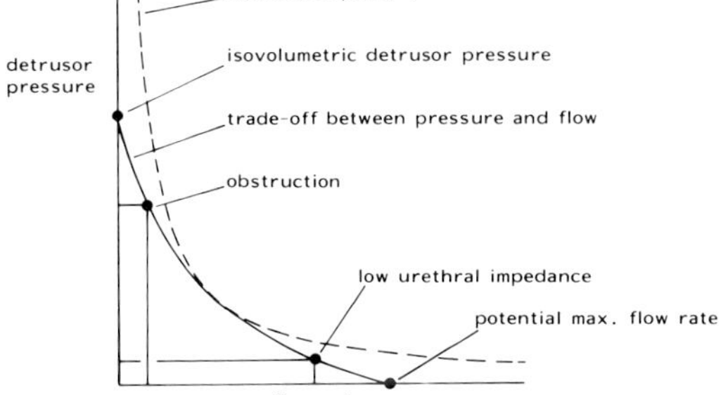

Figure 5–2. *Solid curve:* pressure/flow trade-off for the contracting detrusor. *Broken curve:* constant-power approximation to full curve. As the bladder empties the potential maximum flow rate falls toward zero.

Because the detrusor is a muscle, when stimulated it can either develop force or shorten. There is a trade-off between the force developed and the velocity of shortening. The bladder is a hollow organ; therefore the active force generates a detrusor pressure, and the velocity of shortening is related to the rate of urine flow out of the bladder. Therefore there is a similar trade-off between the detrusor pressure and the urine flow rate generated by an active contraction. The trade-off curve (Fig. 5–2) shows the flow rates and detrusor pressures that potentially can be delivered by a contraction of one particular strength. In a man with an obstructed urethra, for example, a good detrusor contraction may manifest as a high detrusor pressure (e.g., 100 cm H_2O) and a low flow rate (5 ml/s). In a woman with low urethral impedance, however, a contraction of exactly the same strength may yield a low detrusor pressure (e.g., 5 cm H_2O) but a high flow rate (30 ml/s). The detrusor pressure may appear so low that one is tempted to say, wrongly, that there is no detrusor contraction. It is in fact difficult to be sure in women who void at low detrusor pressures if and how strongly the detrusor is contracting.

One method of avoiding such difficulties is to measure the detrusor pressure when there is no flow. The pressure attained under these conditions (known as the isovolumetric detrusor pressure) is the pressure potentially available to drive the flow at that moment (Fig. 5–2). Under a given level of stimulation the pressure appears to depend relatively little on the volume in the bladder (*2*) and is therefore a reasonable reliable indicator of the strength of the detrusor contraction at that moment. In this way one can judge the strength of the contraction: (a) outside the period of voiding proper, e.g., during unstable bladder contractions without leakage, or during contractions against a dyssynergically closed urethral sphincter; and (b) during voiding, by suddenly interrupting the flow so that the detrusor pressure rises to an isovolumetric value (the stop test). In practice, inhibition of the detrusor may cause the strength of the contraction to be lower when the flow has stopped than it was just before the interruption (*3*).

Obviously the main disadvantage of using the isovolumetric detrusor pressure is that one cannot assess the detrusor contraction when one would like to, i.e., during flow. Oher methods have therefore been proposed; each has its disadvantages.

The trade-off between detrusor pressure and flow rate described above resembles a curve of constant mechanical power (P) (Fig. 5–2)

$$P = p_{det} \times Q$$

Thus a contraction of constant strength can be approximately represented by a given power (P) (*4,21*). For example, a contraction might yield a flow rate of 25 ml/s at a detrusor pressure of 20 cm H_2O (P = 500 cm $H_2O \cdot$ml/s = 50 mW) or, if the urethral impedance were higher, a flow rate of 10 ml/s at a detrusor pressure of 50 cm H_2O (P = 500 cm $H_2O \cdot$ml/s = 50 mW). It is therefore tempting to say that a contracting detrusor has a given amount of power available that can manifest as either pressure or flow. The analogy is helpful but of limited value for two reasons, (a) it breaks down at extremely high or low values of the flow; for example, if the flow is interrupted and the pressure rises to a high isovolumetric value, the power generated is then zero (see equation) even though the contraction is still at full strength; (b) for a contraction of given strength the power available depends on the volume in the bladder; as the bladder empties, the flow rate that can potentially be produced decreases (Fig. 5–2) and so the power available decreases.

Computer-based methods of juggling the variables detrusor pressure, flow rate, and bladder volume to arrive at a reliable assessment of the strength of the detrusor contraction are being developed.

IMPEDANCE OFFERED BY THE URETHRA TO THE BLADDER

For micturition the most important property of the urethra is that when bladder pressure is sufficient it allows urine to flow. At a given bladder pressure, what flow rate does it allow to pass? The answer is given by the impedance offered by the urethra to the expulsive action of the bladder (Fig. 5–1). High impedance implies obstruction: low flow rates for high pressures. Low impedance means no obstruction: high flow rates for low pressures. The urethral impedance represents directly the degree of (or lack of) urethral obstruction.*

Urethral impedance can be represented either by a formula (enabling the flow rate to be calculated from the bladder pressure) or graphically (so that the flow rate can be read for any given bladder pressure). In order to obtain such a formula or graph and to shed light on the origin of the urethral impedance, two approaches have been taken: the energy approach (*5–8*) and the distensible-tube approach (*2,9,10,21*).

Energy Approach

The intravesical pressure represents the potential energy of the urine in the bladder available to drive the flow through the urethra. As the urine flows through the urethra, some of this energy is dissipated by turbulence and viscosity into eddying motions and ultimately into heat. What remains appears as the kinetic energy of the urine in the external stream. Because energy is neither created nor destroyed, the intravesical pressure is equal to the energy dissipated plus the residual kinetic energy of the stream as shown in Figure 5–3. (Strictly speaking, the energies are per milliliter of urine.)

The kinetic energy in the stream depends on the stream volocity (v_{str}) and the density of the urine (ρ) and is approximately equal to $\rho v_{str}^2/2$. Because the stream velocity is equal to the urine volume flow rate (Q) divided by the stream cross-section (A_{str}), this kinetic energy is $\rho Q^2/2A_{str}^2$. A_{str} is related but not exactly equal to the area of the external urethral meatus. Therefore the kinetic energy in the stream depends on the (flow rate)^2

* The term "urethral impedance" is used instead of the more common term "urethral resistance" in order to avoid confusion. In the past "urethral resistance" has been used to refer to both urethral impedance and energy dissipation in the urethra; these two concepts are not synonymous, however (see below).

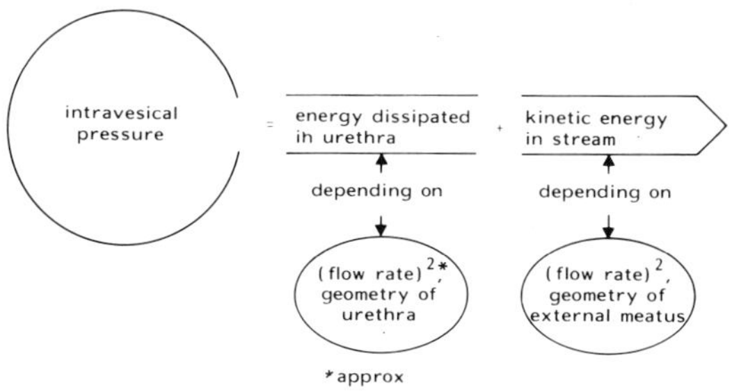

Figure 5–3. Energy balance during voiding.

and the geometry of the external meatus, as indicated in Figure 5–3.

The energy dissipated during the flow of urine through the urethra depends on the properties of the urine, as well as on the rate of flow and the shape of the urethra. For a fixed shape the amount dissipated increases with increasing flow rate; it is often roughly proportional to (flow rate)^2. Thus the energy dissipated depends on the flow rate and the internal geometry of the urethra, as indicated in Figure 5–3.

The complete figure shows that there is a formula linking the intravesical pressure to the flow rate via the geometry of the urethra and meatus. This formula represents the urethral impedance (Fig. 5–1). Because a narrow lumen tends to give high dissipation, and a narrow meatus tends to give high kinetic energy in the external stream, a narrow urethra presents a higher impedance to the bladder than a wide one.

Comparison of Figures 5–1 and 5–3 shows that energy dissipation is not synonymous with urethral obstruction. In obstruction the elevated urethral impedance can be due either to increased dissipation or to increased kinetic energy in the stream.

Intraurethral obstruction is associated with high dissipation and meatal obstruction with high kinetic energy. Measurement of the kinetic energy in the external stream, in addition to the bladder pressure, allows one to calculate the energy dissipation. However, splitting up the bladder pressure in this way (Fig. 5–3) does not give any extra information about the existence of urethral obstruction; at best it may allow one to judge whether obstruction, if present, is meatal or intraurethral. Manipulation of the energy dissipation to yield a resistance factor (e.g., dissipation/Q^2) (*6,7*) or an energy loss factor (dissipation/p_{ves}) (*8*) does not eliminate this basic problem. Such factors are open to the further objection that in normal micturition they are not constant (see Distensible Tube Approach, below), although this objection may have less force in anatomically obstructed micturition.

The energy approach is extremely general in its application. It is technically correct (when a few minor details that we have glossed over are included) for any kind of tube, regardless of whether it is a normal urethra. Such universal validity is an obvious advantage. The corresponding disadvantage is that no account is taken of how any particular tube (e.g., a urethra) behaves. This situation can make it difficult to apply and interpret the energy approach in a particular case. A simple-minded interpretation of Figure 5–3 for example, suggests that:

1. The intravesical pressure is roughly proportional to the (flow rate)^2. (Thus when the flow rate is zero the pressure is zero.)
2. The intrinsic and extrinsic contributions to the intravesical pressure, p_{det} and p_{abd}, are equivalent, as only their sum (p_{ves}) appears in the equations. (Thus detrusor contraction and abdominal straining are equally efficient methods of voiding.)
3. The energy dissipation throughout the whole urethra contributes to the impedance offered to the bladder and therefore to any urethral obstruction that may be present.

None of these conclusions is necessarily correct. For a rigid tube or one that behaves as nearly rigid, the urethral and meatal geometry factors in the figure are essentially fixed, and the conclusions are then essentially correct. For a highly distensible tube, however, the urethral and meatal geometry factors can vary dramatically in automatic response to changes in the flow rate. Although Figure 5–3 and the energy argument remain valid, the real behavior can be totally different from what the simple-minded interpretation suggests.

Distensible Tube Approach

With the distensible tube approach (*2,9,10,21*) changes in urethral geometry occurring in automatic response to changes in flow rate are taken into account *ab initio*. Unlike the energy approach, the theory is not applicable to tubes of any sort, only to those that are indeed highly distensible; whether any particular urethra behaves like this is open to experimental test. This limitation is a disadvantage but the corresponding advantage is that the theory can give much more detailed insight than the energy approach into the mechanical behavior of the urethra.

Of the two contributions to the intravesical pressure, p_{det} is in practice the more significant (see Expulsive Action of the Bladder, above; see also below). The urethral impedance offered to this pressure can be represented by a graph showing the flow rate (Q) produced by each value of p_{det} (see Impedance Offered by the Urethra to the Bladder, above). An approximation to such a graph can be produced experimentally by plotting, throughout a micturition cycle, each measured value of p_{det} against the corresponding, simultaneous value of Q. For any normal, unobstructed micturition a roughly similar curve is always obtained (Fig. 5–4): There is a threshold pressure below which no flow occurs; as soon as P_{det} exceeds the threshold, a large flow rate passes with little further increase in pressure. Because this graph does not resemble one in which pressure is proportional to (flow rate)^2, conclusion b, above, is not valid, and so distensible tube effects must certainly be taken into account.

Because of the shape of the curve, any "resistance" or "impedance" factor, based on the detrusor or intravesical pressure and intended to express the degree of urethral obstruction (e.g., p_{det}/Q^2), depends greatly on the flow rate, and thus no normal value can be defined. High values are obtained if the maximum flow rate is low, e.g., if there is detrusor underactivity, even though there is no obstruction (*11*).

The oft-repeated claim that at maximum flow the normal urethra can be treated as indistensible (e.g., *7*) is certainly incorrect: Pressure/flow plots show that it is just as distensible at maximum flow as at near-zero

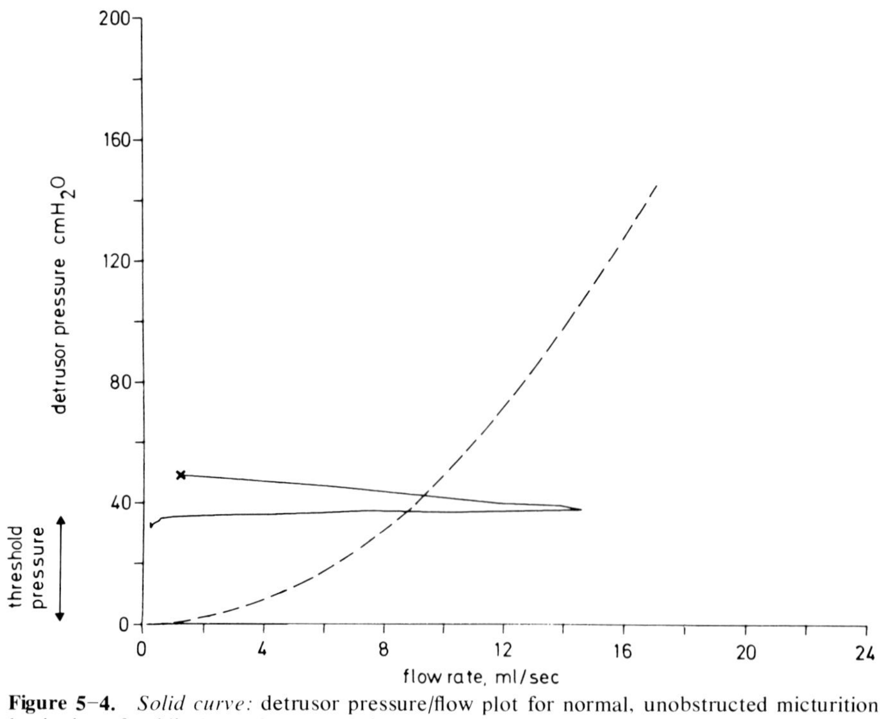

Figure 5–4. *Solid curve:* detrusor pressure/flow plot for normal, unobstructed micturition. (The cross marks the beginning of voiding). *Broken curve:* (hypothetical) relation of detrusor pressure proportional to (flow rate)^2.

flow. There are urethras that behave indistensibly at maximum flow; their pressure/flow plots turn upward at maximum flow to approximate the form pressure proportional to (flow rate)^2 (Fig. 5–5). Such urethras are urodynamically slightly obstructed (see Urethral Obstruction, below).

A fundamental characteristic of distensible tube flow, which distinguishes it from flow through a (near) rigid tube, is the possible existence of a flow-controlling region that governs the impedance presented upstream (e.g., to the bladder) and isolates the bladder from any effect of the more distal parts of the tube (Fig. 5–6) (*2,9,21*). The flow-controlling region has been described as a region of "extrinsic pressure" (*10*) or a "compressive zone." In the vicinity of such a flow-controlling region the tube assumes a characteristic funnel configuration (Fig. 5–7), and there is a corresponding fall (from upstream to downstream) in the static fluid pressure. The narrowing of the tube causes energy dissipation and so a fall in the total pressure as well. Radiographic evidence and measurements during normal voiding (*12,13*) suggest that in women there is a flow-controlling region somewhere in the distal urethra, whereas in men there appears to be one near the distal striated sphincter —thus in both sexes near the distal closure mechanism. The threshold pressure (Fig. 5–4) is simply the "extrinsic pressure" or "compression" referred to above. Its existence indicates that during voiding the closure mechanism continues to compress the urethra with a closure pressure that must be overcome by the detrusor pressure in order to produce any flow. Once that pressure threshold has been exceeded, the rapid increase in flow rate indicates that, once open, the closure mechanism is easily distensible.

The existence of a flow-controlling region accounts for the relatively small effect of abdominal pressure on flow rate (see Expulsive Action of the Bladder, above). If changes in the abdominal pressure were transmitted equally to the bladder and the proximal urethra up to the flow-controlling region,

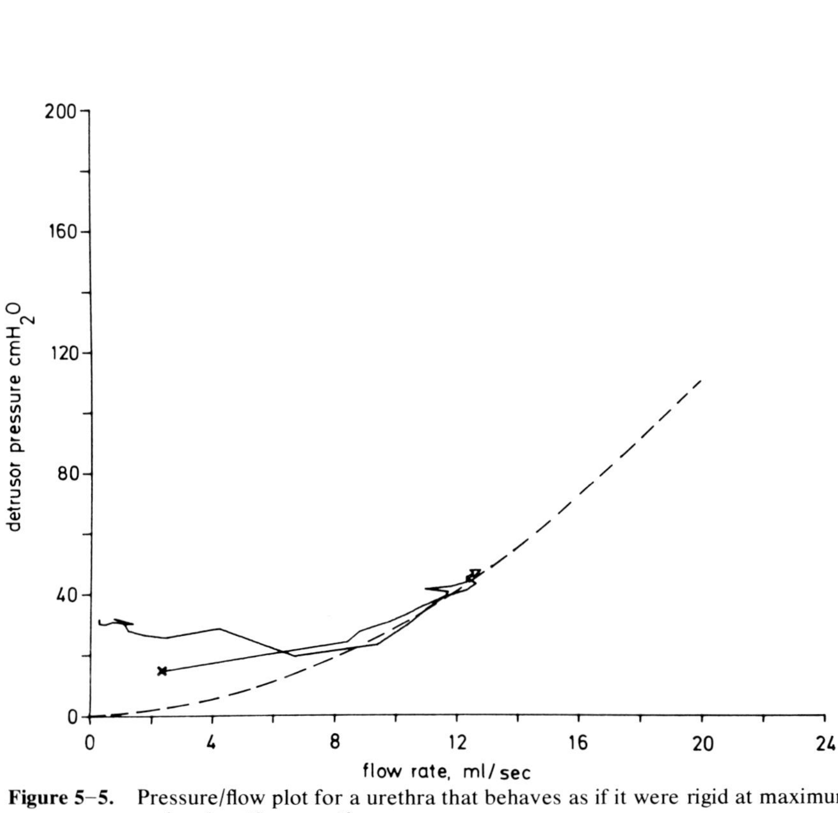

Figure 5–5. Pressure/flow plot for a urethra that behaves as if it were rigid at maximum flow. *Broken line:* detrusor pressure proportional to (flow rate)^2.

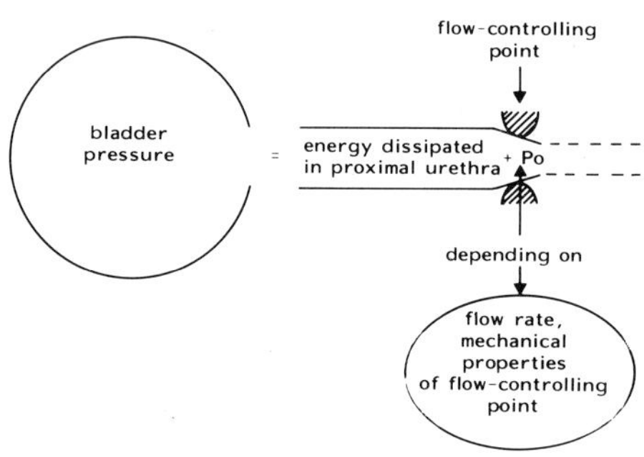

Figure 5–6. Energy balance during voiding, according to the distensible tube approach, when a flow-controlling region is present, p_0 is the total pressure needed locally to overcome the elasticity of the flow-controlling region. The distal parts of the urethra and the external stream (*dotted*) have no effect on p_0 or the proximal parts of the urethra and thus do not contribute to the impedance presented by the urethra to the bladder. Although this diagram is not consistent with the third conclusion of the energy approach, which is based on a simple interpretation of Figure 5–3, there is no real inconsistency: Figure 5–3 merely implies that the energy dissipated in the distal urethra plus the kinetic energy in the external stream are equal to p_0.

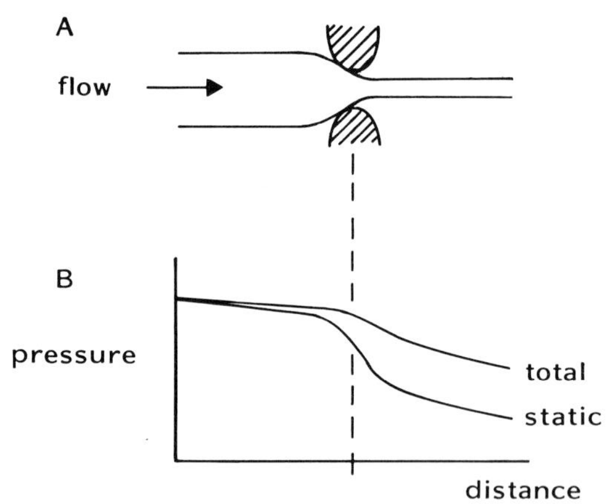

Figure 5–7. Shape (**A**) and urethral pressure (**B**) profiles during voiding, near a flow-controlling region (*shaded*) in a highly distensible urethra. The total pressure (also known as the pressure head or stagnation pressure) can in principle be measured with a catheter with an end-hole facing upstream. The static pressure (which is in fact the ordinary fluid pressure) can in principle be measured with a side-hole catheter lying parallel to the direction of flow. The pressure profiles would of course be identical if the narrowing shown in (**A**) were rigid instead of distensible, provided the shape remained the same. The only difference between the two cases is that a flow-controlling region changes its shape automatically in response to changes of flow rate, whereas a rigid narrowing does not.

there would be a cancellation and no net effect on the flow rate. In practice, such changes are transmitted to both organs but not necessarily equally, so that the cancellation is not equal. The transmission to the bladder is essentially a passive process; that to the urethra has both passive and active (neuromuscularly mediated) components (*14*).

If there is no detrusor contraction, the proximal urethra is normally closed. Transmission to that part of the urethra then ensures that abdominal straining is an extremely inefficient way of producing urine flow.

Urethral Obstruction

During micturition the key property of the urethra is the impedance it presents to the contracting bladder. A urethra is urodynamically obstructed only if its impedance is abnormally elevated (see Impedance Offered by the Urethra to the Bladder, above). When there is anatomic obstruction, the pressure/flow graph is characteristically different from that for a normal unobstructed urethra (Fig. 5–8). At the higher flow rates the relation between pressure and flow rate approaches that expected for a near-rigid tube, i.e., pressure porpotional to (flow rate)^2 (see Energy Approach, above). Under these circumstances the impedance is dominated by the hydrodynamics of the near-rigid narrowing responsible for the obstruction, and distensible tube effects are relatively unimportant. In fact, if the narrowing lies in the distal urethra, and if it is urodynamically obstructive, the increased upstream pressure completely abolishes the flow-controlling region, blowing it open so that there is no longer any funnel configuration. Under these circumstances a "resistance" or "imepedance" factor (e.g., p_{det}/Q^2) may express to a reasonable approximation the degree of obstruction, as its value is relatively independent of the flow rate.

In the vicinity of an obstructive narrowing there is a decrease in static pressure (from upstream to downstream). Energy dissipation associated with local turbulence causes a similar fall in total pressure as well (Fig. 5–7). Measurement of urethral pressure profiles (static or total) during voiding can therefore help locate an anatomic obstruc-

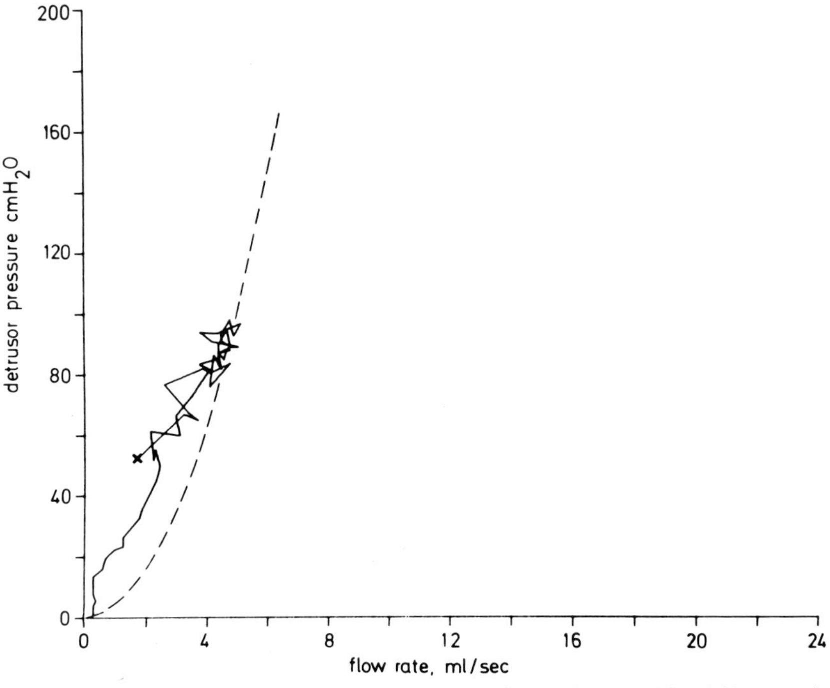

Figure 5–8. Pressure/flow plot for a urethra anatomically obstructed by rigid narrowing. *Broken curve:* pressure proportional to (flow rate)^2.

tion (*15*). (Care must be taken that the measuring catheter does not provoke obstruction at the external meatus; see below.) Such profiles must be compared with those for the normal, unobstructed case, as shown in Figure 5–9. In the normal man a large part of the urethra lies distal to the urethral closure mechanism, which probably forms a flow-controlling region. Although considerable energy dissipation occurs in this distal part, according to Figure 5–6, it does not contribute to the impedance offered by the urethra to the bladder and therefore cannot be considered obstructive. It means that, were the dissipation in the distal urethra to be reduced (e.g., by surgery), there would be no increase in the flow rate—thus contradicting conclusion 3, above (see Fig. 5–3). We believe that energy dissipation is not synonymous with urethral obstruction.

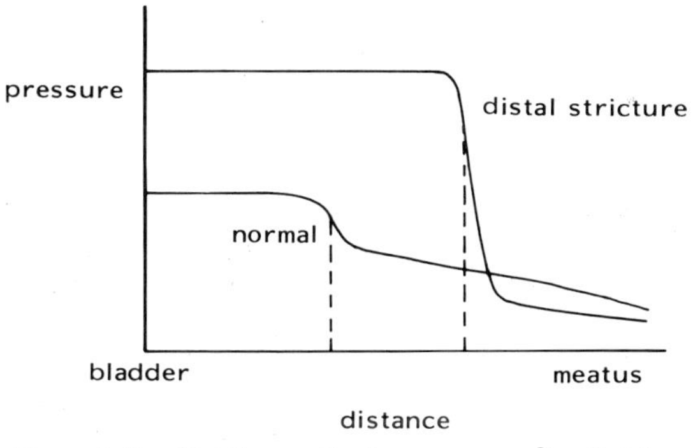

Figure 5–9. Voiding urethral pressure profiles (total or static) for a normal and a distally obstructed male urethra. In the normal case a pressure drop occurs at the flow-controlling region; in the obstructed case it occurs at the distal stenosis.

To summarize, not every decrease in pressure (from upstream to downstream) on a voiding pressure profile indicates obstruction. To diagnose obstruction urodynamically one should first determine if the urethral impedance is elevated in a characteristic way (Fig. 5–8) (put simply, if there is elevated bladder pressure p_{det}). If there is obstruction, then it can be located by means of a voiding pressure profile (static or total (*15*)) or by radiography. Obviously, if there is locally a large fall in total pressure, implying energy dissipation of, for example, more than 40 cm H_2O, the bladder pressure must in any event be elevated, suggesting obstruction. However, the possibility of functional rather than anatomic obstruction must be considered. These abnormalities can be distinguished by the pressure/flow plot: With functional obstruction the plots obtained typically demonstrate an increased threshold pressure (reflecting incomplete relaxation of the urethral closure mechanism) and, more importantly, are variable and complicated in form, reflecting active changes in the degree of obstruction (*2,16,21*). In men urethral obstruction at the bladder neck or in the prostatic urethra has both anatomic and functional aspects. Plots of detrusor pressure against flow rate vary from case to case and may suggest anything from a near-rigid narrowing (Fig. 5–8) to an elevated closure pressure in the proximal urethra (Fig. 5–4 with an elevated threshold pressure) (*4*).

External Meatus

In women the external meatus is considered to be the least distensible part of the urethra. Pressure/flow plots show, however, that the flow-controlling region, even though it may lie quite distally, is highly distensible (Fig. 5–4). Only when there is quite severe meatal or distal urethral stenosis does the pressure/flow relation change to a form that indicates obstruction by near-rigid narrowing (Figs. 5–5 and 5–8). A slightly less severe stenosis, urodynamically nonobstructive in everyday life, can be made obstructive by the presence of a urethral catheter (*17*).

In boys meatal obstruction appears even more easily provoked by a urethral catheter (*18*). In the absence of a catheter, and provided the foreskin does not interfere, the kinetic energy of the external stream at any given flow rate (the "exit pressure") is determined by the meatal part of the urethra (Fig. 5–3) (*2*). It means that the velocity of the stream and the force exerted by the stream against a plate (the momentum flux) are similarly determined. If the meatus is wide, the stream has low velocity, low momentum flux, and low kinetic energy for any given flow rate. If there is meatal stenosis the opposite is true. Measurements of these variables (together with the flow rate) give information about the properties of the meatal portion of the urethra. It has been reported that the stream velocity is abnormally low (for the flow rates observed) in men with underactive detrusor function (*19*), whereas in men with overactive detrusor function the opposite has been suggested (*20*). If true, these reports imply that there is an association between the mechanical properties of the external meatus and the activity of the detrusor. The physiologic basis for such an association is unknown.

INTERPLAY BETWEEN BLADDER AND URETHRA

Up to this point the bladder and the urethra have been treated as separate organs (Fig. 5–1). In reality the behavior of each affects the other. Such interaction can occur directly [e.g., the contracting detrusor may constrict the bladder neck, causing functional obstruction (*9*)] and indirectly. For example, if the urethra is obstructed it offers high impedance to the bladder (see Impedance Offered by the Urethra to the Bladder, above). For a given detrusor pressure it means a reduced flow rate. However, when the flow rate is reduced, the detrusor pressure becomes automatically higher because of the trade-off between pressure and flow (see Expulsive Action of the Bladder, above). Thus the elevated detrusor pressures observed in obstruction represent partly a purely myogenic response to the increased urethral impedance and do not necessarily imply detrusor hypertrophy or any other structural or functional abnormality in the detrusor.

The shapes of the flow curves observed in different circumstances are the result of the interplay of bladder and urethra (*9*). During normal unobstructed micturition the urethral impedance holds the detrusor pressure approximately constant (Fig. 5–4), and the flow rate follows a typical bell-shaped curve that mirrors the behavior of the detrusor. After the peak flow has been passed, the steady fall in flow rate until voiding ceases is related to the decreasing "power" available as the bladder empties (see Expulsive Action of the Bladder, above). The flow rate potentially available decreases; the detrusor pressure potentially available (isovolumetric pressure), however, remains well above the threshold pressure (Fig. 5-4), and so there is no likelihood of residual urine.

In anatomic obstruction the altered urethral impedance (Fig. 5–8) results in a flow curve with a characteristic flat top (a plateau). Provided the detrusor continues to behave normally there is no possibility of residual urine. Typically, however, the detrusor decompensates: The (isovolumetric) pressure potentially available decreases catastrophically before the bladder is empty, leaving residual urine. A similar failure of the detrusor contraction, with residual urine, can be observed in overstretched bladders even in the absence of urethral obstruction, as well as in many types of neuropathy.

In this chapter the expulsive action of the bladder and the impedance offered to it by the urethra have been described in detail. The result of their interplay can be quite simply summarized as follows. Residual urine is typically a sign of abnormal detrusor function, whereas elevated bladder pressure during voiding is a sign of urethral obstruction (in that voiding), either anatomic or functional.

REFERENCES

1. Hasegawa, N., Kitagawa, Y., Takasaki, N., and Miyazaki, S.: The effect of abdominal pressure on urinary flow rate. *J. Urol.* 130:107–111, 1983.
2. Griffiths, D. J.: *Urodynamics: The Mechanics and Hydrodynamics of the Lower Urinary Tract.* Adam Hilger, Bristol, 1980.
3. Coolsaet, B. L. R. A.: Stop-flow test. In Coolsaet, B. L. R., and Van Duyl, W. A., (eds.), *Principles of Bladder Function and Urodynamics.* Lameris, Utrecht, 1981, pp 37–41.
4. Abrams, P. H., and Griffiths, D. J.: The assessment of prostatic obstruction from urodynamic measurements and from residual urine. *Br. J. Urol.* 51:129–134, 1983.
5. Gleason, M. D., Bottaccini, M. R., Perling, D., and Lattimer, J. K.: A challenge to current urodynamic thought. *J. Urol.* 97:935–940, 1967.
6 Whitaker, J., Johnston, G. S., and Lawson, J. D.: Urinary outflow resistance estimation in children: theory, method and results. *Invest. Urol.* 7:127–135, 1969.
7. Smith, J. C.: Urethral resistance to micturition. *Br. J. Urol.* 40:125–156, 1968.
8. Byrne, J. C., Bottaccini, M. R., and Gleason, M. D.: Energy loss during micturition. *Invest. Urol.* 10:221–225, 1972.
9. Griffiths, D. J.: Mechanics of micturition. In Chisholm, G. D., and Innes Williams, D., (eds.), *Scientific Foundations of Urology*, 2nd ed. Heinemann, London, 1982, pp. 411–420.
10. Scott, J. E. S., Clayton, C. B., Dee, P. M., and Simpson, W.: A study of the hydrodynamics of the female urethra. 1. Experiments with models. *J. Urol.* 96:763–769, 1966.
11. Griffiths, D. J.: Uses and limitations of mechanical analogies in urodynamics. *Urol. Clin. North Am.* 6:143–148, 1979.
12. Scott, J. E. S., Clayton, C. B., Dee, P. M. and Simpson, W.: A study of the hydrodynamics of the female urethra. 2. Static pressure profile measurements. *J. Urol.* 96:770–778, 1966.
13. Woodside, J. R.: Micturitional static urethral pressure profilometry in women. *Neurourol. Urodyn.* 1:149–158, 1982.
14. Thüroff, J. W., Bazeed, M. A., Schmidt, R. A., and Tanagho, E. A.: Mechanisms of urinary continence: animal model to study urethral responses to stress conditions. *J. Urol.* 127:1202–1206, 1982.
15. Yalla, S. V., and Fraser, L.: Total and static pressure measurements of the male lower urinary tract. *Neurourol. Urodyn.* 1:159–171, 1982.
16. Griffiths, D. J., and Scholtmeijer, R. J.: Detrusor/sphincter dyssynergia in neurologically normal children. *Neurourol. Urodyn.* 2:27–37, 1983.
17. Griffiths, D. J., and Scholtmeijer, R. J.: Precise urodynamic assessment of meatal and distal urethral stenosis in girls. *Neurourol. Urodyn.* 1:89–95, 1982.
18. Griffiths, D. J., and Scholtmeijer, R. J.: Precise urodynamic assessment of anatomical urethral obstruction in boys. *Neurourol. Urodyn.* 1:97–104, 1982.
19. Gleason, M. D., Bottaccini, M. R., Reilly, R. J., and Byrne, J. C.: The residual stream energy is a diagnostic index of male urinary outflow obstruction. *Invest. Urol.* 10:72–77, 1972.
20. Meyhoff, H. H., Griffiths, D. J., Nordling, J., and Hald, T.: Clinical applications of momentum flux measurements with special reference to detrusor hyperreflexia and meatal stenosis. *Urol. Res.* 8:71–75, 1980.
21. Shäfer, W.: Urethral resistance? Urodynamic concepts of physiological and pathological bladder outlet function during voiding. *Neurourol. Urodyn.* 4:161–201, 1985.
22. Griffiths, D. J., Constantinou, C. E., and Van Mastrigt, R.: Urinary bladder function and its control in normal females. *Am. J. Physiol.* 251:R225–R230, 1986.

Viscoelastic Properties of the Bladder and Urethra

6

JACQUES G. SUSSET, M.D., AND CLAUDE H. REGNIER, M.Sc.

Bladder and urethral viscoelastic property measurements are important clinically because, through simple mechanical tests, they allow derivation of various parameters that relate to the structure and function of the detrusor and urethra. Such measurements, however, depend on the physiologic environment in which they are made. The pressure recorded inside the bladder (or urethra), for instance, results from two basic factors. The first factor is neuromuscular, characterizes the properties of live tissue, and is directly linked to neural inputs, cellular membrane depolarization, and active muscular strength. The second factor is purely mechanical; it depends on the degree of stretch and continues to exist, in a modified form, in dead tissue. The latter factor is directly related to the tissue structure, particularly its collagen content, which in the bladder constitutes an average of 50 percent (*1*).

It appears necessary to differentiate the respective roles of the neuromuscular and mechanical factors involved in pressure measurements. For the bladder it could be an attempt to define bladder "tone" in better terms, as it has never been defined properly. By necessity, "tone" relates to the neuromuscular factor (*2*). On the other hand, the increased intravesical pressure during filling results from the two factors mentioned above and should thus be referred to as bladder "compliance," i.e., change of volume relative to the associated change in pressure. For the time being, however, it is impossible to distinguish between the neuromuscular and mechanical components of detrusor pressure, and it appears that in the passive state bladder and urethral compliance may sometimes be described just in terms of their viscoelasticity.

We have therefore restricted the scope of this chapter to the assessment of vesical and urethral viscoelastic properties. Some basic theoretical concepts are discussed and various measurement techniques are presented. The practical importance of these methods is addressed from a clinical point of view through emphasis on their significance and limitations in patient populations.

BASIC PRINCIPLES

Definitions

Stress. Stress is defined as force per unit area. In a specimen subjected to a given force, stress varies inversely with its thickness. In view of the variability of specimens studied *in vitro* (or even whole bladders and urethras) under different pathologic states, it is more meaningful to use stress than force. Stress can be defined in two ways. Analyzing eulerian stress means using the cross-sectional area of the tissue submitted to a given force in its deformed state—obviously difficult to do experimentally. The advantage of using the lagrangian stress is to use the area of the tissue in its undeformed state. For example, when studying several bladder strips *in vitro*, two or three strips can be fixed in formalin immediately, prior to any elongation, and the corresponding cross-sectional areas determined histologically. The langrangian stress, although less accurate, is definitely more practical. With this approach the measured area is greater than that of the deformed tissue if we assume that the tissue is incompressible; the measured stress is thus underestimated.

In the international system of units, the basic unit of force is the newton (N) and that of length is the meter (m). The basic unit of stress is the pascal (N/m^2). A force of 1 N can accelerate a body mass of 1 kg to 1 m/s^2, and a force of 1 dyne can accelerate a body mass of 1 g to 1 cm/s^2; thus 1 dyne $= 10^{-5}$ N.

Strain. Deformation of a solid that can be related to stresses is described by strain. If a bladder strip of initial length L_0 is stretched to a length L, the change can be described by L/L_0 (λ = stretch ratio), (L − L_0/L_0 (ϵ) or (L − L_0)/L (ϵ'). Such dimensionless ratios eliminate the absolute length from consideration. In live tissues the resting ("reference") state (L_0) is entirely arbitrary and can be defined in different ways; e.g., it can be measured when a given level of measurable force (which obviously depends on the dimensions of the tested specimen) is reached.

Viscoelasticity. When a live tissue or solid is subjected to strain that is initiated suddenly and is maintained at a constant level, the corresponding induced stresses decrease with time. This situation is called "stress relaxation" or simply "relaxation." When the tissue is subjected to a cyclically varying strain of a given frequency and amplitude, the corresponding stress can be expressed during extension and recoil of the tissue; this phenomenon is called "hysteresis," which characterizes the stress–strain relation in the "loading/unloading" process. On the other hand, if the tissue is suddenly stressed, and the stress remains constant afterward, the tissue continues to be deformed; this phenomenon is called "creep." Relaxation, hysteresis, and creep are considered features of viscoelasticity, which is significant only when either stress or strain varies with time.

Methods of Study

Three basic and complementary biomechanical approaches can be followed when studying the mechanical behavior of the bladder and urethra.

Biologic Approach. The biologic approach utilizes observations *in vivo*. For example, when the bladder is subjected to sudden strain, e.g., step-wise increments in filling volume, the resultant stress relaxation curve can be fitted to a mathematic equation; a mechanical model can be derived from such a relation and used for calculating vesical elasticity and viscosity coefficients (i.e., viscoelastic properties). Stress relaxation curves following rapid injection cystometry or rapid stretching of a tissue specimen have been so analyzed in both canine and human bladders and fitted to a third-order exponential equation; a corresponding mechanical model was thereby derived to calculate vesical viscoelastic parameters (*3–12*). Such a quantitative approach proved to be useful for comparing bladders with different collagen contents, as elastic coefficients are directly proportional to collagen content.

"Continuum" Approach. The continuum approach applies a mechanical consideration that can iteratively be adjusted to biologic observations. With this approach theories of general-material mechanics are applied to specific tissue characteristics. Even the smallest volume of any tissue presumably contains a large number of atoms and molecules; it is thus permissible and convenient to consider such tissue, from the mechanical standpoint, as a continuum (i.e., a homogeneous material) and on this basis attempt a macroscopic representation of its properties. The approach of continuum mechanics offers a sound scientific analysis of forces of biologic deformation (*13*). Motion and deformation of the bladder and urethra, and the mechanisms of the forces involved, need to be described. We have applied the continuum approach to the study of elastic behavior of the bladder; a finite strain theory, developed for hollow spherical structures, was used to derive a strain/energy function that can correlate intrinsic energy of the bladder wall with the degree of its muscular stretch during filling (*14,15*).

Microstructural Approach. The microstructural approach contradicts the continuum approach, as it is based on the premise that live tissue is heterogeneous with respect to its contents and the structure of its various load-bearing elements, i.e., collagen, elastin, and smooth muscle. Each of these components can be analyzed structurally and its mechanical characteristics thereby established. A general "constitutive equation" of each tissue can be formulated by combining individual "equations" of the three components. Although collagen, elastin, and smooth muscle can be, and already have been, analyzed and defined separately, the microstructural approach is far from being accurately predictive of viscoelastic properties of the bladder in either normal or pathologic settings.

Biomechanical Steps. Because the above three approaches are complementary, they can be integrated in Fung's proposal (*16*), which comprises the following steps.

1. Study of the morphology of the organism, anatomy of the organ, and both histology and ultrastructure of the tissue under study, to define its architecture and constituent elements.
2. Determination of the mechanical properties of materials or tissue involved in the problem under study. In biomechanics this step is often difficult because isolation of the tissue for testing may not be possible, the size of the procured samples is too small, or keeping the tissue to be tested under normal live conditions is impossible. Furthermore, live tissues are often subject to significant deformations *in vivo* (or even *in vitro*), and their stress/strain relations are usually time-dependent. All of the above limitations, especially the last, make determination of the "constitutive equation" of live tissues a challenging, or even impossible, task. Nevertheless, the mathematic form of such an equation may be determined empirically on the basis of certain numerical parameters obtained by physiologic experiments, as indicated below (steps 6 and 7).
3. Derivation of the governing differential or integral equations based on fundamental laws of physics (conservation of mass, conservation of momentum, conservation of energy, Maxwell's equations, etc.) and the constitutive equation of the material.
4. Understanding the environment in which the organ/tissue under study normally functions in order to define meaningful "boundary" conditions.
5. Solving boundary-value problems analytically or numerically by applying or formulating the differential equations with appropriate boundary conditions.
6. Performing physiologic experiments that test the above-mentioned boundary-value solution and, if necessary, resolve and reformulate the mathematic problem to make sure that the theory used and the experimental observations made do match; i.e., that theory and experiment are testing the same hypothesis.
7. Comparing all experimental and corresponding theoretical results. Through this step it is determined if the initial hypothesis is justified; and if it is, numerical values of coefficients undetermined in the constitutive equation(s) involved are identified.
8. Exploring all practical applications of the theory tested and all experiments such testing involves.

Mechanical Models

Various mechanical models can be used in the "biologic" approach to characterize muscle behavior biomechanically. In the following paragraphs are described the three basic elements used (in combination) to form such models, i.e.,the Hooke, Newton, and Maxwell elements (Fig. 6–1).

The Hooke element characterizes the elasticity of a material; it is represented by a spring in which stress (F) varies linearly with strain (X) according to Hooke's law: $F = E \cdot X$, where E is an elastic coefficient, also known as Young's modulus (*3*). This law, however, is only meaningful when strains are small, i.e., in the order of 1 percent elongations, as encountered in metals (*17*). It is not directly applicable to live tissues because their strains are always greater than unity (e.g., 200–300% for the bladder), and they do not have linear stress/strain relations.

The Newton element characterizes the viscosity of a material; it is represented by a dashpot in which stress (F) varies linearly with the time rate of change in strain (dX/dt), according to Newton's law: $F = \eta(dX/dt)$, where η denotes a viscosity coefficient. In other words, the response of a Newton element depends on the speed of its deformation, also called "strain rate." A common analogy is the force required to pump water

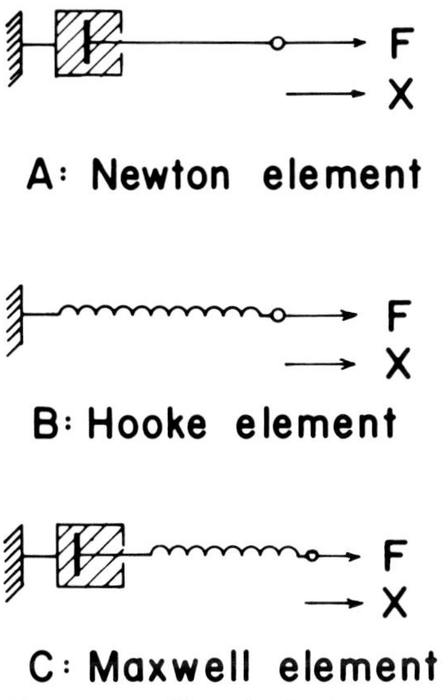

Figure 6–1. Three basic elements used in the mechanical representation of tissue viscoelasticity. The Newton and Hooke elements characterize, respectively, viscosity and elasticity. The Maxwell element represents the stress/relaxation phenomenon encountered in live tissues. (From Kondo, A., *et al.: Invest. Urol.* 10:154–163, 1972. Copyright © 1972, The Williams & Wilkins Co., Baltimore.)

(e.g., from a tank) with a syringe; it is more difficult to fill the syringe quickly than slowly. A material in which stress is proportional to the strain rate is called a viscous material.

The Maxwell element is a combination of Hooke and Newton elements placed in series. It is used to represent the "stress/relaxation" phenomenon that occurs in live tissues and therefore mimics their viscoelasticity. A fast stretch characterizes such behavior by enhancing a high stress followed by progressive relaxation, i.e., a decrease in the stress response. The spring action (elasticity) predominates during stretching of the Maxwell element to create a force that pulls on the dashpot until complete relaxation is achieved and stress becomes zero.

VISCOELASTICITY OF THE BLADDER

Statement of the Problem

The human bladder wall (dry weight) contains 57.4 percent (± 9%) of insoluble proteins, and less than 43 percent of muscle elements (*1*). Aside from collagen and smooth muscle, the bladder contains elastin (2%), reticulin, and the hydrophilic gel "ground substance" that includes mucopolysaccharides and tissue fluid. Distensibility of the bladder may allow it to attain a 200 to 300 percent volume because of the mechanical nature of these constituents, reflecting its properties as a storage organ. The normal bladder can "accommodate" to increasing volumes without significant increase in pressure. The central question is to obtain a method that characterizes such "viscoelastic" behavior. In theoretical terms it can be done by doing either relaxation, hysteresis, or creep experiments. In practical terms, however, only a few techniques have been used clinically. Rapid cystometry is one of these techniques; pressure can be observed after inducing a sudden strain by a stepwise volume increment, corresponding to a stress relaxation experiment. The same technique can be applied *in vitro* by inflating a whole bladder or stretching a bladder specimen. The following paragraphs describe how such techniques have been developed and discuss the clinical significance of their results. They relate essentially to the biologic approach to biomechanical study of vesical behavior.

Methods of Measurement

Rapid Cystometry. Rapid cystometry is defined as the sudden injection of water into the bladder with continuous pressure recording. It is generally performed at an infusion rate of 30 to 35 ml/s using an angiographic injector or manually with a glass syringe. The injections are successive and cumulative until bladder capacity [previously determined by slow (conventional) cystometry] is reached. A Foley catheter can be used for infusion and a separate (6 F. ureteral) catheter for pressure recording. In a normal situation the intravesical pressure increases to a maximum and then progressively decreases (within 1–2 minutes) with relaxation of the detrusor. The stabilized intravesical pressure following every injection never reaches the pressure observed prior to that injection, and it varies in proportion to volume (Fig. 6–2). The rapid cystometry test corresponds to a stress/relaxation experiment because strain

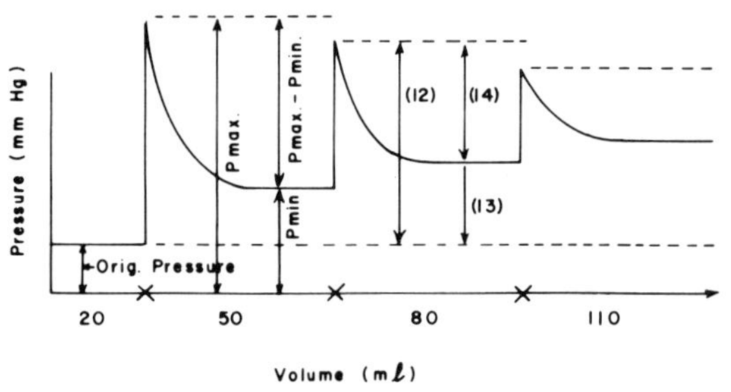

Figure 6–2. Three successive injections in rapid cystometry. Maximal pressure is read at the end of each injection, and minimal pressure 3 minutes after relaxation starts. (From Kondo, A., *et al.*: *Invest. Urol.* 10: 154–163, 1972. Copyright © The Williams & Wilkins Co., Baltimore.)

is suddenly fixed to a given value (volume), and the corresponding stress (pressure) is measured with time. The relaxation phase, i.e., decrease in pressure, is characteristic of viscoelastic behavior of the bladder.

Rapid cystometry experiments have been carried out on both the canine and human bladder (*3–5,8,18*). In one experiment, performed on anesthetized adult female dogs (40–45 lb), 30 ml of saline was injected into the bladder within 1.25 seconds using a Barber-Colman angiographic injector (*3*), and changes in intravesical pressure were observed over 3 minutes. The same injection was repeated two consecutive times without emptying the bladder. Because 20 ml was left initially in the dog's bladder, the maximum volume attained after three injections was 110 ml. The same experiment was repeated *in vitro* after the bladder was taken out and immersed in Ringer-Locke solution. In humans rapid cystometry has been performed by manual injection of 100 ml of saline into the bladder within 3 seconds using a glass syringe (*18*); the same injection was repeated after the intravesical pressure stabilized up to bladder capacity, which had been determined beforehand by a slow cystometrogram.

***In Vitro* Testing of Bladder Strips.** Stretching of bladder strips is an alternative technique for characterizing viscoelastic behavior of the bladder. It is done by immersing detrusor specimens in a muscle bath that contains an oxygenated physiologic solution (e.g., Tyrode's solution) kept at constant temperature. The design of such a bath may vary according to user preferences. In general, the specimen is secured at the bottom of the bath (e.g., with a suture), and the upper portion of the strip is connected to a force transducer that can be moved vertically by hand or through an automatic mechanism. Stretch of the strip can be controlled to provide stepwise increments of variable magnitudes. The speed of stretch, however, determines different types of *in vitro* experiments. In one type, applied to both animal and human bladder specimens (*9,10,12,19*), the length of the specimen is suddenly increased to a fixed value, with simultaneous recording of the corresponding force. It results in a curve whose shape is similar to that of a rapid cystometrogram; the force increases to a maximum and is followed by progressive relaxation. The test is repeated at increasing lengths of the specimen, after its relaxation is complete, until it reaches its elastic limit.

In another type of experiment the specimen is stretched slowly, and the force is recorded only after relaxation is achieved; the values thereby obtained are then plotted against the length of the strip on a graph. This method provides a curve in which force increases exponentially with deformation. The data obtained are characteristic of viscoelastic behavior of the bladder, although its relaxation phase is not expressed on the curve. Slow stretch is actually the preferred method of strip testing because it can be combined with contractility studies and can be standardized easily. Moreover, values of active force can be determined after electric field stimulation and plotted against specimen length, and the effects of a specific drug on both active and passive properties of the detrusor can be tested. All of these measurements are important in any attempt to differentiate between the neuromuscular and mechanical components of vesical behavior. Previous studies using this technique aimed only at defining the effects of alpha- and beta-adrenergic blocking agents on the active force (*20,21*). The same methodology, however, has been used to evaluate the effect of hormones, obstruction, and decentralization on the contractility and passive properties of animal bladders (*22–24*).

Mechanical Model of the Bladder. The stress/relaxation curves obtained from rapid cystometry or rapid stretching of bladder strips *in vitro* may be analyzed mathematically to derive a mechanical model that characterizes detrusor elasticity and viscosity. This has been done in previous work (*3,25*). The phase of relaxation, expressed by the decrease in pressure, was fitted to an equation that contained three exponentials. By using various algebraic and geometric transformations, the analysis led to a mechanical analogy consisting of a parallel arrangement of one Hooke and three Maxwell elements (*vide supra*). The final model (Fig. 6–3) allows interpretation of the stress/relaxation curves obtained in rapid cystometry in biomechanical terms. During the rapid injection, the four springs (Hooke elements) are submitted to deformation (increase of pressure to a maximum value); after the injection the three dashpots (Newton elements) are successively pulled out from the tension exerted by the three springs, allowing restoration of the original length of each spring (relaxation phase); the fourth spring represents the residual pressure observed after relaxation. A simplified representation of this phenomenon, including only one Maxwell element, is presented in Figure 6–4.

It is possible from the various equations used in this model to derive four elastic constants (one for each spring) and three viscous coefficients (one for each dashpot) that are characteristic of the curve. For practical purposes, however, it appears that the sum of the four elastic constants provides a sufficient measure of detrusor elasticity. Such sum can be determined directly from the maximum pressure obtained at the end of a

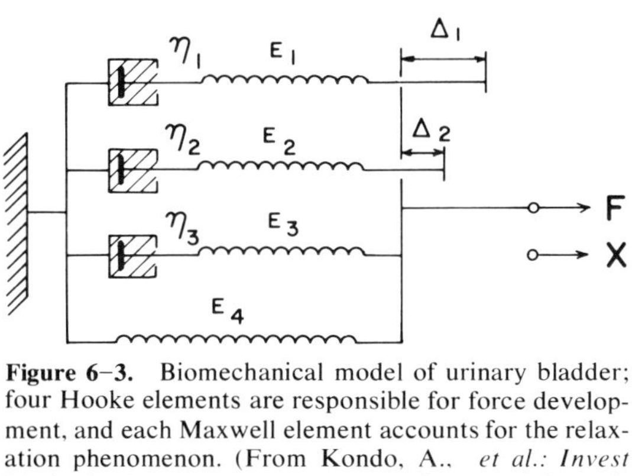

Figure 6–3. Biomechanical model of urinary bladder; four Hooke elements are responsible for force development, and each Maxwell element accounts for the relaxation phenomenon. (From Kondo, A., *et al.*: *Invest Urol.* 10:154–163, 1972. Copyright © The Williams & Wilkins Co., Baltimore.)

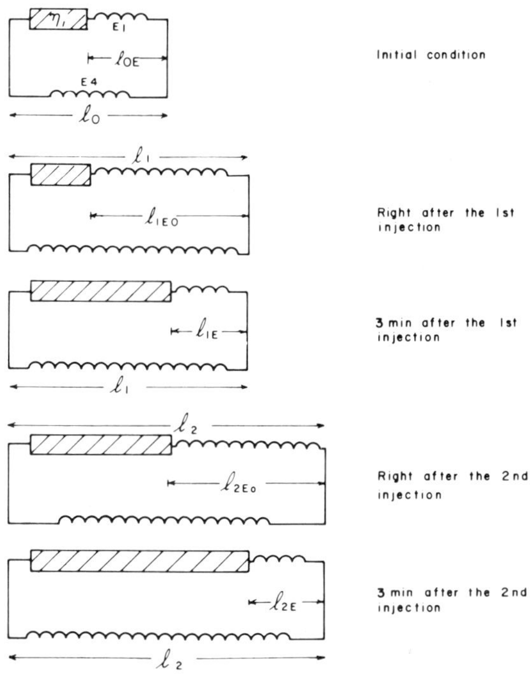

Figure 6–4. Mechanical representation of bladder relaxation following two successive stepwise volume increments. Elongation of spring E_1 is proportional to the difference between the last and a previous deformation; elongation of spring E_4 is the difference between the last and the initial deformation. (From Kondo, A., *et al.*: *Invest. Urol.* 10:154–163, 1972. Copyright © The Williams & Wilkins Co., Baltimore.)

given injection. It also appears convenient to measure detrusor viscosity as the half-decay time (HDT), which is defined as the time required for the pressure to decrease 50 percent from its maximum value (at the end of the rapid injection) to the one measured 3 minutes afterward.

Viscoelasticity of the bladder may thus be expressed by various elastic and viscous coefficients, which can be determined from a biomechanical model derived from rapid cystometry experiments. Such a model has been confirmed by *in vitro* studies (*9,10,19*) and appears to offer a sound explanation of vesical biomechanical behavior.

Clinical Applications of the Biomechanical Viscoelastic Model

Importance of Collagen Content and Muscle Cell Mass for Determining Viscoelastic Parameters. Various studies indicate a relation between structure and mechanical properties of the detrusor. A practical way to verify this thesis is to quantify the amount of collagen present in the bladder wall through measurement of its content of hydroxyproline (*26*) and correlate such amounts with the viscoelastic parameters derived from rapid cystometry (or *in vitro* testing of bladder strips). Estimation of collagen content, however, is meaningful only when associated with estimation of the muscle cell mass to provide a collagen/muscle ratio. There is indeed evidence that collagen proliferation may not necessarily indicate an increase of this ratio. In humans a 10 percent increase in the collagen/muscle ratio was observed in women 50+ years old compared to a 3 percent decrease of the same ratio in men in the same age group; the difference was attributed to concomitant hypertrophy of the detrusor secondary to prostatic hypertrophy in men (*1*). A study of vesical outlet obstruction in the rat confirmed this observation (*27*); in these obstructed bladders the total amount of detrusor collagen was increased fourfold, but the collagen concentration (collagen/muscle ratio) was decreased to one-third of normal because of a significant (12-fold) increase in detrusor weight.

It is important to interpret the above findings in biomechanical terms. The bladder wall is composed essentially of muscle and collagen. In situations where collagen is increased in proportion to muscle, e.g., following muscular hypertrophy, the detrusor becomes thicker. If it occurs in a 1:1 proportion, the measured elastic and viscous parameters of the bladder should remain unchanged because the bladder maintains the same muscle/collagen ratio. This phenomenon can be explained simply, as follows. In a bladder specimen of cross-sectional area A that is subject to a given force F, stress can be calculated as force/unit area (F/A); in a specimen composed of the same tissue elements with cross-sectional area 2A, subject to a force 2F, the stress (2F/2A = F/A) remains the same. In other words, parallel increases in collagen and muscle mass are likely to enhance higher forces in the bladder wall, but the viscoelastic parameters remain unaltered. Consequently, when the collagen mass is greater than that of muscle, the elastic and viscous coefficients of the detrusor are increased and vice versa. Figure 6–5 illustrates the case of a fibrotic bladder in which an increase of the collagen/muscle ratio can account for high force development and reduction of relaxation.

It thus appears that measured viscoelastic parameters in the bladder reflect variations in collagen content of the detrusor relative to its muscle cell mass. The following paragraphs discuss various experimental results that illustrate and confirm this view.

Effect of Vesical Outlet Obstruction. In one study a series of dogs underwent obstruction of the vesical neck (*4,28*). Rapid

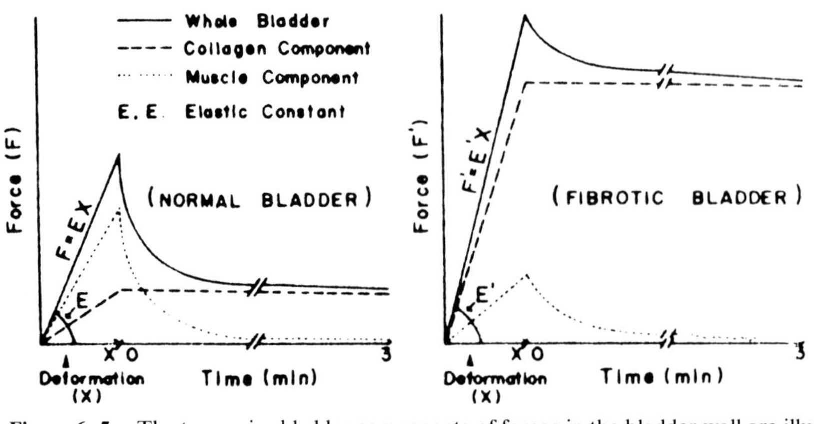

Figure 6–5. The two major bladder components of forces in the bladder wall are illustrated in a fibrotic bladder. An increase of the collagen/muscle ratio is responsible for elevation of the total elastic coefficient. (From Kondo, A., and Susset, J.: *Invest. Urol.* 11:459–465, 1974. Copyright © 1974, The Williams & Wilkins Co., Baltimore.)

cystometry and determination of collagen versus muscle content of the detrusor were carried out prior to and 3 months following the procedure. Table 6–1 shows the changes in collagen content and muscle mass obtained in this group, in contrast to other pathologic conditions. Differences in the viscoelastic parameters were not statistically significant (p > 0.005) because little increase in the collagen/muscle ratio was observed (*4*). This finding was verified by various *in vitro* studies in obstructed rabbits; detrusor "stiffness" was actually decreased in moderate obstruction owing to predominant detrusor muscle hypertrophy, relative to collagen proliferation, as determined histologically (*23*). It appeared, however, that the degree of obstruction had a significant impact on vesical biomechanical properties, as the opposite finding was observed in the severely obstructed detrusor (Fig. 6–6), i.e., increased collagen/muscle ratio. These findings therefore confirm that detrusor muscular hypertrophy occurs in some models of experimental chronic obstruction (*28*).

It can therefore be stated that the type of structural changes in the detrusor following obstruction of the vesical outlet affects viscoelastic behavior of the bladder. When muscle hypertrophy predominates, the bladder wall is more compliant because it contains proportionally less collagen. On the other hand, when collagen predominates, viscoelasticity of the bladder is significantly increased. All of these changes seem to depend on the degree and duration of the obstruction. It thus becomes necessary to develop methods to quantify the degree of outlet obstruction in order to assess the clinical significance of the above experimental findings.

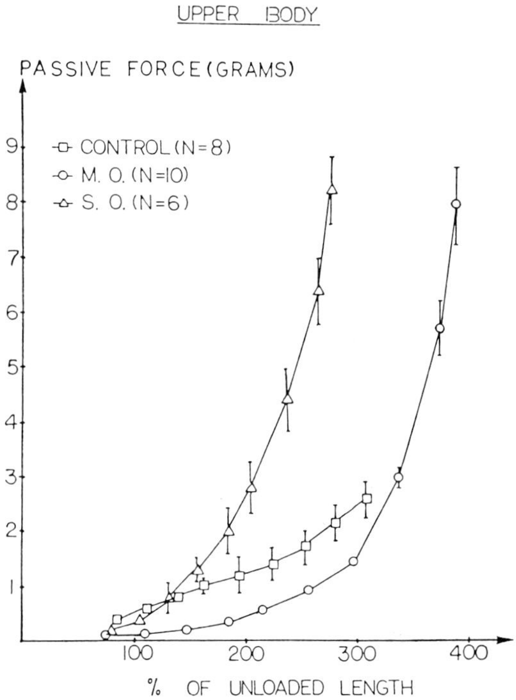

Figure 6–6. Passive properties of the rabbit urinary bladder following vesical outlet obstruction. The degree of obstruction affects the detrusor elasticity; the predominance of muscular hypertrophy in moderate obstruction accounts for the right shift of the curve. From Ghoniem. G. *et al.*: *J. Urol.* 135:1284–1289, 1986. Copyright © 1986, The Williams & Wilkins Co., Baltimore.)

Table 6–1. Relative Increase of Collagen in Relation to Muscle in Three Experimental Dog Groups*

CONDITION	COLLAGEN WEIGHT (GM)	MUSCLE WEIGHT (GM)	COLLAGEN/MUSCLE *Ratio*	COLLAGEN/MUSCLE *% Increase*
Normal ($n = 20$)	4.9	11.5	0.42	
Decentralization ($n = 8$)	17.2 ($p < 0.01$)	23.1 ($p < 0.01$)	0.74 ($p < 0.01$)	76
Sclerosing Agent ($n = 5$)	10.5 ($p < 0.02$)	10.1 ns	1.03 ($p < 0.001$)	145
Bladder Neck obstruction ($n = 7$)	7.6 ($p > 0.05$)	15.0 ($p > 0.05$)	0.51 ($p > 0.05$)	19

*The elastic and viscous parameters determined from rapid cystometry reflect the collagen/muscle ratio. The increase of the ratio is significantly higher in decentralized and sclerosed bladders (Student's *t*-test).

Effect of Bladder Decentralization. Following complete sacral (dorsoventral) rhizotomy in female dogs, there was a significant increase of viscoelastic coefficients and collagen/muscle ratio in the detrusor, with a 244 percent increase in collagen content in contrast to a 100 percent increase in muscle mass (*4,28*). An *in vitro* study of the decentralizated male dog bladder confirmed the above finding (*24*). In this study increased stiffness of the bladder wall (Fig 6–7) and predominant collagen infiltration associated with an increased number of smooth muscle nuclei were observed in all layers of the bladder wall.

It thus appears that decentralization of the bladder results in a drastic increase of the collagen/muscle ratio, so that the detrusor becomes a somewhat "rigid" structure. Viscoelastic parameters derived from rapid cystometry in such bladders reflect these changes, attesting to their probable clinical significance.

Effect of Other Factors. Conditions other than obstruction and decentralization may induce increased detrusor collagen content and thereby affect its biomechanical properties. Long-standing chronic infection or infestation of the bladder may lead to excessive collagen deposits in the detrusor, as exemplified (in severe form) by tuberculous or schistosomal cystitis (*30*). Aging may be another factor, although in men the collagen/muscle ratio in the detrusor decreases because of a proportionate increase in muscle mass (*1*). In some patients the etiology of structural detrusor abnormality is simply unkown. Although the exact mechanism of collagen deposition in the detrusor is not completely understood, it clearly has an important impact on detrusor biomechanical behavior.

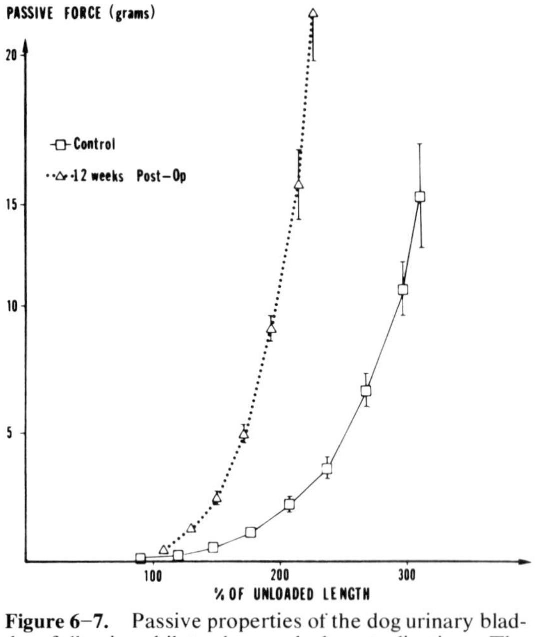

Figure 6–7. Passive properties of the dog urinary bladder following bilateral sacral decentralization. The increased collagen/muscle ratio accounts for the left shift of the curve due to significant detrusor stiffness. (From Ghoniem, G.M., *et al.: Neurourol. Urodynam.* 3:32–33, 1984. Copyright © Alan R. Liss, Inc., New York.)

Significance of Abnormal Detrusor Viscoelasticity

Relation Between Detrusor Viscoelasticity and Contractility. The previous paragraphs have shown that rapid cystometry allows one to derive elastic and viscous parameters that reflect the collagen/muscle ratio. It can be postulated that a high muscular content relative to collagen enhances detrusor contraction and vice versa. This postulate was actually verified experimentally in rabbit bladders; the upper body was found to be the most contractile part of the bladder and the base, rich in collagen, the least contractile (*23*). A number of other studies confirmed the observation that collagen deposition is associated with reduction of bladder contractility (*23,24,27,31*).

The mechanism by which collagen deposition reduces contractility is unclear, but morphologic studies point to a possible hypothesis. Because only one of seven to ten detrusor muscle cells is directly innervated, synchronized detrusor contraction is largely explained by electrotonic spread between cells at their intercellular junctions. One study supports this hypothesis (*32*). Three specimens obtained at the time of bladder surgery from heavily trabeculated bladders in older men were compared to seven from nontrabeculated detrusors. In trabeculated bladders, heavy collagen deposits occupied the intercellular spaces, enlarging, sometimes considerably, the distance between cells; cell junctions were absent. Furthermore, numerous fibroblasts were present, and muscle cells were hypertrophied. The effect that collagen deposits may have on detrusor contractility may thus become understandable; as collagen invades the bladder, cell junctions are lost, rendering nonfunctional the noninnervated muscle cells. These findings were confirmed by Gosling and Dixon (*33*).

It can thus be said that the "quality" of detrusor contraction depends in part on the collagen/muscle ratio. Conditions causing an increase in collagen, e.g., aging, obstruction, decentralization, and chronic inflammation, do indeed impair detrusor contractility. The proposed viscoelastic model of the bladder to some extent allows evaluation of collagen versus muscle in the bladder wall. Nevertheless, factors that reduce bladder contractility do not necessarily affect the collagen/muscle ratio (*22,34,35*).

Limitations of Rapid Cystometry. It was initially thought that rapid cystometry can be used to determine, at the clinical level, the amount of collagen relative to muscle and thereby analyze changes in muscular strength to determine the mechanical component of bladder compliance during filling. There is, however, a major obstacle to interpreting the results obtained clinically. Detrusor inflammation, so frequently encountered in patients on catheter drainage, may cause alteration of the mechanical model and render its results insignificant. The test therefore is applicable only to patients with no bladder inflammation.

In a study on 70 male patients, it appeared that rapid cystometry might be more useful as a clinical tool in the diagnosis of neurogenic vesical dysfunction (*18,36*). In patients with peripheral nerve lesions affecting the bladder, contractions of short amplitude and duration were always present, following the rapid rise in intravesical pressure (Fig. 6–8). Such contractions appeared only occasionally and were inconsistent in normal patients, but they were also observed in patients with prostatic obstruction who have detrusor distension and high residual urine, suggesting the vesical distension may lead to intramural "denervation."

VISCOELASTICITY OF THE URETHRA

Statement of the Problem

The urethra has some structural similarities to the bladder; it contains collagen, smooth muscle, and elastin. Its embryologic origin, geometry, and function, however, are markedly different from those of the bladder. The urethra is not a storage organ, and thus its distensibility is limited. Because the urethra carries a flow of liquid (urine) during micturition, the problem of assessing urethral mechanical properties has often been approached from the fluid dynamic point of view. Various techniques based on pressure/flow studies during voiding have been developed to derive a simple form of "urethral resistance" and thereby determine (indirectly) abnormal patterns of flow rate, e.g., in obstruction (*37,38*). It seems, however, that the flow of a liquid in a collapsible (compliant) tube such as the urethra involves interaction between liquid and solid.

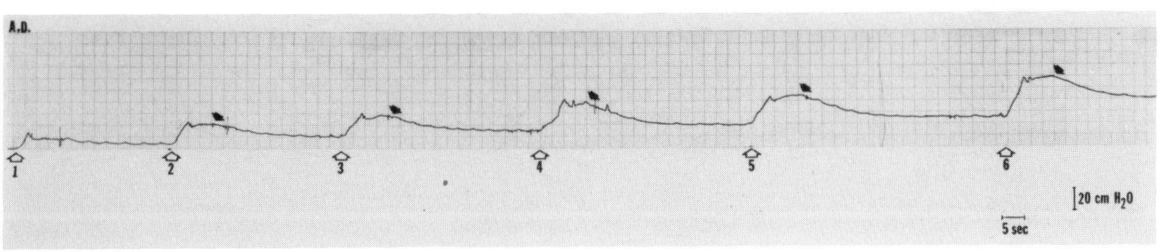

Figure 6–8. Rapid cystometry in a patient with a cauda equina lesion. An active contraction appears after every injection and becomes more pronounced as injections are repeated; these waves are characteristic of peripheral bladder "denervation." (From Susset, J., and Ghoniem, G.: *J. Urol.* 132:705–706, 1984. Copyright 1984, The Williams & Wilkins, Co., Baltimore.)

Theoretically, the quantitation of urethral viscoelastic behavior would allow one to derive various parameters and determine which segment or region along the urethra is mostly controlling (limiting) the outflow under particular conditions. In practical terms, little is known in this regard. We limit the scope of this section to a description of the various techniques that have been used to measure urethral compliance. Such a measurement provides quantitative data on urethral distensibility in the passive state. As in the bladder, relaxation, hysteresis, and creep experiments may be performed. They can be done using an appropriate device that, when inserted in the urethra, measures the mechanical properties. Clinical data are available, but their interpretation remains complex and has not reached the point where an appropriate mechanical model to derive and calculate viscoelastic parameters is possible.

Methods of Measurement

Catheters of Increasing Size. With one approach, urethral pressure is measured at various diameters. It can be done, for instance, using catheters of different size. A urethral pressure profile is performed with each catheter, according to the Brown and Wickham technique (*39*), and the pressures obtained from a given urethral location are reported on a graph plotted against catheter diameter. Several graphs may thus be obtained to "map" compliance along the urethra. For each location, a "compliance index" is calculated as the percentage of pressure change from one catheter size to another of a larger diameter; a high index corresponds to urethral rigidity.

Urethral compliance may also be measured using the multisize probe illustrated in Figure 6-9 (*40*); urethral pressure is successively recorded (typically from 5F to 25F, in 5F increments) as the catheter is advanced. The measurements are made at the striated sphincter level or as a complete profile. Data on urethral pressure are plotted against catheter diameter. Because the number of measurements are often greater than in the previous technique, the curve may be analyzed differently by fitting a mathematic equation to the recorded pressure values. This equation is characterized by two parameters that relate to urethral closure pressure and the rate at which pressure increases as higher diameters are introduced into the urethra.

Impedance Changes. Urethral wall "softness" can be measured using a special measuring catheter; the probe is made of plexiglass with two cone-shaped stainless steel electrodes (*41*). The principle of indirect compression between the electrodes is then used to detect abnormal rigidity. Compression of the tissue creates a change in the electrode area, which is detected by a change in the measured voltage between the elec-

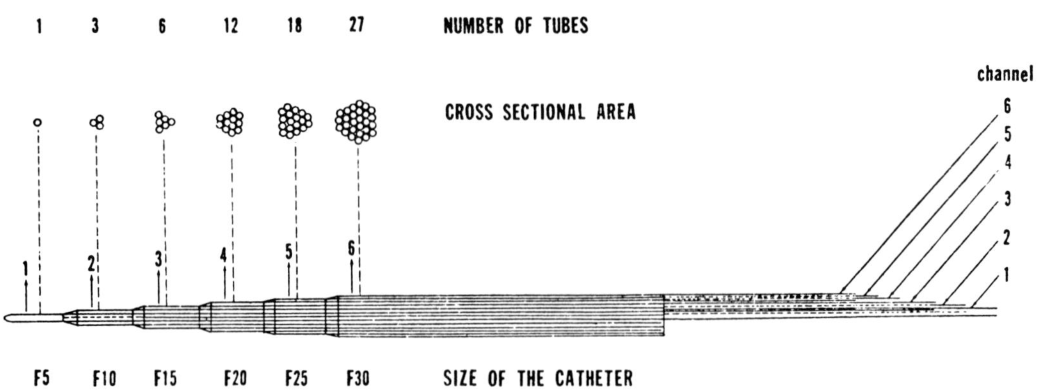

Figure 6–9. Measurement of urethral compliance using a multisize probe. Pressure is recorded at each diameter and reported on the pressure/diameter graph; data are analyzed in terms of the urethral closure pressure (catheter-free) and the rate of pressure increase as higher diameters are introduced into the urethra. (From Regnier, C.H., *et al.*: *J. Urol.* 129:1060–1062, 1983. Copyright © 1983, The Williams & Wilkins Co., Baltimore.)

trodes. In reality, this method measures the compliance of the urethral mucosa. It is likely, however, that a close relation exists between compliance of the whole urethral wall and mucosal softness, but it has not yet been demonstrated.

Related Values of Pressure and Cross-Sectional Area. The probe developed by Colstrup *et al.* allows recording of related values of pressure and cross-sectional area in the resting urethra (*42*). The probe consists of a 9F polyvinyl catheter with a small balloon that can be inflated at low pressures (Fig. 6–10). The cross-sectional area of the balloon is measured according to the field gradient principle (*43*). The probe is used in a manner that allows pressure to be increased in steps of 10 cm H_2O, distending the urethra up to a given value. Recordings can be performed at 5-mm steps along the urethra. Pressure can also be recorded as the balloon is deflated along the same steps as inflation, thereby obtaining hysteresis cycles.

Various parameters can be derived from the curves obtained with this technique to describe closure function in terms of urethral rigidity, outlet closure pressure of the noninstrumented urethra, capabilities of isometric and isotonic contraction, muscular function, and power of the closure mechanism.

Clinical Application of Urethral Compliance Measurements

Normal Urethral Compliance in Women. Urethral compliance was measured in young nulliparous female volunteers using a multisize probe (*40*). The measurements were made at the level of striated sphincter during its relaxation. The results showed that little increase in urethral pressure (range 60–80 cm H_2O) occurs for the size range of 5F to 25F. The urethra can easily "accommodate" increasing diameters in that range because of its viscoelasticity. With diameters larger than 25F, however, the urethral wall reaches its elastic limit, and the sphincter contracts, resulting in high pressures.

Abnormal Urethral Compliance in Female Incontinence. Two studies have reported abnormal urethral compliance in relation to incontinence in women. In a series of 160 female patients presenting with frequency (37%), nocturia (56%), difficulty of voiding (37%), and stress incontinence (55%) or urge incontinence (54%), the urethral pressure profile was measured successively with catheters of different size (Susset, unpublished data). An average of 40 percent of these patients had an abnormal compliance index (>25%); most of these presented with pure stress incontinence. On the other hand, 50 percent of the patients in that same series, who had an average of four childbirths, had an abnormally low pressure at 12F that did not increase at larger diameters; this was described as high urethral compliance (also called hyperlaxity). Urethral compliance was also found to decrease with age, which confirmed the fact that urethral pressure is lower in the older age group (*44*).

In a second series of 57 patients presenting with similar lower urinary tract symptoms, urethral compliance was measured

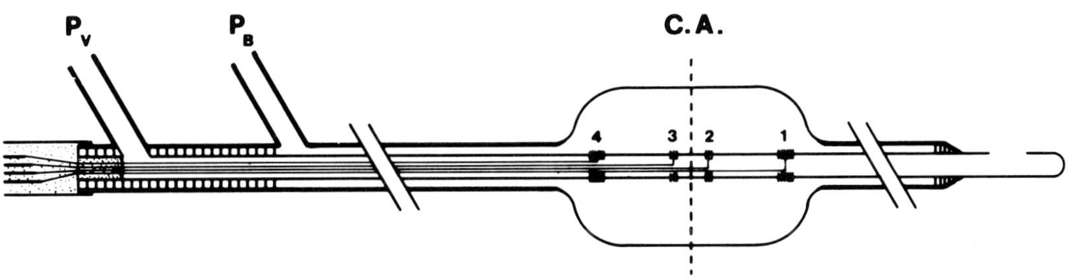

Figure 6–10. Probe used for measuring related values of intraurethral pressure, and cross-sectional area (*C.A.*) measured at the dotted line, based on the field gradient principle. Platen windings (*1* and *4*) are used as generating electrodes; detecting electrodes are marked *2* and *3*. Pressure in the balloon is measured at P_B and pressure in the bladder at P_V. Such recordings are useful to detect locally obstructive areas in the urethra. (From Colstrup, H., *et al.*: *J. Urol.*, 130:507–511, 1983. Copyright © 1983, The Williams & Wilkins Co., Baltimore.)

with a multisize probe (*45*). Fifty percent of the patients demonstrated urethral rigidity; the urethral closure pressure (catheter-free) was significantly lower than normal, and the rate of increase in pressure as the catheter diameter increased exceeded the normal range. Twenty percent of the patients in the same series demonstrated urethral hyperlaxity; the initial pressure was low, as in rigidity, but the rate of pressure did not differ significantly from normal.

It appears that the aforementioned two techniques for measurement of urethral compliance, based on the same principle of recording urethral pressure at different diameters, allow differentiation of two primary types of abnormal compliance, i.e., urethral rigidity and hyperlaxity. The results so far obtained have some clinical significance and indicate that abnormal compliance can be an important factor in female incontinence. Analysis of the data, however, remains incomplete and does not reflect differences in urethral geometry. It is possible that rigidity and hyperlaxity result from a common structural abnormality, e.g., collagen deposition, in which case the above results would mainly express changes in urethral geometry. Indeed, a rigid urethra may have a large caliber and present high pressures at diameters exceeding those used in the measurements. Pressure/diameter curves should be "normalized" acording to a "reference state" (diameter) at which the urethra becomes under tension. This parameter, however, would be arbitrary, may be inaccurate, and may introduce artifacts.

Distal Urethral Stenosis in Women. Meatal stenosis or abnormality can objectively be demonstrated by performing urethral pressure profiles with catheters of different size. Using this technique, an abnormal rise in distal urethral pressure may appear at a given diameter and increase proportionately with the size of the testing catheter.

In a series of 49 patients meatoplasty performed on the basis of abnormal distal urethral compliance gave good results in 80 percent of the patients (*46*). The operation consisted in resecting a V-shaped wedge of the urethral meatus from 3 to 9 o'clock. The length of resection was 5 to 10 mm, depending on the length of distal urethra with abnormal compliance as measured on the urethral pressure profile. It was concluded that such measurement is useful in the diagnosis of urethral stenosis and is more objective than the bougie à boule used to detect urethral stenosis by resistance encountered when pulling it out through the urethral meatus.

Mechanical Vesical Outlet Obstruction in Men. To detect locally obstructive areas of the urethral wall, it is preferable to define the relation between urethral pressure and cross-sectional area (*vide supra*). The technique of using catheters of different size does not allow such definition because the urethral wall is "forced" by the catheter to a precise diameter, and the pressure is read afterward. Although no data for the male urethra are available as yet, significant results obtained in normal women confirmed that changes in urethral pressure are not significant for cross-sectional areas that correspond to 5F to 25F catheter sizes (*47,48*).

The advantage of using the pressure/cross-sectional area relation is that it allows determination of regional values of "hydrostatic compliance," which is defined as the change in area for a given change in pressure. This problem was analyzed extensively in collapsible tubes subjected to unsteady fluid flow (*49,50*); the results were expressed by a theoretical law and were used to determine the segment or region along the tube that most controls (limits) fluid outflow under specific conditions.

Significance of Abnormal Urethral Compliance

Relation Between Flow Rate and Urethral Compliance. It is possible to hypothesize that impaired flow rate in women is due to an insufficient urethral opening secondary to structural rigidity. Indeed, a rigid tube neither opens nor closes well, thereby preventing its proper funneling during micturition. The mechanism by which rigidity occurs, however, is not completely clear.

In young women the urethra has sufficient elasticity to become funneled smoothly during micturition. Because the urethra is of the same embryologic origin as the vagina, it is understandable that E_2-hypoestrogenism (e.g., during and after menopause) may change the urethra in the same manner as it affects the vagina. Tissue dryness and collagen deposits resulting in tissular rigidity may therefore occur in the urethra, preventing normal urethral funneling with subsequent relative obstruction of urinary flow. Similar changes may occur as a result of chronic urethritis. The distal female urethra is known to have outlying glands (Skene's glands) that are the homologue of the prostate. It is possible that the abnormal estrogenic milieu of menopause can induce sufficient "enlargement" of these glands to cause urethral "obstruction." Although acute urethritis is rare in women, it can be assumed that chronic nonspecific urethritis is common. It is likely that fibrosis is the end result of the chronic inflammatory process, with poor urethral opening due to the resultant tissue rigidity. Although this idea has not been confirmed, it remains a probability. Periurethral or vaginal surgery is yet another cause of periurethral fibrosis that may affect voiding similarly.

The etiology of urethral hyperlaxity in women is not clear. Multiparity is a known cause of muscular "decompensation," which in turn may explain abnormal urethral "tone." Urethral muscular decompensation or hypotonia may be manifested by a dilated urethra on radiographic films taken at peak flow during a voiding cystourethrogram (*51*); in such a case the flow rate is better than normal because the urethra is widely opened. Periurethral muscles may also decompensate as a result of aging, resulting in high compliance. In men, outlet obstruction is likely to reduce urethral compliance of the urethral wall, but the lack of clinical studies obviates any meaningful conclusion in this regard.

Urethral Compliance as a Factor in Female Incontinence. Of 200 female patients presenting with incontinence or "urethral syndrome," a large number had a reduced flow rate; urethral dilatation or internal urethrotomy in such cases resulted in significant improvement of the flow rate as well as alleviation of the symptoms (*51*). Postoperative improvement in flow rate and symptoms was confirmed in another study on 300 flow curves prior to, and 500 curves 3 to 12 months following, urethral dilatation or urethrotomy (*52*). Improvement was less in patients who had undergone periurethral surgery.

Urethral dilatation, internal urethrotomy, and meatotomy have been performed for years in most women presenting with what has been called the urethral syndrome. This term, however, has been loosely defined, without any real attempt to define its exact pathogenesis; many such patients were considered psychotic. Indications for the operative procedures often were purely empirical and carried out at random with a high rate of failure.

The fact remains that abnormal urethral compliance does occur in women. It is important that urethral rigidity is assessed before proposing or ruling out any treatment, even urethral dilatation. Measurement of urethral compliance by one of the above-described techniques can provide the urologist with information on which to base sound therapeutic recommendations. It should be emphasized, however, that neither disease nor syndrome is the result of a single factor, especially in women with voiding dysfunctions, and that all etiologic factors that are known or even suspected must be evaluated carefully before therapeutic recommendations are made.

REFERENCES

1. Susset, J. G., Servot-Viguier, D., Lamy, F., Madernas, P., and Black, R.: Collagen in 155 human bladders. *Invest. Urol.* 16:204–206, 1978.
2. Ruegg, J. C.: Smooth muscle tone. *Physiol. Rev.* 51:1, 1971.
3. Kondo, A., Susset, J. G., and Lefaivre, J.: Viscoelastic properties of bladder. I. Mechanical model and its mathematical analysis. *Invest. Urol.* 10:154–163, 1972.
4. Kondo, A., and Susset, J. G.: Viscoelastic properties of bladder. II. Comparative studies in normal and pathologic dogs. *Invest. Urol.* 11:459–465, 1974.
5. Kondo, A., and Susset, J. G.: Physical properties of the urinary detrusor muscle: a mechanical model based upon the analysis of stress relaxation curve. *J. Biomech.* 6:141–151, 1973.
6. Alexander, R.: Mechanical properties of urinary bladder. *Am. J. Physiol.* 220:1413, 1971.
7. Alexander, R : Viscoplasticity of smooth muscle of urinary bladder. *Am. J. Physiol.* 224:618, 1973.
8. Coolsaet, B. L. R. A., Van Duyl, W. A., van Mastrigt, R., and van Der Zwart, A.: Stepwise cystometry of urinary bladder. *Urology* 2:255–257, 1973.
9. Coolsaet, B. L. R. A., Van Duyl, W. A., van Mastrigt,

R., and Van Der Zwart, A.: Viscoelastic properties of the bladder wall. *Urol. int.* 30:16–26, 1975.
10. Coolsaet, B. L. R. A., Van Duyl, W. A., van Mastrigt, R., and Huygen, R. E.: Viscoelastic properties of bladder wall strips at constant elongation. *Invest. Urol.* 13:435–440, 1976.
11. Van Mastrigt, R., Coolsaet, B. L. R. A., and Van Duyl, W. A.: Passive properties of the urinary bladder in the collection phase. *Med. Biol. Eng. Comp.* 16:471, 1978.
12. Apter, J., Mason, P., and Lang, G.: Urinary bladder wall dynamics. *Invest. Urol.* 9:520, 1972.
13. Pipkin, A. C.: Non-linear phenomena in continua. In: *Non-linear Continuum Theories in Mechanics and Physics and Their Applications.* Edizioni Tremonese, Rome, 1970, pp. 51–150.
14. Regnier, C. H., Kolsky, H., Richardson, P. D., Ghoniem, G. M., and Susset, J. G.: The elasticity of the urinary bladder for large deformations. In Saha, S. (ed.), *Biomedical Engineering; Recent Developments.* Pergamon Press, Oxford, 1982, pp. 183–186.
15. Regnier, C. H., Kolsky, H., Richardson, P. D., Ghoniem, G.M and Susset, J. G.: The elastic behavior of the urinary bladder for large deformations. *J. Biomech.* 16:915–922, 1983.
16. Fung, Y. C.: *Biomechanics. Mechanical Properties of Living Tissues.* Springer-Verlag, Berlin, 1981, pp. 12–13.
17. Fung, Y. C.: Biorheology of soft tissues. *Biorheology* 10:139–155, 1973.
18. Susset, J. G., Ghoniem, G. M., and Regnier, C. H.: Rapid cystometry in males. *Neurourol. Urodyn.* 1:319–327, 1982.
19. Susset, J. G., and Regnier, C. H.: Viscoelastic properties of bladder strips: standardization of a technique. *Invest. Urol.* 18:445–450, 1981.
20. Ghoniem, G. M., Regnier, C. H., Biancani, P., and Susset, J. G.: Receptor changes of rat urinary bladder after estradiol treatment and/or castration. In *Proceedings 78th Annual AUA Meeting,* Las Vegas, 1983.
21. Ghoniem, G. M., Regnier, C. H., Biancani, P., Johnson, L., and Susset, J. G.: Morphology, contractility, and pharmacology studies in parasympathetically denervated dog bladders. In *Proceedings 13th Annual ICS Meeting,* Aachen, 1983.
22. Ghoniem, G. M., Regnier, C. H., Biancani, P., and Susset, J. G.: Effect of diethylstilbestrol on bladder contractility in male rats. *J. Urol.* 129:865–868, 1983.
23. Ghoniem, G. M., Regnier, C. H., Biancani, P., Johnson, L., and Susset, J. G.: Effect of vesical outlet obstruction on detrusor contractility and passive properties in rabbits. *J. Urol.* 1985, 135: 1284–1289.
24. Ghoniem, G. M., Regnier, C. H., Biancani, P., Johnson, L., and Susset, J. G.: Effect of bilateral sacral decentralization on detrusor contractility and passive properties in dogs. *Neurourol. Urodyn.* 3:23–33, 1984.
25. Kondo A.: Viscoelastic Properties of the Bladder. *Ph.D. thesis.* University of Sherbrooke, Canada, 1971.
26. Woessner, J. F.: The determination of hydroxyproline in tissue and protein samples containing small proportions of this amino acid. *Arch. Biochem. Biophys.* 93:440, 1961.
27. Uvelius, B., Persson, L., and Mattiasson, A.: Smooth muscle cell hypertrophy and hyperplasia in the rat detrusor after short-time infravesical outflow obstruction. *J. Urol.* 131:173–176, 1984.
28. Kondo, A., and Susset, J. G.: Collagen content in detrusor muscle and ratio of bladder weight to body weight. *Acta Urol. Jpn.* 9:683–687, 1973.
29. Brent, L., and Stephens, F. D.: The response of smooth muscle cells in the rabbit urinary bladder to outflow obstruction. *Invest. Urol.* 12:494–502, 1975.
30. Mayo, M. E., and Hinman, F.: Structure and function of the rabbit bladder altered by chronic obstruction or cystitis. *Invest. Urol.* 14:6–9, 1976.
31. Mattiasson, A., and Uvelius, B.: Changes in contractile properties in hypertrophic rat urinary bladder. *J. Urol.* 128:1340, 1982.
32. Clermont, A.: Etude Ultrastructurale du Muscle Vésical Chez L'Homme. M.D. thesis, University of Nice, France, 1976.
33. Gosling, J. A., and Dixon, J. S.: Structural changes associated with obstruction of the urinary tract: a comparison between upper and lower systems. In Zinner, N. R., and Sterling, A. M. (eds.), *Female Incontinence.* Alan R. Liss, New York, 1981, pp. 283–284.
34. Levin, R. M., Shofer, F. S., and Wein, A. J.: Estrogen-induced alterations in the autonomic responses of the rabbit urinary bladder. *J. Pharm. Exp. Ther.* 215:614–618, 1980.
35. Levin, R. M., Brendler, K., Van Arsdalen, K. N., and Wein, A. J.: Functional response of the rabbit urinary bladder to anoxia and ischemia. *Neurourol. Urody.* 2:233–244, 1983.
36. Susset, J. G., and Ghoniem, G. M.: Rapid cystometry and sacral evoked response in the diagnosis of peripheral bladder and sphincter denervation. *J. Urol.* 132:704–707, 1984.
37. Schäfer, W.: The contribution of the bladder outlet to the relation between pressure and flow rate during micturition. In Hinman, F., (ed.), *Benign Prostatic Hypertrophy.* Springer-Verlag, New York, 1983, pp. 470–496.
38. Griffiths, D.: *Urodynamics. The Mechanics and Hydrodynamics of the Lower Urinary Tract.* Adam Hilger, Bristol, 1980.
39. Brown, M., and Wickham, W. E.: The urethral pressure profile. *Br. J. Urol.* 51:211–214, 1969.
40. Regnier, C. H:, Susset, J. G., Ghoniem, G. M., and Biancani, P.: A new catheter to measure urethral compliance in females: normal values. *J. Urol.* 129:1060–1062, 1983.
41. Plevnik, S., and Vrtacnik, P.: How to measure inner urethral wall softness? In Zinner, N. R., and Sterling, A. M. (eds.), *Female Incontinence* Alan R. Liss, New York, 1981, pp. 253–258.
42. Colstrup, H., Mortensen, S. O., and Kristensen, J. K.: A new method for the investigation of the closure function of the resting female urethra. *J. Urol.* 130:507–511, 1983.
43. Mortensen, S., Djurhuus, J. C., and Rask-Andersen, H.: A system for measurement of micturition urethral cross-sectional areas and pressures. *Med. Biol. Eng. Comput.* 21:482, 1983.

44. Edwards, L., and Malvern, J.: The urethral pressure profile:theoretical considerations and clinical application. *Br. J. Urol.* 46:325, 1976.
45. Susset, J. G., Regnier, C. H., and Ghoniem, G. M.: Abnormal urethral compliance in females; diagnosis, results and treatment: preliminary study. *J. Urol.* 129:1063–1065, 1983.
46. Susset, J. G., Regnier, C. H.: Compliance anormale de l'urèthre distal chez la femme. In *Procedings 8th Annual Société Internationale Francophone d'uro-Dynamique Meeting,* Bordeaux, France, 1985.
47. Colstrup, H.: Rigidity of the resting female urethra. I. Static measurements. *J. Urol.* 132:78–81, 1984.
48. Colstrup, H.: Rigidity of the resting female urethra. II. Dynamic measurements. *J. Urol.* 132:82–86, 1984.
49. Shapiro, A.: Steady flow in collapsible tubes. *J. Biomech. Eng.* 99:126–147, 1977.
50. Kamm, R., and Shapiro, A.: Unsteady flow in a collapsible tube subjected to external pressure or body forces. *J. Fluid Mech.* 95:1–78, 1979.
51. Susset, J. G., Shoukry, I., Schlaeder, G., Cloutier, D., and Dutartre, D.: Stress incontinence and urethral obstruction in women: values of uroflowmetry and voiding urethrography. *J. Urol.* 120:504–513, 1974.
52. Susset, J. G., Toppercer, A., Ghoniem, G. M., and Regnier, C. H.: Objective basis for urethral dilatation, internal urethrotomy or meatotomy in females. In *Proceedings 76th Annual AUA Meeting,* Boston, 1981, p. 154.

7

Basic Research Models and Methods in Neuromuscular Studies of the Lower Urinary Tract

ROBERT M. LEVIN, Ph.D., S. BRUCE MALKOWICZ, M.D., AND ALAN J. WEIN, M.D.

In urology, as in other clinical specialties, there has been significantly increased interest in applied basic research—as indicated by the marked increase in the number of basic research studies presented at American Urological Association meetings. This increased interest of clinical urologists in basic science is reflected also by the increase in the number of basic scientists holding appointments in urology departments.

It is the purpose of this chapter to present information on basic research techniques and animal models that are presently utilized for the study of neuromusculature of the lower urinary tract. It is hoped that this information will be useful to the academic urologist who has an interest in developing an animal research program in this area.

We first present a general classification of basic research models followed by a detailed discussion of one or two examples from each classification. Following this methodologic section, we discuss methods of data anaylsis and presentation.

There are four major species utilized for research purposes: dog, cat, rabbit, and rat. Each has specific advantages and disadvantages to their use. The urinary bladders of the cat and dog are structurally similar to that of man. The urinary bladders of the rat and rabbit are thin-walled structures and contain significantly less connective tissue than do those of the cat, dog, or man. The cost of cats and dogs ($150–250 each) and the space required to house these species prevent their use in research projects that require large numbers of research animals. The rat is a popular species for research purposes, but the small size of the bladder in rats prevents its functional evaluation. The rabbit has a moderately large bladder (65-ml capacity), the cost is reasonably low ($15 each), and rabbits can be stored in large quantities in most animal facilities. Thus the rabbit is becoming an increasingly attractive research animal for urologic projects.

There are four major subdivisions of research models presently utilized in urological research.

1. *In vivo whole animal preparations.* These models are used to study the neurophysiology of the intact bladder. Such models have the advantage of preserving intact central innervation to the bladder and are widely utilized for identifying spinal and supraspinal reflexes involved in the control of micturition. In addition, these preparations are used to determine the effects of specific drugs on intravesical pressure generation and voiding function. The mechanisms of drug action include both direct effect on the urinary tract smooth muscle and reflex action via the neuronal innervation.

2. *In vitro bladder-strip and whole-bladder preparations.* The bladder is excised from the experimental animal and suspended in an isolated muscle bath. These preparations are

utilized for determining the response of the isolated smooth muscle to specific pharmacologic agonists and antagonists, electric field stimulation, and metabolic inhibitors. Although these preparations are devoid of extrinsic neuronal innervation, the neuronal synapses and intramuscular neuronal elements are still present. Thus the response of this preparation to pharmacologic and electric stimulation (and inhibition) can be attibuted to direct action on the smooth muscle elements, indirect action via effects on the neuronal synapses, and local neuronal elements.

3. *Tissue homogenates or subcellular membrane preparations.* With these techniques bladder tissue from specific regions of the urinary tract are homogenized in physiologic buffers, and subcellular membrane fractions are obtained by differential centrifugation. These homogenates and membrane preparations are utilized to determine the presence of specific autonomic receptors, the content of specific substances such as neurohumoral transmitters, intracellular ATP, and neuropeptides, the specific activities of a variety of enzymes, etc.

4. *Histologic and histochemical preparations.* For these studies specific regions of the urinary tract are excised and fixed by a variety of specific techniques for histologic study. Such studies include: light microscopy for identification of gross cellular and subcellular structure; histochemistry and histofluorescence for identification and location of adrenergic and cholinergic innervation; immunohistofluorescence for the identification and location of specific neuropeptides such as substance P, endorphins, and vasoactive intestinal polypeptide (VIP); and electron microscopy for the identification of subcellular structures.

IN VIVO WHOLE-ANIMAL PREPARATIONS

All of the previously mentioned species have been employed for *in vivo* studies; however, the cat and dog have been more often utilized because of their size, general heartiness, and the wealth of background information that exists in regard to their neuroanatomy, neurophysiology, and urodynamics.

Cats and dogs are now moderately expensive depending on the purchase source and local regulatory control; therefore these species are not suitable for screening-type experiments, which require a large number of animals. Their central and peripheral neuroanatomy is well defined, and their pelvic neuroanatomic structures are relatively easy to isolate intraoperatively. These animals can be well controlled on inhalational anesthetics via intubation or tracheostomy. This form of anesthesia also allows better control of oxygenation and ventilation. Although inhalational anesthesia is superior, both cats and dogs can tolerate unintubated intravenous barbiturate anesthesia without difficulty.

The anatomic structure of the urologic organs of the dog and cat more closely resemble those of man than do the same organs of the rat and rabbit. In addition, the autonomic nerves that innervate the bladder are easily accessible to surgical isolation and modification. Hence these species have been extensively utilized to investigate the neurophysiology of bladder control and function (1–3). Because of the size of these animals isolation of specific autonomic and spinal nerves is feasible, whereas the rat and rabbit are too small for these studies.

Catheterization of the carotid and femoral arteries and veins is technically easy and can be utilized for blood pressure monitoring and drug administration. It is helpful to monitor respiration during surgical procedures and to maintain the animal's body temperature with a heating pad.

Although it can be performed, bladder catheterization of the male cat is often difficult and can be obviated if the study design permits placement of a transducer catheter through the bladder body followed by adequate stabilization using suture ligatures. When employed, Silastic pediatric Foley catheters (6–10F) are durable and easily incorporated into an intravesical pressure monitoring system.

In neuropharmacologic studies the cat has been extensively utilized for identifying the spinal reflexes that control bladder function. In this regard, access to the spinal cord is obtained through a standard laminectomy incision. When both abdominal and dorsal exposures are necessary, the animal can tolerate long-standing placement on its side. Specific electrophysiologic techniques are described in the references of other reports (*1–3*).

When studying pressure–volume relations relative to various physiologic or pharmacologic manipulations, it should be noted that the method and rate of fluid instillation can affect the cystometric curve obtained. Intermittent rapid filling of the bladder, although time-saving, results in steep curves and can easily initiate spontaneous sustained contractions. Slow continuous filling through a Harvard pump system affords the advantages of semiautomation, reproducibility, and a lesser incidence of sustained spontaneous contractions (*4*). Urethral dynamics may also be studied in the cat. A variety of catheters with lateral perfusion sites may be employed as well as transducer-tipped pressure catheters. Catheter withdrawal may be accomplished manually or mechanically (*5,6*).

Studies that involve measuring the response of the intact bladder to pharmacologic agents must take several factors into account when analyzing the data: (a) method of administration; (b) absorption and distribution of the drug; (c) penetration of the blood–brain barrier; (d) reflex actions via activation of spinal or supraspinal reflexes; (e) reflex actions via cardiovascular effects; and (f) activity of metabolic products of metabolism. The above factors limit the ability to perform accurate dose-response curves in the intact preparation (*7,8*).

IN VITRO BLADDER-STRIP AND WHOLE-BLADDER PREPARATIONS

Muscle-Strip Preparation

Although muscle-strip preparations can be used with any of the four species of experimental animal, cat and dog bladders are rather thick structures and often produce inconsistent results. Moreover, the high expense of these species makes them financially impractical for studies requiring a large number of animals.

The bladders from the rat and rabbit are thin-walled structures and are well suited for isolated strip preparations. The relatively inexpensiveness for these species allows their use for screening studies. The rat bladder can be separated into at most three strips: one strip from the bladder base and two from the bladder dome. Each rabbit bladder can be easily separated into six to eight strips: two from the bladder base and four to six from the bladder dome. A detailed description of the rabbit preparation is given below (*9–11*).

Male New Zealand white rabbits (2.5 kg) are anesthetized with intramuscular ketamine/xylazine (25 mg ketamine, 6 mg xylazine per kilogram). The urinary bladder is removed rapidly and dissected free of fat and serosa. Longitudinal smooth muscle strips of bladder body and base (1.0 X 0.5 cm) are placed in individual muscle baths containing 30 ml of Tyrode's solution (NaCl 125 mM, KCl 2.7 mM, NaH_2PO_4 0.4 mM, $CaCl_2$ 1.8 mM, $MgCl_2$ 0.5 mM, and $NaHCO_3$ 23.8 mM) and glucose (1 mg/ml) equilibrated with a gas mixture of 95% O_2/5% CO_2 and maintained at 37°C. Contractility is monitored with a Grass force displacement transducer connected to a four-channel Beckman recorder.

After equilibrating for 20 minutes, a tension of 1.0 gm is placed on each strip and the strips are maintained in the oxygenated buffer for an additional 10 minutes. Drugs dissolved in deionized water are added in 50-μl aliquots. Dose-response curves to specific pharmacologic agents are generated via the cumulative addition of drug to the muscle bath at 5-minute intervals. Drug concentrations are expressed as the total concentration in the bath with a minimum of six concentrations for each curve.

It is important to note that the responses one gets depends on several factors, e.g., the location of the bladder strip (base or body), the direction from which the strip is taken (longitudinal or horizontal), and the length of the strip. It is important to be internally consistent in these factors. Figures 7–1 to 7–5 display the contractile response of sequential strips (from bladder base to bladder body) of rabbit bladder to the following specific autonomic agonists: methoxamine (alpha-adrenergic), isoproterenol (beta-adrenergic), epinephrine (alpha- and beta-adrenergic), bethanechol (muscarinic cholinergic), and ATP (purinergic) (*10*). Table 7–1 gives the pharmacologic characteristics of a variety of

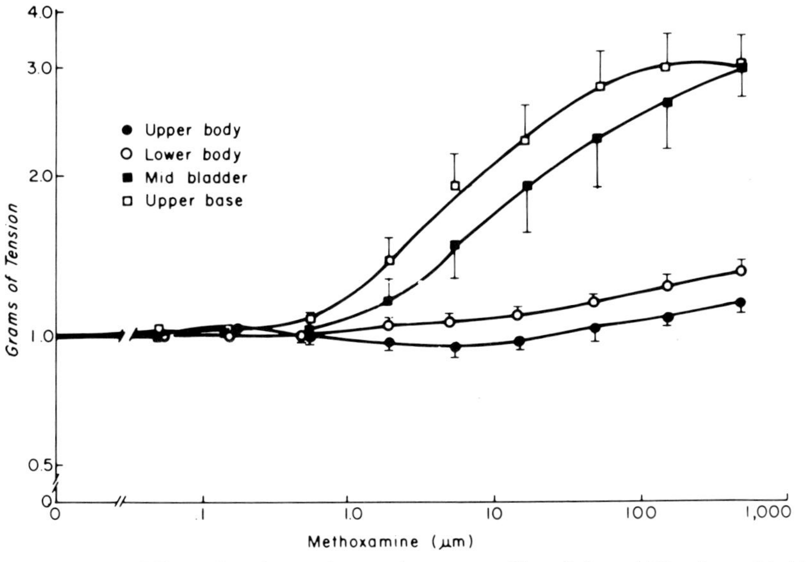

Figure 7–1. Effect of methoxamine on the contractility of the rabbit urinary bladder.

specific drugs utilized to either stimulate or inhibit smooth muscle strips.

From these studies it is clear that the response observed for bladder strips depends on the site from which the strip was taken. The bladder body responds preferentially to beta-adrenergic, muscarinic cholinergic, and purinergic stimulation, whereas the bladder base responds preferentially to alpha-adrenergic stimulation.

The muscle strip preparation can also be used to study the contractile response to both field and direct electric stimulation (*14,15*). Field stimulation is produced by placing the electrodes on either side of the tissue and then stimulating between the electrodes. The tissue responds with a strong contraction. This contraction is mediated by a combination of the release of neurohumoral transmitters by synaptic nerve endings

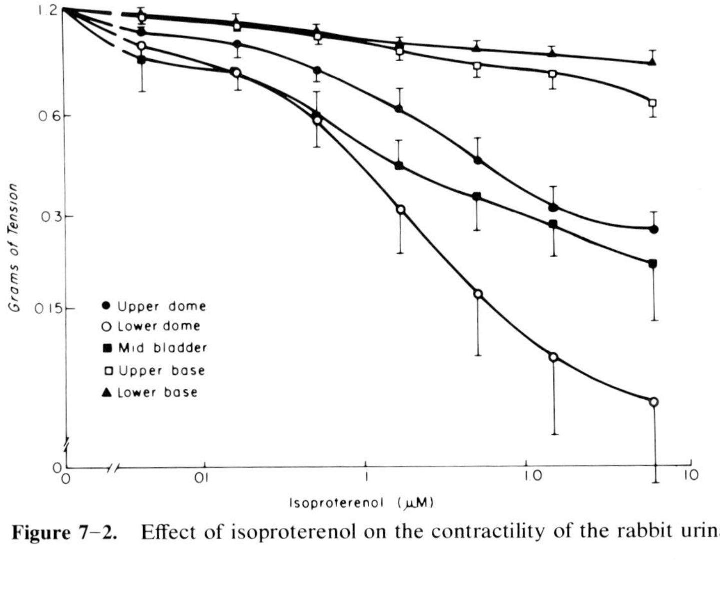

Figure 7–2. Effect of isoproterenol on the contractility of the rabbit urinary bladder.

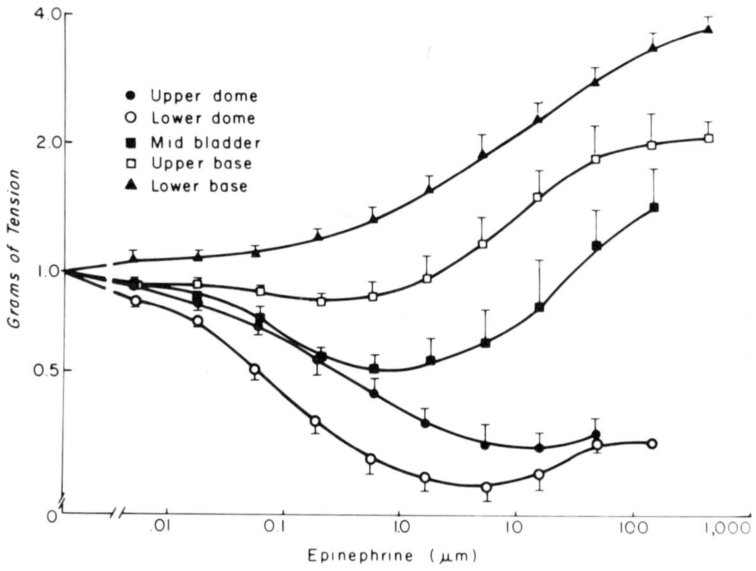

Figure 7–3. Effect of epinephrine on the contractility of the rabbit urinary bladder.

and by direct depolarization of the smooth muscle fibers. Through the use of specific neurohumoral antagonists and by altering the electric parameters, one can demonstrate a nonadrenergic, noncholinergic component of bladder contraction that is not a result of direct muscle stimulation (*15*). Tetrodotoxin, one of the most potent poisons known, specifically inhibits neuronal action potentials by blocking the sodium channels of excitable membranes. Using a dose of tetrodotoxin that does not inhibit direct muscle stimulation but completely inhibits nerve stimulation, Downie and Dean (*15*) demonstrated that low-frequency field stimulation of bladder muscle stimulated contraction via the activation of intramural nerve fibers. This contractile response is believed to be mediated by the release of a specific neurotransmitter substance, possibly ATP (purinergic). Direct

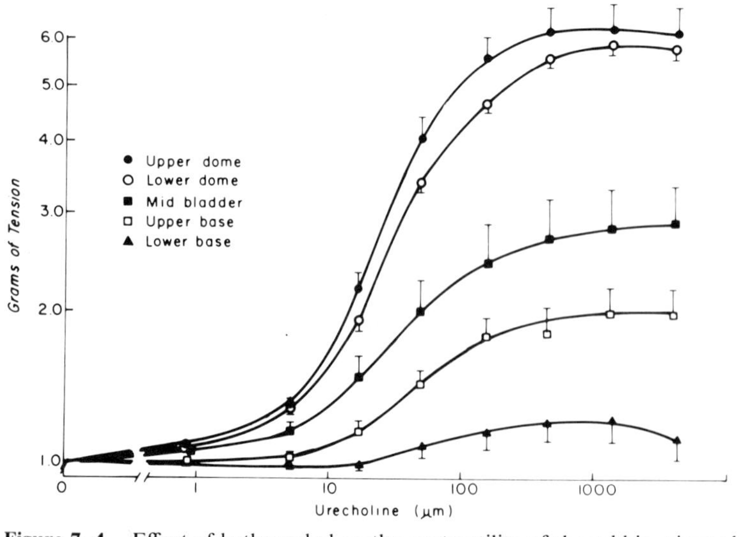

Figure 7–4. Effect of bethanechol on the contractility of the rabbit urinary bladder.

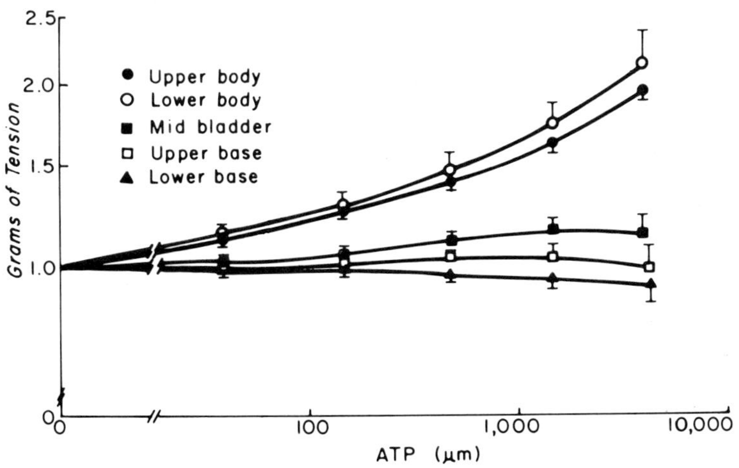

Figure 7–5. Effect of ATP on the contractility of the rabbit urinary bladder.

stimulation is produced by placing the electrodes on the smooth muscle strips and stimulating the muscle.

Whole-Bladder Preparation

Muscle strip preparations generate significant information on the contractile response of specific bladder sections to pharmacologic agents. One major limitation of these methods is that they provide no functional information on bladder integrity. It was to overcome this limitation that we developed the whole-bladder model of bladder function (*16,17*).

The bladder of an anesthetized rabbit is exposed through a midline incision, the ureters tied, and the bladder excised as low on the urethra as possible. The bladder is

Table 7–1. Pharmacologic Agents Utilized in Isolated Bath Techniques

DRUG	CLASSIFICATION	ACTION ON THE BLADDER
Methoxamine	Alpha-adrenergic agonist	Stimulates contraction
Isoproterenol	Beta-adrenergic agonist	Reduces isometric tension
Norepinephrine	Alpha- and beta-adrenergic agonist	Contracts bladder base, reduces tension of body
Epinephrine	Alpha- and beta adrenergic agonist	Contracts bladder base, reduces tension of body
Bethanechol	Muscarinic cholinergic agonist	Stimulates contraction
ATP	Putative purinergic agonist	Stimulates contraction
Phentolamine	Alpha-adrenergic blocker	Antagonizes alpha stimulation
Propranolol	Beta-adrenergic blocker	Antagonizes beta stimulation
Atropine	Muscarinic blocker	Antagonizes muscarinic stimulation
Imipramine	Blocks norepinephrine uptake	Increases response to norepinephrine
	Direct smooth muscle relaxant	Decreases isometric tension: inhibits contractile response to bethanechol
Physostigmine	Inhibits acetylcholinesterase	Increases response to acetylcholine
Tetrodotoxin	Inhibits nerve stimulation via inhibition of sodium channels	Inhibits neuronally mediated field-stimulated contraction
Diltiazem	Inhibits calcium channels	Inhibts contractile effects of drugs
Nifedipine	Inhibits calcium channels	Inhibits contractile effects of drugs
Verapamil	Inhibits calcium channels	Inhibits contractile effects of drugs

emptied and the urethra cannulated with a saline-filled transducer-tipped catheter. The bladder is mounted in a 300-ml isolated bath chamber containing Tyrode's solution equilibrated with 95% O_2/5% CO_2 and maintained at 37°C (Fig. 7–6).

As shown in Figure 7–6, the catheter is connected by way of a three-way valve to either a saline-filled graduated burette, which can be rapidly moved up or down, or a saline-filled bag resting on top of an electronic pan balance. The balance is mounted on a platform that can also be raised or lowered. With the valve open to the burette, the level of saline in the burette is set at the same level as the bladder base; at this point the pressure is set at zero (volume = 0). After a 30-minute equilibrium period, the burette is raised in 10-ml (6 cm) increments. After each increment the bladder is allowed to equilibrate as the saline enters (5 minutes). At equilibrium the volume that entered the bladder and the pressure are recorded. Using this methodology the volume–pressure relation (cystometry) for the isolated bladder can be determined, which is of course independent of all neuronal influences (Fig. 7–7).

For pharmacologic studies one of two systems can be used.

1. *Closed system.*" The bladder is filled to a specific volume by raising the burette as described above. After equilibration at the specific volume, the three-way valve is rotated so that the bladder is "closed" to the burette or saline bag. Thus bladder volume cannot change. The drug is then added to the bath in a cumulative manner at 5-minute intervals. In this system the volume of the bladder cannot change, and thus isometric (isovolumic) contraction is measured as a rise in intravesicular pressure.

2. *Expulsion system.* The bladder is filled to a specific volume by raising the burette as previously described. After equilibration the burette valve is closed and the saline-filled expulsion tube is connected to the system as pictured in Figure 7–6. The top of the saline reservoir bag is set equal to the saline level in the burette, thereby maintaining the same pressure in the system. The bladder is opened to the saline bag so that saline can move freely between the bladder and the bag. Drugs are then added to the bath as previously described. In this system the static pressure is constant, and smooth muscle response to pharmacologic agents is reflected in a change in bladder volume. These changes in bladder volume are re-

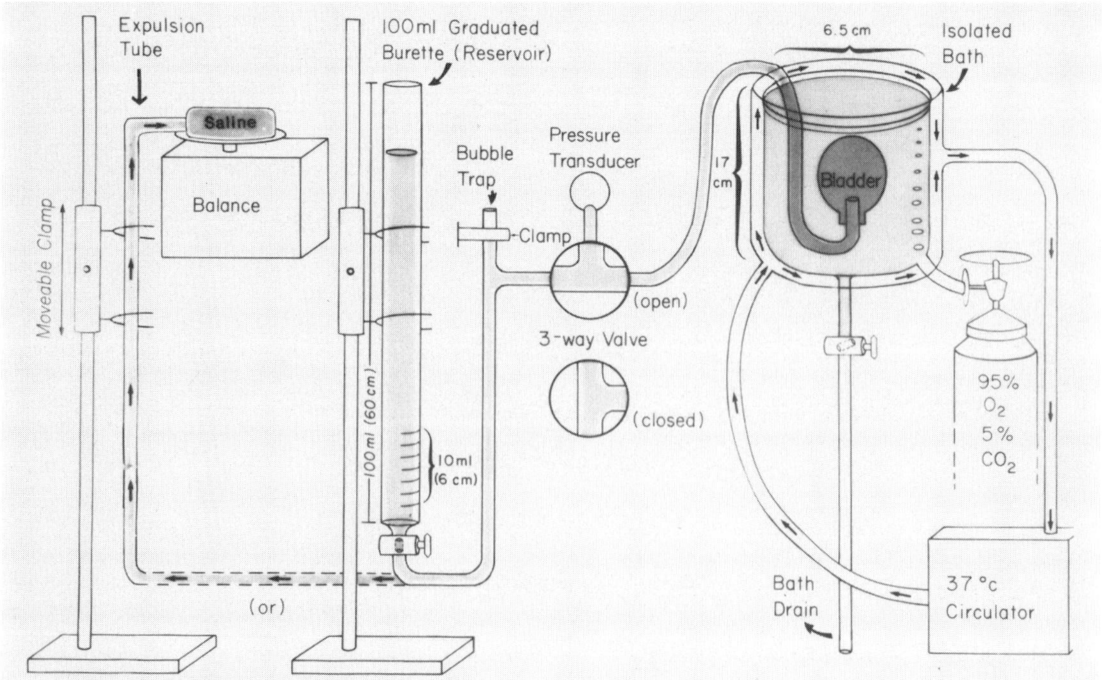

Figure 7–6. Whole-bladder apparatus.

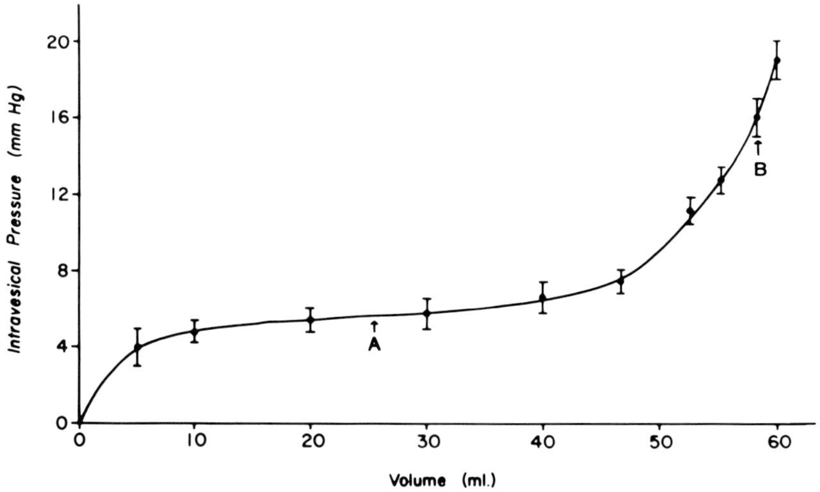

Figure 7–7. Volume–pressure relation of the whole-bladder model.

flected in changes in the weight of the saline bag. The digital electronic balance is connected via an analog converter to a Grass polygraph and recorded along with the intravesical pressure.

The following is a brief summary of the comparison of the whole-bladder model with the isolated strip. Using the closed system (in which the volume is constant), bethanechol produced a dose-response curve (Fig. 7–8) that is similar to the response of isolated strips (both having similar ED_{50} values). The maximum effect of several agents is presented in Figure 7–9. Isoproterenol, which produces a marked relaxant effect on isolated strips, produced only a mild decrease in intravesical pressure.

Using the expulsion system at low and intermediate volumes (which allows the bladder to change volume in response to drugs), bethanechol completely emptied the bladder at concentrations significantly lower than the concentration required for maximum pres-

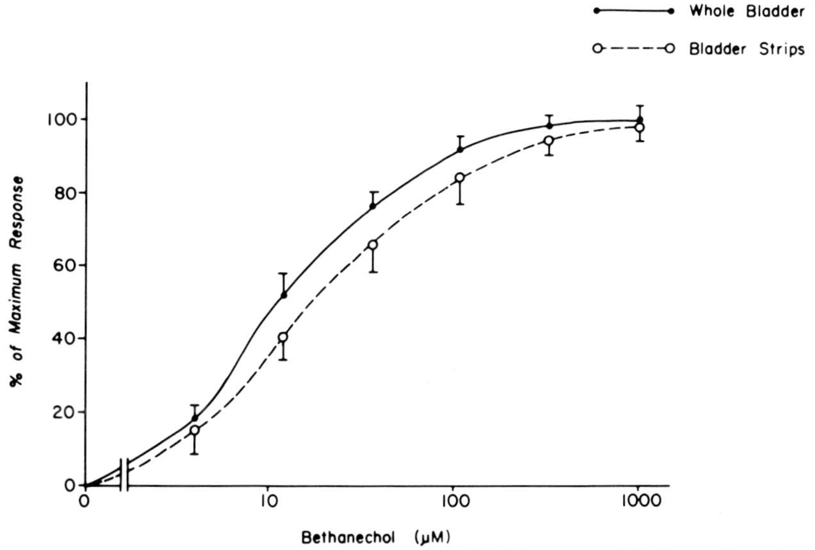

Figure 7–8. Effect of bethanechol in the whole bladder versus bladder strips (closed system).

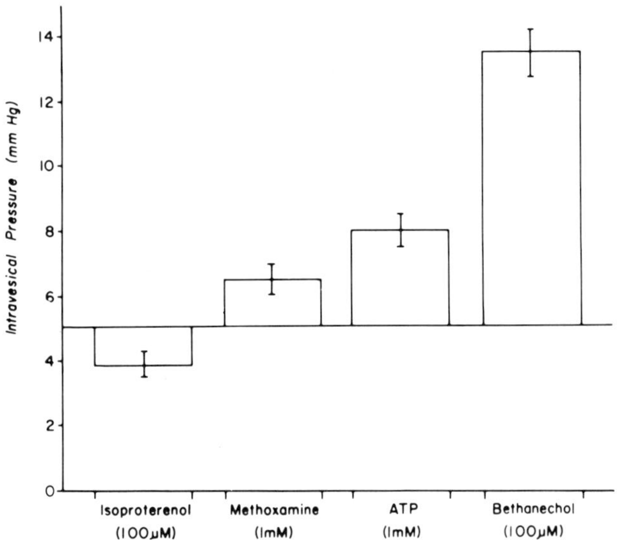

Figure 7–9. Effect of autonomic agonists in the whole-bladder model.

sure generation (Fig. 7–10). Whereas isoproterenol produced only a mild decrease in intravesical pressure in the closed system, in the whole-bladder system the bladder responded to isoproterenol with a significant increase in volume (Fig. 7–11). Results from these comparative studies include the following: (a) The whole-bladder system is capable of displaying a functional response to pharmacologic stimulation. (b) In response to bethanechol, the bladder completely empties at concentrations of bethanechol that produce only mild changes in bladder pressure. It is a reflection of the "reserve capacity" of the bladder. (c) Using this model, one can evaluate the functional integrity of the bladder.

The responses of these *in vitro* models to pharmacologic agents are considerably less complicated to analyze than are the response of *in vivo* models. Because the tissues mounted are devoid of extrinsic nerves and vasculature, the concentrations of drugs the bladders are exposed to can be exactly calculated. The response of the bladder can involve the following mechanisms: (a) action on the smooth muscle membrane directly; (b) action on the intrinsic neuronal elements

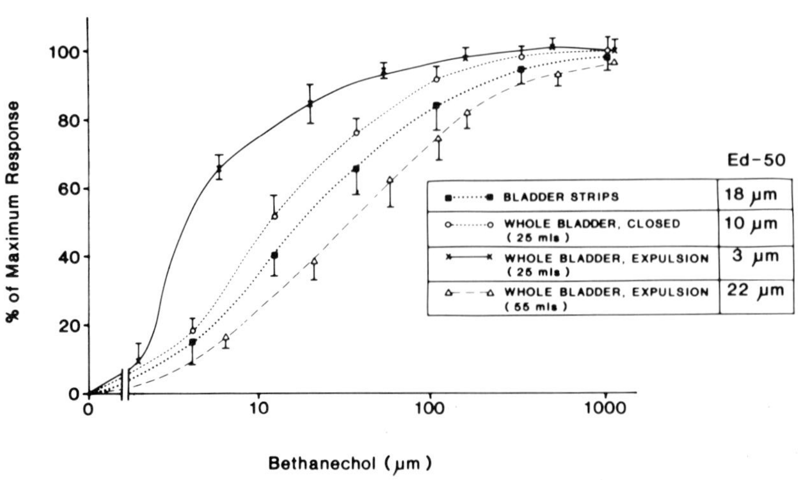

Figure 7–10. Effect of bethanechol in the whole bladder versus bladder strips (expulsion system).

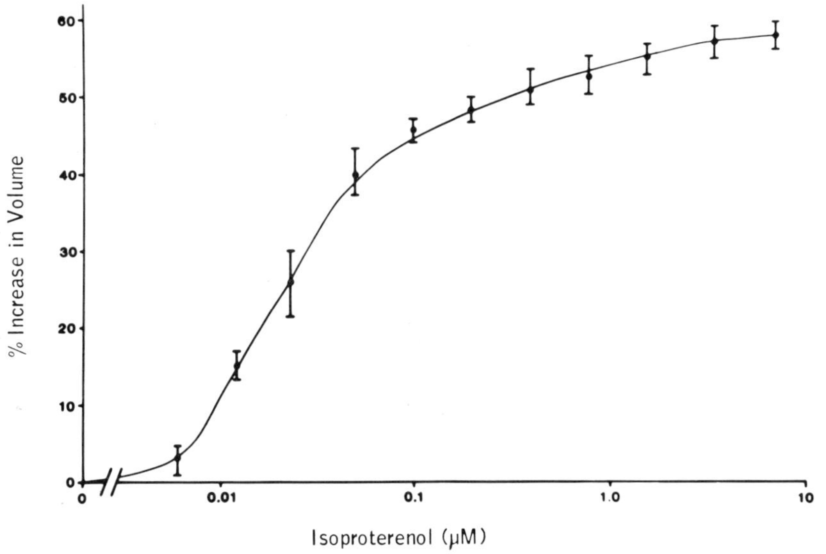

Figure 7–11. Effect of isoproterenol in the whole-bladder model.

(synaptic structures) to release transmitter substances; and (c) action directly on autonomic receptor sites on the bladder smooth muscle. These mechanisms of drug action can be differentiated using specific pharmacolgic agents.

Although the pharmacologic response of the bladder in these *in vitro* systems may be more easily ascribed to specific mechanisms, one must be careful when attempting to relate these findings to the clinical usefulness of the drugs. As previously mentioned, the action of a drug given *in vivo* is dependent on both direct and indirect actions. In some cases a drug that can be shown to have a direct action on bladder muscle *in vitro* may have either no action or the opposite action *in vivo* (via reflex activity). Similarly, there is no reason to believe that the potency of a series of agents on bladder muscle strips would be the same *in vivo*, especially if these agents are taken orally.

In summary, the isolated strip methodology can evaluate the response of specific sections of the urinary bladder to specific pharmacologic stimulation. Thus one can indirectly determine if an experimental condition has altered the distribution of autonomic receptors in the bladder. In this regard, estrogen administration has been demonstrated to significantly increase the response of the bladder body to alpha-adrenergic stimulation (*18*). The whole-bladder model has the advantage of being able to evaluate the functional integrity of the bladder.

STUDIES UTILIZING TISSUE HOMOGENATES OR SUBCELLULAR MEMBRANE PREPARATIONS

Autonomic Receptor Radioligand Binding Assays

The use of specific radioligands to quantitate the density of autonomic receptors is well established. The theory behind these methods is quite easy to understand. First, one must prepare a tissue homogenate or subcellular membrane preparation. Second, this membrane preparation is placed into two groups of test tubes. In the first set of test tubes the membranes are incubated with a radioactive substance that specifically binds to one type of receptor. In the second group of tubes, the membranes are incubated in the same concentration of radioligand and a substantially higher concentration of a nonradioactive compound that also specifically binds to the specific receptor under study. This nonradioactive substance completely prevents the specific binding of the radioligand but does not inhibit a small amount of nonspecific binding to the membranes. Thus the amount of radioactivity bound to the membranes in the first series of tubes (total binding) consists in both specific binding to the receptors and nonspecific binding, whereas in the second group of tubes the amount of radioactivity bound to the membranes consists only in the nonspecific binding. The specific binding to the membranes is calculated by subtracting the nonspecific binding from the total binding. By calculating the specific binding at increasing concentrations of radioligand, one can calculate both the maximum receptor density in the tissue and the affinity of the membranes for the radioligand. The following is a detailed description of the radioligand assay for muscarinic cholinergic receptors (*10*).

Adult male white New Zealand rabbits were anesthetized with ketamine–xylazine as previously described. The urinary bladder was rapidly removed, sectioned into three sections (bladder base, mid-bladder, and bladder dome), and frozen in liquid nitrogen in 250-mg sections.

Each frozen section was rapidly weighed and homogenized in ice-cold 50 mM phosphate buffer, pH 7.4 (75 mg/ml). The homogenate was passed through a double layer of gauze and was used immediately for the receptor binding assay.

The homogenate (250 μl) was incubated in the presence and absence of 10 μM atropine (the nonradioactive competitor) and varying concentrations of ^{3}H-QNB (quinuclidinyl benzylate, the specific radioligand) ranging from 0.03 to 40.00 nM (in a total volume of 350 μl). The mixture was incubated for 1 hour at 25°C. The reaction was stopped with the addition of 4 ml of ice-cold buffer, and the mixture was rapidly filtered through a whatman GF/C glass fiber filter. The filter was washed with three 5-ml portions of cold buffer. The filters were then placed in scintillation vials with 5 ml scintillation fluid, and the radioactivity was determined by liquid scintillation spectrometry. The specific binding at each concentration of ^{3}H-QNB was determined by subtracting the amount of radioactivity bound in the presence of atropine (nonspecific binding) from the total binding, which is the amount of radioactivity in the absence of atropine. The dissociation constant (Kd) and maximum receptor density were calculated by Scatchard analysis. As is discussed in a later section, the Scatchard analysis is a mathematic method of linearizing binding data and thus extrapolate the theoretical binding at high ligand concentrations (which would be equal to the theoretical maximum receptor density-B_{max}).

The relation between total, nonspecific, and specific binding is presented in Figure 7–12. Figure 7–13 presents the specific binding in the three sections of rabbit urinary bladder, and the Scatchard analysis of the data is presented in Figure 7–14. As can be seen, the density of muscarinic receptors is significantly higher in the bladder body than in the bladder base. This finding correlates well with the isolated smooth muscle strips that demonstrated that the bladder body responds preferentially to muscarinic stimulation by bethanechol.

Assays for adrenergic alpha- and beta-

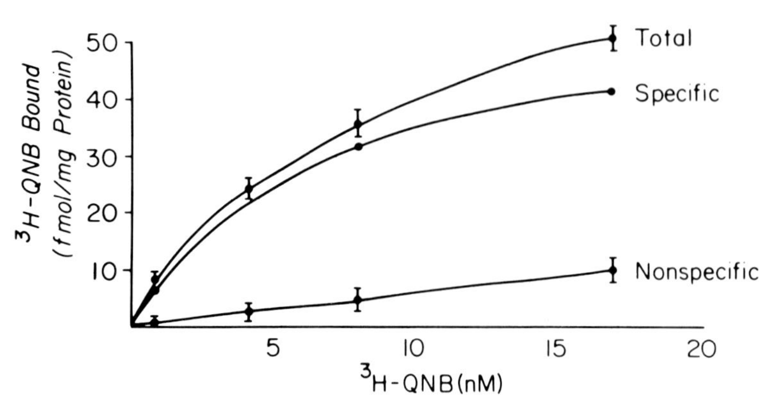

Figure 7–12. Binding of ^{3}H-QNB to homogenates of rabbit urinary bladder.

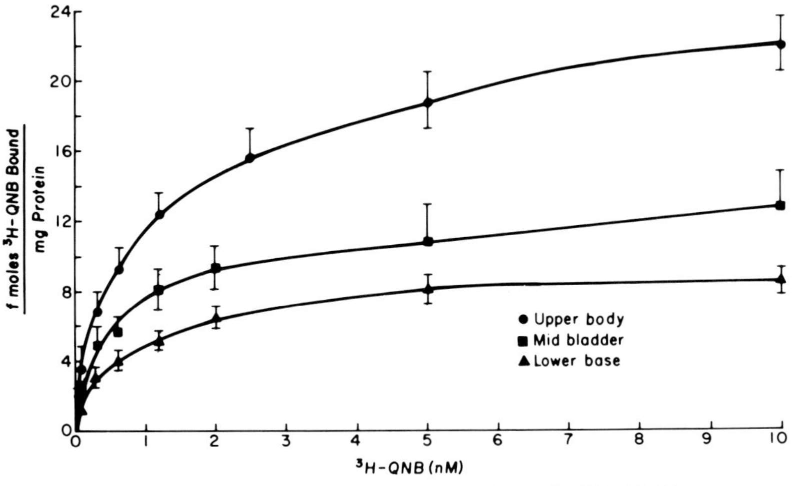

Figure 7–13. Specific binding of ^{3}H-QNB to sections of rabbit bladder.

adrenergic receptors are performed in a manner similar to that presented for the muscarinic receptor, except: (a) the buffer is 50 mM Tris, pH 7.5, containing 10 mM Mg^{2+}; (b) the incubation is carried out for 15 minutes at 30°C; (c) the radioligand for the beta assay is ^{3}H-DHA (dihidroalprenolol) and for the alpha assay ^{3}H-DHE (dihydroergocryptine); and (d) the nonradioactive competitive agents are propranolol for the beta assay and phentolamine for the alpha assay.

Results demonstrate that the beta-receptor density of the bladder body is significantly greater than that of the bladder base, whereas the density of alpha-receptors is greater in the bladder base than in the body. This finding correlates well with the response of the bladder strips to alpha- and beta-adrenergic agents. This differential distribution of both autonomic receptor density and specific response to autonomic agonists is similar for all species tested including rat, cat, dog, rabbit, and man.

The methodologies described above use tissue homogenates for the determination of receptor densities. Because autonomic receptors are localized to the synaptic regions of cell membranes, it is easy to use purification methodologies to prepare membrane fractions that are rich in synaptic membranes. One commonly utilized methodology uses differential centrifugation to prepare synaptic-rich membrane preparations: Tissue is homogenized as previously described in ice-cold buffer. The homogenate is centrifuged at 900 X g for 10 minutes. The supernate is separated from the pellet and centrifuged again for 10 minutes at 900 X g. The pellet fractions containing the crude membrane debris are combined. The supernate is centrifuged at 10,500 X g for 20 minutes and then separated from the pellet. The supernate is again centrifuged at 10,500

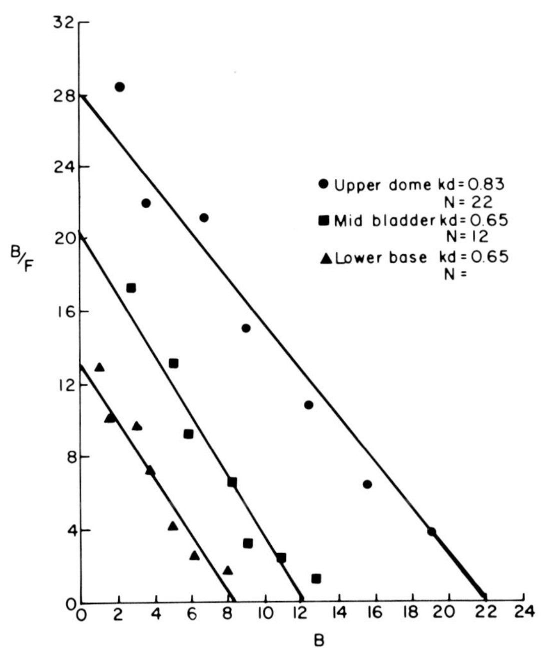

Figure 7–14. Scatchard analysis of ^{3}H-QNB bonding.

X g, and the pellet is combined with the first 10,500 X g pellet. This pellet is the mitochondrial fraction. The supernate is then centrifuged at 100,000 X g for 1 hour. The pellet is separated from the supernate and resuspended in cold buffer to its original volume. This pellet is the microsomal and synaptic vesicle fraction. In general, this final pellet should have the highest density of autonomic receptors, and the 900 X g pellet should have the lowest density.

Studies Measuring Intracellular Components

There are literally hundreds of important intracellular substances that can be quantitated from tissue preparations. There are some general principles that can be applied to these methods. First, the substance under investigation must be separated from components that may either interfere with its determination or enzymatically inactivate or metabolize the substance. Separation techniques include differential centrifugation, chromatographic techniques, and chemical extraction techniques. Once the substance has been isolated from interfering compounds, it can either be assayed directly or reacted in such a way that it can be quantitated.

One such intracellular component that we measure routinely is intracellular ATP (*19*). For these studies bladder tissue is rapidly homogenized in 0.625 M perchloric acid. Homogenization in acid denatures all protein and inactivates all enzymes including those that metabolize ATP. The homogenate is centrifuged at 900 X g for 20 minutes, and the pellet is separated from the supernate. The pellet is dissolved in 1 N sodium hydroxide and analyzed for protein concentration. The supernate is neutralized and analyzed for ATP using the luciferin–luciferase assay (*20*). In this assay, 100 μl of neutralized supernate is incubated for 10 minutes at 37°C with 50 μl of Dupont Luciferin–luciferase preparation. The luciferin binds specifically to ATP with the generation of an exact amount of light. The amount of light generated is directly proportional to the amount of ATP present and is quantitated using a Dupont biometer. This assay can be used to quantitate any reactions that can be linked to ATP, e.g., the quantification of intracellular ADP and AMP. In this case we incubate the neutralized supernate in the 50 mM glycyl-glycine buffer, pH 8.0, containing phosphoenolpyruvate (PEP), myokinase (MK), and pyruvate kinase (PK); all the ADP and AMP present in the supernate is converted to ATP and can be assayed by luciferin–luciferase as previously described. Thus if we analyze two sets of tubes—one containing just the supernate plus luciferin–luciferase, which measures ATP, the second containing PEP, MK, and PK, which measures the combination of ATP, ADP, and AMP—the ADP–AMP concentration is determined by subtracting this value from the first. Figure 7–15 demonstrates the effect of anoxia on intracellular adenine nucleotide concentration (*19*).

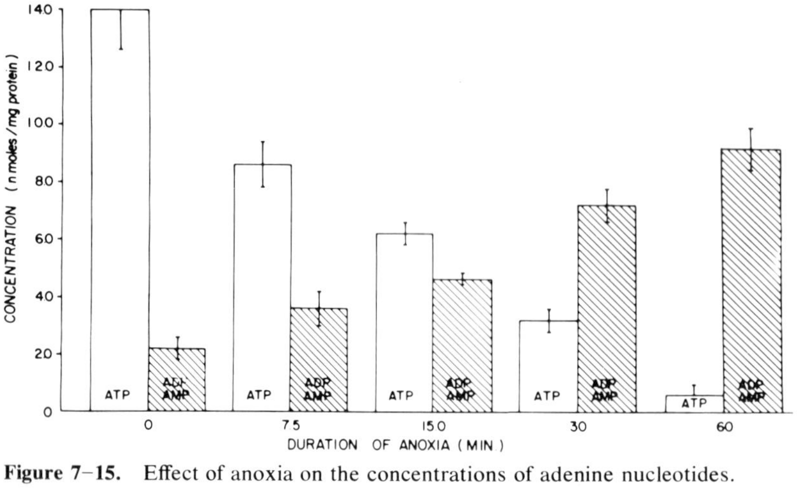

Figure 7–15. Effect of anoxia on the concentrations of adenine nucleotides.

Studies Measuring Intracellular Enzyme Activity (21,22)

There are far too many important intracellular enzymes to give details on their measurements. In general, one must be able to isolate the specific enzyme under evaluation from other enzymes that act on its substrate or product as well as from substances that can interfere with enzyme's activity. In addition, there must be a method available for quantification of the product of enzymatic activity. The following preliminary studies must be performed to establish the methodology: (a) enzymatic activity of increasing concentrations of enzyme (tissue concentration); (b) enzymatic activity at increasing times of incubation; (c) enzyme activity using several buffer systems at various pH levels and temperatures; and (d) the effect of specific ions and cofactors on enzymatic activity.

From the above preliminary experiments, the conditions required for maximal enzyme activity are determined. Only after these conditions have been determined can the enzyme activity be characterized. Figures 7–16 and 7–17 display the substrate concentration curves for phosphodiesterase activity in the canine external sphincter and urinary bladder dome. Kinetic analysis of the phosphodiesterase activity of the external sphincter demonstrate that the activity follows the law of mass activity; that is, the Lineweaver-Burk plot (1/velocity plotted against 1/substrate concentration) is linear. Kinetic activity of the urinary bladder, on the other hand, demonstrates that the enzyme activity is nonlinear. The Hill plot, which demonstrates that the enzyme activity shows positive cooperativity. Further studies demonstrated that cyclic GMP acts as an allosteric activator of bladder phosphodiesterase, as evidenced by conversion of the nonlinear kinetics of the bladder phosphodiesterase, to linear kinetics in the presence of cyclic GMP (Fig. 7–18, 21).

Although it is easy to establish an enzymatic assay and measure activity, it is an involved procedure to fully characterize the enzyme activity and ensure that what one measures is a true reflection of the intracellular activity of that enzyme.

HISTOLOGY AND HISTOCHEMISTRY

It is beyond the scope of this chapter to give specific details of the wide variety of methodologies available for the histologic study of the urinary tract structures. Thus we present only an overview of the various techniques utilized.

Light Microscopy

The tissue to be studied must be obtained by dissection and then fixed in order to stop intracellular processes and "fix" them in the cell in such a way as to allow their identification. The actual methods employed for fixation depend on the structures and sub-

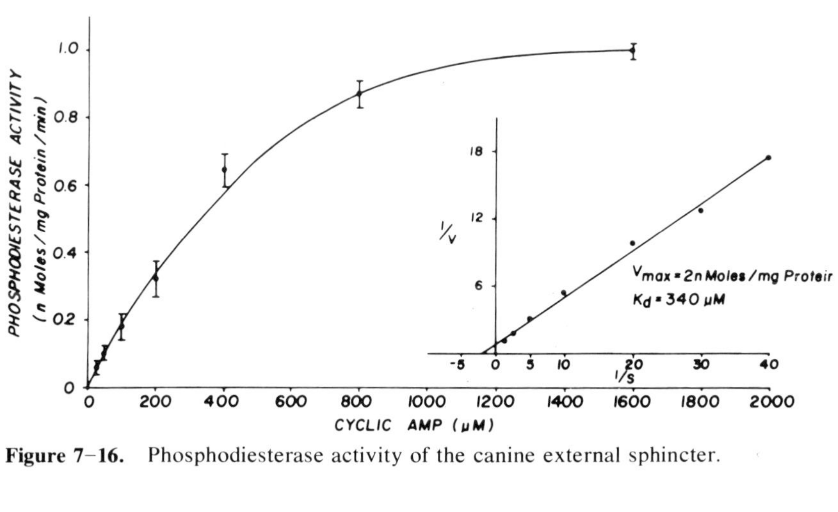

Figure 7–16. Phosphodiesterase activity of the canine external sphincter.

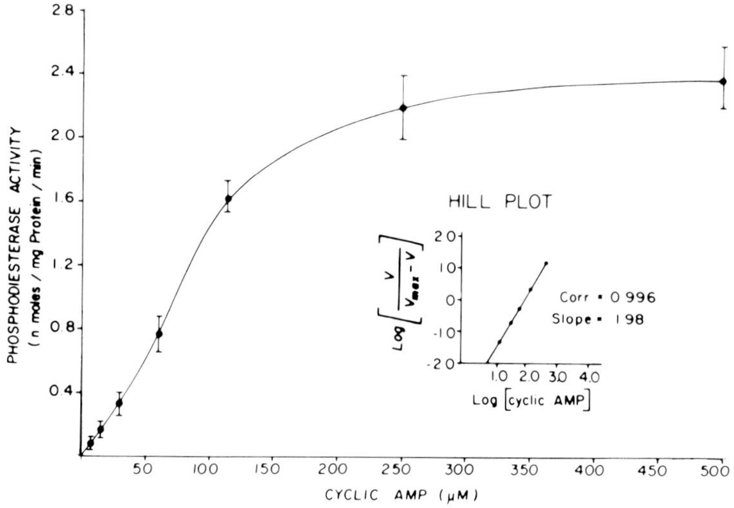

Figure 7–17. Phosphodiesterase activity of the canine bladder body.

stances that are to be studied. Thus if one wishes to study the nuclear organization of a cell, the fixation procedures are completely different from the methods utilized if one wishes to study the carbohydrate distribution.

After fixation, the tissue sample is embedded in paraffin or other material and sectioned into thin specimens and mounted on glass slides. The sections are then stained in such a way as to allow microscopic identification of the intracellular structures the investigator wishes to study. Hematoxylin and eosin are the most common stains. They allow identification of nuclear, cytoplasmic, and cartilagenous structures. A large number of specific stains exist for the identification of specific intracellular structures and substances.

Histofluorescence and Histochemical Methods

Histofluorescence techniques utilize light at one wavelength to illuminate (at the exciting wavelengh) the specimen. The secondary emitted light from the specimen is observed via a series of filters (which allow only the emission wavelength to be viewed). Histofluorescence visualization of adrenergic nerves and synapses has been widely utilized. Two basic methods have been em-

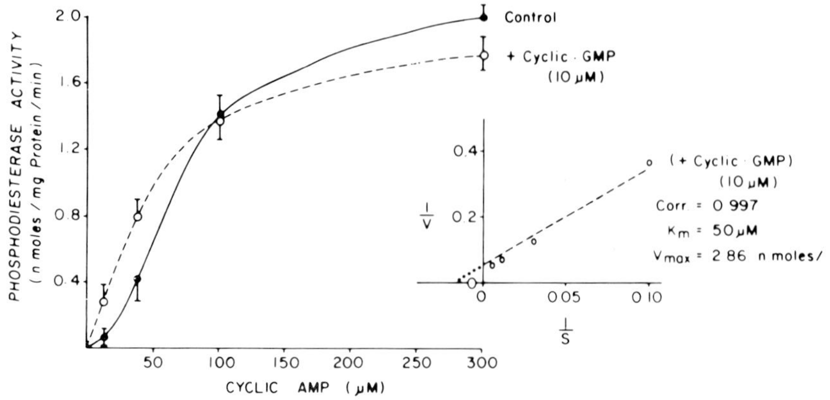

Figure 7–18. Effect of cyclic GMP on phosphodiesterase activity.

ployed in these studies: The first method, developed for the visualization of biogenic amines, utilized formaldehyde-induced histofluorescence (*23*). These methods employ freeze-dry fixation followed by formaldehyde vapor exposure. The tissue specimen is then embedded in paraffin and sectioned. Biogenic amines fluoresce when exposed to ultraviolet irradiation. These methodologies have been used to map adrenergic nerve fibers and synapses in many tissues, including those isolated from the urinary tract.

A second method to identify adrenergic structures via histofluorescence uses glyoxylic acid condensation (*24*). This technique does not require the use of freeze-dried tissue and is much more rapid than the formaldehyde method. Figure 7–19 displays the adrenergic innervation of the rabbit bladder base and body (*25*).

The use of fluorescence microscopy is becoming increasingly more important in the localization of specific bioactive polypeptides via immunohistofluorescence (*26*). These methods use specific antibodies that have been produced to bind to specific proteins (e.g., substance P, VIP, Endorphins). It is quite easy to link a fluorescent dye to the immunoglobulins and then react the antibodies with histologically sectioned tissue. Fluorescence microscopy is then utilized to visualize the distribution and density of the specific substances.

Histochemical microscopy uses specific enzymatic activity to produce a product that can be microscopically identified. One of the most common uses for histochemical microscopy is in the identification of cholinergic nerves via specific acetylcholinesterase staining techniques (*27,28*). Figure 7–20 demonstrates the cholinergic innervation of the rabbit bladder base and body.

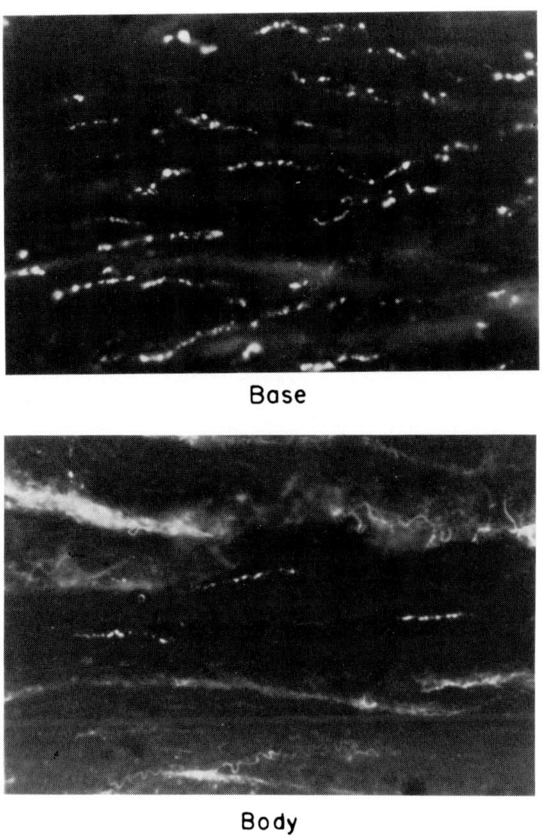

Figure 7–19. Adrenergic innervation of the rabbit urinary bladder.

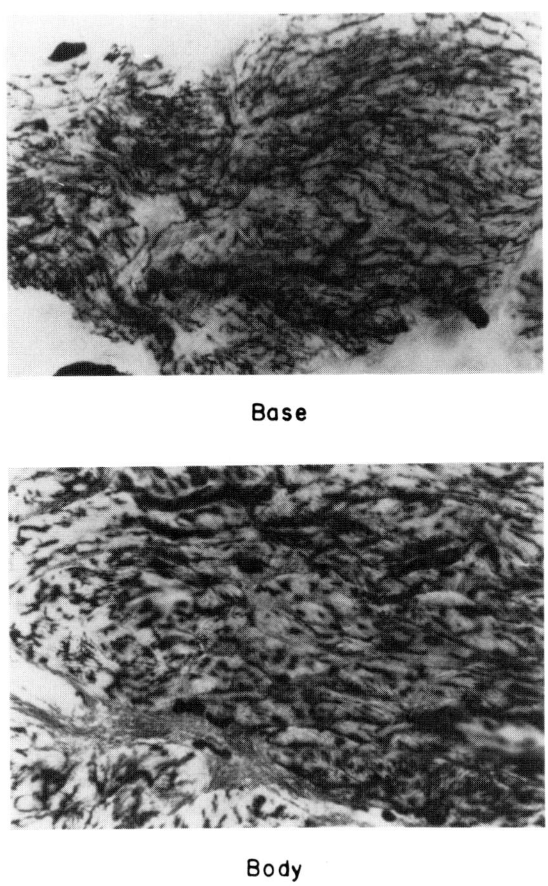

Figure 7–20. Cholinergic innervation of the rabbit urinary bladder.

Electron Microscopy

Electron microscopy (*29,30*) is utilized to identify intracellular structure at the level of individual intracellular membranes. These techniques can identify subtle changes in membrane structures and location. Scanning electron microscopy can show the surface structure of a cell, whereas transmission electron microscopy displays actual intracellular structure.

RELATING EXPERIMENTAL MODELS WITH CLINICAL MEDICINE

The therapeutic effect of a drug that can affect bladder function (as an example) depends on a variety of factors including route of adminstration, absorption, distribution, excretion, and drug metabolism. In addition to the above pharmacologic factors, personal factors can markedly affect the therapeutic effect of a drug. These factors include whether the person takes the drug as prescribed, the weight (and fat content) of the person, and the presence of other systemic disease (e.g., renal or liver disease can markedly alter a drug's effectiveness). The mechanism of action can include direct action on the bladder, indirect action via spinal and/or supraspinal reflexes, direct action on the central nervous system, and the placebo effect, which can vary markedly from patient to patient.

The more sophisticated the experimental model, the fewer are the factors involved in relating drug concentration with a specific biologic action. Thus in acute whole-animal models, route of administration, absorption, and distribution are involved in the magnitude of response observed. The mechanisms of action may include direct action at the site, indirect actions via spinal and supraspinal reflexes, and direct central action.

Using *in vitro* muscle bath methodology, factors that determine a drug's effectiveness include solubility, penetration to the sites of action, metabolism by the tissue, direct action on specific receptors, and indirect action via altering the membranes' permeability to ions (i.e., local anesthetics).

Using tissue homogenates, the effectiveness of a drug to either bind to a purified membrane preparation or to stimulate specific enzyme activities is directly related to the affinity of the drug to the specific receptor.

As stated above, the clinical efficacy of a drug depends on a variety of factors and may involve several mechanisms of action. One must be careful when trying to relate the potency of a drug in particular research model with clinical efficacy of the drug. Keeping this fact in mind, it is best to approach a problem using a variety of research models, including both *in vivo* and *in vitro* preparations. Additionally, one should always keep in mind species specificity; that is, the response of one species to a drug may not be characteristic of all species. Species variability should be kept in mind when trying to relate the results of animal studies to clinical medicine.

METHODS OF DATA PRESENTATION

In virtually all methodologies that involve measuring the response of a biologic system to a drug, the data are presented in some graphic form. The following is a brief discussion of the dose-response theory and the various methods that one can use for presentation of dose-response data.

We begin the discussion by defining some commonly used and misused pharmacologic terms.

Receptor: that portion of a cell that specifically binds to a particular agent, the combination of which produces the characteristic response to that agent.

Binding site: an area on a biologic membrane that binds to an agent without necessarily producing a biologic response. Although all receptors are binding sites, not all binding sites are receptors.

Agonist: a drug that when combined with a receptor produces a pharmacologic effect.

Antagonist: a drug that reduces or abolishes the response to an agonist. A *pharmacologic antagonist* is an antagonist that acts at the same receptor as the agonist. A *physiologic (functional) antagonist* is an antagonist that acts at a site other than the agonist's receptor.

ED_{50}: the effective dose that produces 50 percent of the maximum response. *Kd* (dissociation constant): the dose of a drug that produces 50 percent receptor occupancy. These two terms are not interchangeable.

I_{50}: the dose of an antagonist that reduces the maximum effect of an agonist by 50 percent. K_i (dissociation constant for inhibitor): the dose of an antagonist that produces 50 percent receptor occupancy. These two terms are not interchangeable.

Efficacy: a measure of the intrinsic ability of a drug to produce an effect. Efficacy relates to the magnitude of the effect produced.

Potency: relates to the concentration at which a particular effect is elicited. It is not related to the magnitude of the effect.

There are two important parameters when analyzing agonist dose response curves: the ED_{50} (the effective dose that gives 50 percent of the maximum response) and the E_{max} (maximal effect of the agonist). The ED_{50} is a measure of the potency of a drug, whereas the E_{max} is a measure of the efficacy.

The most common method of data presentation is simply to graph the drug concentration against the response. As an example we use the contractile response of a tissue to a contractile agonist. Figure 7–21 presents a linear–linear dose-response curve that presents the actual tension at the various drug concentrations. As noted, the basal tension (at zero drug) is 2.0 gm. It is a common practice to present this type of data as the contractile response (increase in tension) rather than the actual tension; it is depicted in Figure 7–22. In cases where the response is graphed, the basal tension (or basal condition) should always be given as well.

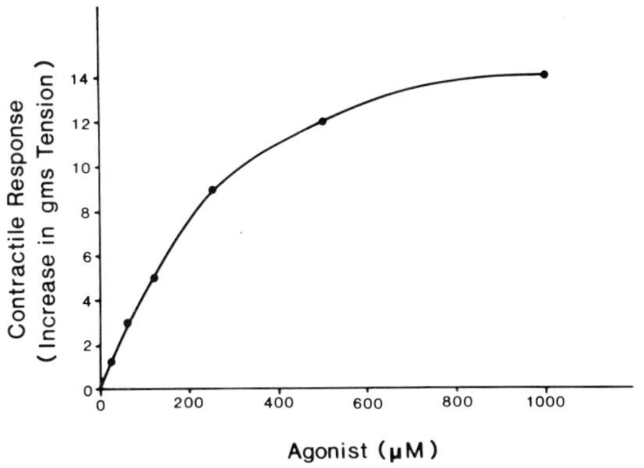

Figure 7–22. Linear–linear dose response curve of an agonist (response).

Figure 7–23 presents the same contractile response data graphed as a log function of the drug concentration (linear–log plot). This type of graph allows visualization of a dose-response curve that covers several orders of magnitude. In addition, the linear–log graph allows comparison of dose-response curves that have widely different ED_{50} values, as in the data presented in Figure 7–24.

It is often desirable to compare the effects of two or more drugs in one system. Figure 7–25 displays the effect of drugs A and B on the contractile response of a smooth muscle strip. It is clear that drug A has a much greater maximal effect than drug B. In order

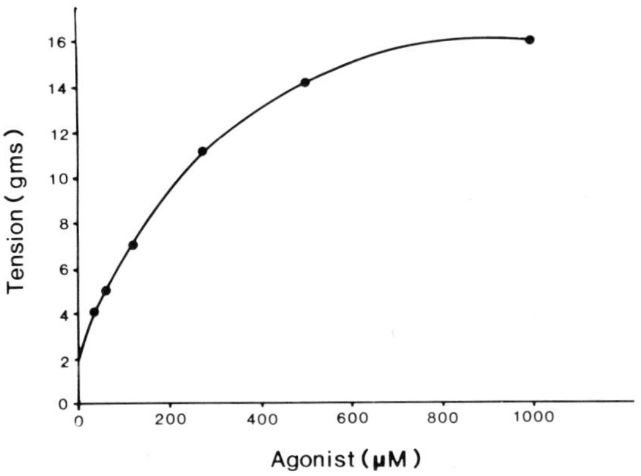

Figure 7–21. Linear–linear dose response curve of an agonist (from baseline).

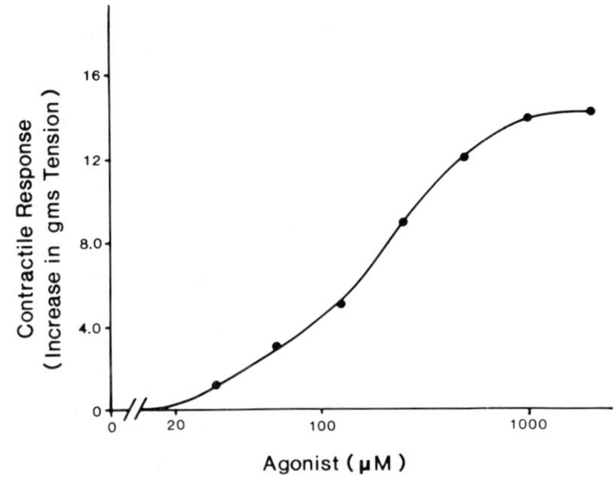

Figure 7–23. Linear–log dose response curve of an agonist (response).

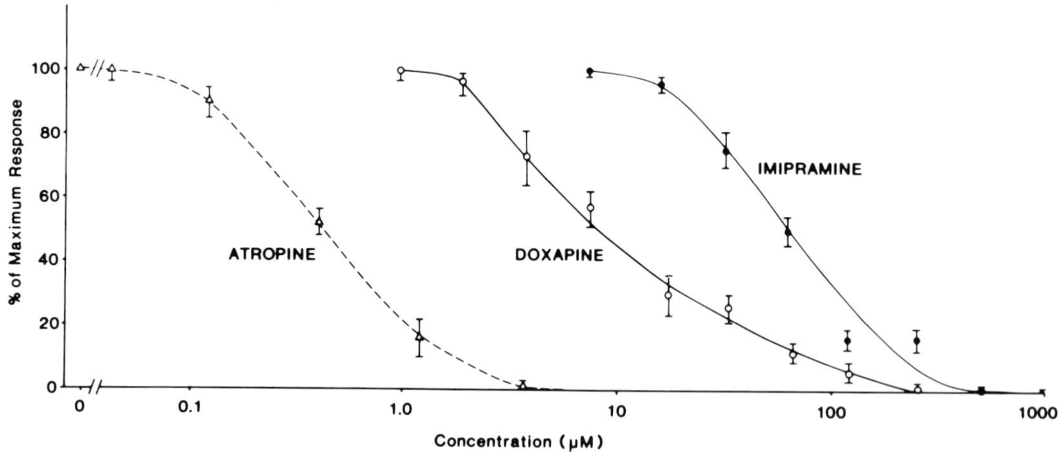

Figure 7–24. Inhibition of bethanechol stimulation by atropine, imipramine, and doxepine.

to compare the potency, one can normalize the data to 100 percent of the maximum response for each drug. Figure 7–26 presents the above data as the percent of the maximum response. From this curve it appears that drug A is more potent than drug B. This curve may be misleading because of the extremely small maximum response to drug B. In cases in which an investigator presents normalized data, it is mandatory to give both the basal level and the maximum effect in real units in the text. In cases that compare the effect of one drug in several systems, one must present the data normalized to 100 percent maximum in each system. An example is presented in Figure 7–10: the response of isolated muscle strips and the whole-bladder model to bethanechol. Again it is mandatory to present both the basal values and the values for 100 percent in each system.

There are primarily two methods of determining the effects of antagonists. The most widely used procedure is to give a maximal dose of an agonist and then obtain a dose-response curve for the antagonist. Figure 7–24 presents data for the inhibition of bethanechol stimulation by atropine, doxepine, and imipramine. From this study one can determine that atropine is considerably more potent than either doxepine or imipramine. Although relative potencies can be determined by this type of experiment, one cannot determine whether the inhibition is competitive or noncompetitive. The second method is to obtain dose-response curves to the agonist in the presence of several con-

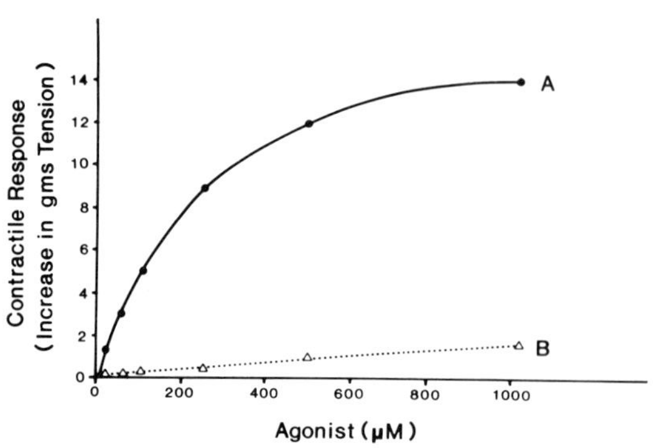

Figure 7–25. Comparative response of two agonists on one tissue.

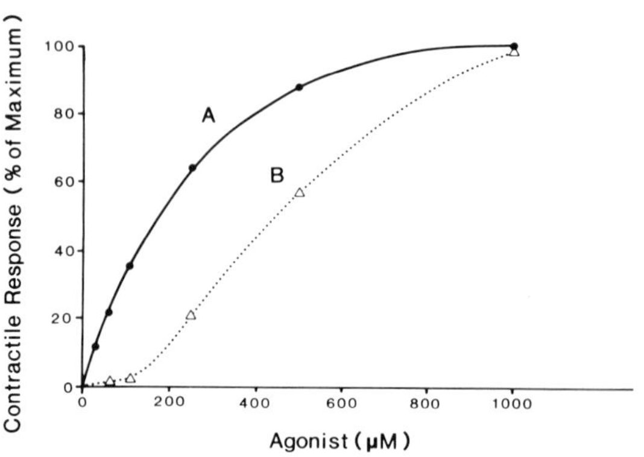

Figure 7–26. Comparative response of two agonists normalized to 100 percent of maximum response.

centrations of the antagonist. Figure 7–27 demonstrates that the dose-response curve to bethanechol is shifted to the right by atropine (ED_{50} increases), whereas the maximum response to bethanechol is unchanged; thus atropine inhibition is of a competitive nature. Figure 7–28 demonstrates that the maximum response to bethanechol in the presence of desmethylimipramine (DMI) is reduced, whereas the ED_{50} is not markedly altered; this finding indicates that DMI inhibition is noncompetitive.

When studying the interaction of a drug with its receptor using molecular pharmacologic methodologies, more sophisticated methods of analysis are generally utilized. Radioligand receptor binding methodologies and enzyme kinetic studies are examples of research methods that utilize the "Law of mass action" as a basis for analysis. In its simplest form the law of mass action is as follows.

$$D + R = DR$$

$$K_{eq} = \frac{DR}{D+R}$$

where D = drug
R = receptor
K_{eq} = equilibrium constant
DR= drug–receptor complex

The response must be proportional to the drug–receptor complex.

If there is only one type of receptor and the response that one measures is proportional to the DR, graphing D (concentration of drug) versus DR (the response) gives a hyperbolic curve. Two examples of reactions that follow the law of mass action are (a) the radioligand binding curve of ^{3}H-QNB to bladder receptors (Fig. 7–13) and (b) the enzymatic activity of phosphodiesterase in the canine external sphincter (Fig. 7–16).

Without giving the mathematic derivations, data that follow the law of mass action can be linearized by several means. The Scatchard analysis is utilized frequently to linearize radioligand binding data. Graphically, the DR = d 3y-axis) is plotted against DR (X-axis). As displayed in Figure 7–14, Kd is equal to the inverse slope, and B_{max} is equal to the *x*-intercept.

Enzymatic kinetics utilize two graphic means for linearizing data. The Hofstee plot uses the inverse of the Scatchard plot, i.e.: DR (*y*-axis) versus DR/D (*x*-axis) to linearize data. The Lineweaver-Burk (double reciprocal) analysis plots 1/DR (*y*-axis) against 1/D (*x*-axis). An example of this form of analysis is given in Figure 7–16 for the phosphodiesterase activity of the canine external sphincter. The *x*-intercept is the negative inverse of the Kd, and the *y*-intercept is the inverse of the B_{max}.

The above equations and graphic methodology are valid only if there is a single receptor site and no cooperativity (i.e., the binding of the drug to the first receptor does not alter the binding of the drug to the next receptor). Such interactions or the presence of a second or third receptor site are graphically represented by nonlinear Scatchard, Hofstee, or Lineweaver-Burk plots. An extensive dis-

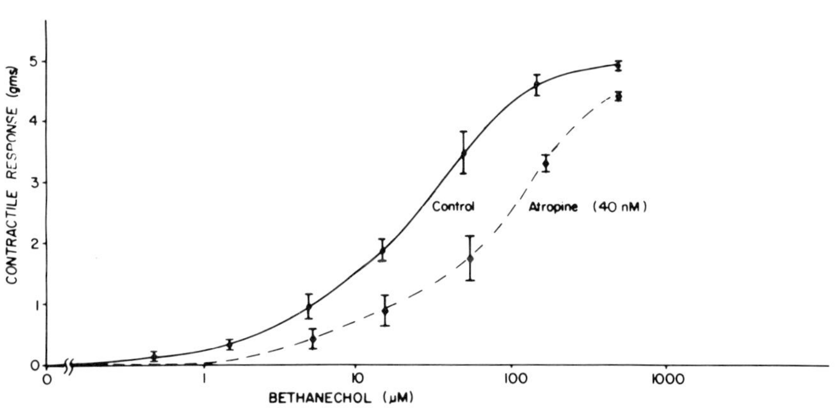

Figure 7–27. Effect of bethanechol in the presence and absence of atropine.

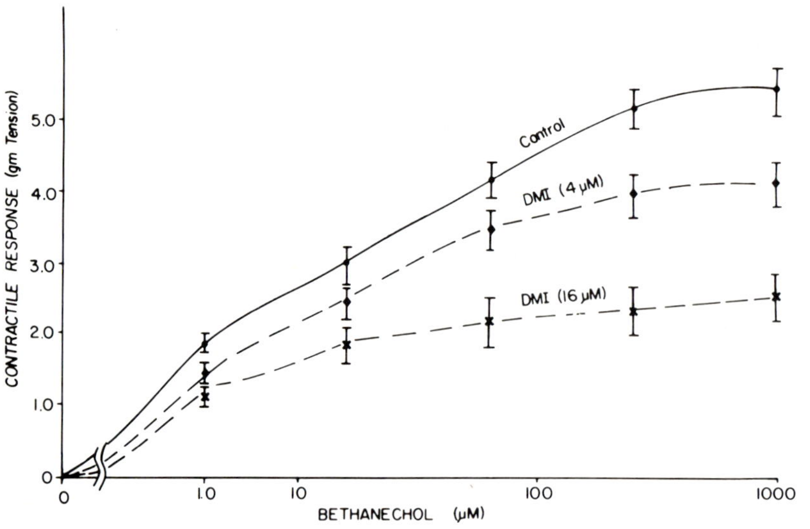

Figure 7–28. Effect of bethanechol in the presence and absence of DMI.

cussion of this topic can be found elsewhere (*31*).

SUMMARY

When organizing a research program, it is best to first pick an area to investigate and then choose two or three approaches to the investigation. For example, if an investigator wishes to study the effect of bladder obstruction on bladder function, he should choose (a) an animal model of obstruction, (b) an *in vivo* preparation to evaluate the effect of the obstruction on bladder function (c) an *in vitro* model to demonstrate the effect of the obstruction on bladder, smooth muscle, and (d) histologic evaluation of structural changes that accompany functional changes. It is always best to approach a problem using diverse techniques rather than to investigate a variety of problems with one technique.

REFERENCES

1. DeGroat, W. C., and Lalley, P. M.: Reflex firing in the lumbar sympathetic outflow to activation of vesical afferent fibres. *J. Physiol. (Lond.)* 226:289–309, 1972.
2. DeGroat, W. C., and Saums, W. R.: Synaptic transmission in parasympathetic ganglia in the urinary bladder of the cat. *J. Physiol. (Lond.)* 256:137–158, 1976.
3. Torbey, K., and Leadbetter, W. F.: Innervation of the bladder and lower ureter: studies on pelvic nerve section and stimulation in the dog. *J. Urol.* 90:395–404, 1963.
4. Klevmark, B.: Motility of the urinary bladder in cats during filling at physiologic rates: intravesical pressure patterns studied by new methods of cystometry. *Acta Physiol. Scand.* 90:565–577, 1974.
5. Sogbein, S. K., Downie, J. W., and Awad, S. A.: Urethral response during bladder contraction induced by subcutaneous bethanechol chloride: elicitation of a sympathetic reflex urethral constriction. *J. Urol.* 131:791–795, 1984.
6. McGuire, E. J.: Experimental observations on the integration of bladder and urethral function *Invest. Urol.* 15:303–307, 1978.
7. Bruschini, H., Schmidt, R. A., and Tanagho, E. A.: The male genitourinary sphincter mechanism in the dog. *Invest. Urol.* 15:284–287, 1978.
8. Creed, K. E.: The role of the hypogastric nerve in bladder and urethral activity of the dog. *Br. J. Pharmacol.* 65:367–375, 1979.
9. Levin, R. M., and Wein, A. J.: Distribution and function of adrenergic receptors in the urinary bladder of the rabbit. *Mol. Pharmacol.* 16:441–448, 1979.
10. Levin, R. M., Shofer, F., and Wein, A. J.: Cholinergic, adrenergic, and purinergic response of sequential strips of rabbit urinary bladder. *J. Pharmacol. Exp. Ther.* 212:536–540, 1980.
11. Levin, R. M., Staskin, D. R., and Wein, A. J.: The muscarinic cholinergic binding kinetics of the human urinary bladder. *Neurourol. Urodyn.* 2:221–225, 1983.
12. Levin, R. M., Staskin, D. R., and Wein, A. J.: Analysis of the anticholinergic and musculotropic effects of desmethylimipramine on the rabbit urinary bladder. *Uro. Res.* 11:259–262, 1983.
13. Levin, R. M., and Wein, A. J.: Comparative effects of five tricyclic compounds on the rabbit urinary bladder. *Neurourol. Urodyn.* 3:127–132, 1984.

14. Paton, W. D. M.: The response of the guinea-pig ileum to electrical stimulation by coaxial electrodes. *J. Physiol. (Lond.)* 127:40P–41P, 1955.
15. Downie, J. W., and Dean, D. M.: The contribution of cholinergic postganglionic neurotransmission to contractions of rabbit detrusor. *J. Pharmacol. Exp. Ther.* 203:417–425, 1977.
16. Levin, R. M., Brendler, K., and Wein, A. J.: Comparative pharmacological response of an in-vitro whole bladder preparation (rabbit) with the response of isolated smooth muscle strips. *J. Urol.* 30:377–381, 1983.
17. Levin, R. M., Goldman, M., and Wein, A. J.: Effect of isoproterenol and EGTA on the volume-pressure relationship of the in-vitro whole bladder preparation. *Neurourol. Urodyn.* 3:133–140, 1984.
18. Levin, R. M., Shofer, F., and Wein, A. J.: Estrogen-induced alterations in autonomic responses of the rabbit urinary bladder. *J. Pharmacol. Exp. Ther.* 215:614–618, 1980.
19. Levin, R. M., High, J., and Wein, A. J.: Metabolic and contractile effects of anoxia on the rabbit urinary bladder. *J. Urol.* 128:194–196, 1982.
20. Lemasters, J. J., and Hackenbrock, L. R.: Firefly luciferase assay for ATP production by mitochondria. *Methods Enzymol.* 57:36–50, 1978.
21. Levin, R. M., Einstein, R., and Wein, A. J.: Phosphodiesterase activity of the lower urinary tract. *J. Urol.* 128:615–617, 1982.
22. Levin, R. M.: Jacoby, R., and Wein, A. J.: Effect of adenosine triphosphate on contractility and adenosine triphosphatase activity of the rabbit urinary bladder. *Mol. Pharmacol.* 19:525–528, 1981.
23. Falck, B., Hillarp, N. A., Thieme, G., and Trop, A.: Fluorescence of catecholamines and related compounds condensed with formaldehyde. *J. Histochem. Cytochem.* 10:348–354, 1962.
24. DelaTorre, J. C., and Surgeon, J. W.: A methodological approach to rapid and sensitive monoamine histofluorescence using a modified glyoxylic acid technique: the SIG method. *Histochemistry* 49:81–93, 1976.
25. Levin, R. M., Malkowicz, S. B., Jacobowitz, D., and Wein, A. J.: The ontogeny of the autonomic innervation and contractile response of the rabbit urinary bladder. *J. Pharmacol. Exp. Ther.* 291:250–257, 1981.
26. Hökfelt, T., Johansson, O., Ljungdahl, A., Lundberg, J., and Schultzberg, M.: Peptidergic neurons. *Nature* 284:515–521, 1980.
27. Koelle, G.: The histochemical identification of acetylcholinesterase in cholinergic, adrenergic, and sensory neurons. *J. Pharmacol. Exp. Ther.* 114:167–184, 1955.
28. Elbadawi, A., and Schenk, E.: Histochemical methods for separate, consecutive and simultaneous demonstrations of acetylcholinesterase and norepinephrine in cryostat sections. *J. Histochem. Cytochem.* 15:580–588, 1967.
29. Dixon, J. S., and Gosling, J. A.: Histology and fine structure of the muscularis mucosae of the human urinary bladder. *J. Anat.* 136:265–271, 1983.
30. Elbadawi, A.: Ultrastructure of vesicourethral innervation. I. Neuroeffector and cell functions in the male internal sphincter. *J. Urol.* 128:120–128, 1982.
31. Tallarida, R. J., and Jacob, L. S.: *The Dose Response Relation in Pharmacology.* Springer-Verlag, New York, 1979.

Section Two
Armamentarium, Techniques, and Methods of Assessment

8

Terminology and Abbreviations

JERRY G. BLAIVAS, M.D.

The following glossary is a compilation of the most common terms used in this book. In most instances the terminology conforms with recommendations of the International Continence Society (*1*) and the recommendations of the Urodynamic Society (*2*). Whenever the terminology differs from that of the International Continence Society, it is marked by an asterisk. For a complete description of urodynamic terminology see Figure 8–1.

Average Flow Rate (Q_{ave}). The average flow rate is derived by dividing the voided volume by the total voiding time.

Accommodation. The ability of the bladder to accept increases in its volume without significantly increasing its pressure.

Bladder Capacity. Bladder capacity is the maximum volume at which the patient feels a strong urge to void or the volume at which incontinence occurs.

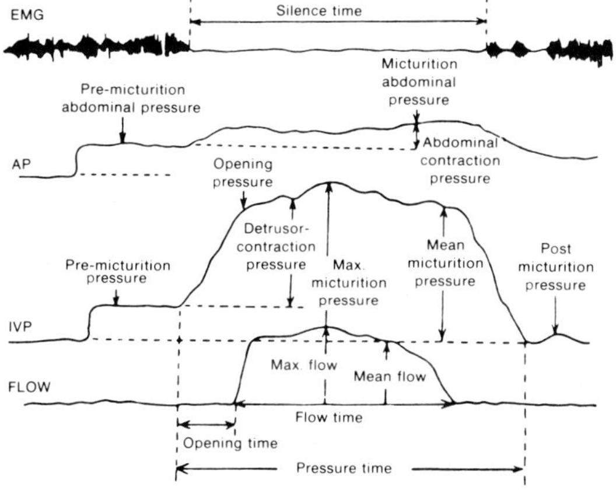

Figure 8–1. Schematic illustration of urodynamic parameters. (From Frimødt-Moller, Scand. J. Urol. Nephrol., 6(15) 153, 1972.)

Compliance. Technically speaking, compliance is the change in volume for a given change in pressure. In practice, however, compliance is measured by determining the change in detrusor or intravesical pressure during bladder filling (a change in volume). The numerical values for compliance and the shape of the cystometric curve are intimately dependent on the rate of bladder filling. A low-compliance bladder is one that has a steep filling curve. A high-compliance bladder accepts a large volume without significant rise in pressure.

Cystometry. Cystometry (CMG) is the graphic representation of intravesical pressure as a function of volume.

Cystometric Capacity. Cystometric capacity is the volume at which the patient has a strong urge to void or develops urinary incontinence.

Decentralization. Decentralization occurs when a central neurologic lesion is present but the peripheral neurons remain anatomically intact. For example, parasympathetic decentralization refers to a lesion of the conus medullaris or cauda equina in which the postganglionic parasympathetic neurons are anatomically intact.

Detrusor Acontractility. Detrusor acontractility is the failure of the detrusor to contract during a cystometric examination although the bladder being filled to capacity.

Detrusor Areflexia. Detrusor areflexia is detrusor acontractility due to a neurologic lesion involving the nerve supply to the detrusor.

Detrusor Instability. An unstable detrusor is one that is shown objectively to develop involuntary detrusor contractions either spontaneously or during provocation. Detrusor instability may be asymptomatic, and its presence does not necessarily imply a neurologic disorder.

Detrusor-Sphincter Dyssynergia. Detrusor-sphincter dyssynergia denotes an inappropriate contraction of the "sphincter" during a detrusor contraction. Detrusor-external sphincter dyssynergia is a well-defined condition characterized by an involuntary contraction of the striated urethral sphincter during an involuntary detrusor contraction. It is seen almost exclusively in patients with neurologic lesions of the spinal cord. Inasmuch as there is some disagreement in the literature about the usage of this term, it is discussed in more detail in the section on electromyography. Detrusor-vesical neck dyssynergia refers to contraction of the smooth muscle of the proximal urethra during micturition, but it has not yet been documented that this condition is a cause of vesical neck obstruction.

Detrusor Stability. A stable detrusor is one that accommondates to increasing bladder volume without a significant increase in detrusor pressure and without involuntary detrusor contractions.

Detrusor Pressure. Detrusor pressure (p_{det}) is that component of the intravesical pressure that is due to active and passive forces in the bladder wall. It is determined by subtracting intraabdominal pressure from intravesical pressure (in the absence of a contraction of the rectum).

Enuresis. Enuresis is synonymous with urinary incontinence. It is usually used to denote incontinence during sleep, but when used in this fasion it should always be preceded by "nocturnal."

Flow Time. Flow time is the time over which urinary flow occurs. When flow is continuous and has a clearly defined end point, measurement of flow time is straightforward. However, when flow is interrupted or there is postvoid dribbling, measurement of flow time may be impossible.

Functional Urethral Length. The functional urethral length is that portion of the urethra wherein the urethral pressure is greater than the intravesical pressure.

Incontinence. The involuntary loss of urine.

Intraabdominal Pressure. Intraabdominal pressure (p_{abd}) is the pressure surrounding the bladder. It is usually estimated by measuring rectal pressure.

Intravesical Pressure. Intravesical pressure (p_{ves}) is the total pressure inside the bladder. It consists in three components: p_{det}, p_{abd}, and the hydrostatic pressure due to the weight of urine in the bladder.

Involuntary Detrusor Contraction. An involuntary detrusor contraction is defined as a sudden rise in detrusor pressure that is not volitional. The patient may perceive the contraction as an urge to void, suprapubic pain, or dysuria; or he may be completely unaware of it. He may or may not be able to supress its onset or abort it once it starts. Although involuntary detrusor contractions are usually described as having more than 15 cm H_2O pressure, they are often of lesser magnitude and may require electronic subtraction of intraabdominal pressure for ease of detection.

Maximum Urethral Pressure. Maximum urethral pressure ($p_{ura\ max}$) is the highest pressure measured during the urethral closure pressure profile (UCPP).

Maximum Urethral Closure Pressure. The maximum urethral closure pressure is the difference between $p_{ura\ max}$ and p_{ves}.

Maximum Urinary Flow Rate. Maximum urinary flow rate (Q_{max}) is the highest instantaneous flow recorded during a single micturition.

Maximum Voiding Pressure. The maximum voiding pressure is the highest pressure (intravesical or detrusor) obtained during urinary flow.

Motor Urgency. Motor urgency is a strong urge to void caused by involuntary detrusor contractions.

Opening Time. The opening time is the interval from the onset of the detrusor contraction to the onset of urinary flow.

Opening Pressure. The opening pressure is the pressure in the bladder (intravesical or detrusor) at the onset of urinary flow.

Sensory Urgency. Sensory urgency is a strong urge to void unassociated with involuntary detrusor contractions.

Sphincteric Incontinence. Sphincteric incontinence (SI) is a condition that occurs when the urethral sphincter mechanism no longer maintains a watertight seal, and leakage of urine occurs either by gravity or with the slightest provocation.

Stress Urinary Incontinence. Stress urinary incontinence (SUI) may be a symptom, a sign, or a condition. The symptom is the involuntary loss of urine associated with coughing, sneezing, or other forms of physical activity. The sign is visualization of urinary loss from the urethra during such physical activity.

The condition of stress incontinence is characterized by the involuntary loss of urine that occurs when, in the absence of a detrusor contraction, a sudden increase in intraabdominal pressure exceeds maximum urethral pressure. When the term stress incontinence is used, it is implied that the urethral sphincter mechanism is capable of maintaining a watertight seal, but it is unable to withstand the sudden increase in pressure.

Urethral Pressure. Urethral pressure (p_{ura}) is the pressure within the urethra.

Urethral Closure Pressure Profile. The urethral closure pressure profile (UCPP) is the intraluminal pressure, measured along the length of the urethra, with the bladder at rest.

Urge Incontinence. Urge incontinence (UI) is the involuntary loss of urine associated with an uncontrollable urge to void. It is further classified as motor urge and sensory urge incontinence.

Urinary Flow Rate. The urinary flow rate (Q) is the volume of fluid expressed from the urethra per unit time expressed in milliliters per second.

REFERENCES

1. Bates, C. P., Bradley, W. E., Glen, E., Griffiths, D., Melchior, H., Rowan, D., Sterling, A., Zinner, N., and Hald, T.: The standardization of terminology of lower urinary tract function. *J. Urol.* 121:551, 1979.
2. Blaivas, J. G., Awad, S. A., Bissada, N., Khanna, O. P., Krane, R. J., Wein, A. J., and Yalla, S.: Urodynamic procedures: recommendations of the Urodynamic Society. I. Procedures that should be available for routine practise. *Neurourol. Urodyn.* 1:51, 1982.

9

Neurourologic Examination

ANANIAS C. DIOKNO, M.D.

Urodynamic research has brought to light exciting information about lower urinary tract anatomy and physiology as well as new diagnostic modalities and therapeutic approaches to the care of patients with neurogenic bladder and sphincter dysfunction. Knowledge of the basic neurourologic history and thorough physical examination are necessary if one is to apply these diagnostic and therapeutic modalities to the patient. Although history and physical examination alone may not be sufficient to make an accurate diagnosis, the information gathered from the initial evaluation is the cornerstone to proper selection of the appropriate urodynamic test that would lead to specific diagnosis. One has to remember that successful therapy rests on accurate diagnosis.

In any neurourologic evaluation, the major goals of the examiner are (a) to establish the specific bladder or sphincter dysfunction, (b) identify the etiology of the disturbance, and (c) outline a specific therapy to cure or control the dysfunction.

MICTURITION HISTORY

Because the major function of the urinary bladder is storage and evacuation of urine, the presenting complaint of patients with voiding disturbance should revolve around those functions. Specifically, the complaint could be related to urinary incontinence, retention, a combination of the two, or other symptoms related to voiding.

The onset of the complaint is of paramount importance. The symptom can be acute or chronic. If chronic, it can be acquired or congenital. In cases of nontraumatic neurologic bladder dysfunction, e.g., multiple sclerosis, tabes dorsalis, diabetic neuropathy, and spinal cord tumors, the insidious onset of most symptoms alerts one to seemingly trivial complaints.

Symptoms related to bladder emptying generally include hesitancy, poor caliber and strength of the urinary stream, interrupted stream, straining to void, and a feeling of incomplete bladder emptying. Men may describe their technique of voiding as sitting or grunting, and women may describe unorthodox positions such as bending over, straddling the toilet bowl, or even using Credé's maneuver to empty their bladders. These symptoms, although suggestive of evacuation problems, are not discriminatory of detrusor or outlet dysfunction. A hypotonic or areflexic bladder, an outlet obstruction, or both can produce these symptoms. However, it should serve as a clue for the examiner to search for other signs and guide him to the next most appropriate study.

Irritative bladder symptoms generally include urinary frequency, urgency, dysuria, nocturia, and suprapubic pain or discomfort. Urinary frequency usually develops when a person perceives bladder fullness and is unable to voluntarily suppress the urge to void. Dysuria is painful voiding, and nocturia is nighttime voiding. This group of symptoms suggests inflammation with or without associated infection as observed in cases of bacterial and nonbacterial cystitis. The most common causes of nonbacterial cystitis include interstitial cystitis, radiation cystitis, cytoxan cystitis, and occasionally carcinoma in situ. However, psychogenic disturbances, and at times outlet obstruction, cannot be ruled out with this symptomatology.

Infrequent voiding or lack of bladder perception of distension is not an unusual complaint. The infrequency of voiding may be an acquired habit. In women it is ascribed to avoidance of public restrooms or simply a busy work schedule. However, pathologic sensory loss may be seen in cases of diabetic neuropathy or tabes dorsalis, and in some patients with syringomyelia. Infrequent voiding can lead to detrusor hypotonia manifested by bladder emptying symptoms.

Involuntary urine loss, or urinary incontinence, presents in a variety of ways. The time spent gathering the specifics of the mechanism of urine loss is always time well spent. Descriptive types of urinary incontinence include urge, stress, overflow, and total.

Urge urinary incontinence is the involuntary loss of urine in a person who has a desire to void but insufficient control to prevent bladder emptying. Emptying can range from a few drops to complete bladder empyting with an excellent urinary stream. This type of incontinence is usually associated with detrusor hyperreflexia or instability, as commonly seen in patients with chronic cerebrovascular accidents and multiple sclerosis. In patients who have lost the sensory bladder component, the sensation of urgency preceding voiding is absent, although precipitate incontinence is still a major complaint. This is typically seen in patients with transverse myelitis above the sacral cord segments. Such incontinence is usually described as reflex incontinence or reflex voiding.

Stress urinary incontinence is described as loss of urine with exertion, e.g., coughing, laughing, or lifting objects. In typical cases the patient is continent in the supine position and many times in the sitting position. Incontinence develops upon assuming an upright position or whenever the patient exerts or increases the intraabdominal pressure. In severe cases, however, urine loss can be expected with minimal exertion, even in the supine position. The manifestation of stress urinary incontinence may be due to several conditions. The most common cause in women is urethral sphincter incompetence secondary to pelvic relaxation; the urethral wall is anatomically intact, but the proximal urethra has lost the support necessary to keep it in the retropubic intraabdominal position. In men, the most common cause is injury to the sphincter mechanism following prostatectomy; other causes of stress urinary incontinence include neurogenic sphincter dysfunction (e.g., paralysis of the periurethral striated muscle or the proximal urethra) and cases of noncompliant urethra from previous multiple instrumentations or operations.

Overflow urinary incontinence, also known as paradoxical incontinence, is characterized by constant dribbling of urine as a result of bladder overdistension and high intravesical pressure overcoming urethral resistance. This situation is commonly seen in patients with outlet obstruction, as in prostatism, and is also observed in patients with a paralytic or hypoactive detrusor.

Total incontinence exists when one is constantly wet with urine. In this condition there is no associated urgency, although normal voiding may be possible. Conditions related to this type of incontinence include ectopic ureter orifice and various fistulas, e.g., vesicovaginal, ureterovaginal and vesicouterine. In patients with severe loss of sphincteric resistance, as sometimes is seen in myelomeningocele and extensive injury to the membranous urethra, total incontinence may be observed.

NONVOIDING HISTORY

Bowel symptomatology may parallel bladder symptoms and should actively be pursued. As in the urinary bladder, problems with bowel evacuation, e.g., chronic constipation or obstipation, should be investigated. The presence of fecal incontinence may be the major complaint. Such symptoms are of great significance, as innervation to the rectum is derived from the same segments in the spinal cord that innervate the urinary bladder and urethral sphincter. Sexual history should also be explored as impotence and ejaculatory dysfunction may be of neurogenic origin.

A significant history includes neurologic diseases, previous urologic, gynecologic, or neurosurgical procedures, chronic use of medications, and chronic heavy ingestion of alcohol. Previous neurologic diseases (e.g., neurosyphilis, poliomyelitis or parkinsonism, or encephalitis) may be the etiology of the bladder and sphincter dysfunction. Long-term medication with tranquilizers is known to cause hypotonic bladders. Other drugs that affect bladder function include anticholinergics, sympathomimetics, and cholinergics. Chronic alcoholics are known to develop peripheral neuropathy, which also can affect micturition.

PHYSICAL EXAMINATION

In addition to a general physical examination, emphasis should be placed on the urogenital and neurologic examination. In men the penis is examined for evidence of phimosis and meatal stenosis that may produce obstructive symptoms. The prostate is palpated to identify any abnormal findings, e.g., hard nodules suggestive of prostatic carcinoma or a tender, fluctuant prostate as in prostatitis or prostatic abscess. An enlarged prostate gland on rectal examination has no meaning in itself unless it is associated with obstructive signs and symptoms. Obstruction can occur in the presence of a large or unenlarged prostate gland. Many large glands on rectal examination are totally asymptomatic and not associated with obstruction. The size of the gland is helpful to the urologic surgeon only when the plan is to remove the prostate gland, and to determine the route to use for removal. Small glands are removed transurethrally, whereas large glands are removed suprapubically.

In women, a vaginal examination includes inspection of the urethral meatus and anterior vaginal wall. The use of a posterior vaginal retractor is helpful for palpating and visualizing the urethra through the anterior vaginal wall in order to locate fistulas and urethral diverticula. The urethra should always be palpated, since in the presence of a diverticulum, purulent discharge may be seen to exude at the urethral meatus. This maneuver also demonstrates the degree of cystocele if one is present. By reversing the retraction and applying the retractor anteriorly, the degree of a rectocele, if any is present, can also be evaluated.

A uroneurologic examination includes sensory and motor testing as well as examination of pertinent reflexes. For those with an obvious spinal cord lesion, it is important to determine whether the cord lesion is complete or incomplete. Sensory and motor levels should be established because in general, bladder and sphincter dysfunction follow a certain pattern, depending on the level of the cord lesion (*1*).

The spinal cord center for micturition is in sacral segments 2, 3, and 4 ($S_{2\text{-}4}$). It is now believed that in a normal setting the pontine mesencephalic center in the brainstem is the major micturition reflex center (*3*). However, in cases of high spinal cord transection, the sacral segments below the injury probably take over and discharge impulses to the bladder and urethral sphincter independent of the higher center.

Because of the location of the spinal cord reflex center at $S_{2\text{-}4}$, confusion has arisen about the finding of a lower motor neuron spinal cord lesion to the lower extremity with upper motor neuron findings in the bladder. A student of neurology will remember that flaccidity of the lower extremities, absence of deep tendon reflexes, and a positive Babinski reflex are signs that suggest a lower motor neuron lesion to the lower extremity. However, one should remember that these structures are innervated by low lumbar segments and that the $S_{2\text{-}4}$ segments may be preserved, giving the bladder an upper motor neuron picture manifested by detrusor hyperreflexia and a positive bulbocavernosus reflex. An upper motor neuron lesion to the extremity manifests with hyperactivity of the deep tendon and muscle reflexes, skeletal muscle spasticity, and a positive Babinski sign. The patellar reflex arc involves the second to the fourth lumbar segments, and the ankle reflex involves the fifth lumbar to the second sacral segments.

Reflexes of interest to the urologist include the bulbocavernosus reflex and the anal wink. The anal sphincter and the bulbocavernosus muscles are innervated by segments $S_{2\text{-}4}$. Testing of these reflexes therefore is a good way of testing their reflex arcs. The bulbocavernosus reflex is tested by inserting a finger into the anus to detect anal sphincter contraction when the glans penis is squeezed, the clitoris is pressed against the pubis, or an indwelling Foley urethral catheter is pulled gently (Fig. 9-1). The anal wink is a visible contraction of the anal sphincter immediately after a pinprick stimu-

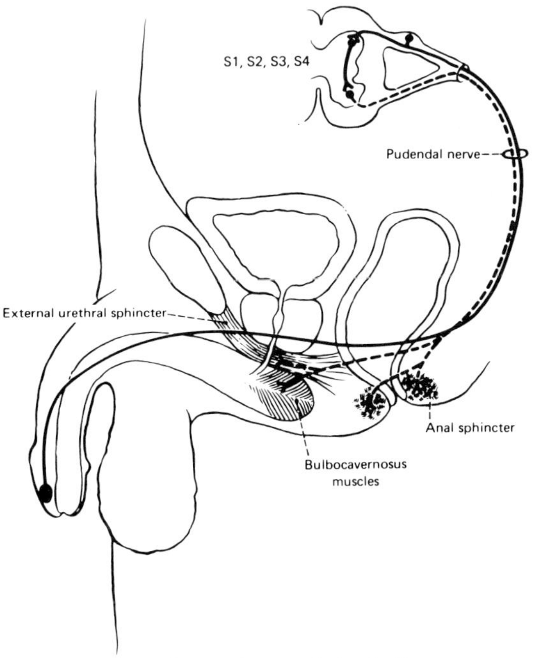

Figure 9–1. Reflex pathway of the bulbocavernosus reflex. Solid line-afferent; dotted line-efferent.

lus is applied to the mucocutaneous junction of the anus.

Sensory testing of the saddle area is extremely important. Unfortunately, access to this area is difficult unless one is placed in the lithotomy or frog-leg position. This problem should not deter the examiner from completing this important uroneurologic examination. Anesthesia of a portion of or the entire perineal area suggests disturbance of the afferent tract of the pudendal nerve. Patients have been encountered in whom this abnomality is the only neurologic deficit observed in association with their bladder dysfunction.

When performing a rectal examination, one should assess the tone of the anal sphincter. Although a patulous anus may suggest paralysis of the anal sphincter, previous anal sphincter surgery or chronic overstretching from severe constipation should be ruled out. In the same setting, the patient should be asked to voluntarily contract the anal sphincter to test for integrity of the corticoregulatory tract.

LABORATORY TESTS

Laboratory tests should include urinalysis and evaluation of renal function. Urinalysis identifies the pH and the presence or absence of albumin and glucose. Microscopic studies of the urine sediment should include noting the presence or absence of pyuria, hematuria, casts, bacteriuria, and crystalluria. Persistent or recurrent urinary tract infection may be a reflection of neuropathic bladder and sphincter dysfunction. Blood urea nitrogen and serum creatinine are generally sufficient initial tests of renal function.

URORADIOGRAPHIC STUDIES

Uroradiographic studies that are helpful in assessing the nature and effects of bladder and sphincter dysfunction include excretory urography and cystourethrography. Excretory urography can identify hydronephrosis and hydroureter and calculus disease, each of which can be due to bladder dysfunction. In neuropathic bladder dysfunction, ureteral obstructions usually occur at the level of the bladder wall because of smooth muscle hypertrophy or chronically elevated intravesical pressure. Ureteral dilatation may also result from vesicoureteral reflux, which can be diagnosed by cystourethrography. Cystography may also identify abnormal bladder configuration due to smooth muscle hypertrophy (trabeculation) and mucosal outpouchings outside the bladder wall (diverticula). A common radiographic finding called "Christmas tree bladder" because of its shape is usually attributed to neuropathic bladder dysfunction (Fig. 9–2). However, this finding is not pathognomonic of neuropathic dysfunction. Whenever a neurogenic bladder and/or sphincter dysfunction is suspected in the absence of obvious neurologic disease, vertebral radiography and electromyography of the lumbosacral myotomes should be considered (*4*). Radiographic study may reveal bony abnormalities such as collapsed vertebral bodies, congenital defects, or metastatic lesions. Electromyography of the lumbosacral myotomes, when positive for denervation, has a high correlation with bladder and sphincter-dysfunction.

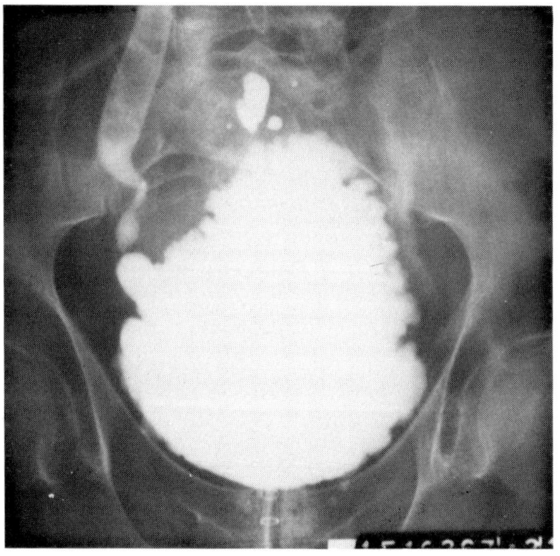

Figure 9–2. Typical "Christmas tree" bladder on cystogram.

ENDOSCOPIC STUDIES

Endoscopy entails visual evaluation of the urethra and the bladder using a cystourethroscope. This procedure can be performed under topical anesthesia, although general or regional anesthesia have been used in some patients with intact sensation.

Endoscopic evaluation of the urethra and urinary bladder is indicated in patients with hematuria, recurrent urinary tract infections, lower urinary tract obstructive symptoms, and urinary incontinence. The major objective of this study is to identify any anatomic abnormalities that may explain the symptoms or signs. Specifically, this procedure can identify the presence of bladder or urethral tumors, calculi strictures, false passages, urethral diverticulum, urethral trauma, prostatic enlargement, abnormalities of the ureteral orifices, and various fistulae. The diagnosis of vesical neck contracture by endoscopy is extremely subjective unless one is dealing with a truly fibrous pinpoint vesical neck as a consequence of previous vesical neck resection. One also has to remember that prostatic enlargement showing visual occlusion on endoscopy may be significant only if it is associated with obstructive symptoms and other signs of obstruction, e.g., trabeculation, diverticula formation, and residual urine.

SPECIALIZED NEUROUROLOGIC STUDIES

Neurogenic bladder can be diagnosed by cystometrography, and the neurogenic external sphincter can be identified by needle sphincter electromyography. However, to assess the function or dysfunction of the bladder and sphincter, dynamic studies such as uroflowmetry, combined cystometry, sphincter electromyography, urethral pressure profilometry, combined bladder, urethral, and abdominal pressures with uroflowmetry and, voiding cystourethrography can be performed. These urodynamic studies not only can define the specific dysfunction but should guide the urologist to the appropriate therapy.

REFERENCES

1. Comarr, A. E.: Diagnosis of the traumatic cord bladder. In Boyarsky, S. (ed.), *The Neurogenic Bladder.* Williams & Wilkins, Baltimore, 1967, pp. 147–152.
2. Lapides, J., and Diokno, A. C.: Urine transport, storage and micturition. In Lapides, J. (ed.), *Fundamentals of Urology.* Saunders, Philadelphia, 1976, pp. 705–713.
3. Bradley, W. E., Timm, G. W., and Scott, F. B.: Innervation of the detrusor muscle and urethra. *Urol. Clin. N. Am.* 1:3, 1974.
4. Sonda, L. P., Kogan, B. A., Koff, S. A., and Diokno, A. C.: Neurologic disease masquerading as genitourinary abnormality. The role of urodynamics in diagnosis. *J. Urol.* 129:1174–1178, 1983.

10

Techniques of Evaluation

JERRY G. BLAIVAS, M.D.

From a clinical standpoint, the purpose of urodynamic testing is to measure and record various physiologic variables while the patient is experiencing those symptoms that constitute his usual complaints. In this context urodynamic studies may be considered to be provocative tests of vesicourethral function. Thus it is the responsibility of the examiner to ensure that the patient's symptoms are in fact reproduced during the study. When the patient does experience his symptoms at the time of the examination, the resulting physiologic data provide the substrate for understanding the etiology of the patient's complaint. However, when the symptoms are not reproduced during the urodynamic investigation, the data so obtained often prove to be irrelevant and, in many instances, misleading. For example, when a patient complains of urinary frequency, urgency, and urge incontinence, and cystometry reveals involuntary detrusor contractions that exactly reproduce the symptoms, the diagnosis is straightforward. However, when a patient complains only of stress incontinence and the cystometrogram demonstrates low-magnitude involuntary detrusor contractions of which she is completely unaware and which do not reproduce her symptoms, one would be misled to conclude that the etiology of her incontinence is detrusor instability.

The widespread availability of many urodynamic techniques and parameters may confound the practicing urologist, but in principle there are only five: cystometry, uroflowmetry, sphincter electromyography, urethral profilometry, and radiographic visualization of the lower urinary tract. To these techniques may be added the measurement of intra-abdominal pressure.

The variables chosen for a particular study depend on a number of factors: the complexity of the clinical problem, the availability of electronic equipment, the ease with which the study can be performed, and the interest and expertise of the urodynamicist. The Urodynamic Society has recommended that in most clinical settings it is practical and cost-effective to screen patients by performing cystometry, uroflowmetry, and measurement of post-void residual urine volume. More sophisticated studies may be indicated when (a) these simple diagnostic procedures have proved inconclusive, (b) the patient has persistent symptoms despite what appears to be appropriate treatment, (c) the patient has a preexisting condition known to be associated with complex urodynamic abnormalities, and (d) the history and physical examination suggest neurologic pathology that requires more elaborate investigation for diagnosis. The need for multichannel studies should be assessed individually for each patient; one should not generalize and conclude that all patients with a particular disorder require elaborate investigation. On the other hand, lower urinary tract symptoms in certain conditions, e.g., spinal cord injury, multiple sclerosis, and after radical pelvic surgery, are accompanied by bizarre and unpredictable pathology often enough to warrant multichannel studies routinely when the clinical setting demands urodynamic investigation.

CYSTOMETRY

Cystometry is the "reflex hammer" of the neurourologist. In simple terms it may be defined as the graphic representation of bladder pressure as a function of filling volume. It is unfortunate that the end result of cystometry is reduced to a paper tracing from a strip chart recorder because it conveys the false impression that, like an electrocardiogram, the cystometrogram can be interpreted by "reading the graph." Nothing could be further from the truth. The examination must be interpreted at the time of the study by maintaining close verbal contact with the patient. It is not enough to note changes in intravesical pressure; it must be determined whether the observed changes are due to a detrusor contraction, an increase in intra-abdominal pressure, or a viscoelastic property of the bladder. If a detrusor contraction is observed, it must be ascertained whether it is voluntary or involuntary, if the patient is aware of it, and if he/she is able to inhibit it. Moreover, it is of crucial importance to understand whether the observed cystometric abnormalities seem to bear any relation to the patient's symptoms.

Despite the fact that detrusor contractions are often elicited during cystometry, the cystometrogram should not be thought of as a test to determine if the bladder is capable of contraction, because many otherwise normal patients are unable to generate a voluntary detrusor contraction in the setting of a cystometric examination—probably due to the psychic inhibition that occurs because of the embarrassing and unphysiologic manner in which the test is performed. Thus the absence of a detrusor contraction during cystometry should not necessarily be considered abnormal.

Physiologic Considerations

Conceptually, the cystometric curve may be divided into three segments (Fig. 10–1): (a) The initial pressure rise represents the first segment (T1). (b) The long, flat segment that occurs during further bladder filling is referred to as the tonus limb (T2). (c) A third terminal segment (T3) has been attributed to stretching of the collagen fibers in the bladder wall (*1*). The first two segments are usually apparent, but the third segment is

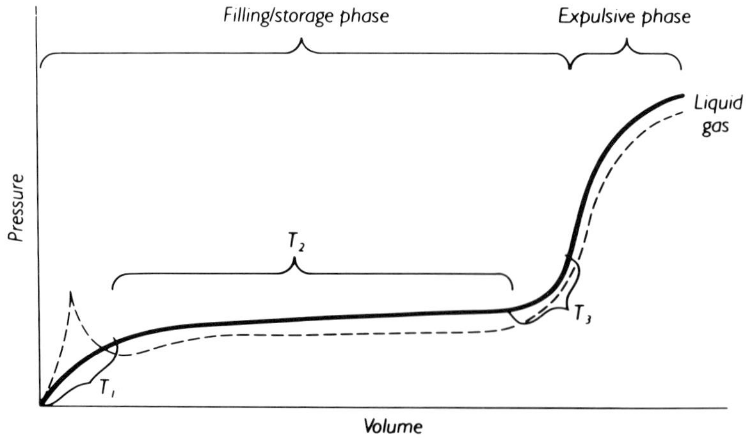

Figure 10–1. Idealized cystometrogram. During bladder filling there is an initial rise in pressure (T_1) that is due to the resting intravesical pressure and the viscoelastic response of the bladder to stretch. As the bladder is filled, it accommodates to increasing volume by increasing its wall tension and the intravesical pressure remains fairly constant (T_2). The third segment (T_3) is a sudden rise in intravesical pressure due to stretching of the bladder to its physiologic limit. (From Blaivas, J. G.: Urodynamic testing. In Raz, S. [ed.], *Female Urology*. Saunders, Philadelphia, 1983.)

often not appreciated. During air cystometry, a T3 segment was observed in 58 percent of 158 patients (*1*), but in our experience it is difficult if not impossible to distinguish T3 from the onset of a detrusor contraction; accordingly, we do not find T3 to be a useful cystometric parameter.

When fluid is instilled into the empty bladder there is an initial rise in pressure (T1) that may have two components. The first component is a purely passive viscoelastic response to stretch, the magnitude of which is related to the degree and speed of the stretch, i.e., the rate and volume of filling (*2–4*). The second response, also due to stretch, is an active contraction of the detrusor, which is discussed more fully below (*5,6*). At slow rates of fill, as is usually accomplished with liquid, the T1 pressure is usually low (0–5 cm H_2O). However, at high rates of fill, as is usual with gas cystometry, the T1 pressure may be high (100 cm H_2O) and may simulate a detrusor contraction (Fig. 10–2).

After the initial viscoelastic response to bladder stretch, more bladder filling usually results in little further change in recorded pressure. This second segment of the cystometric curve is called the tonus limb (T2). The fairly stable pressure observed during the tonus limb is possible because the bladder accommodates to increasing volume by increasing its wall tension at the expense of pressure (*2*).

In an important study, Klevmark clearly demonstrated the effect of rate of fill on the tonus limb of the cystometrogram (*2*). He laboriously and meticulously performed cystometry on cats using a method of investigation he termed "controlled slow cystometry" (CSC). During CSC fluid is instilled into the bladder at some multiple of the normal rate at which urine is delivered to the bladder by the kidneys. He called the normal physiologic rate the hour diuresis (HD). During cystometry there was no change in detrusor pressure when the bladder was filled at rates up to 2.4 HD; i.e., the tonus limb was horizontal. In different experimental preparations, a pressure increase was observed at rates varying from 2.4 to 7.0 HD. If the cystometrogram was begun at one rate (above 2.4 HD) and the filling rate was then reduced, the pressure fell but remained at a higher level than would have been attained if filling had been continued at the initial rate. Klevmark called it the "pressure accumulation phenomenon."

From a theoretical standpoint the pressure accumulation phenomenon may have importance because it provides a mechanism for increased bladder wall tension, at a given bladder volume, based on the rate of fill, e.g., during diuresis. Wall tension is approximated by the LaPlace law for a thin-walled sphere:

$$\text{Tension} = \text{pressure} \times \text{radius}/2.$$

Since the radius of the bladder is the same for any given volume, wall tension is determined primarily by the intravesical pressure, which is dependent on the rate of bladder filling and the pressure accumulation phenomenon.

Klevmark subsequently determined that these rate-dependent intravesical pressure patterns obtained during cystometry were preserved in animals who had undergone ex-

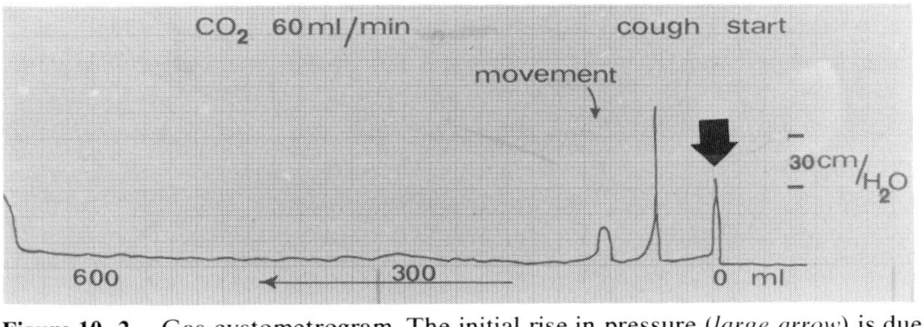

Figure 10–2. Gas cystometrogram. The initial rise in pressure (*large arrow*) is due to the viscoelastic properties of the bladder and is not related to a detrusor contraction. The tracing moves from right to left.

tensive denervation procedures (*7*). Although the basal (T1) intravesical pressure was increased after parasympathetic decentralization by about 5 cm H_2O, there was no change in the rate-dependent intravesical pressure patterns. Sympathetic decentralization had no effect on either the T1 pressure or the tonus limb.

Prior to Klevmark's studies, Ruch and Tang (*8,9*) had also shown that the slope of the tonus limb is independent of neural control. They performed cystometric studies on cats who had undergone denervation procedures including decerebration, spinal transection, ganglionic blockade, and section of the anterior sacral and coccygeal roots, as well as on intact animals immediately after death. None of these conditions changed the slope of the tonus limb. However, fibrosis of the detrusor does alter the tonus limb by changing the viscoelastic properties of the bladder such that it cannot maintain its low pressure during filling. The resulting low-compliance tonus limb is characterized by a steep rise in pressure. Bradley *et al.* performed cystometry in dogs before and after injecting a sclerosing agent into the wall of the bladder (*10*). A marked increase in the slope of the tonus limb was seen after injection of the sclerosing agent. There was a 300 to 400 percent increase in hydroxyproline content (a constant component of collagen) in the low-compliance bladders, but the expected fibrosis of the detrusor was not demonstrated by histologic sections. It was suggested that the hydroxyproline content is a more sensitive index of fibrosis than histologic sections. Kondo and Susset performed similar studies in dogs and found a marked increase in the elastic constant calculated from the pressure-decay curve obtained after rapid-injection cystometry (*11*). This diminished compliance of the bladder wall was also accompanied by an increase in collagen content as measured by hydroxyproline content (*11*). From a clinical standpoint, a hypertonic tonus limb may be encountered in conditions associated with fibrosis, e.g., radiation and tuberculous cystitis, long-term use of indwelling catheters, and parasympathetic nerve damage.

Kondo and co-workers introduced the concept of rapid-injection cystometry as a more precise means of evaluating viscoelastic properties (*3-5*). A mechanical model of the bladder composed of viscous and elastic elements was developed. In *in vivo* and *in vitro* experiments the bladders of female cats were filled incrementally by injecting 30 ml of saline over a period of 1.25 seconds. The resulting pressure decay curves were mathematically analyzed. The maximum bladder pressure obtained after rapid injection was thought to characterize the elastic behavior of the bladder. The speed of pressure decay was a measure of bladder viscosity. It was found that the viscous and elastic coefficients thus obtained were directly related to the percentage of collagen present in the bladder wall (*11,12*). The higher the collagen content, the higher was the maximum pressure attained after rapid injection and the slower was the speed of decay of the pressure curve, i.e., the "stiffer" was the bladder.

Coolsaet *et al.* devised another means for evaluating the viscoelastic behavior of the bladder. They performed "stepwise cystometry" by incrementally filling the bladder, and they found that it was necessary to wait 15 minutes between injections for equilibration (*13,14*). They defined at least two viscoelastic coefficients, suggesting at least two functional components of the bladder. Furthermore, they noted that the cystometrogram, as it is currently performed by continuous filling, does not provide useful information about the viscoelastic properties of the bladder.

These studies clearly document that the shape of the cystometric curve is intimately dependent on the rate at which the bladder is filled, and that the viscoelastic properties of the bladder wall itself are independent of neuromuscular control. From a clinical standpoint, it is thus meaningless to consider the slope of the cystometric curve or the compliance of the bladder unless one does so in a standardized fashion in which the bladder is filled at a constant and predetermined rate.

In Klevmark's studies and those of Ruch and Tang, micturition could be elicited at different bladder volumes and pressures, depending on the rate of infusion (*2,8,9*). Although the tonus limb was uninfluenced by denervation, the timing and appearance of detrusor contractions were shown to be under neural control. In general, reflex detrusor contractions were elicited at lower bladder volumes in cats with suprasacral spinal cord lesions and were abolished in those with sectioned sacral roots. These data confirm the well-known clinical findings of detrusor hyperreflexia in patients with suprasacral neurologic lesions and detrusor "areflexia" in those with lower motor neuron disease (*15–18*).

An unexpected outcome of rapid-injection cystometry was the observation that rapid distension of the bladder could elicit several kinds of detrusor contraction (Fig. 10-3), some of which were not seen during routine cystometry (*5,6*). Although it is hoped that the characteristics of these contractions will ulimately be shown to have clinical significance, convincing data to substantiate this hope have not been presented.

Nathan (*19*) and Bradley *et al.* (*20*) have described two kinds of bladder sensation: proprioception and exteroception. *Proprioception* includes the first sensation of bladder filling, the sense of fullness, the urge to void, and the feeling that micturition is imminent. There is also a vague abdominal sensation of fullness that may be preserved even after extensive denervation of the bladder. Although the precise sensory neurologic pathways have not been well described, it is likely that there are at least two kinds of proprioceptive receptors in the bladder. Volume receptors are stimulated by stretch only, whereas tension receptors, because they are in series with muscle fibers, probably respond to both passive stretch and active muscle contraction. The impulses from volume and tension receptors probably are transmitted to higher centers by the parasympathetic and sympathetic divisions of the central nervous system.

Exteroceptive sensations consist in pain, temperature, and touch. The neural impulses from these receptors are transmitted by the pelvic nerve to reach neurons in the posterior root ganglion, cross to the contralateral side and ascend in the lateral spinothalamic tract to the thalamic nuclei and then are projected upon the sensory cortex.

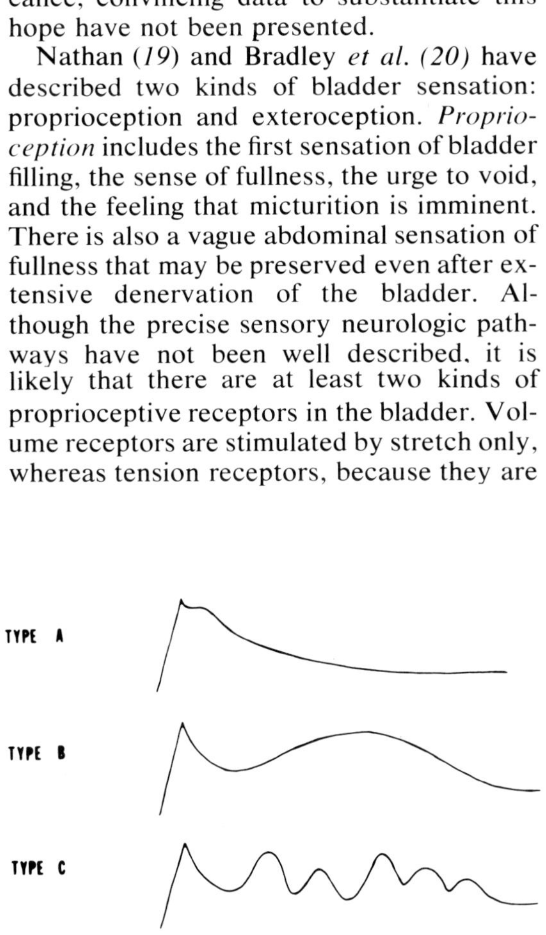

Figure 10–3. Rapid injection cystometry. Three types of detrusor contraction have been described. Type A contractions are brief, low-grade contractions that occur almost immediately after the nadir of the viscoelastic response. Type B contractions are sustained, coordinated contractions. Type C are polyphasic in configuration. (From Susset, J. G., *et al.*: *Neurourol. Urodyn.* 1:319, 1982.)

Cystometers. The simplest "cystometer" consists of a catheter connected to a fluid reservoir such as the barrel of a 50-ml catheter tip syringe with the plunger removed (Fig. 10–4). Fluid may be instilled into the bladder by gravity and the intravesical pressure determined by lowering or raising the height of the barrel until fluid ceases to flow. The height of the meniscus above the symphysis pubis represents the intravesical pressure. Detrusor contractions may be detected by observing changes in the level of the meniscus or a slowing of the infusion rate. The cystometric curve may be approximated by plotting the intravesical pressure as a function of volume.

Such a cystometer is adequate for observing obvious involuntary detrusor contractions and for approximating cystometric capacity, but it has certain disadvantages. The height of the barrel must be moved in order to measure the intravesical pressure, and a constant or predetermined infusion rate is impossible to attain. Because pressure can be measured only intermittently, contractions occurring between measurements may not be detected, and low-magnitude detrusor contractions may be difficult to appreciate.

To combat these inherent deficiencies, commercially available electronic cystometers usually provide (a) a constant rate of infusion, (b) electronic subtraction of the pressure head due to infusion from the total intravesical pressure, (c) an instantaneous and continuous graphic display of the cystometric curve, (d) a pressure cutoff valve to protect against continued infusion when intravesical pressure becomes too high, and (e) automatic pressure calibration.

Catheters. For routine cystometry the

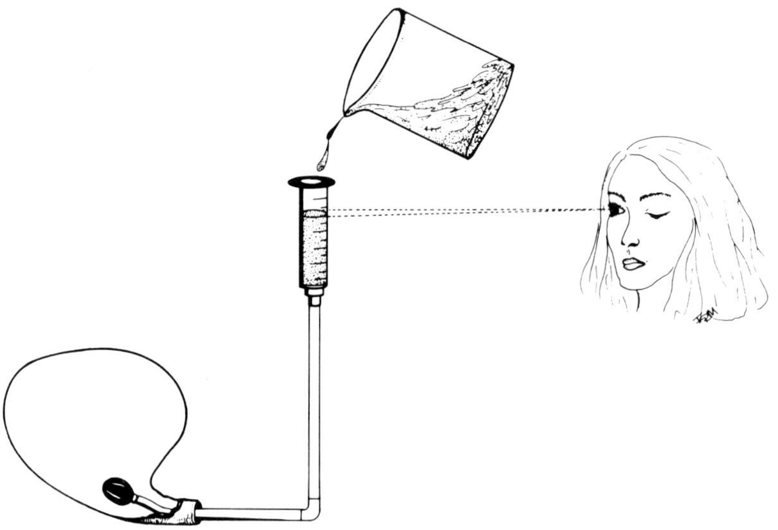

Figure 10–4. Simple "cystometer." The simplest cystometer can be constructed by removing the barrel from a large syringe and attaching it to the end of a catheter that is placed in the bladder. The bladder is filled by pouring fluid into the syringe, and the height of the fluid meniscus at which flow stops measures the intravesical pressure.

type of catheter makes little difference with respect to the results; but obviously the smaller the catheter, the less is the discomfort that is experienced by the patient and the easier it is for him/her to void around the catheter if necessary. Catheters that are too small limit the rate at which fluid can be instilled and may be difficult to insert transurethrally. In practical terms, 12F to 16F Foley catheters are most often used.

Special catheters have been designed for multichannel urodynamic studies. The simplest type is a double-lumen catheter of about 8F to 10F. The larger lumen opens at the end of the catheter and is used for bladder filling; the smaller lumen opens several centimeters proximal to the first and is used to record intravesical pressure. A triple-lumen catheter adds a third channel for measuring urethral pressure. The location of the urethral measuring port may vary, but one positioned approximately 7 cm from the intravesical port is practical for measuring urethral pressures in both sexes (Fig. 10–5). These catheters provide reasonably precise and accurate data; their main disadvantage is that they are cumbersome because they require separate tubing and fluid for each channel. In addition, in order to measure urethral pressure, fluid must be instilled through the urethral measuring channel at a slow rate (approximately 2–10 ml/min) in order to prevent the urethral wall from occluding the lumen.

A four-channel membrane catheter has been devised to obviate the need for urethral infusion (*21,22*). One channel is used for bladder filling and opens at the tip of the catheter. A second channel ends in a side hole 1 cm proximal to the tip and is used for measuring intravesical pressure. The third and fourth channels are used to transduce urethral pressure. They end in side holes 1 cm apart located 7 cm from the tip. They are covered by a thin latex membrane and marked by metal rings.

Microtip transducer catheters have been introduced to incorporate the transducers for measuring pressures into the catheter itself, thereby avoiding the need for separate tubing and fluid for each pressure channel (*23–26*). They are available from several manufacturers in one- to three-sensor catheters for measuring as many as three pressures simultaneously. A separate channel may be added for bladder filling. Currently available microtip transducers are expensive, and some are also fragile and sensitive to temperature. Some are rather stiff, which may cause difficulty when inserting the catheter in male urethra.

There is one important difference between

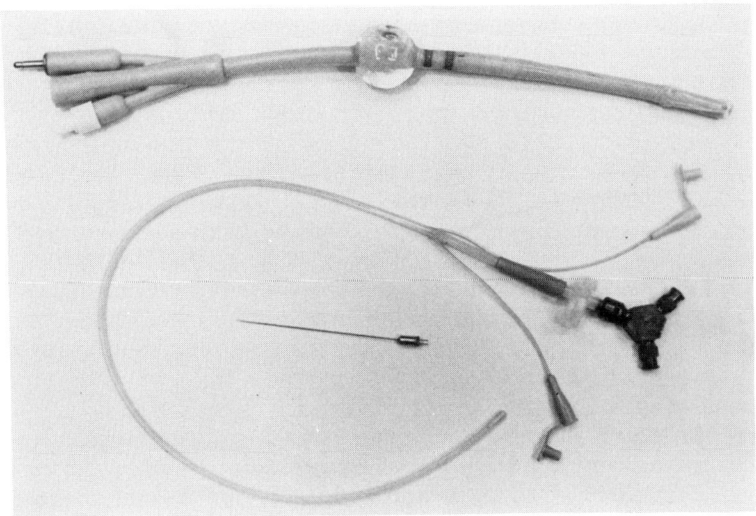

Figure 10–5. Urodynamic equipment. Triple-lumen urodynamic catheter for simultaneous measurement of intravesical and intraurethral pressure (*middle*), concentric needle electrode for electromyography (*bottom*), and rectal pressure monitoring catheter with mounted surface electrodes for anal sphincter electromyography (*top*). See text for details.

microtip transducers and conventional recording techniques that must be taken into account when interpreting the results of pressure studies. When the transducer is located outside the bladder, the zero reference point, by convention, is atmospheric pressure measured at the symphysis pubis. Thus neither movement of the catheter tip within the bladder nor the weight of the fluid within the bladder affects the recorded pressure. When the transducer is located at the tip of the catheter, the transducer tip becomes its own zero reference point. Accordingly, the weight of the fluid within the bladder affects the measurement of total intravesical pressure. In the supine position, this factor has a relatively small effect on recorded pressure unless the bladder capacity is large, but in the sitting or standing position there may be a difference of 15 cm H_2O or more depending on whether the catheter tip is at the bottom or the top of the column of fluid in the bladder.

Technique and Interpretation

Immediately prior to cystometry the patient is asked to void, and the urinary flow rate is determined. The bladder is catheterized and the post-void residual urine measured. The size of the catheter does not affect the results of cystometry, but if simultaneous flow rates are to be determined a catheter no larger than 10F is usually required. At some laboratories two catheters are placed: one for filling the bladder and a second smaller one for measuring intravesical pressure. If voiding is anticipated, the larger catheter may be removed after the filling phase has been completed.

After passage of the catheter the purpose of the cystometric examination is reiterated to the patient. He is instructed to neither void nor attempt to suppress micturition but simply to report his sensations to the examiner. The bladder is filled at a predetermined rate depending on the nature of the patient's symptoms. Periodically during filling the patient is asked to cough and strain in order to provoke involuntary detrusor contractions and to check that the cystometer is working properly. The bladder volume at which the following events occur is noted: (a) the first sensation of bladder filling; (b) the first sensation of fullness; (c) the urge to void; (d) the feeling that micturition is imminent; and (e) the occurrence of involuntary detrusor contractions. Abnormal sensations such as suprapubic or back pain are noted. Cystometric bladder capacity is recorded as the volume at which the patient is uncomfortably full or voids (voluntarily or involuntarily). The slope of the tonus limb (compliance) is noted, but it must be reemphasized that the shape of this curve is very much dependent on the rate of bladder filling as discussed above. Normal cystometrograms are depicted in Figures 10–2 and 10–6.

When the patient experiences the feeling that micturition is imminent, he/she is asked to try to "let it come out by itself." If he is unable to generate a detrusor contraction, the examination is terminated unless involuntary detrusor contractions are suspected as being part of his/her problem. In that case the examination is repeated sitting, standing, or walking in place. If the urge to void is accompanied by a detrusor contraction, the examination is repeated, but this time the patient is instructed to try to inhibit the onset of micturition. If he/she is unable to do so, the resulting detrusor contraction is considered to be involuntary. If an involuntary detrusor contraction occurs during the course of bladder filling, the patient is asked to try to stop it, and his/her ability to do so is noted.

An involuntary detrusor contraction is defined as a sudden rise in detrusor pressure that is not volitional. The patient may perceive the contraction as an urge to void, as suprapubic pain, or as dysuria; or he/she may be completely unaware of it. He/she may or may not be able to supress its onset or abort it once it starts. Although involuntary detrusor contractions are usually described as being more than 15 cm H_2O, they are often of lesser magnitude and may require electronic subtraction of intraabdominal pressure for ease of detection (Fig. 10–7). If involuntary detrusor contractions are suspected but not demonstrated, provocative maneuvers such as coughing (Fig. 10–8), straining, sitting, and walking in place are performed (Fig. 10–9).

When the patient develops a strong urge to void or when capacity is attained, he/she is asked to try to urinate in his/her normal manner. Many patients initiate micturition with abdominal straining, and in these instances it is often impossible to distinguish a detrusor contraction from the effects of straining unless intraabdominal pressure is measured simultaneously. Since all cystometers measure intravesical pressure, which is the sum of detrusor and intraabdominal pressure, any rise in intraabdominal pressure is recorded as a rise in intravesical pressure and may be mistaken for a detrusor contraction (Fig. 10–10 and 10–11). Moreover, many otherwise normal patients are unable to generate a voluntary detrusor contraction in the presence of an examiner. This situation is thought to be due to the embarrassing and unphysiologic setting in which the urodynamic studies are performed. Thus the absence of a detrusor contraction during cystometry is not considered to be abnormal unless there are other clinical or urodynamic findings to substantiate the presence of either lower motor neuron disease or detrusor muscle abnormalities. Accordingly, the proper term for describing a bladder that does not contract during cystometry is detrusor acontractility, not detrusor areflexia. The latter term is used only to connote an acontractile bladder that is due to neurologic abnormalities.

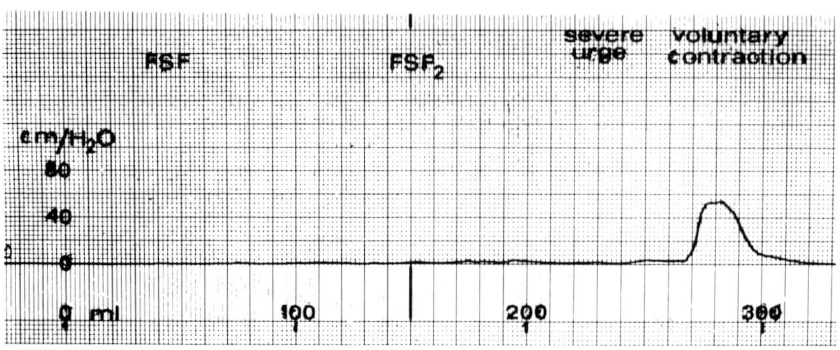

Figure 10–6. Normal (liquid) cystometrogram. *FSF* = first sensation of bladder filling. FSF_2 = urge to void. (From Blaivas, J. G.: Urodynamic testing. In Raz, S. [ed.], *Female Urology*. Saunders, Philadelphia, 1983.)

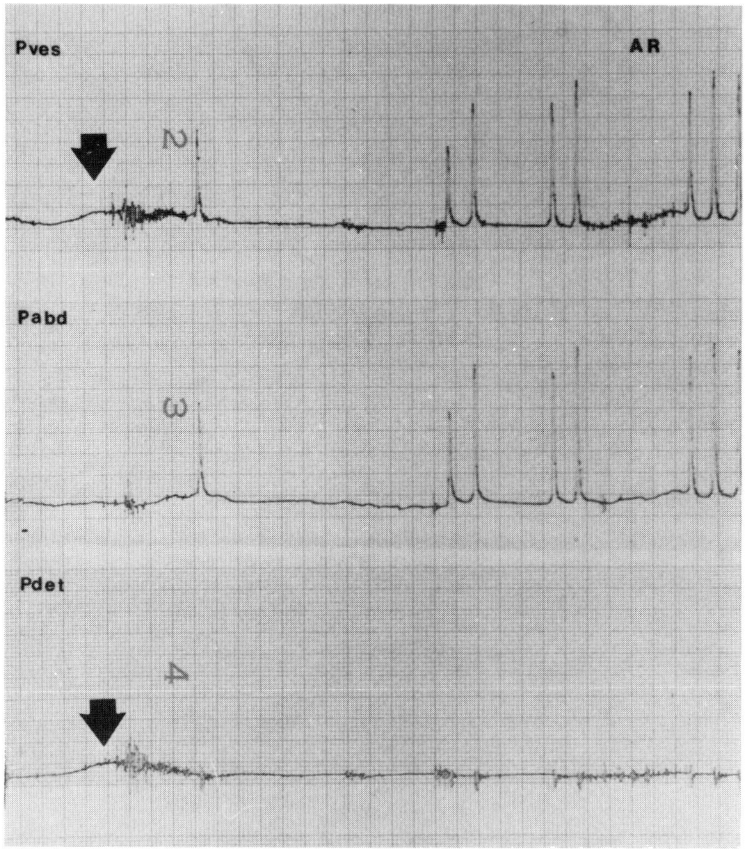

Figure 10–7. Low-magnitude involuntary detrusor contraction. At the arrow there is an involuntary detrusor contraction of only 9 cm H_2O. The sudden rises in pressure are due to coughs. Without rectal pressure monitoring and electronic subtraction, this detrusor contraction may not have been appreciated. Each large division on the vertical scale = 15 cm H_2O.

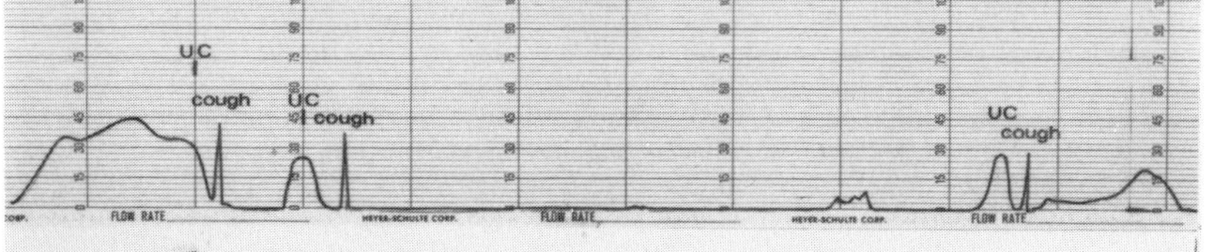

Figure 10–8. Provocative cystometry. Involuntary detrusor contractions initiated by cough. *UC* = involuntary detrusor contraction. (From Blaivas, J. G.: A critical appraisal of specific techniques. In Krane, R. J., and Siroky, M. B. [eds,], *Clinical Neurourology*. Little, Brown, Boston, 1979.)

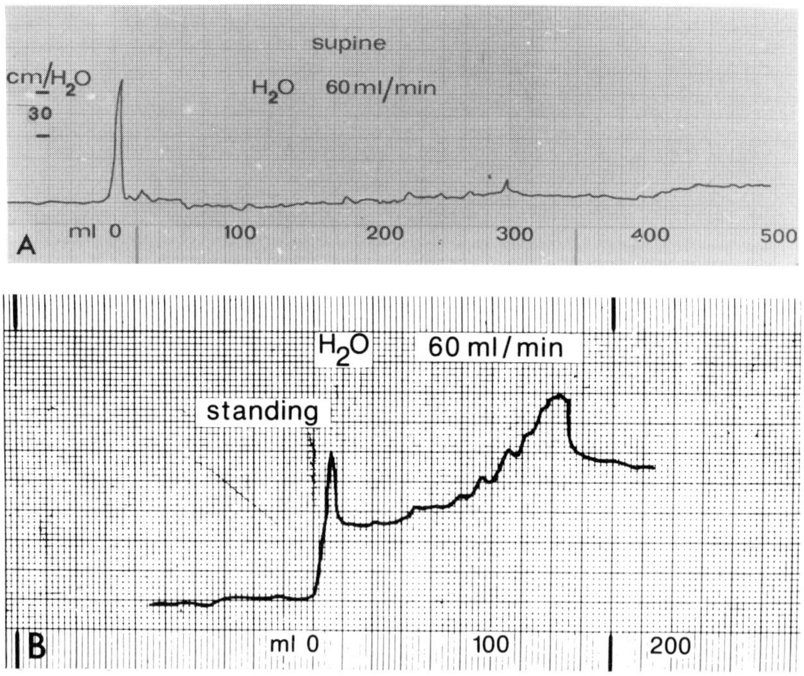

Figure 10–9. Provocative cystometry. **A.** In the supine position there are no involuntary detrusor contractions. **B.** The same patient in the standing position has an obvious involuntary detrusor contraction. (From Blaivas, J. G.: Urodynamic testing. In Raz, S. [ed.], *Female Urology*. Saunders, Philadelphia, 1983.)

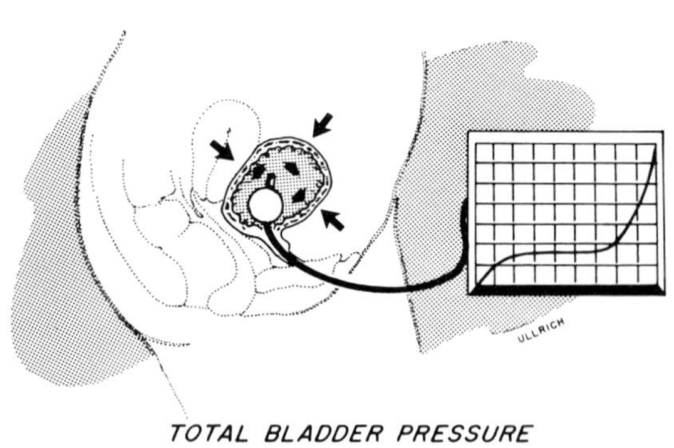

Figure 10–10. All cystometers measure intravesical pressure, which is the sum of detrusor pressure and intraabdominal pressure. (From Blaivas, J. G.: A critical appraisal of specific techniques. In Krane, R. J., and Siroky, M. B. [eds.], *Clinical Neurourology*. Little, Brown and Co., Boston, 1979.)

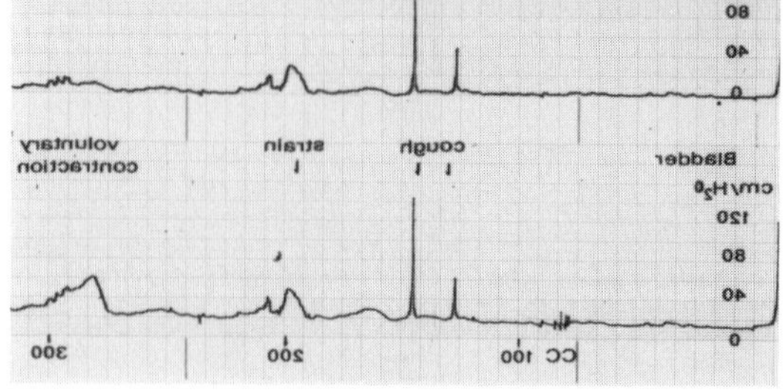

Figure 10–11. Effect of increased intraabdominal pressure on intravesical pressure. Each increase in intraabdominal pressure is transmitted to the bladder. If intraabdominal pressure is not measured, the rise in intravesical pressure might simulate a detrusor contraction. *EUS EMG* = electromyography of the external urethral sphincter. (From Blaivas, J. G.: In Hinman, F., Jr. [ed.], *Benign Prostatic Hypertrophy*. Springer-Verlag, New York, 1983.)

Pharmacologic Tests

Probanthine Test. When involuntary detrusor contractions have been demonstrated during cystometry, it may be desirable to test the efficacy of an anticholinergic drug in abolishing them in order to predict the outcome of pharmacologic treatment. Propantheline bromide is the prototype anticholinergic used for this purpose (*27*). Propantheline bromide (15 mg) is administered parenterally after a baseline cystometrogram has revealed involuntary detrusor contractions. The cystometrogram is repeated whenever the pharmacologic effects of the drug are apparent (dry mouth or blurred vision). It usually occurs within 20 minutes of the injection. A positive response to the anticholinergic is defined as the complete abolition of involuntary detrusor contractions or a 200 percent increase in the bladder volume at which they occur. If the parenteral dosage of propantheline is effective, a favorable clinical response to the orally administered dose can be expected in most patients provided an adequate dosage can be tolerated without untoward side effects (*27,28*).

For the last several years parenteral propantheline bromide has been commercially unavailable in the United States. As a substitute, the anticholinergic glycopyrrolate (Robinul) has been suggested (*29,30*). The usual parenteral dosage is 0.2 mg, which is available in a 1-ml vial for injection. To date, however, there have been no reports to document the efficacy of this drug in either test situations or clinical trials.

Bethanechol Test. The bethanechol test has long been advocated as a means of distinguishing neurogenic from nonneurogenic causes of detrusor acontractility and for evaluating the therapeutic efficacy of the drug (*31–36*). The test is based on Cannon's law of denervation, which states that a smooth muscle deprived of its innervation becomes hypersensitive to certain chemical substances, especially its own neurotransmitter (*37*). As originally described by Lapides *et al.* (*33*), the test is performed in the following manner.

A cystometrogram is performed with liquid at medium fill, and the intravesical pressure at 100 ml volume is recorded. The bladder is emptied via the catheter, and 2.5 mg bathanechol is administered subcutaneously. The bladder is again filled to 100 ml and the pressure measured at 10, 20, and 30 minutes after administration of the drug. A rise in pressure of more than 15 cm H_2O over the control is considered to be a positive response.

Our experience with the denervation supersensitivity test in its original form has been disappointing. We prospectively evaluated a group of patients in whom the test was most critical—those with an equivocal diagnosis of a lower motor neuron lesion involving the bladder who demonstrated an acontractile bladder during cystometry. All patients had careful neurologic evaluation, including myelography in all of those in whom the diagnosis of lower motor neuron lesions could not otherwise be made. We found a false-positive rate of 50 percent and a false-negative rate of 26 percent (*38*). Other authors have documented false-positive results in normal patients and those with cystitis or emotional stress (*32,35*). False-negative results are much less common and are usually found in patients with neurologic conditions of recent onset.

Several authors have modified the original methodology and reported improvement in diagnostic accuracy. Merrill and Rotta supplanted liquid infusion with air and reported equally good results (*35*). Pavlakis *et al.* (*36*) suggested using 5.0 mg rather than 2.5 mg bethanechol and reported no false positives and a false-negative rate of only 2 percent. Glahn administered 2.5 mg bethanechol with the bladder filled to 100 ml and measured the pressure continuously without emptying it (*32*). She considered a pressure rise of less than 15 cm H_2O to be normal, a rise between 15 and 20 cm H_2O to be equivocal, and a rise of more than 20 cm H_2O to be indicative of a neurologic lesion. Seventeen percent of neurologically normal patients had equivocal values (false-positive results according to Lapides' criteria), and 9 percent had a false-negative response. Glahn suggested a number of factors that may affect the results (*32*).

1. Excessive bladder volume. This may cause a falsely elevated value. There may be an unexpectedly large bladder volume if the bladder was not emptied completely at the time of catheterization or if there is a large diuresis during the examination.

2. Emotional stress. A false-positive result may occur in patients who experience excessive anxiety during the test.

3. Myogenic failure. Repeated overdistension of the bladder or other myopathic processes may result in a detrusor that simply cannot contract, resulting in a false-negative response.

4. Poor absorption of bethanechol. Extremely obese patients or those with poor circulation may not completely absorb the drug, resulting in a false-negative test.

5. Timing after neurologic insult. The bethanechol test usually becomes positive within several weeks after an acute neurologic event. Occasionally, however, an interval of 6 months or more is required for the test to become positive.

The use of subcutaneous bethanechol to test the therapeutic efficacy of the drug in promoting micturition has also led to equivocal results. Downie *et al.* found that in order for the drug to be effective, sacral reflex pathways must be intact (*39*). Moreover, they noted that the subcutaneous route is far more efficacious than the oral route of administration. Wein and co-workers found no correlation between a positive bethanechol test and the clinical efficacy of the drug in promoting micturition (*40*). In that series of patients, all of whom had a positive test, 5 mg bethanechol administered subcutaneously failed to improve either the urinary flow rate or the residual urine. Yalla *et al.* found that bethanechol actually enhanced the obstructive effects of the urethra in patients with spinal cord injury (*41*).

Uroflowmetry

The assessment of urinary flow rate has been widely accepted as one of the most useful screening urodynamic procedures. It is noninvasive, simple, inexpensive, and cost-effective, yet it provides important information about the integrated function of the detrusor and bladder outlet. Nevertheless, the clinical assessment of urinary flow rate has been beset with problems similar to those encountered with other urodynamic procedures. Some patients are unable to relax sufficiently to void in their normal fashion for accurate measurement of uroflow. Many patients do not void in a sufficient volume; others void in an interrupted stream, which makes interpretation of the flow curve difficult. Moreover, there may be a considerable discrepancy between the first and subsequent measures of uroflow (*42*); therefore multiple samples are most efficient for enhancing an accurate assessment. Most flowmeters require at least 100 ml voided volume for accurate measurement, yet as many as one-third of patients do not void that amount during the setting of a uroflow examination (*43*). The actual numerical values of flow depend on bladder volume, age, and sex. Accordingly, it is important to interpret the uroflow data in conjunction with the clinical setting and other urodynamic parameters.

The simplest estimation of uroflow is made by observation of the voided stream. The presence of an obviously normal or an obviously impaired stream provides useful information that, in most clinical situations, is sufficient for an accurate diagnosis to be made. However, when the adequacy of the stream is not obvious, further clinical observations may be misleading. For example, observation and even measurement of the cast distance of the urinary stream has been suggested as a measure of urinary flow (*44*). The cast distance, however, is dependent not only on the flow rate but also on the height of the urethra from the ground and the velocity of the urinary stream. The narrower the urethral meatus, the greater is the velocity (and cast distance) for any given flow rate. Thus a patient with meatal stenosis may have a cast distance far in excess of that of a patient with normal flow.

Von Garrelts was the first to record an estimation of instantaneous flow (*45*). He measured the change in pressure at the base of a collecting cylinder and recorded it on a photokymograph as a function of time. Electronic derivation of the flow curve provided a calculated estimate of instantaneous flow that was recorded simultaneously on the graph along with voided volume and abdominal pressure. This method had wide clinical applicability but proved inaccurate at low flow rates and in patients with an interrupted urinary stream. Moreover, the instrument itself was quite sensitive to temperature and pressure changes. Nevertheless, the impetus provided by the pioneering work of von Garrelts continues to the present time and serves as a fertile substrate for continued improvements in urodynamic technology and thought.

Another means of determining uroflow is the momentum exchange flowmeter. The voided stream is directed at a rotating disk that is maintained at a constant velocity. As the urine strikes the disk, the increased electrical current necessary to maintain a constant velocity is proportional to urine flow (*46*). A potential error of up to 10 percent underestimation may be recorded depending on where the urine strikes the disk (*47*).

A pneumatic, nonelectric flowmeter powered by a carbon dioxide reservoir has also been developed (*48*). In this system carbon dioxide flows through a separate circuit at a predetermined rate. Voided urine strikes a loading ramp that blocks the flow of carbon dioxide. The change in carbon dioxide flow is directly related to urine flow and, after calibration, is displayed on a strip chart recorder.

All of the techniques discussed so far provide an indirect measurement of instantaneous flow; i.e., the volume-versus-time curve is electronically differentiated to obtain a calculated value of instantaneous flow. Although these indirect methods are more than adequate for routine clinical puposes, it may be necessary to measure instantaneous flow directly in certain research conditions.

Cardus *et al.* reported on the use of an electromagnetic flowmeter, adapted from a blood flowmeter, that measures instantaneous flow directly (*49*). The principle of operation required that the flow transducer be immersed in electrolyte-containing fluid, and that the subject be directly connected to the probe by a column of fluid. These requirements made this type of flowmeter cumbersome and subject to artifacts. Any motion of the patient was transmitted to the transducer, causing a movement artifact. Moreover, the adapter used to connect the patient to the system sometimes constricted the urethral meatus, impeding flow or causing discomfort. The adapters are cumbersome, difficult to apply, and time-consuming. If the subject is not directly connected to the system, he voids into a funnel, but the introduction of air bubbles causes potential artifacts. This method also requires an underdamped system to keep the resistance to flow at a minimum. Accordingly, rapid changes in flow tend to be overestimated. For all these reasons, the use of an electromagnetic flowmeter never became clinically applicable.

Susset *et al.* described a flowmeter based on a system of air displacement (*50*). A constant flow of air was used to cool a hot wire. Voided urine displaced a proportionate amount of air, and the urine flow was recorded as a derivative of the amount of electrical power necessary to maintain the wire at exactly 180°F.

Other flowmeters that have been devised are based on audio recordings of the urinary stream (*51,52*), high-speed cinematography, (*53*), and drop spectrometry (*54*), but none has achieved widespread clinical usage.

Normal Flow Curve

A normal flow curve is depicted in Figure 10–12. There is normally a rapid rise to maximal flow that consumes approximately one-third of the total voiding time, a period of fairly stable flow centered about the nadir, and a decrease in flow that produces a slightly less steep curve than the initial rise. Urinary flow rate is influenced by voided volume, initial bladder volume, sex, and age. There is a positive relation between initial bladder volume, voided volume, and maximum flow rate (*43,50,55–58*). Maximum flow increases in a nonlinear fashion up to a voided volume of approximately 500 ml, after which there is a slight decrease. Nomograms have been constructed relating voided volume to maximum and mean flow in order to facilitate comparisons between patients who void different volumes (*43,57,59*) and are discussed in more detail below.

Interpretation

Most flowmeters record instantaneous flow by electronically integrating the volume-versus-time curve. Thus the time interval over which this calculation is made influences the shape and accuracy of the curve. If the time interval is too short, artifactually high values may be obtained. The patient may inadvertently strike or move the flowmeter, causing a movement artifact. If flow is interrupted or urine momentarily collects in

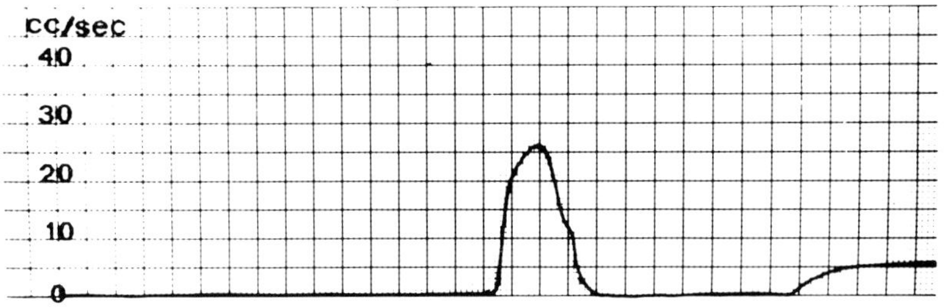

Figure 10–12. Normal uroflow. Voided volume = 100 ml. (From Blaivas, J. G.: A critical appraisal of specific techniques. In Kane, R. J., and Siroky, M. B. [eds.], *Clinical Neurourology*. Little, Brown, Boston, 1979.)

the funnel, there may be a sudden artifactual surge that reaches the transducer all at once, causing a falsely elevated value of instantaneous flow.

In most instances, visual inspection of the instantaneous flow curve is sufficient for a clinical judgment to be made without the need for precise measurements. An impaired uroflow is usually apparent from the shape of the curve; but, as discussed in the section on pressure-flow studies, the clinician should not equate poor uroflow with bladder outlet obstruction. Poor flow may be caused by a poor detrusor contraction or obstruction, but current technology does not permit this distinction to be made on the basis of flow alone (Fig. 10–13). Nevertheless, measurement of serial uroflows has proved to be an excellent noninvasive method of following the progress of patients with bladder outlet obstruction before and after treatment (*60–62*).

Many authors have analyzed various char-

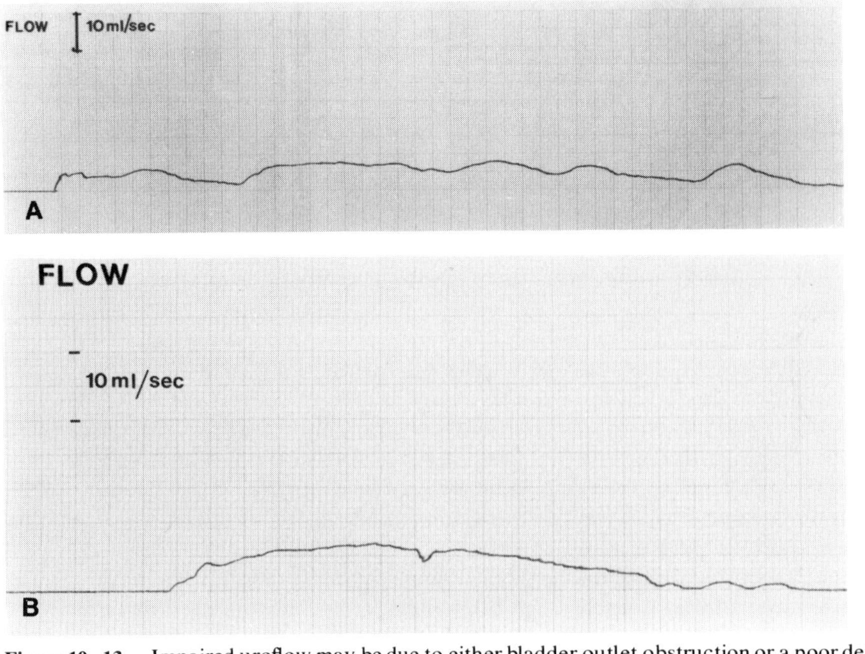

Figure 10–13. Impaired uroflow may be due to either bladder outlet obstruction or a poor detrusor contraction. **A.** Impaired uroflow due to poor detrusor contraction. Voided volume = 230 ml. **B.** Impaired uroflow due to vesical neck obstruction. Voided volume = 190 ml.

acteristics of the flow curve (*50,63,64*). The following parameters have been suggested for routine clinical usage.

Maximum Flow Rate

The maximum flow rate (Q_{max}) is the highest instantaneous flow recorded during a single micturition. Normally, Q_{max} ranges from 12 to 30 cm H_2O depending on the sex, age, and urine volume. Many authors have documented the interrelation between voided volume and Q_{max} (*43,50,55–58*). Von Garrelts found a nearly linear relation between voided volume and the square root of Q_{max} up to a voided volume of approximately 300 ml (*50*). Other investigators have suggested linear (*65*), square root (*66*), exponential (*67*), hyperbolic (*43*), and quadratic (*64*) equations to more accurately describe the relation between flow and voided volume. However, only hyperbolic and quadratic equations approximate the relation throughout the full range of voided volumes. Because of the dependency of Q_{max} on voided volume, nomograms have been constructed to facilitate comparison of one voiding event to another (*57*) (Fig. 10–14). They have been modified further to include age and sex (*59*) (Fig. 10–15).

The dependence of Q_{max} on initial bladder volume is even greater than the dependence on voided volume. It has been suggested that when there is considerable residual urine the use of flow nomograms based on voided volume, rather than initial bladder volume, may grossly overestimate the adequacy of the patient's flow (*57*).

Normal women have a higher Q_{max} than normal men, usually on the order of magnitude of 5 ml/s for a given volume (*42,43*). Moreover, there is a greater increase in Q_{max} per unit volume in women than in men. In Drach *et al.*'s series (*43*), Q_{max} increased 5.6 ml/s voided volume in normal women but only 2.5 ml/s voided volume in normal men. They also found a decrease in Q_{max} with advancing age in men (a fall in Q_{max} by 2 ml/s for every 10 years of age) but not in women. Women with stress incontinence and recurrent urinary tract infection tend to have a lower Q_{max} than normals (*43*).

When two populations of patients were compared, i.e., those with normal and those with "abnormal" micturition, it was found

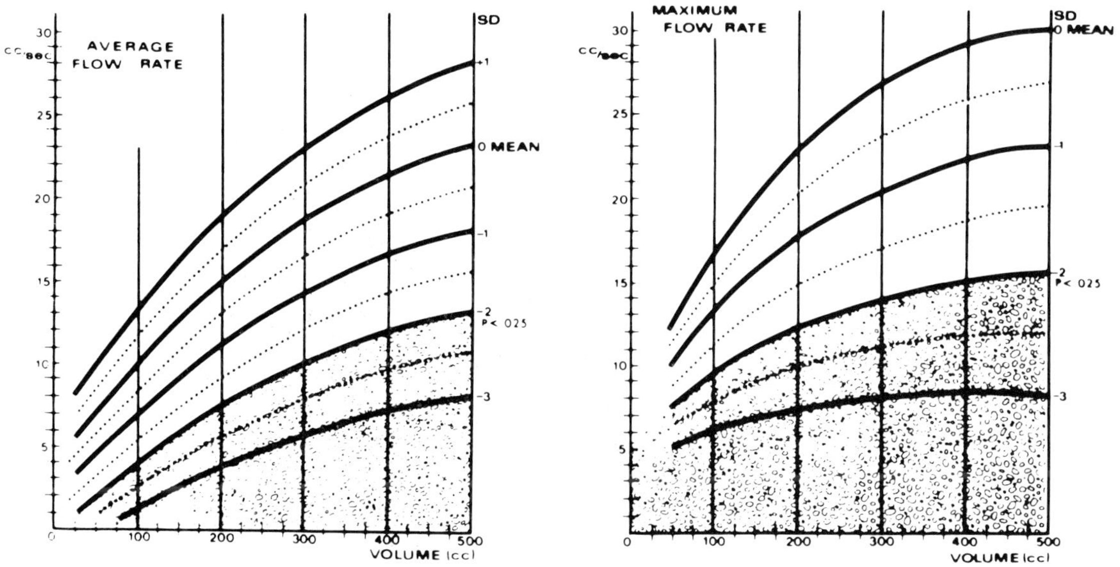

A **B**

Figure 10–14. Flow rate nomogram relating average flow (**A**) and maximum flow (**B**) to voided volume. (From Siroky, M. B., *et al.*: *J. Urol.* 122:665, 1979. Copyright © 1979, The Williams & Wilkins Co., Baltimore.)

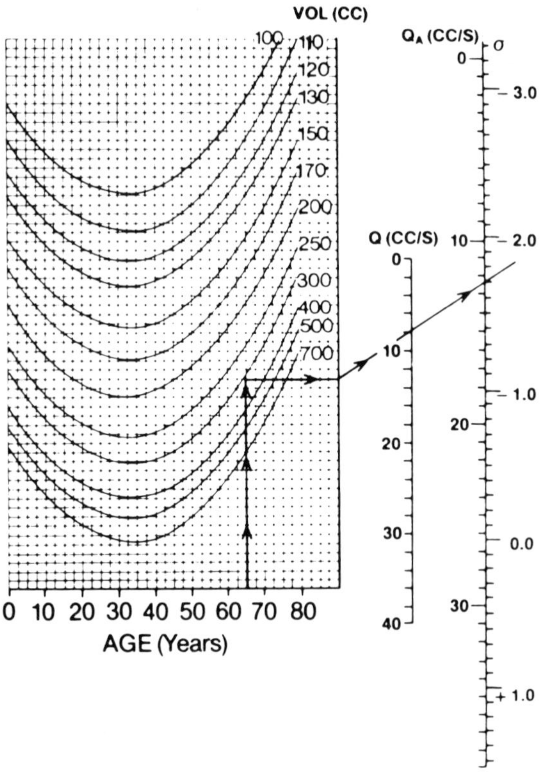

Figure 10–15. Flow rate nomogram relating maximum flow, voided volume and age. (From Drach, G. W., *et al.*: *J. Urol.* 128: 960, 1982. Copyright © 1982, The Williams & Wilkins Co., Baltimore.)

that there was an overlap of approximately 16 percent in the mean values of Q_{max} (*68*). Thus it may be impossible on the basis of flow alone to determine if an individual patient is normal with respect to flow.

Since instantaneous flow is electronically derived from the volume-time curve, the numerical value of Q_{max} depends on the time interval over which the calculation is made. If the time interval is too short, artifactually high values may be obtained. Flowmeters that measure instantaneous flow directly may show marked fluctuations that are difficult to interpret. Such findings are due to the fact that as the stream leaves the meatus it breaks up into droplets that strike the transducer of the flowmeter. If the time constant is too short, the resulting irregular curve may be difficult to decipher. This situation may be avoided by electronically damping the system by increasing the time constant.

Average Flow Rate

The average flow rate (Q_{ave}) is derived by dividing the voided volume by the total voiding time. However, because the precise end of micturition is often difficult to ascertain, Q_{ave} is beset with technical difficulties. Patients with interrupted streams or terminal dribbling have no clearly definable voiding time, and for this reason Q_{ave} cannot be accurately determined (Fig. 10–16). Accordingly, Q_{ave} is of most clinical use when a clearly definable end point of micturition is apparent. In order to overcome these obstacles it has been suggested that Q_{ave} be based on a certain percentage of the voided volume. For example, one might define Q_{ave} as 95 percent of the voided volume divided by the time over which that volume of urine was voided. This calculation eliminates the problems due to terminal dribbling but does not address the issue of an interrupted stream. The interrelationship of Q_{ave}, urine volume, sex, and age is similar to that observed for Q_{max}, and flow nomograms relating these parameters have been contructed (*50,57,59,63,64*). Average flow varies from approximately 6 to 25 ml/s depending on the voided volume. When divided into normal and abnormal patients, there was a 36 percent overlap in the mean values of Q_{ave}; thus Q_{ave} is even less reliable than Q_{max} in distinguishing normal from abnormal micturition (*68*).

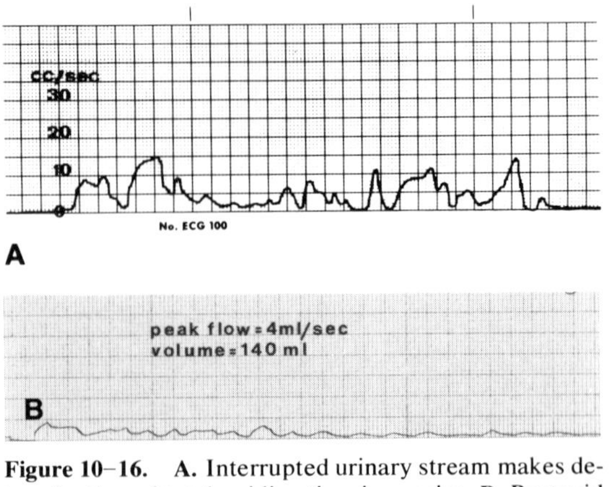

Figure 10–16. **A.** Interrupted urinary stream makes determination of total voiding time imprecise. **B.** Postvoid dribbling makes determination of total voiding time imprecise.

Voiding Time

As mentioned above, precise measurements of voiding time (T_v) may be impossible when flow is interrupted or there is terminal dribbling. When accurate measurements are possible, it has been determined, as one would expect, that voiding time bears a linear relation to voided volume. Voiding times vary from approximately 10 to 20 seconds at a voided volume of 100 ml to 25 to 35 seconds for a volume of 400 ml (*50,57,63,64*).

Time to Maximum Flow

The time from onset of flow until T_{max} is attained bears a linear relation to voided volume and does not appear to change significantly with outflow obstruction, although this parameter has not been extensively studied (*50,63*). Normally, T_{max} is approximately one-third of T_v.

SYNCHRONOUS PRESSURE–FLOW STUDIES

Screening uroflowmetry has been heralded as a major advance in the diagnosis of bladder outlet obstruction, yet it is not widely appreciated that a poor urinary flow rate may also be caused by an impaired detrusor contraction. The distinction between bladder outlet obstruction and poor detrusor contractility is a crucial one because surgical relief of obstruction is almost always curative, whereas when symptoms are due to impaired detrusor contractility empirical surgery designed to reduce outlet resistance is usually of no help and often makes the condition worse.

From a practical standpoint, bladder outlet obstruction may be defined as a poor urinary flow rate in the presence of an "adequate" detrusor contraction (Fig. 10–17). For an individual patient, however, it may be difficult to determine if the detrusor pressure is "adequate" with respect to the flow rate, and for this reason many investigators have attempted to formulate a mathematical definition of bladder outlet obstruction. Resistance coefficients were constructed using the formulas $R = P_{ves}/Q$ (*69*) and $R = P_{ves}/Q^2$ (*70,71*). Using the latter formula the normal urethral resistance coefficient was determined to be 0.26 ± 0.19, with values above 0.45 being indicative of obstruction.

However, the hydrodynamic principles from which these resistance coefficients are dervied assume that the bladder behaves as a geometric sphere and that the urethra behaves as a rigid tube. Since this is clearly not the case, the clinical usefulness of these formulas must be correlated with other findings. It is my opinion that when they are most necessary (in equivocal bladder outlet obstruction) these formulas are least accurate, and therefore they are of little use in their present form (*72*).

Further attempts to clarify the complex relation between pressure and flow were made by the innovative work of Griffiths and Scholtmeijer (*73–78*) and Schäfer (*79*). They measured detrusor pressure and flow simultaneously and plotted the values on an X-Y recorder. Griffiths (*73–75*) fitted a curve to the recorded values of pressure and flow and constructed an idealized "bladder output relation" that compared the actual detrusor contraction to a calculated maximum isometric contraction derived from extrapolation of the idealized curve. Similarly, a "urethral resistance relation" defined outlet resistance. Further anaylses of the pressure–flow curve and plots of detrusor pressure versus velocity of muscle shortening has resulted in refinements in the diagnostic accuracy of distinguishing bladder outlet obstruction from poor detrusor function (*76–78*).

Schäfer developed a slightly different way of analyzing pressure–flow data (*79*). He constructed a curve derived from a computer program that approximates the pressure–flow curve during the period of lowest urethral resistance. The resulting time-independent curve displays the contribution of the passive morphologic factors responsible for the minimum outlet resistance and does not depend on detrusor pressure; hence it is a method of assessing the presence or absence of outlet obstruction independent of the inherent strength of the detrusor. The normal passive urethral resistance relation (PURR) has a steep slope and relatively low

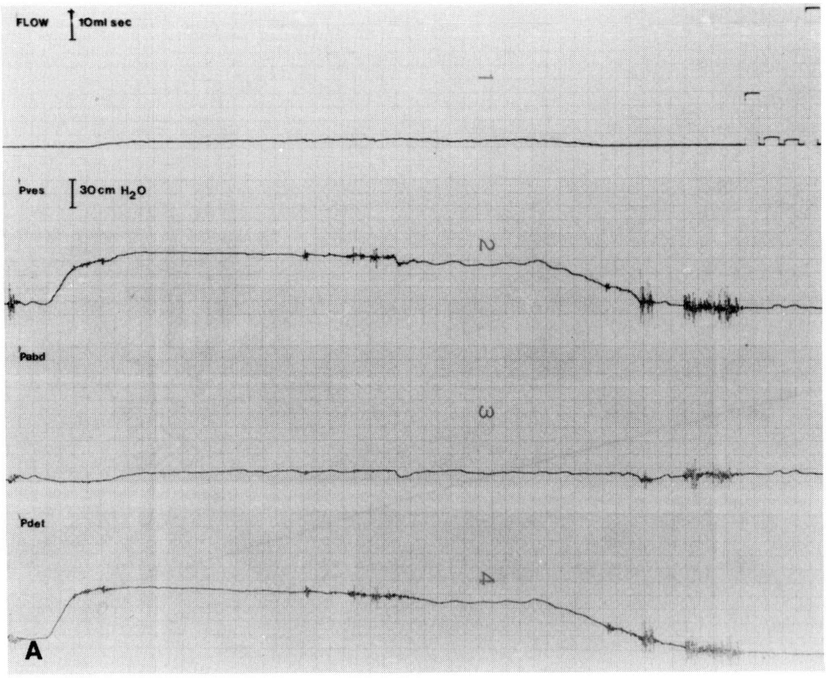

Figure 10–17. A poor urinary flow rate may be caused by either bladder outlet obstruction or impaired detrusor contractility. **A.** Bladder outlet obstruction is defined by an impaired urinary flow rate (Q_{max} = 5 ml/s) in the presence of a sustained detrusor contraction ($p_{det\ max}$=75 cm H_2O).

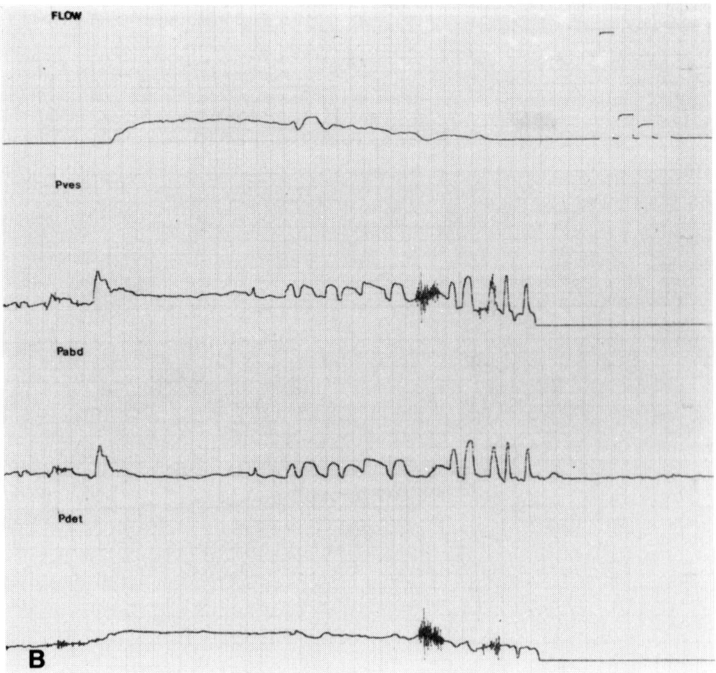

Figure 10–17. B. Impaired uroflow due to poor detrusor contraction. Q_{max} = 4ml/s; $P_{det\ max}$ = 30 cm H_2O. (from Blaivas, J. G.: *Urology* 23:421, 1984.)

detrusor pressure (Fig. 10–18). Two types of bladder outlet obstruction were described: compressive obstruction and constrictive obstruction. Compressive obstruction is characterized by a normal-appearing slope with a shift to the right of the curve; that is, the flow rate attains a normal or near-normal value but at the expense of a much higher detrusor pressure. The implication of this type of obstruction is that a much higher detrusor pressure is necessary to open the urethra and initiate flow; but once flow has begun, the urethra attains a normal or near-normal cross-sectional area. A constrictive obstruction is characterized by a decrease in the slope of the PURR; that is, the flow rate never assumes a normal value despite a high detrusor pressure. The implication of this type of obstruction is that there is a diminished cross-sectional area of the urethra throughout micturition. Most patients with bladder outlet obstruction have mixed constrictive and compressive obstruction.

If one plots the raw values of pressure and flow, after compensating for the 0.5- to 0.7-second delay in the recording of flow, it is possible to evaluate any segment of the curve and obtain useful physiologic information. At any given point, the slope of the curve may be either positive or negative. A positive slope (d/Q/dp) indicates that both the flow and detrusor pressure are increasing. This situation occurs during periods of relatively constant outlet resistance. The steeper the slope, the lower is the outlet resistance; conversely, the more gradual the slope, the greater is the resistance. A negative slope indicates an active change in outlet resistance (Fig. 10–19).

The dynamic urethral resistance relation (DURR) plots changes in outlet resistance as a function of time. Because rapid increases in resistance are usually due to sphincter contractions and a rapid decrease to sphincter relaxation, the DURR describes the contribution of muscular changes in outlet resistance over time and as such is analogous to sphincter electromyography (Fig. 10–20). If one considers that the PURR is representative of the minimum urethral resistance (which occurs at the left-hand side of the pressure–flow curve), all deviations from the PURR may be considered to be due to active changes in resistance.

The technique of synchronous pressure–flow studies requires the use of either a transurethral or a suprapubic catheter. When transurethral catheters are used they must be of small diameter (10F or less), and it must be recognized that even this size catheter

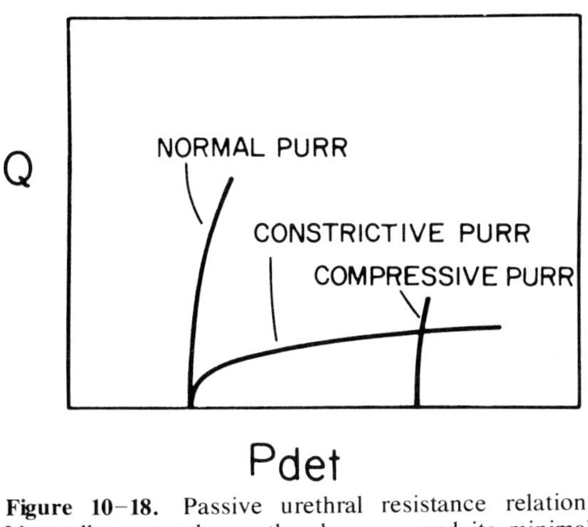

Figure 10–18. Passive urethral resistance relation. Normally, once the urethra has assumed its minimal resistance, there is little further change in detrusor pressure despite an increasing flow rate. A compressive obstruction is characterized by a normal-shaped curve that is "shifted to the right" and does not attain a normal peak flow. A constrictive obstruction only increases its flow at the expense of markedly increasing the detrusor pressure. (Modified from Schäfer, W.: In Hinman, F., Jr. [ed.], *Benign Prostatic Hypertrophy*. Springer-Verlag, New York, 1983.)

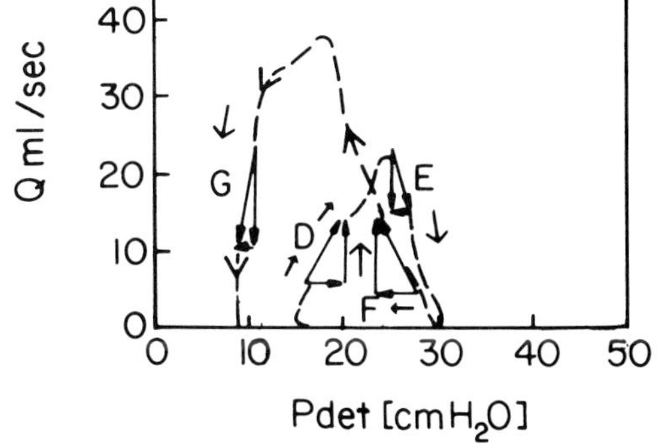

Figure 10–19. Detailed analysis of detrusor pressure-flow curve. (Modified from Schäffer, W.: In Hinman, F., Jr. [ed.], *Benign Prostatic Hypertrophy*. Springer-Verlag, New York, 1983.)

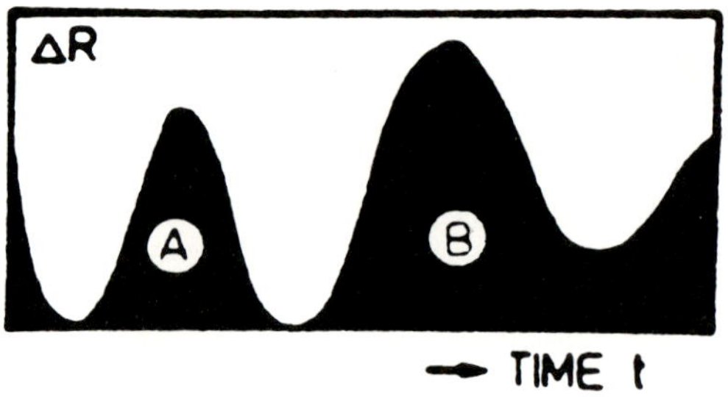

Figure 10–20. Dynamic urethral resistance relation (DURR). The DURR plots changes in urethral resistance as a function of time. At *A* an external urethral sphincter contraction momentarily increases outlet resistance. At *B* another contraction interrupts the stream, after which the detrusor contraction abates and the "resting" urethral resistance is achieved. (Modified from Schäfer, W.: In Hinman, F., Jr. [ed.], *Benign Prostatic Hypertrophy*, Springer-Verlag, New York, 1983.)

often causes a relative outlet obstruction and thus impedes flow (*80*). Preliminary data suggest that even when flow is impaired by the presence of the catheter, useful diagnostic information may still be obtained. In fact, Griffiths and Scholtmeijer (*76*) suggested that subtle bladder outlet obstruction may best be diagnosed by noting the effect of increasing catheter size on the pressure–flow curve. They hypothesized that the obstructive effects of an intraurethral catheter would be more pronounced in patients with preexisting obstruction than in those without obstruction, and their data seem to bear this hypothesis out (Fig. 10–21). Thus synchronous pressure–flow studies obtained with a transurethral catheter may be more sensitive than those obtained with a suprapubic one.

SPHINCTER ELECTROMYOGRAPHY

Sphincter electromyography (EMG) plays a dual role in urodynamic testing. It provides kinesiologic information about the external sphincter and perineal floor musculature, and it provides objective documentation concerning the integrity of the innervation of these muscles. We believe that EMG is most useful as an aid to neurologic diagnosis and, as such, is necessary only when a neurologic disorder is suspected. However, in order to make a neurologic diagnosis, EMG should be performed by an experienced elec-

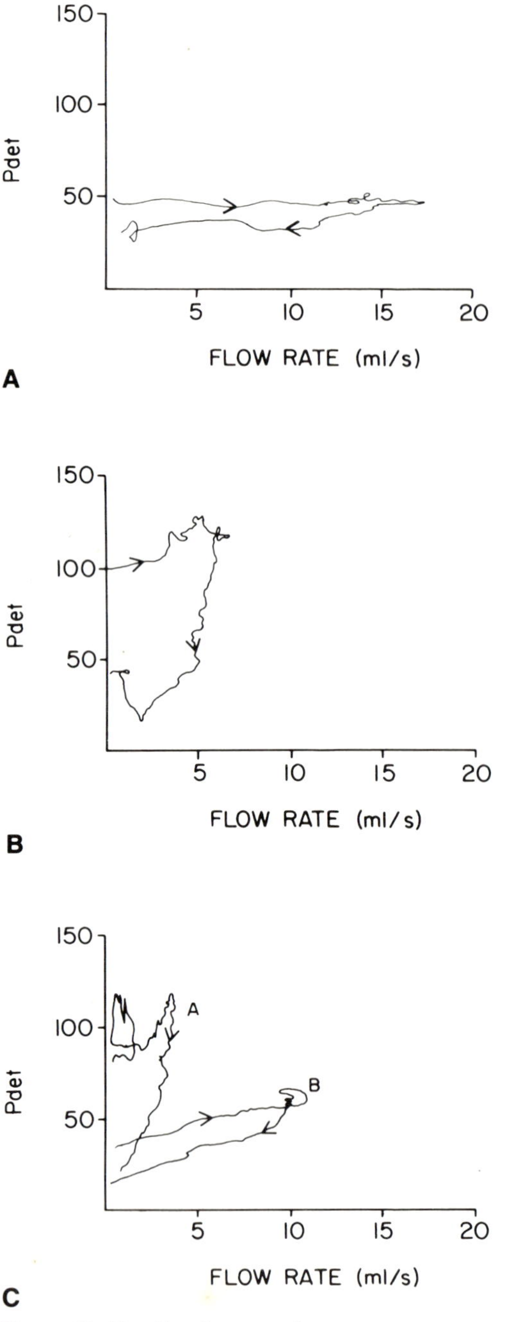

Figure 10–21. Synchronous detrusor pressure versus flow curve. **A.** Normal. Flow is initiated at a pressure of 50 cm H_2O, and the flow rate increases to almost 20 ml/s with no further appreciable rise in pressure. **B.** Bladder outlet obstruction. Flow is not initiated until a detrusor pressure of 100 cm H_2O, and despite a further rise in detrusor pressure maximum flow attains only 6 ml/s. **C.** Effect of catheter size on pressure–flow relation. With two urethral catheters in place (3.5F and 8.0F) the curve (*A*) shows definite obstruction. When the larger catheter is removed, the curve (*B*) is near normal. (From Griffiths, D. J., and Scholtmeijer, R. J.: *Neurourol. Urodyn.* 1:97, 1982.)

tromyographer using needle electrodes and oscilloscopic or audiographic control so that individual motor unit action potentials and recruitment patterns may be observed. EMG using surface electrodes is capable only of kinesiologic information, and with commercially available equipment, the recordings are so riddled with artifact that it makes their overall clinical usefulness of questionable value. Moreover, most of the necessary kinesiologic information can be obtained with simple clinical and fluoroscopic observations. In contrast, needle EMG provides not only kinesiologic but also specific neurologic and myologic information about the individual muscles of the pelvic floor. It should be remembered, however, that there is not necessarily a precise relation between sphincter EMG activity and effective muscular contraction as measured by urethral pressure. For example, a urethral stricture results in fibrosis and poor compliance of the urethral wall. Contraction of the striated muscle of the external sphincter around such a stricture results in a marked increase in EMG activity, but there may be no rise in urethral pressure at all because of the stiffness of the wall.

Theory

With the bladder empty, the perineal floor muscles are electrically quiescent; zero to two action potentials fire per second (81-84). There may be some high frequency, irregular discharges in the vicinity of the motor end-plate. These discharges are called end-plate noise. Their amplitude is usually less than 100 μV, and their duration is between 0.5 and 2.0 ms (*85–87*).

During bladder filling there is a gradual increase in EMG activity that reaches a maximum just prior to voiding. A normal micturition reflex is initiated by complete electrical silence (relaxation of the external urethral sphincter). The latency between sphincter relaxation and the onset of the rise in detrusor pressure varies from several milliseconds to as long as 20 to 30 seconds. There is a marked increase in EMG activity in response to a number of stimuli including cough, Credé and Valsalva maneuvers, the bulbocavernosus reflex, and the command to stop voiding (Fig. 10–22) (*81,83,88–90*).

Neuropathic and myopathic pathology results in characteristic abnormalities of the sphincter EMG. Immediately after a lower

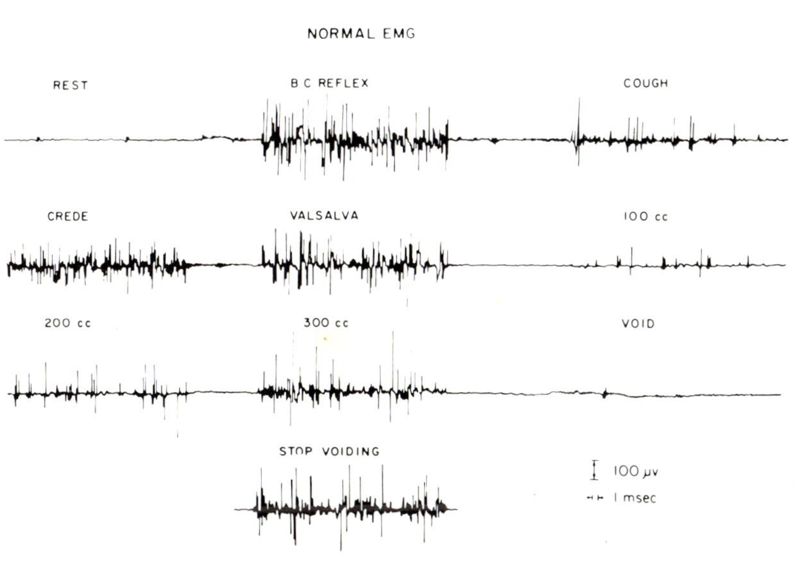

Figure 10–22. Normal sphincter electromyogram. With an empty bladder there are few sporadic motor units firing (rest). During bladder filling there is a gradual increase in EMG activity. Note the abrupt increase in activity in response to cough, Credé, or Valsalva maneuver, bulbocavernosus reflex, and the command to stop voiding. During a micturition reflex there is complete electrical silence. (From Blaivas, J. G., *et al.*: *J. Urol.* 117:773, 1977. Copyright © 1977, The William & Wilkins Co., Baltimore.)

motor neuron lesion is sustained, voluntary and reflex activity in the involved muscles is abolished. Within 2 to 4 weeks spontaneous EMG activity in the form of positive sharp waves or fibrillation potentials is usually apparent. A fibrillation potential is characterized by its short duration (1-5 ms), its form (bi- or triphasic), an amplitude between 50 and 300 μV, and a characteristic sound on the loudspeaker that is similar to the puttering of an outboard motorboat. Occasionally fibrillations are polyphasic in form. A positive sharp wave is a characteristic biphasic action potential whose initial major deflection is down (positive) with only a small component that rises above the baseline. Neurologic recovery is characterized by reinnervation and the appearance of polyphasic action potentials that have more than four deflections. Normally, polyphasic action potentials comprise less than 15 percent of the potentials recruited from a given muscle. With diseases of the upper motor neuron, individual motor unit action potentials are usually normal, but the striated muscle is hyperreflexic and may no longer be under voluntary control (*85–87*).

On occasion, myotonic or pseudomyotonic discharges are encountered during sphincter EMG. These bizarre, high-frequency action potentials are often evoked by movement of the electrode. The form of the individual motor unit action potential may be normal, or it may resemble positive sharp waves or fibrillations. The frequency of the discharge waxes and wanes, producing a characteristic "dive-bomber" sound from the loudspeaker. Myotonic discharges are thought to be a disorder of the muscle fiber membrane; they are seen primarily in patients with myotonic disorders and only rarely in those with other neurologic disorders (*85*-87). Pseudomyotonic discharges, also called repetitive complex discharges, are similar in form to myotonic discharges except that the frequency of discharge is quite regular (Fig. 10–23). They are thought to represent nonspecific membrane irritability and have been seen in a variety of neurologic and nonneurologic disorders (*85,91,92*).

Technique

Electrode Application and Insertion. A variety of surface electrodes are available for EMG investigations. Most consist of a metallic (platinum) contact embedded within a self-adhesive material that can be applied directly to the skin. Because of the possibility of EMG artifacts due to poor contact of the elctrode with the skin, it is necessary to wash the sampling site and dry it thoroughly before applying the electrode. Some authors recommend that the skin also be painted with benzoin to ensure a better contact. The electrode is best applied on a smooth, flat surface in the perineum or on the buttocks with the patient in the dorsal lithotomy position.

Needle electrodes are inserted in the following fashion: In the male patient, with an examining finger in the rectum, the needle is inserted percutaneously 2 cm lateral to the midline halfway between the anus and the

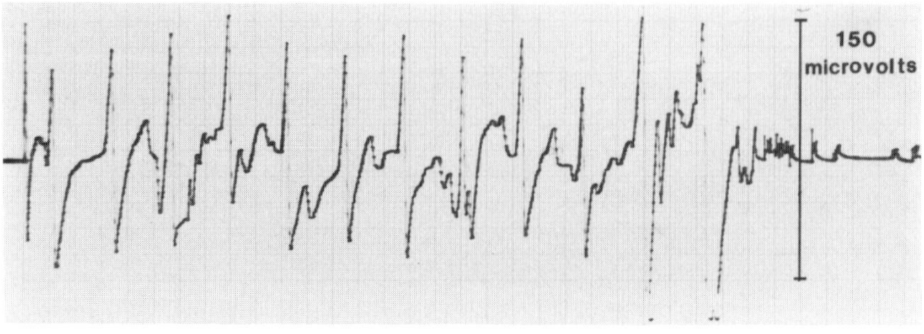

Figure 10–23. Complex repetitive discharges (pseudomyotonic discharges). See text for details. (From Blaivas, J. G.: *Neurourol. Urodynam.* 2:269, 1983.)

lower border of the scrotum. The needle is advanced obliquely toward the apex of the prostate until individual motor unit action potentials characteristic of skeletal muscle are detected audibly or are visualized on the oscilloscope screen. In some instances the needle inadvertently traverses the bulbocavernosus muscle prior to reaching the external urethral sphincter. Because this muscle is thin, it is readily distinguished from the external urethral sphincter by the fact that motor unit action potentials can be recruited for a distance of only several millimeters, whereas action potentials can be detected for several centimeters in the external urethral sphincter. Sometimes it is desirable to sample the bulbocavernosus muscle separately. The bulbocavernosus muscle lies around the corpus spongiosum of the urethra and may be identified at its origin by palpating the ischial tuberosity. Because the bulbocavernosus muscle is usually electrically silent at rest, it may be necessary to squeeze the glans and elicit the reflex in order to identify the proper position of the needle.

In women the needle is inserted just lateral to the urethral meatus in a slightly ventral and medial direction. The periurethral musculature is much thinner in women and may be much more difficult to locate. In general, when difficulty is encountered the muscle is usually found to be more anterior than anticipated.

The anal sphincter is easy to identify in both sexes by passing a 2.50- to 3.75-cm (1.0- to 1.5-in.) needle electrode approximately 1 cm lateral to the anus until the characteristic motor unit action potentials are detected.

Recording Equipment. Most commercially available urodynamic equipment is ill-equipped for performing sophisticated EMG. At best, these units are capable of displaying integrated EMG data on a strip chart recorder or loudspeaker; and the inherent artifacts, as discussed above and below, are a continuing source of difficulty. EMG units designed to provide accurate neurologic information must have certain electrical characteristics. A high input impedance is necessary to prevent loss of the EMG signal. The overall recording system should have a frequency response of approximately 2,000 to 10,000 Hz, and there should be a mechanism to alter the frequency response in order to exclude electrical noise or interference. A detailed discussion of technique factors related to EMG recording devices has been presented by Guld *et al.* (93).

There are important differences between the oscilloscopic or audible display of EMG potentials and ordinary strip chart recordings. During maximal muscle contraction individual motor units may fire hundreds or thousands of times per second. Because most strip chart recorders run at several millimeters or centimeters per second, they display only a small fraction of the available electrical information. At these slow recording rates it is difficult to quantitatively analyze EMG activity. In fact, it is often difficult even to distinguish complete electrical silence from low-level electrical interference or maximal activity from alternating current interference or movement artifact. On an oscilloscope screen EMG information can be displayed at recording speeds as high as 25 m/s. At these speeds technical artifacts can be easily recognized and avoided (Fig. 10–24). In order to minimize the inaccuracy of paper strip chart recorders, many EMG untis are equipped with electronic devices to average or integrate the EMG data. Although this setup is an improvement over evaluating the raw data, it is my opinion that the EMG information so obtained is still too crude and unreliable for routine clinical application.

Method of Investigation. Electromyography should always be performed with simultaneous cystometry. After placing a needle electrode, the presence or absence of insertional or spontaneous activity is noted (see above). Recruitment patterns are recorded during bladder filling, and the patient is asked to contract and relax the sphincter, cough, strain, and perform the Credé maneuver. When a detrusor contraction occurs, the temporal relation to sphincter activity is observed.

When evaluating EMG responses it is essential to distinguish voluntary from involuntary activity. Since the striated perineal floor muscles can be activated at will, each time there is an abrupt change in EMG activity it must be immediately ascertained (by talking to the patient) whether the response was voluntary, involuntary, or reflex in nature.

When a neurologic lesion is suspected but not confirmed, it may be necessary to repeat

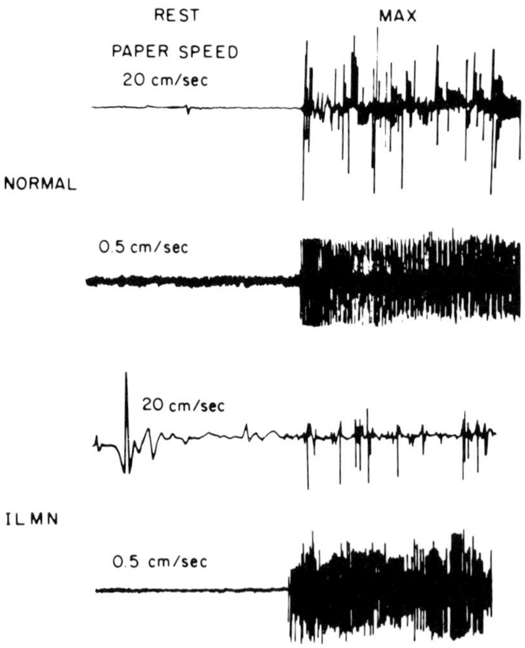

Figure 10–24. Discrepancy between oscilloscopic and strip chart recordings. The top tracing are recordings as they appear on an oscilloscope screen. On the bottom are the tracings as they appear on a strip chart recorder. On the left the sphincter is at rest. On the right there is maximal contraction. Top two tracings- Normal. Bottom two tracings- Incomplete lower motor neuron lesion (ILMN). On the strip chart recording it appears as if there is a greater response at maximum contraction in the patient with the lower motor neuron lesion that in the normal patient, whereas on the oscilloscope screen it is clear that the normal patient has a much more complete contraction. See text for details. (From Blaivas, J. G., *et al.*: *J. Urol.* 117:773, 1977.) Copyright © 1977, The Williams & Wilkins Co., Baltimore.)

the examination at multiple sampling sites within the perineal floor and in muscles of adjacent dermatomes. It is not unusual for incomplete neurologic lesions to affect some and spare other portions of the perineal floor musculature (*15*).

Single-fiber EMG is a diagnostic modality that has had only limited application in neurourology (*94,95*). With this technique the number of muscle fibers belonging to a motor unit is quantitatively determined by calculating the mean fiber density from a number of sampling sites. In 14 normal patients fiber density of the external anal sphincter ranged from 1.3 to 1.8 with a mean of 1.5. Fiber density increased with advancing age, and there was increased fiber density in patients with stress urinary incontinence (*94*). It is stressed, however, that these data are preliminary and that much more clinical work is necessary before the role of single-fiber EMG can be determined.

Diagnostic Formulation

Normal Sphincter EMG. The external urethral sphincter is usually electrically silent at rest, although one or two motor unit action potentials may fire per second. During bladder filling there is usually a gradual increase in EMG activity that reaches a maximum just prior to voiding. Individual motor unit action potentials are of normal configuration, but as many as 15 percent may be polyphasic. Spontaneous potentials (fibrillations and positive sharp waves) are never seen. The initiation of a voluntary detrusor contraction is heralded by complete relaxation (electrical silence) of the external urethral sphincter. This relaxation usually occurs immediately before the detrusor contraction but may precede it by as much as 20 to 30 seconds (Fig. 10–25). When a patient strains to initiate voiding, there is often a momentary increase in EMG activity fol-

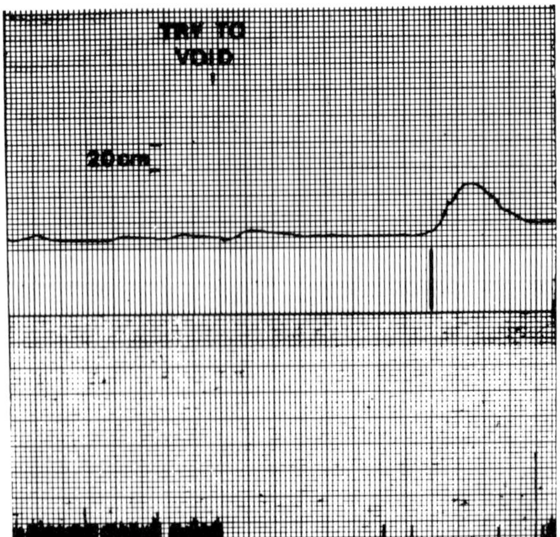

Figure 10–25. Normal (CMG)-EMG. There is complete relaxation of the external urethral sphincter 4 seconds prior to the onset of the detrusor contraction. (From Blaivas, J. G.: Cystometry. In Raz, S. [ed.], *Female Urology*. Saunders, Philadelphia, 1983.)

lowed by electrical silence. Sphincter relaxation persists throughout the detrusor contraction, and at the end of voiding EMG activity resumes. Not infrequently there is a strong contraction of the external urethral sphincter just at the end of the detrusor contraction. If the patient is asked to voluntarily stop voiding, there is an abrupt increase in EMG activity that represents a voluntary sphincter contraction (Fig. 10–26). An increase in EMG activity accompanies any sudden increase in abdominal pressure such as cough or movement (Fig. 10–27). Elicitation of the bulbocavernosus reflex results in a marked increase in EMG activity (*81,96*).

Lower Motor Neuron Lesion. Damage to the anterior horn cell is called a lower motor neuron lesion. If all of the neurons innervating a certain segment are involved, the lesion is complete; if only some are involved, it is incomplete. With a complete lesion there is neither motor nor sensory function in the involved segment. With incomplete lesions motor and sensory functions are variable. Immediately after a complete lower motor neuron injury is sustained there is neither voluntary nor reflex activity of the involved muscles, and sensation is lost. Within 2 to 6 weeks spontaneous potentials appear in the form of fibrillations and positive sharp waves. If the lesion is incomplete, reinnervation is marked by the appearance of polyphasic potentials. Reflex activity returns but is incomplete, and a full interference pattern is usually not seen with maximal muscle contraction (Fig. 10–28). Lower motor neuron lesions involving the sacral micturitional pathways are relatively uncommon but may be seen with myelodysplasia, diabetes, tumors and injuries to the conus medullaris or cauda equina, herniated disks, and anterior spinal artery occlusion.

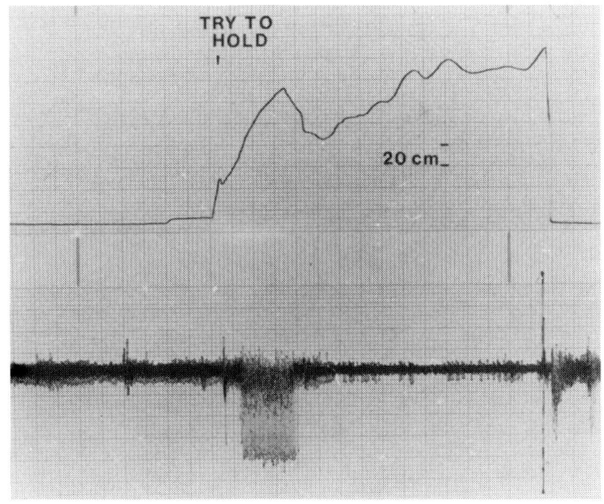

Figure 10–26. CMG–EMG. This patient is trying to inhibit an involuntary detrusor contraction by contracting the external urethral sphincter. If the examiner does not know what the patient is trying to do, this tracing might be misinterpreted as detrusor–external sphincter dyssynergia. (From Blaivas, J. G.: Cystometry. In Raz, S. [ed.], *Female Urology*. Saunders, Philadelphia, 1983.)

Upper Motor Neuron Lesion. With upper motor neuron disease there is a neurologic lesion that interrupts the connections between higher centers and the anterior horn cell, but the anterior horn cell and its peripheral connections are intact. All of the urethral reflexes are intact, and the EMG is normal except for a lack of voluntary control. When the neurologic lesion is above the brainstem, there is usually detrusor hyperreflexia associated with complete relaxation of the external urethral sphincter. Thus in a physiologic sense these patients void nor-

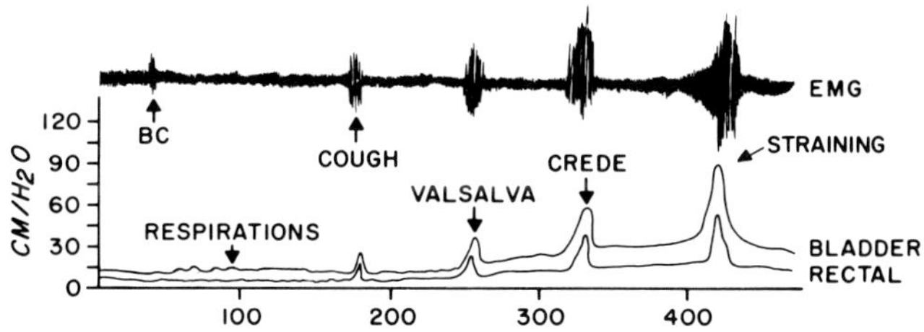

Figure 10–27. Anything that increases intraabdominal pressure usually results in a reflex increase in EMG activity. *BC*=bulbocavernosus reflex. (From Blaivas, J. G.: *Neurourol. Urodyn.* 2:269, 1983.)

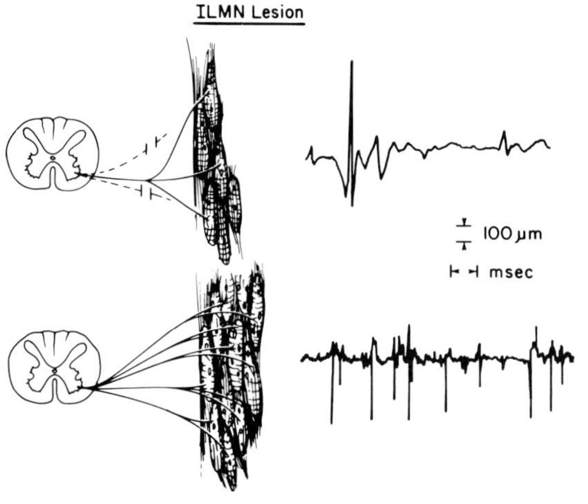

Figure 10–28. With incomplete lower motor neuron (ILMN) lesions certain motor units are destroyed. Some muscle fibers undergo atrophy, and others become reinnervated by axons that formerly innervated other anterior horn cells. Muscle fibers formerly supplied by three anterior horn cells are now supplied by one. The resulting motor unit action potential has a polyphasic configuration and is of increased amplitude and duration. At maximal contraction only a partial interference pattern is seen because of fewer functioning units. (From Blaivas, J. G.: *J. Urol.* 117:773, 1977.) Copyright © 1977, The Williams & Wilkins Co., Baltimore.)

mally; they simply lack control (*15*) (Fig. 10–29). When the neurologic lesion is between the brainstem and the sacral spinal cord, there is usually a discoordination between the detrusor and external sphincter. In the mildest cases the detrusor contractions are simply weak and poorly sustained; at the other extreme is detrusor–external sphincter dyssynergia (Fig. 10–30).

Detrusor–External Sphincter Dyssynergia. Detrusor-external sphincter dyssynergia (DESD) is a pathologic condition wherein micturition is uncoordinated. It is characterized by an involuntary contraction of the external urethral sphincter during an involuntary detrusor contraction (*15, 83,84,97-101*). In this context, DESD is always due to a neurologic lesion of the spinal cord (*15,97,100*). DESD has been classified into three main categories on the basis of the temporal relation between the detrusor and external sphincter contractions (*98*). With type I DESD there is an increase in EMG activity that reaches its maximum at the height of the detrusor contraction. At that point there is sudden and complete relaxation of the external sphincter, and voiding occurs as the detrusor pressure is falling (Fig. 10–31). Type II dyssynergia is characterized by sporadic increases in EMG activity throughout the detrusor contraction (Fig.10–32). With type III DESD there is a crescendo–decrescendo pattern of EMG activity that parallels the rise and fall in detrusor pressure (Fig. 10–33).

It is essential that during the EMG examination it is determined whether sphincter contractions are truly involuntary or are merely the conscious attempt of the patient to voluntarily inhibit micturition. This fact can easily be ascertained at the time of the study by maintaining close verbal contact with the patient. Moreover, DESD must be differentiated from other conditions, which

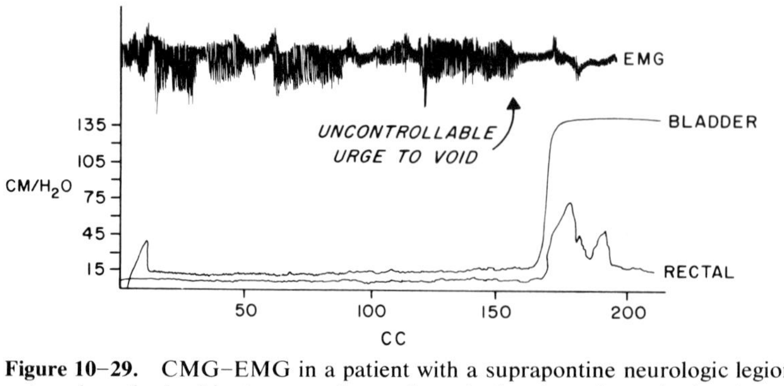

Figure 10–29. CMG–EMG in a patient with a suprapontine neurologic legion. There is complete relaxation of the external urethral sphincter preceding and continuing throughout the involuntary detrusor contraction.

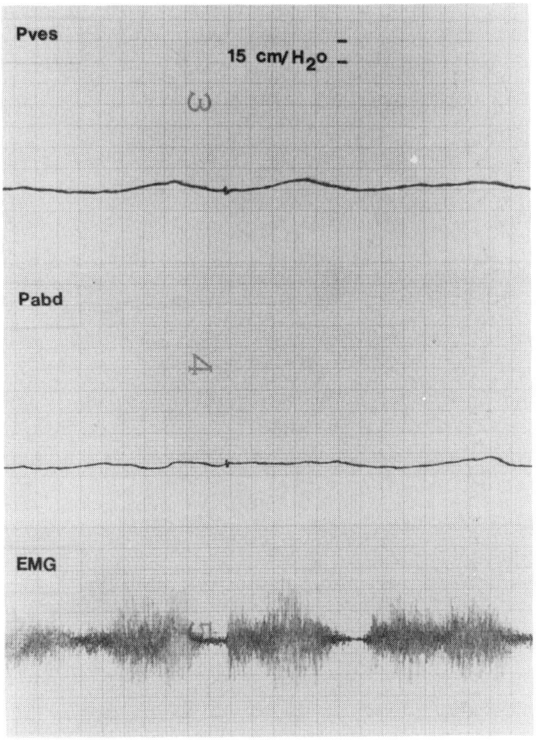

Figure 10–30. CMG–EMG in a patient with an incomplete cervical spinal cord lesion. Note the weak, poorly sustained detrusor contractions and associated detrusor–external sphincter dyssynergia.

have also been called DESD, in which there is increased EMG activity (as measured by a surface electrode) during voluntary attempts to void. These syndromes are encountered most often in women with "urethral syndrome" (*102,103*), men with "abacterial prostatitis or prostatodynia," and children with enuresis or recurrent urinary tract infection (*104,105*). There are two main abnormalities detected under these circumstances. There may be failure of the pelvic floor musculature to relax during attempts to void with abdominal straining (Fig. 10-34) or intermittent contractions of the pelvic floor during voiding (Fig. 10–35). Both of these phenomena are thought to be due to psychological or learned behavior.

Summary

When performed with needle electrodes and oscilloscopic or audiographic control (or both), sphincter EMG is a sophisticated method of evaluating the integrity of the innervation to the striated perineal floor muscles and the supraspinal neurologic pathways involved in lower urinary tract function. As yet, however, there is no objective, quantitative method for evaluating the innervation of the detrusor per se. In general, it is reasonable to assume that when a neurologic lesion is found to affect the striated perineal floor muscles it is likely that that same process also involves the detrusor, as both the pudendal and parasympathetic nuclei lie in the sacral spinal cord practically adjacent to one another. Nevertheless, certain neurologic disorders (e.g., multiple sclerosis, myelodysplasia, ruptured intervertebral disk, diabetic neuropathy) often involve one portion of the nervous system and spare another. With these disorders reliance on abnormalities of the striated musculature may provide misleading information concerning the status of the smooth muscle of the detrusor, vesical neck, and proximal urethra.

When performed with surface electrodes, sphincter EMG provides, at best, a gross assessment of the overall electrical activity of the pelvic floor musculature. The relation between pelvic floor electrical activity and sphincteric activity has not been well studied and needs further clarification before the clinical utility of this method can be determined. At present, it is too riddled with artifacts to be clinically useful.

SACRAL EVOKED RESPONSES

Measurement of the latency of an electrically evoked bulbocavernosus reflex (BCR) is an outgrowth of sphincter EMG (*89,106–109*). Clinically, the bulbocavernosus reflex may be elicited by briskly squeezing the glans penis or clitoris or by pulling the balloon of a Foley catheter against the vesical neck and observing or feeling a reflex contractile response of the external anal sphincter or bulbocavernosus muscle. The BCR is detectable in almost all normal men and in approximately 80 percent of normal women. Absence of the reflex is strongly suggestive of a sacral neurologic lesion, but it is present in approximately 50 percent of patients with an incomplete lower motor neuron lesion (*96*). Because it is difficult to

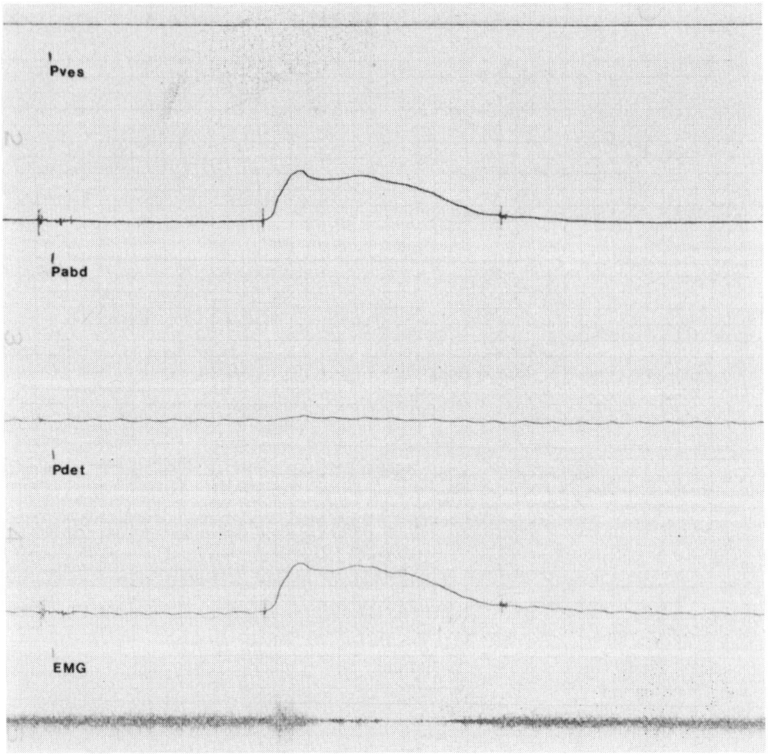

Figure 10–31. Type 1 detrusor–external sphincter dyssynergia. There is an increase in EMG activity coincident with the onset of the involuntary detrusor contraction. At the peak of the contraction there is sudden and complete electrical silence as voiding occurs. Each large division on the vertical scale = 15 cm H_2O.

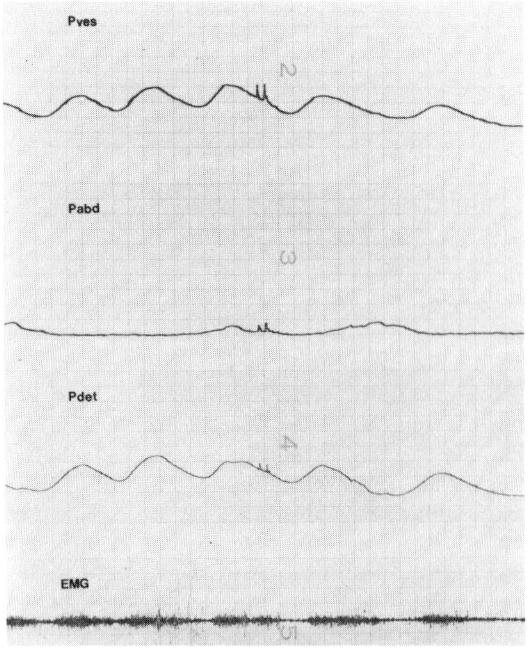

Figure 10–32. Type 2 detrusor–external sphincter dyssynergia. During the involuntary detrusor contraction there are sporadic contractions of the external urethral sphincter. Note the rise in detrusor pressure that occurs each time the external sphincter contracts and the fall in pressure as it relaxes. Each large division on the vertical scale = 15 cm H_2O.

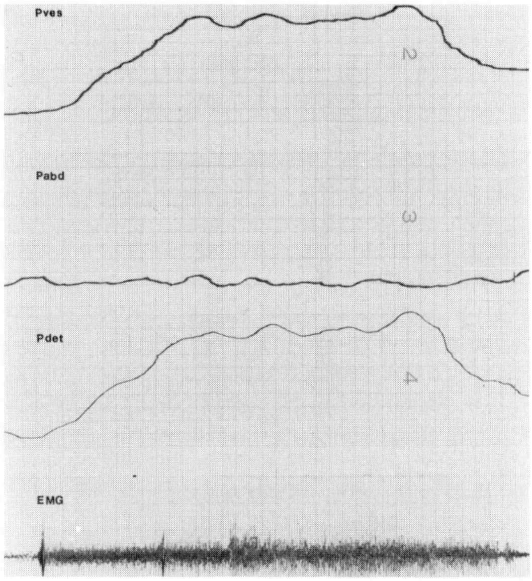

Figure 10–33. Type 3 detrusor–external sphincter dyssynergia. There is a marked increase in EMG activity that persists throughout the detrusor contraction and that parallels the rise and fall in detrusor pressure. Each large division on the vertical scale = 15 cm H_2O.

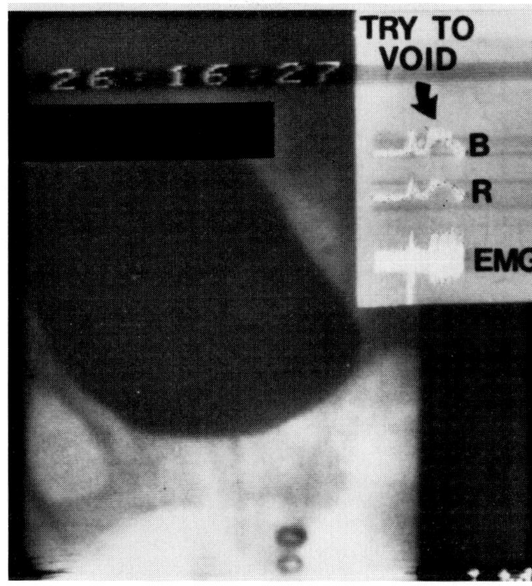

Figure 10–34. "Pseudodyssynergia." Video/pressure/EMG study. This woman strained during the attempt to void, increasing intraabdominal and intravesical pressure. The increased EMG activity is a normal response to straining, but it may simulate detrusor–external sphincter to the inexperienced examiner. $p_{ves\ max}$ during straining was 56 cm H_2O. *B* = intravesical pressure. *R* = intraabdominal pressure.

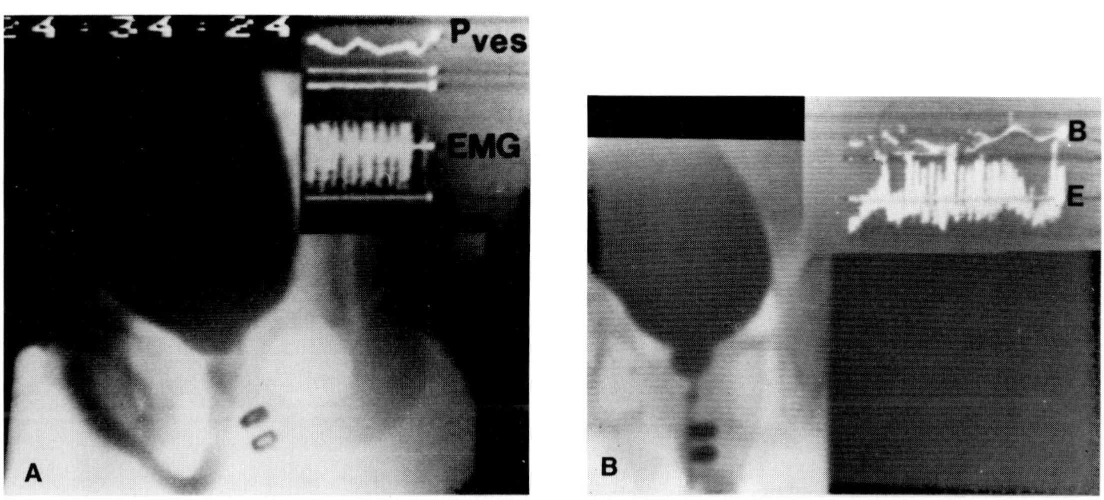

Figure 10–35. "Pseudodyssynergia." Video/pressure/EMG study. There are intermittent contractions of the external urethral sphincter throughout the detrusor contraction. Voiding occurs during periods of sphincter relaxation (*A*). When the external sphincter contracts, it obstructs micturition. *B* = intravesical pressure. *E* = EMG.

grade the reflex clinically, measurement of the bulbocavernosus reflex latency offers a more quantitative means of evaluating the sacral reflex arcs.

The BCR is a crossed reflex. When one side of the penis is stimulated, there is a bilateral contractile response in the bulbocavernosus muscle (*89,107,108*). The afferent limb of the reflex is mediated by small-diameter, myelinated fibers of the pudendal nerve whose conduction velocity is approximately 20 m/s (*109*). The efferent limb consists of pudendal motor fibers whose conduction velocity is 50 to 60 m/s (*110*). Preliminary data suggest that the reflex is polysynaptic, traversing at least several spinal cord segments (*108*).

Technique

The technique is shown in Figure 10-36. Two concentric needle electrodes are inserted on either side of the midline into the bulbocavernosus muscle, external urethral sphincter, or external anal sphincter as described in the section Electrode Application and Insertion. A surface stimulating electrode is placed on the glans, and a rectangular pulse of 0.5 to 1.0 ms duration with a frequency of 0.5 to a 1.0 stimulations per second is applied. The stimulating current is adjusted by gradually increasing the voltage until the patient first experiences the sensation of the stimulation. This voltage (or amperage if it is available) is recorded as the sensory threshold. The voltage is increased further until each stimulation causes a consistent depolarization wave on the oscilloscope. This voltage is recorded as the stimulation threshold voltage. The voltage is then further increased until just below the pain threshold, and the latency of the refex is measured at this supramaximal voltage (Fig. 10–37). The frequency, duration, and amplitude of the stimulus may affect the latency. Determination of the onset of the evoked response requires considerable expertise because of the possibility of interference from motor units, which are firing either randomly or because of anxiety. In order to overcome this problem, most authors have recommended that the evoked response of 20 to 30 stimulations be electronically averaged (Fig. 10-38) (*89,106,108*). However, because the bulbocavernosus reflex is a polysynaptic one, the shortest latency, rather than the average, is a more specific means of evaluating the sacral segments.

Since the bulbocavernosus reflex is a crossed response, it is possible to stimulate on one side and record simultaneously from both the ipsilateral and contralateral bulbocavernosus muscles. It requires that separate needle electrodes be placed into the muscle on either side of the midline. Normally, the crossed responses are almost identical to the ipsilateral responses, but with certain conditions (e.g., a herniated disk) there may be asymmetrical involvement of the different limbs of the reflex arc. Subtle abnormalities that affect only a single afferent or efferent pathway may be detected with this technique (*107,108*).

The normal bulbocavernosus reflex latency varies from approximately 30 to 40 ms, but the exact values vary slightly from one laboratory to another (*83,89,107–109*). Any neurologic process that interferes with the integrity of the reflex arc results in a prolonged latency. Common disorders that result in prolonged latencies include diabetic

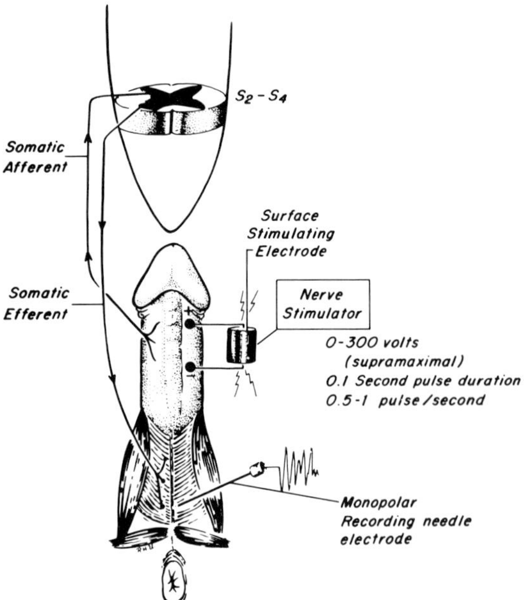

Figure 10–36. Measurement of the bulbocavernosus reflex latency. See text for details. (From Blaivas, J. G.: *et al.: Vasculogenic Impotence.* Charles C Thomas, Springfield, IL, 1980.)

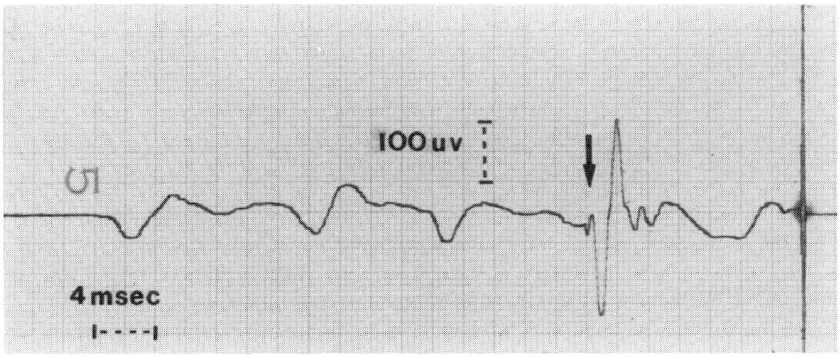

Figure 10–37. Bulbocavernosus reflex latency. Normal evoked potential from the bulbocavernosus muscle (*arrow*). Stimulus occurs at the far left, but the stimulus artifact is not seen. (From Blaivas, J. G.: In Barrett, D. M., and Wein, A. M. [ed.], *Controversies In Neurourology*. Churchill Livingstone, New York 1983.)

neuropathy, alcoholic neuropathy, and ruptured disks. Less commonly, a prolonged latency may be an early manifestation of a spinal cord tumor or multiple sclerosis.

Bulbocavernosus reflex latencies may also be obtained by stimulating the proximal urethra or vesical neck (*106,108,111*). A ring surface electrode mounted on a Foley catheter (*108*) is inserted into the bladder transurethrally, and the needle electrodes are positioned in the bulbocavernosus muscle as described above. Pulses of approximately 50 mA with a duration of 0.2 second and a frequency of five per second are usually sufficient to obtain a consistent reflex response. Latencies obtained with this technique are more prolonged than those obtained by stimulating the penis because the afferent limb of the reflex is an unmyelinated autonomic fiber. In the few published studies to date normal values have ranged from approximately 50 to 70 ms (*106,108,111*). Because latencies obtained from stimulating the vesical neck are much longer than those obtained by stimulating the glans, it is likely that these two techniques evaluate two reflexes that share a common efferent pathway (the pudendal nerve). When the glans is stimulated, the pudendal nerve supplies both afferent and efferent pathways of the reflex. The longer latencies associated with vesical neck stimulation suggest that the afferent

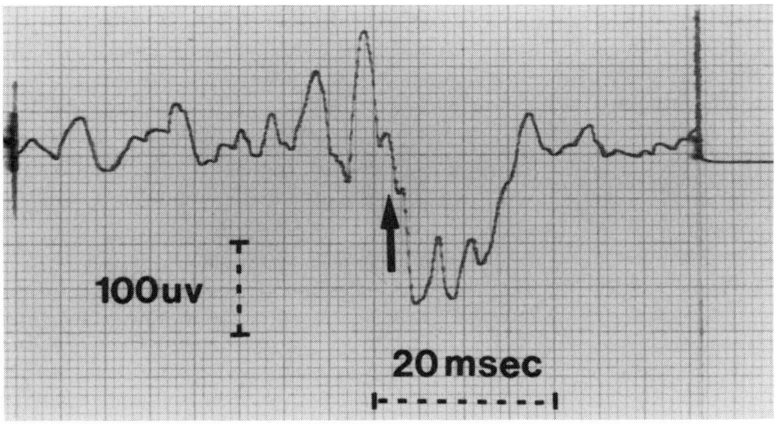

Figure 10–38. Bulbocavernosus reflex latency. *Arrow* points to the averaged response of 30 stimulations. (From Blaivas, J. G.: Electromyography: Other uses. In Barrett, D. M., and Wein, A. M. [eds], *Controversies in Neurourology*. Churchill Livingstone, New York, 1983.)

pathway is autonomic. Whether the pathway is sympathetic or parasympathetic is not known.

SOMATOSENSORY EVOKED POTENTIALS

Another application of electrophysiologic techniques to the lower urinary tract is the use of somatosensory evoked potentials. With this technique a peripheral nerve is stimulated, and the evoked potential is recorded from the spinal cord or cerebral cortex. Neurologic lesions that interrupt or impair nerve conduction result in absent or delayed latencies. For example, when the posterior tibial nerve is used, a stimulating surface electrode is placed on the skin overlying the nerve. A stimulus with the following characteristics is applied: square wave pulse of 0.2 ms duration, frequency of 4 to 5 Hz, and whatever amplitude is necessary to cause a visible twitch in the foot. The evoked potentials are recorded from the spinal cord with a gold-plated cup electrode placed over the spine. Potentials from the cerebral cortex may be detected with ordinary electroencephalography (EEG) electrodes. However, because of the small amplitude of the potentials, computerized averaging of approximately 1000 stimuli is necessary to ensure an accurate determination. It should be remembered, however, that the neuroanatomic pathways involved in somatosensory stimulation are of somatic origin and hence traverse the spinal cord in the dorsal columns. The pathways for the micturition reflex are in the lateral horns. Accordingly, it is possible for a neurologic process, e.g., a plaque of multiple sclerosis, to involve one pathway and spare the others. In order to overcome this obstacle, several investigators have begun preliminary investigations of eliciting evoked potentials by stimulating the vesical neck, proximal urethra, and bladder.

URETHRAL PRESSURE PROFILE

The urethral pressure profile (UPP) is a graphic representation of intraluminal pressure along the length of the urethra. When the pressure measurements are obtained with the bladder empty and "at rest," the graph denotes the urethral closure pressure profile (UCPP) (*112*). When simultaneous measurements of intravesical and intraurethral pressures are obtained during stress, the curve is called the stress urethral pressure profile (SUPP). When simultaneous urethral and intravesical pressures are measured during micturition, it is called the micturitional urethral pressure profile (MUPP).

From its inception it was hoped that measurement of urethral pressure would aid in the diagnosis of urinary incontinence and bladder outlet obstruction, but from a clinical standpoint this hope has not been realized for several reasons. First, bladder outlet obstruction is not necessarily associated with a high urethral closure pressure. Second, sphincteric incontinence is not necessarily accompanied by a diminished urethral closure pressure or a short functional urethral length. Most importantly, however, the clinical diagnosis of both bladder outlet obstruction and sphincteric incontinence can be made in a much more straightforward manner: by evaluating pressure–flow curves for the former and by clinical examination for the latter. Thus, although urethral pressure measurements are of considerable interest to both basic science and clinical research, the UCPP and the SUPP have little role to play in clinical urodynamics. The MUPP, on the other hand, is useful for defining not only the presence of bladder outlet obstruction but the site of the obstruction as well. Unfortunately, this technique requires expensive equipment (at least three pressure channels and simultaneous fluoroscopy) and considerable expertise in performing the procedure and interpreting the results. Accordingly, at the present time only a few urodynamic laboratories are equipped to perform the MUPP.

Because of the inherent limitations of urethral profilometry, investigations have sought to devise techniques that will prove clinically useful in diagnosing equivocal cases of sphincteric incontinence and bladder outlet obstruction. One such method is a probe mounted on a catheter that measures cross-sectional area and pressure simultaneously at discrete points in the urethra (*113*). The urethral lumen is incrementally distended by known pressures, and a number of parameters are recorded that permit more precise description of the urethral closure mechanism. Of particular importance is the ability of this technique to evaluate the rigidity and compliance of the urethral lumen.

History

The first report that recorded measurement of urethral pressure was published in 1923 by Bonney. He devised a crude method of measuring the pressure necessary to force fluid through the urethra into the bladder. It was thought that this pressure represented maximum sphincteric resistance. Bors and Comarr (*114*) refined this technique by using a Lewis cystometer to record and display the sphincterometric curve. Despite its initial appeal, sphincterometry never became an accepted or widespread procedure. Its most obvious drawback is the fact that it measures maximum pressure at an unknown point in the urethra. Moreover, because the technique requires manual manipulation of the distal urethra to ensure a good seal, voluntary or reflex contractions of the striated perineal floor muscles might well interfere with test results.

Simons (*115*) measured urethral pressure utilizing a catheter-mounted fluid-filled balloon connected to an external transducer; and other investigators have modified this technique (*116–118*). A major disadvantage has been the technical difficulty of eliminating all air from the system. Trapped air bubbles can cause considerable artifact by damping the pressure response.

In 1960 Lapides *et al.* described an infusion technique for measuring urethral pressure that was the forerunner of most currently utilized methods (*119*). A fluid-filled water manometer was connected to a whistle-tip catheter positioned in the proximal urethra. When flow through the catheter ceased, the height of the fluid column equaled the urethral pressure. The catheter was withdrawn at 1-cm intervals, and a UCPP was recorded. Refinements in technique were accomplished by replacing the water manometer with a pressure transducer and recording the pressures on a strip chart recorder (*120,121*).

Brown and Wickham devised a drip chamber to provide constant flow of fluid via a specially designed catheter with multiple side holes positioned 5 cm from the occluded tip (*122*). They theorized that at slow infusion rates the pressure necessary to permit flow into the urethra would approximate the pressure exerted by the urethral wall against the catheter. Harrison and Constable modified the technique further by adding an X-Y recorder that displayed urethral pressure as a function of distance from the vesical neck—a direct recording of the UCPP (*123*). Gleason *et al.* adapted a constant-infusion pump to mechanically withdraw the urethral catheter at a constant rate (*124*).

Membrane and ballon techniques for measuring urethral pressure were first described by Enhörning (*117*). He fashioned a fluid-filled balloon catheter by tying a soft rubber balloon over the lumen of a multilumen urethral catheter. The balloon channel was filled with fluid and connected to an external transducer; urethral pressures were measured at 0.5-cm intervals along the urethra. A second balloon channel measured intravesical pressure simultaneously, and a UCPP was thus recorded. Tanagho and Jonas further modified this technique by utilizing a thin Silastic membrane over three of the lumens of a four-channel catheter. One channel was used for measuring intravesical pressure, two channels measured urethral pressure at 2-cm intervals, and the fourth channel was used for bladder filling (*21,22*).

A number of other investigators substituted gas for liquid infusants and used conventional cystometers for recording and displaying the UCPP curves (*125–127*). Although the gas UCPP has been said to be reliable, there are several potential sources of artifact that must be considered. Gas is much more compressible than liquid and must be infused at rapid rates in order to obtain reproducible results. Hence there are rapid changes in intravesical volume during the performance of the UCPP that cannot be ignored. Under these circumstances involuntary detrusor contractions may be evoked and, if unrecognized, may be misconstrued as reflecting changes in urethral pressure.

Catheter-mounted microtip transducers have gained in popularity for use in clinical urodynamics (*23–26*). In the beginning these catheters were quite expensive, fragile, and temperature-sensitive. Although still expensive, some commercially available microtip transducers are much more durable, and when the price of disposable catheters is considered they are fast becoming cost-effective.

Technique and Interpretation

There are three basic techniques for measuring urethral pressures: (a) perfusion, (b) ballon–membrane catheters, and (c) microtip transducers. Perfusion techniques measure the total resistance to the escape of infused fluid into the urethra. Thus the recorded pressure reflects the cumulative effect of the pressure exerted by the urethral walls against the catheter lumen and the resistance to flow (due to such factors as turbulence and friction) both proximal and distal to the hole through which the perfusate escapes. Membrane or balloon catheters and microtip transducer catheters measure the pressure exerted by the urethral walls at a discrete point in the urethra.

The specifics of the technique vary depending on the particular catheter and recording device used. Generally, the patient is asked to report to the urodynamic laboratory with a full bladder, and a urinary flow rate is obtained. He is placed in the dorsal lithotomy position, the bladder is catheterized, and postvoid residual urine is measured. It is best to perform the UCPP with a partially filled bladder so that the catheter can be moved in and out without causing discomfort by hitting the back wall of the bladder. The manometer is zeroed at the level of the symphysis pubis to atmospheric pressure. The resting intravesical pressure is measured, and the catheter is slowly withdrawn, either manually or by a mechanical puller. The urethral pressure is measured at 1-cm intervals and recorded as a function of distance. An idealized UCPP is shown in Figure 10–39; actual tracings are depicted in Figure 10–40. Figure 10–41 shows the SUPP.

When infusion techniques are utilized it is necessary to have a Y-tube connector, which permits the infusion channel to be directly connected to the transducer. Catheter sizes ranging from 8F to 12F do not significantly affect the results nor do withdrawal speeds of 1 to 40 cm/min (*122,123,128,129*). Errors due to tubing compliance and resistance may cause an artifactually high pressure to be recorded. There is a rise in pressure of approximately 1 cm H_2O for each milliliter per minute increase in infusion rate (*130*). Thus at an infusion rate of 10 ml/min. the recorded urethral pressure is approximately 10 cm H_2O higher than the real pressure. Moreover, infusion techniques have a relatively slow response to increasing pressures (*131*).

When microtip transducer catheters are used, the technique is slightly different. Only custom-made catheters have a filling channel incorporated in the design; accordingly, in most instances the bladder must be emptied and filled with an ordinary catheter, which is then replaced with the microtip catheter.

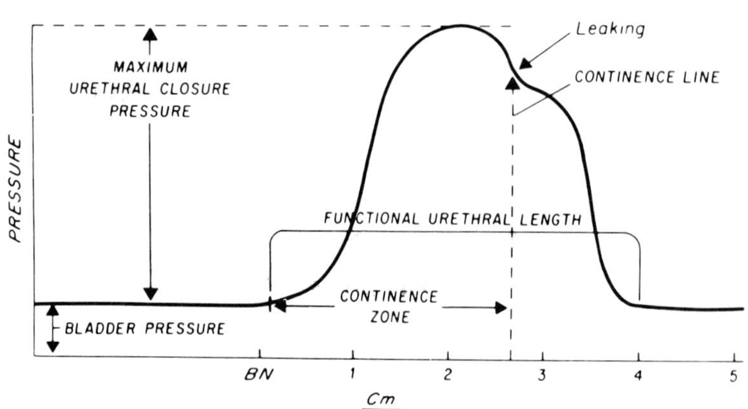

Figure 10–39. Idealized urethral pressure profile. *BN* = bladder neck. Numbers refer to distance from bladder neck in centimeters. (From Blaivas, J. G.: A critical appraisal of specific techniques. In Krane, R. J., and Siroky, M. B. [eds.]. *Clinical Neurourology*. Little, Brown, Boston, 1979.)

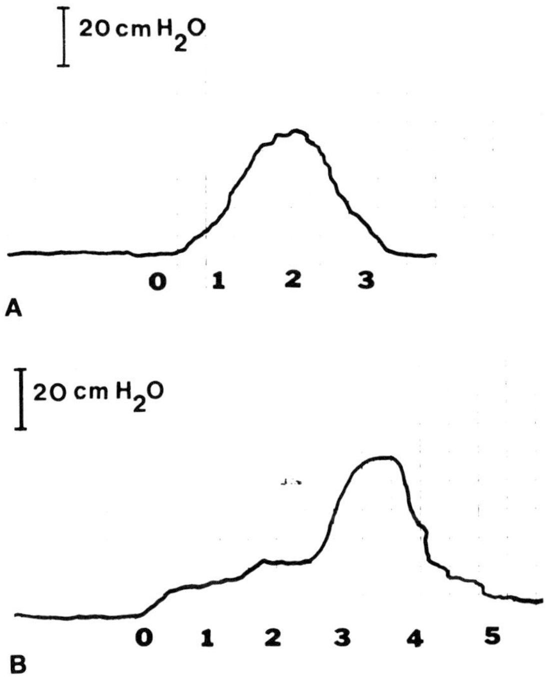

Figure 10–40. Urethral pressure profile. A. Normal woman. B. Normal man. Numbers refer to the distance from the vesical neck in centimeters.

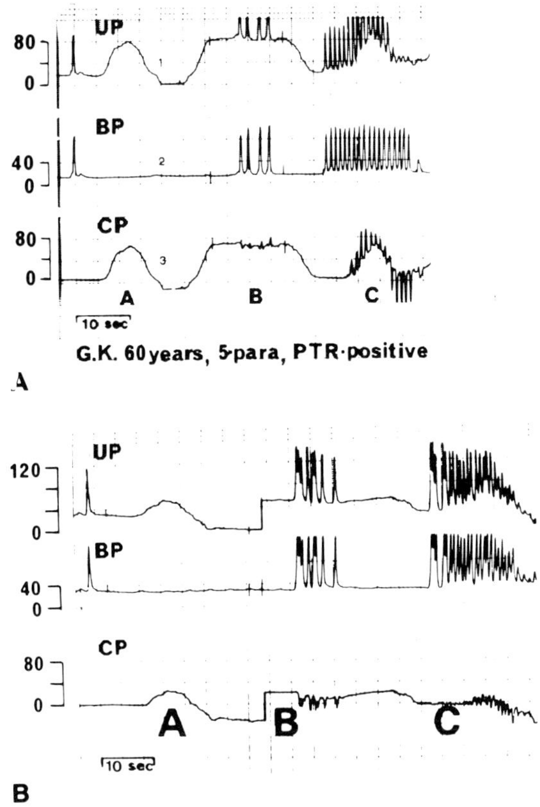

Figure 10–41. Stress urethral pressure profile. A. Normal woman. In section A, a UCPP is performed. In section B, p_{ura} is measured at the site of $p_{ura\ max}$ on the UCPP while the patient repeatedly coughs. In section C, p_{ura} is measured throughout the profile length during successive coughs. In the normal patient the closure pressure is positive throughout the proximal urethra. B. patient with stress incontinence. Note the negative closure pressure in the proximal urethra during coughing with the pressure sensor held at maximum urethral pressure. *UP* = urethral pressure. *BP* = intravesical pressure. *CP* = closure pressure (*UP* – *BP*). (From Rud, T.: The striated pelvic floor muscles and their importance in maintaining urinary continence. In Zinner, N.R., and Sterling, A.M. [eds.]: *Female Incontinence*. Alan R. Liss, New York, 1981.)

Orientation of the position of the pressure sensor in the radial axis of the urethra may affect the results. In general, all pressure measurements are increased and urethral length measurments decreased when the transducer membrane is oriented anteriorly compared to laterally or dorsally (*132,133*). Moreover, because the microtip transducer serves as its own reference point, all pressure measurements are increased by the hydrostatic pressure of the fluid. This factor is negligible when the UCPP is performed in the supine position but may be a significant factor when the profile is done with the patient sitting or standing.

There may be a high degree of variability when the UCPP is performed serially during the same session, particularly among the first few profiles performed (*23,133–136*). Plante and Susset attributed this variability to activation of the periurethral striated musculature and external urethral sphincter, presumably due to anxiety (*137*). Accordingly, they recommended that the lowest profile be recorded. Others have recommended averaging a series of profiles (*23,134,136*), and Obrink *et al.* (*135*) suggested using the third recording only. Toguri *et al.* (*138*) found a large variability in UCPP using fluid, and Wein *et al.* (*139*) found an even larger variability using gas perfusion techniques.

Regardless of the recording technique, when urethral pressures are measured without fluoroscopic control it is impossible to determine the site of the anatomic vesical neck. Thus when the proximal urethra is nonfunctioning, as in the case of prostatectomy or type III stress urinary incontinence, the first rise in pressure may not occur until the region of the membranous urethra is reached (Fig. 10–42) (*140*). Because pressures in this area are usually much higher than those in the more proximal urethra, one may conclude wrongly that it represents a vesical neck obstruction.

SYNCHRONOUS VIDEO/PRESSURE/FLOW/EMG

Simultaneous measurement of pressure in the bladder, urethra, and rectum combined with urinary flow rate, sphincter EMG, and radiographic visualization of the lower urinary tract provides the most artifact-free, precise display of normal and abnormal physiology (*141–145*). The time, effort, and expense required to operate such a urodynamic facility is considerable; nevertheless, we believe that these studies offer unique advantages to patients with complicated problems and in the long run are both necessary and cost-effective.

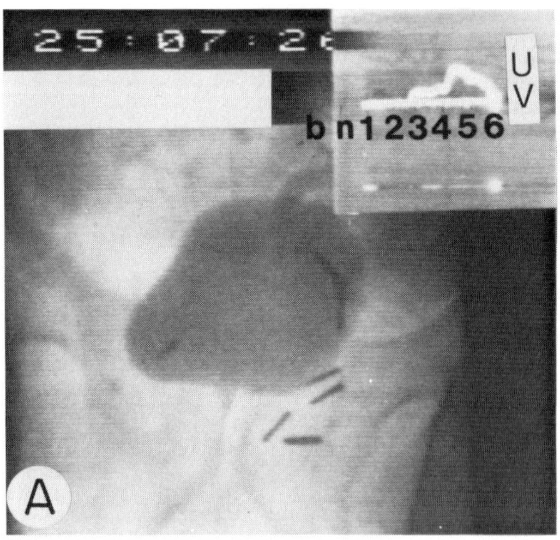

Figure 10–42. Nonfunctional proximal urethra after abdominoperineal resection of the rectum in a 62-year-old man. Video urethral pressure profile. Note that the configuration of the urethral pressure profile is normal, as is the maximum urethral pressure. However, the onset of urethral pressure does not occur until almost 3 cm from the anatomic vesical neck. (From Blaivas, J. G., and Barbalias, G. A.: *J. Urol.* 129:84, 1983. Copyright © 1983, The Williams & Wilkins Co., Baltimore.)

A block diagram of the basic video/urodynamic unit is seen in Figure 10–43. Radiographic contrast is used as the infusant for cystometry, and urodynamic parameters are transduced and displayed on a storage oscilloscope. A television camera scans the oscilloscope screen and sends the information to a television monitor, where it is mixed with the video image from fluoroscopic visualization of the bladder and urethra. Recently, computerized techniques have been developed that supplant the need for a television camera and storage oscilloscope. Optical images from the fluoroscope are digitized and stored in the computer memory along with the digitized data from the urodynamic tracings. The digitized signals can be displayed on a television screen or printed on paper.

The advantages of such a system are obvious. By simultaneously measuring multiple urodynamic variables one gains a better insight into the underlying pathophysiology. Moreover, because all variables are visualized simultaneously one can better appreciate their interrelations and identify artifacts with ease. For example, alternating current interference usually simulates an increase in EMG activity. If this increase is unaccompanied by either a rise in urethral pressure or narrowing of the urethra on the fluoroscope, the nature of the "increased EMG activity" is obvious.

Technique

The patient is asked to report to the examination with a full bladder. Urinary flow rate is obtained, and the bladder is catheterized with a triple-lumen urodynamic catheter for measuring intravesical and urethral pressures simultaneously. Rectal pressure is monitored via a fluid-filled balloon catheter. Sphincter EMG is performed as outlined in the previous section. Radiographic contrast is instilled into the bladder at a rate determined by the clinical setting. In most instances medium-fill cystometry is performed; but if sensory urgency or a small capacity bladder is suspected, a slow filling rate is utilized. All pressures are zeroed to atmospheric pressure at the level of the symphysis

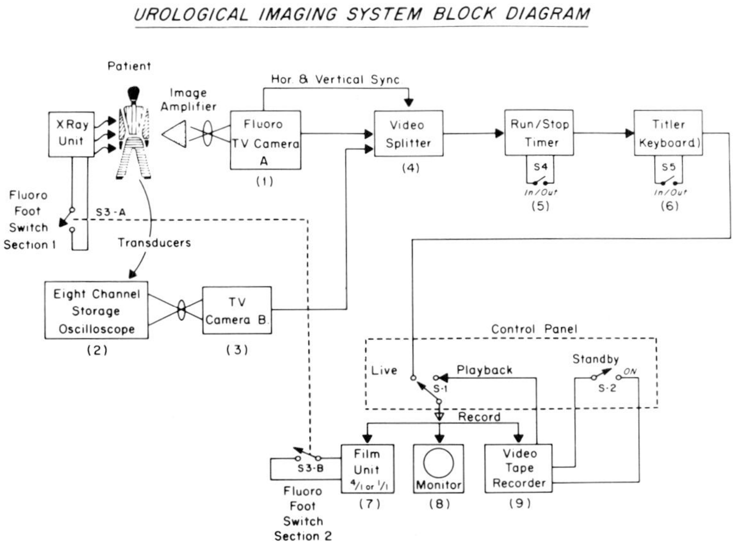

Figure 10–43. Block diagram of basic video/urodynamic unit. (From Blaivas, J. G., *et al.*: *J. Urol.* 125:693, 1981. Copyright © 1981, The Williams & Wilkins Co., Baltimore.)

pubis; the zeros for urethral and intravesical pressure are superimposed on one another, so that when the pressure in the bladder and urethra are equal only one line is visualized on the recorder; when they are different, two lines are seen.

With the patient in a semioblique position, a scout film is recorded on videotape. Radiographic contrast is instilled until the location of the vesical neck is obvious; this usually requires approximately 50 ml of contrast. With the urethral and bladder recording channels in the bladder, the catheter is slowly withdrawn and a urethral pressure profile obtained with fluoroscopic control (Fig. 10–44). The radiopaque marker of the urethral measuring port is positioned at the point of highest urethral pressure; the patient is asked to contract his sphincter; and the pressure rise and EMG response are recorded (Fig. 10–45). The responses to cough, Credé and Valsalva maneuvers, and the commands to start and stop voiding are noted.

With the patient in his usual voiding position (lying, sitting, or standing), bladder filling is begun. The urethral pressure monitoring port is positioned at the point of maximum urethral pressure. The patient is instructed to neither void nor inhibit micturition, but to report his sensations to the examiner. A normal study is seen in Figure 10–46. If involuntary detrusor contractions occur, it is determined if the patient was aware of them and if he could inhibit their onset or abort them once they started. Most importantly, it is determined if they are part of the usual symptoms the patient experiences. The events are recorded periodically on videotape, and the bladder is emptied and filling begun again. This time the patient is

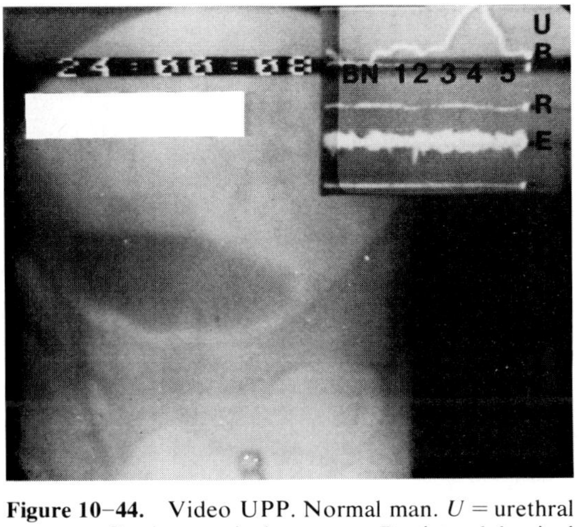

Figure 10–44. Video UPP. Normal man. *U* = urethral pressure. *B* = intravesical pressure. *R* = intraabdominal pressure.

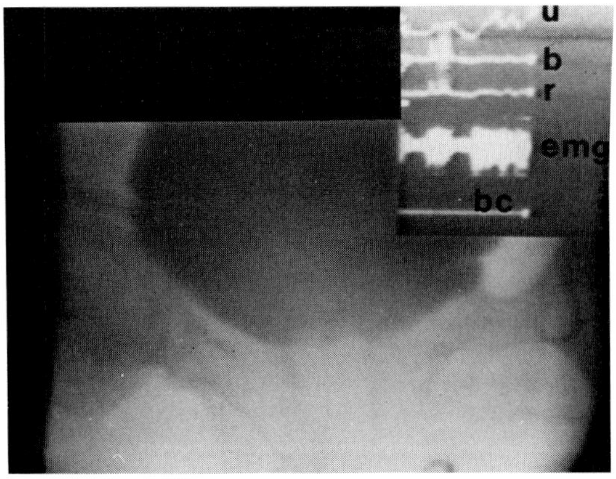

Figure 10–45. Video urodynamic demonstration of the bulbocavernosus reflex. *bc* = bulbocavernosus reflex. *u* = urethral pressure. *b* = intravesical pressure. *r* = intraabdominal pressure. (From Blaivas, J. G., *et al.*: *J. Urol.* 126:197, 1981. Copyright © 1981, The Williams & Wilkins Co., Baltimore.)

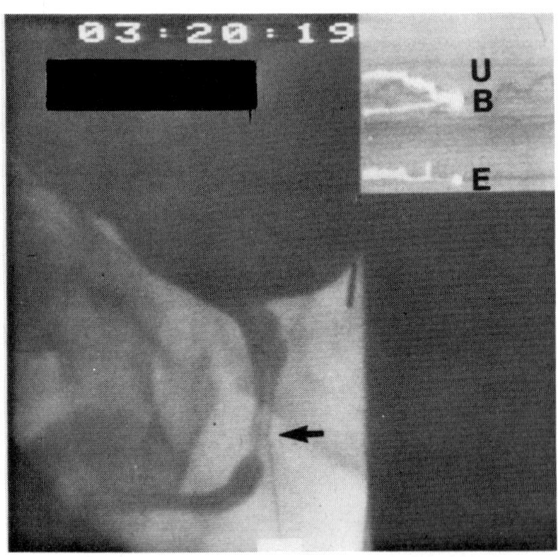

Figure 10–46. Normal video urodynamic study. Note the fall in urethral pressure accompanied by complete relaxation of the external urethral sphincter just prior to and throughout the detrusor contraction. During micturition the entire proximal urethra is isobaric with the bladder. The arrow points to the site in the urethra where urethral pressure is being measured. *U* = urethral pressure. *B* = intravesical pressure. *E* = sphincter electromyogram. Urethral and intravesical pressures have the same baseline.

asked to try to inhibit micturition, and his ability to do so is recorded as well as the cystometric bladder capacity. If involuntary detrusor contractions are suspected but not demonstrated, the examination is repeated at faster filling rates in the upright position. The patient is asked to cough and strain and sometimes to walk or jump in place to see if detrusor instability can be provoked. When involuntary detrusor contractions are demonstrated, it is important to exclude concomitant bladder outlet obstruction as the cause.

If involuntary detrusor contractions do not occur, the bladder is filled until the patient has a strong urge to void. Particular note is made of the EMG activity during attempts to void. Normally, EMG activity increases during straining in an attempt to void, but it becomes quiescent immediately prior to the detrusor contraction.

If the patient complains of urinary incontinence and involuntary detrusor contractions are not detected as the cause, the integrity of the vesical neck and proximal urethra is assessed and their position in relation to the symphysis pubis is noted at rest and in response to coughing and straining. However, it should be noted that with mild and moderate degrees of stress urinary incontinence radiographic visualization of leakage is often not accomplished even though the anatomic substrate (descent of the urethra and opening of the vesical neck) is apparent. Direct visualization of the urethral meatus during these provocative maneuvers, especially once the catheter is removed, may provide visual evidence of urinary incontinence and is an essential part of the examination that should not be omitted.

If bladder outlet obstruction has been diagnosed or is suspected but the site of obstruction is not clear, a MUPP usually provides a definitive answer (*146*). The examination is performed by slowly withdrawing the urethral port of the catheter through the proximal urethra during micturition. Normally, the bladder and entire proximal urethra are approximately isobaric during micturition (Fig. 10–47). At the level of the membranous urethra there is usually a variable drop in urethral pressure, but the magnitude of this decrease has not been well defined. A fall of pressure proximal to the membranous urethra, especially when ac-

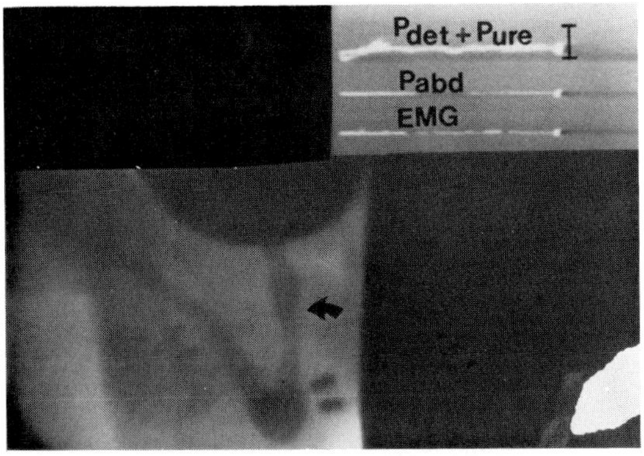

Figure 10–47. Normal micturitional urethral pressure profile. The entire proximal urethra is isobaric with the bladder during micturition. The patient is voiding voluntarily with a detrusor contraction of 38 cm H_2O. Urethral and detrusor pressure are zeroed to the same baseline. When the pressures are equal, only one line is seen. During micturition the urethral sensor is moved up and down the prostatic urethra, and at every point the pressure in the urethra is seen to be the same as that in the bladder. The *arrow* points to the site in the urethra where pressure is being measured at this instant in time.

companied by radiographic evidence of narrowing, is indicative of an obstruction between the bladder and the site of the fall in urethral pressure (Fig. 10–48).

Specific indications for video urodynamics have not been delineated. However, they are particularly useful in the following situations:

1. *Bladder outlet obstruction versus poor detrusor contractility.* Impaired uroflow may be caused by either bladder outlet obstruction or an inadequate detrusor contraction. Although simple pressure flow analysis may make this distinction, unless pressures are measured simultaneously in the bladder and urethra it may be difficult to determine the exact site of obstruction. Moreover, in some patients obstruction coexists with impaired detrusor contractility (Fig. 10–49).

2. *Detrusor-external sphincter dyssynergia versus "pseudodyssynergia."* Detrusor-external sphincter dyssynergia is char-

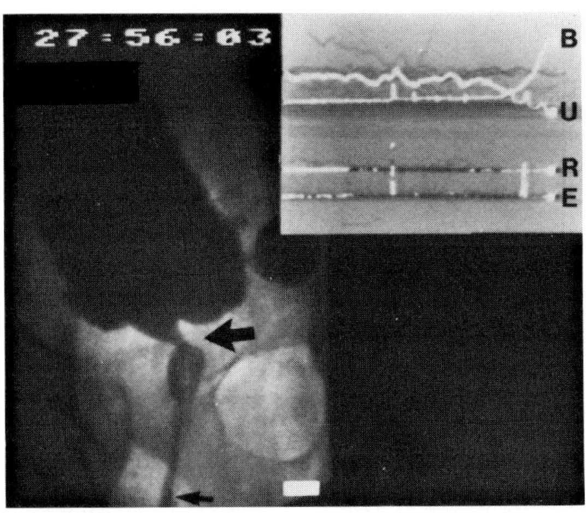

Figure 10–48. Micturitional urethral pressure profile of vesical neck obstruction. The *large arrow* depicts the site of obstruction approximately 1 cm distal to the anatomic vesical neck. The small arrow shows the point in the urethra where pressure is being measured. Urethral pressure distal to the point of obstruction (20 cm H_2O) is much lower than the detrusor pressure (150 cm H_2O). Urethral and intravesical pressures were zeroed to the same baseline, and the urethral pressure sensor was held stationary at the site of highest urethral pressure on the resting UPP until voiding occurred. During micturition the catheter was moved up and down the urethra to measure the profile. B = intravesical pressure. U = urethral pressure. R = intraabdominal pressure. E = sphincter electromyogram. (From Blaivas, J. G.: In Hinman, F., Jr. [ed.], *Benign Prostatic Hypertrophy.* Springer-Verlag, New York, 1983.)

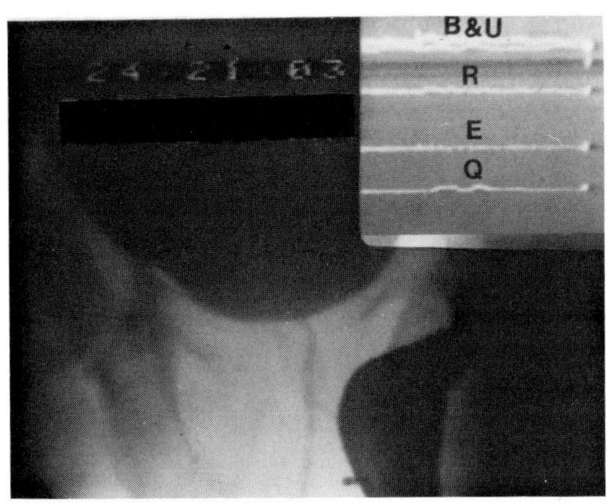

Figure 10–49. Micturitional urethral pressure profile. Bladder neck obstruction coexisting with impaired detrusor contractility. During micturition maximum detrusor pressure is only 21 cm H_2O, demonstrating impaired detrusor contraction. Urethral pressure, measured 1 cm distal to the vesical neck, was 10 cm during voiding, showing an obstruction at the vesical neck. Urethral and intravesical pressure were zeroed to the same baseline, and the urethral pressure sensor was held stationary at the site of highest urethral pressure on the resting UPP until voiding occurred. During micturition the catheter was moved up and down the urethra to measure the profile. U = urethral pressure measured at the *arrow*. B = intravesical pressure. R = intraabdominal pressure. E = sphincter electromyogram. Q = uroflow. (From Blaivas, J. G.: *Urology,* 23:421, 1984, with permission.)

acterized by involuntary contraction of the external urethral sphincter during involuntary detrusor contractions (*97*). There are three types of dyssynergia depicted in Figures 10–50 to 10–52 (*96*). With pseudodyssynergia the increase in EMG activity may be voluntary (or subconscious) and accompanied by contraction of the external urethral sphincter with a rise in intraurethral pressure and interruption of the stream (Fig. 10–35B). Alternatively, there may be increased EMG activity unassociated with either a rise in urethral pressure or interruption of the stream.

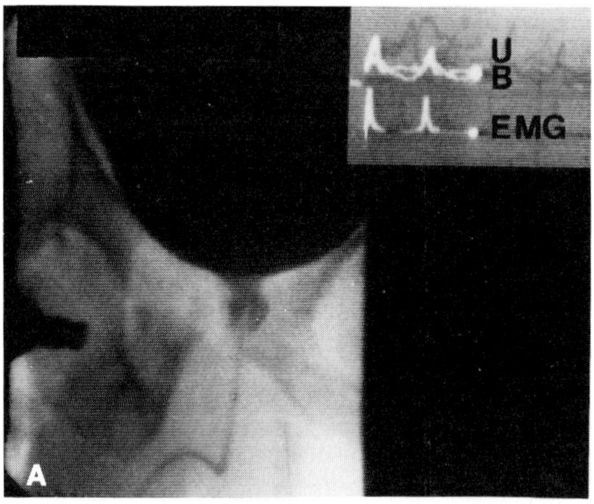

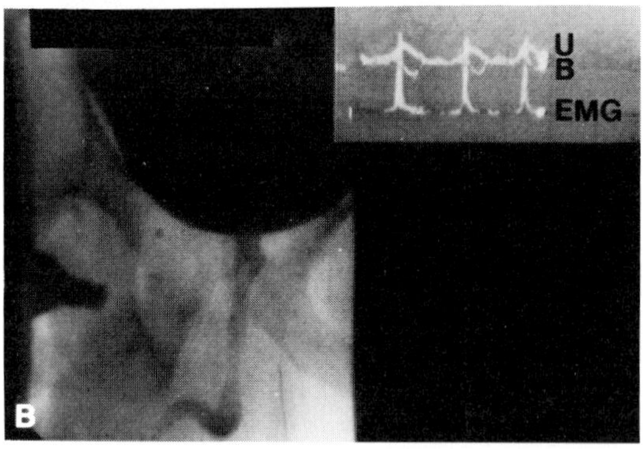

Figure 10–50. Type 1 detrusor–external sphincter dyssynergia. **A.** At the onset of each detrusor and sphincter contraction there is complete obstruction at the level of the external sphincter. **B.** Immediately after the peak of the detrusor contraction there is complete relaxation of the external sphincter, and voiding ensues. U = urethral pressure at the membranous urethra. B = intravesical pressure. Urethral and intravesical pressure are zeroed at the same baseline. (From Blaivas, J. G.: *Urology*, 23:421, 1984.)

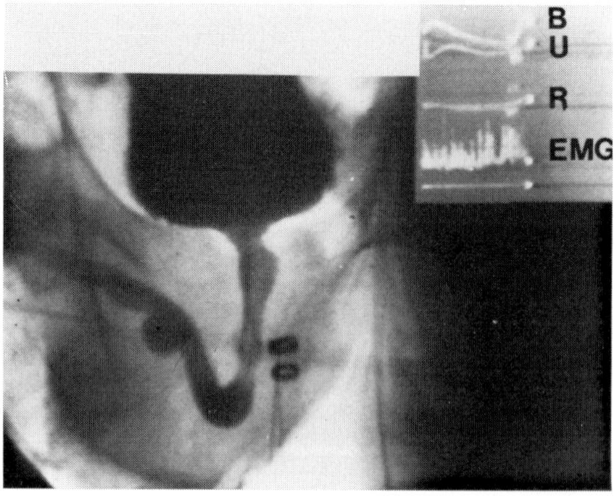

Figure 10–51. Type 2 detrusor–external sphincter dyssynergia. Note the sporadic increase in EMG activity throughout the detrusor contraction. U = urethral pressure. B = intravesical pressure. R = abdominal pressure. (From Blaivas, J. G.: *J. Urol.* 125:545, 1981. Copyright © 1981, The Williams & Wilkins Co., Baltimore.)

3. *Stress incontinence versus a nonfunctioning urethral sphincter.* Patients who have failed multiple operations for stress urinary incontinence may be left with a fibrotic, rigid urethra that no longer functions as a sphincter (*140,147,148*). Similarly, patients with denervation of the smooth muscle of the proximal urethral (particularly myelodys-

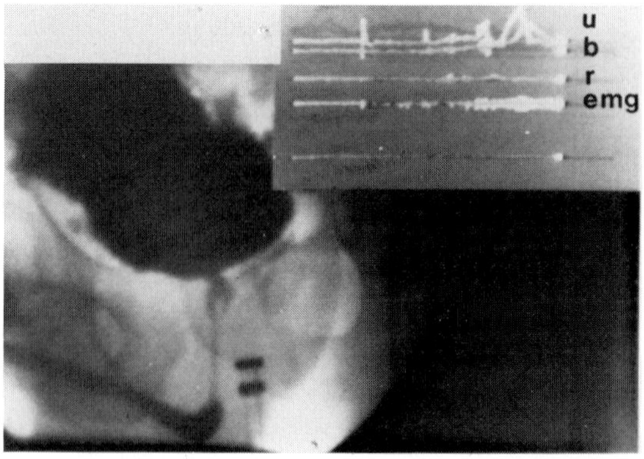

Figure 10–52. Type 3 detrusor–external sphincter dyssynergia. Crescendo–decrescendo pattern of EMG activity during detrusor contraction. u = urethral pressure measured at membranous urethra. b = intravesical pressure. r = abdominal pressure. (From Blaivas, J. G.: *J. Urol.*, 125:545, 1979. Copyright © 1979, The Williams & Wilkins Co., Baltimore.)

plastic patients and those who have had abdominoperineal resection of the rectum or radical hysterectomy) develop nonfunction of the proximal urethral sphincteric mechanism that may be confused with stress incontinence (*140,149*).This condition is termed type III stress incontinence and is readily diagnosed by the video/urodynamic demonstration of an open vesical neck during bladder filling and a proximal urethra that is isobaric with the bladder (Fig. 10–42).

REFERENCES

1. Merrill, D. C., Bradley, W. E., and Markland, C.: Air cystometry. II. A clinical evaluation of normal adults. *J. Urol.* 108:85, 1972.
2. Klevmark B.: Motility of the urinary bladder in cats during filling at physiologic rates. I. Intravesical pressure patterns studies by a new method of cystometry. *Acta Physiol. Scand.* 90:565, 1974.
3. Kondo, A., Susset, J. G., and Lefaivre, J.: Viscoelastic properties of bladder. I. Mechanical model and its mathematical analysis. *Invest. Urol.* 10:154, 1972.
4. Kondo, A., and Susset, J. G.: Physical properties of the urinary detrusor muscle: a mechanical model based upon the analysis of stress relaxation curve. *J. Biomech.* 6:141, 1973.
5. Kondo, A., Susset, J., and Lefaivre, J.: Viscoelastic properties of bladder. II. Comparative studies in normal and pathological dogs. *Invest. Urol.* 11:459, 1974.
6. Susset, J., Ghoniem, G. M., and Regnier, C. H.: Rapid cystometry in males. *Neurourol. Urodyn.* 1:319, 1982.
7. Klevmark, B. J.: Motility of the urinary bladder in cats during filling at physiologic rates. II. Effects of extrinsic bladder denervation on intramural tension and on intravesical pressure patterns. *Acta Physiol. Scand.* 101:176, 1977.
8. Ruch, T. C., and Tang, P. C.: The higher control of the bladder In Boyarsky, S. (ed.), *The Neurogenic Bladder*. Williams & Wilkins, Baltimore, 1967.
9. Tang, P. C., and Ruch, T. C.: Non-neurogenic basis of bladder tone. *Am. J. Physiol.* 181:249, 1955.
10. Bradley, W., Chou, S., Markland, C., and Swaiman, K.: Biochemical assay technique for estimation of bladder fibrosis. *Invest. Urol.* 3:59, 1965.
11. Kondo, A., and Susset, J.: Collagen content in detrusor muscle and ratio of bladder weight to body weight. *Acta Urol. Jpn.* 19:683, 1973.
12. Susset, J., Servot-Viguier, D., Lamy, F., Madernas, P., and Blascj, R.: Collagen in 155 human bladders. *Invest. Urol.* 16:204, 1978.
13. Coolsaet, B. L. R. A., Van Duyl, W. A., Van Mastrigt, R., and Van Der Zwart, A.: Stepwise cystometry. *Urology* 2:255, 1973.
14. Coolsaet, B. L. R. A.: *Stepwise cystometry*. Doctoral thesis, Erasmus University, Rotterdam, 1977.
15. Blaivas, J. G.: The neurophysiology of micturition: a clinical study of 550 patients, *J. Urol.* 127:958, 1982.
16. Fletcher, T. F., and Bradley, W. E.: Neuroanatomy of the bladder-urethra. *J. Urol.* 119:153, 1978.
17. Kuru, M.: Nervous control of micturition. *Physiol. Rev.* 45:425, 1965.
18. Nordling, J., Meyhoff, H. H., and Hald, T.: Neuromuscular dysfunction of the lower urinary tract with special reference to the influence of the sympathetic nervous system. *Scand. J. Urol. Nephrol.* 15:7, 1981.
19. Nathan, P. W.: Sensations associated with micturition. *Br. J. Urol.* 28:126, 1956.
20. Bradley, W. E., Timm, G. W., and Scott, F. B.: Cystometry. V. Bladder sensation. *Urology* 6:654, 1975b.
21. Tanagho, E. A., and Jonas, U.: Membrane catheter: effective for recording pressure in lower urinary tract. *Urology* 10:173, 1977.
22. Tanagho, E. A.: Urethral pressure profile: membrane catheter. In Barrett, D. M., and Wein, A. J. (eds.), *Controversies in Neurourology*. Churchill Livingstone, New York, 1984.
23. Asmussen, M., and Ulmstein, U.: Simultaneous urethrocystometry and urethral pressure profile measurement with a new technique. *Acta Obstet. Gynecol. Scand.* 54:385, 1975.
24. Bruskewitz, R., and Raz, S.: Urethral pressure profile using microtipped catheter in females. *Urology* 14:303, 1979.
25. Leach, G. E., Farsaii, A., and Raz, S.: New dual-channel microtipped transducer catheter for urethral pressure profile and cystometry, *Urology* 20:555, 1982.
26. Miller, G. W., and Baker, L. E.: A stable ultraminiature catheter tip pressure transducer. *Med. Biol. Eng.* 11:86, 1973.
27. Blaivas, J. G., Labib, K. B., and Scott, R. M.: Urodynamic evaluation as a test of sacral cord function. *Urology* 9:682, 1979.
28. Gibaldi, M., and Grundhofer, B.: Biopharmaceutic influences on the anticholinergic effects of propantheline. *Clin. Pharmacol. Ther.* 18:457, 1975.
29. Mirakhur, R. K., Dundee, J. W., and Jones, C. J.: Evaluation of the anticholinergic actions of glycopyrronium bromide. *Br. J. Clin. Pharmacol.* 5:77, 1978.
30. Wein, A. J.: Nonsurgical treatment of lower urinary tract dysfunction. In Raz, S. (ed.), *Female Urology*. Saunders, Philadelphia, 1983.
31. Diokno, A. C., Davis, R., and Lapides, J.: Urecholine test for denervated bladders. *Invest. Urol.* 13:233, 1975.
32. Glahn, B. E.: Neurogenic bladder diagnosed pharmacologically on the basis of denervation supersensitivity. *Scand. J. Urol. Nephrol.* 4:13, 1970.
33. Lapides, J., Friend, C. R., Ajemian, E. P., and Reus, W. S.: Denervation supersensitivity as a test for neurogenic bladder. *Surg. Gynecol. Obstet.* 114:241, 1962.

34. Melzer, M.: The urecholine test. *J. Urol.* 108:728, 1972.
35. Merrill, D. C., and Rotta, J.: A clinical evaluation of detrusor denervation supersensitivity using air cystometry. *J. Urol.* 111:27, 1974.
36. Pavlakis, A. J., Siroky, M. B., and Krane, R. J.: Neurogenic detrusor areflexia: correlation of perineal electromyography and bethanechol chloride supersensitivity testing. *J. Urol.* 129:1182, 1983.
37. Cannon, W. B.: Law of denervation. *Am. J. Med. Sci.* 198:737, 1939.
38. Blaivas, J. G., Labib, K. B., Michalik, S. J., and Zayed, A. A. H.: Failure of bethanechol denervation supersensitivity as a diagnostic aid. *J. Urol.* 123:199–201, 1980.
39. Downie, J. W., Moochhala, S. M., and Bialik, J. G.: The role of reflexes in modifying the response to bethanechol chloride: A basis for selectivity of action on the bladder. *Neurourol Urodyn.* 2:301, 1983.
40. Wein, A. J., Raezer, D. M., and Malloy, T. R.: Failure of the bethanechol supersensitivity test to predict improved voiding after subcutaneous bethanechol administration. *J. Urol.* 123:202, 1980.
41. Yalla, S. V., Rossier, A. B., and Fam, B.: Dyssynergic vesicourethral responses during bladder rehabilitation in spinal cord injury patients: effect of suprapubic percussion, Credé method and bethanechol chloride. *J. Urol.* 115:575, 1976.
42. Backman, K. A.: Urinary flow during micturition in normal women. *Acta Chir. Scand.* 130:357, 1965.
43. Drach, G. W., Layton, T. N., and Binard, W. J.: Male peak urinary flow rate: relationship to volume voided and age. *J. Urol.* 122:210, 1979.
44. Ballenger, E. G., Elder, F., and McDonald, H. P.: Voiding distance decrease, an important early symptom of prostatic obstruction. *South Med. J.* 25:863, 1932.
45. Von Garrelts, B.: Analysis of micturition: a new method of recording the voiding subjects. *Acta Chir. Scand.* 112:326, 1956.
46. Tammren, H.: Miktiograph 7005. *Acta Medicotechn.* 19:10, 1971.
47. Rowan, D., McKenzie, A. L., McNee, S. G., and Glen, E. S.: A technical and clinical evaluation of the Disa flowmeter. *Br. J. Urol.* 49:285, 1977.
48. Corlett, R. C., and Roy, S.: Carbon dioxide uroflowmetry. *J. Urol.* 122:512, 1979.
49. Cardus, D., Quesada, E. M., and Scott, F. B.: Use of an electromagnetic flowmeter for urine flow measurements. *J. Appl. Physiol.* 18:845, 1963.
50. Sussett, J. G., Picker, P., Kretz, M., and Jorest, R.: Critical evaluation of uroflowmeters and analysis of normal curves. *J. Urol.* 109:874, 1973.
51. Keitzer, W. A., and Huffman, G. C.: The voiding audiograph: a new voiding test. *J. Urol.* 96:404, 1966.
52. Lyons, R. P., and Smith, D. R.: Distal urethral stenosis. *J. Urol.* 89:414, 1963.
52a. Maizels, M., and Firlit, C. F.: Pediatric urodynamics: a clinical comparison of surface versus needle pelvic floor/external sphincter electromyography. *J. Urol.* 122:518, 1979.
53. Zinner, N. R., Ritter, R. C., Sterling, A. M., and Harding, D. C.: High speed cinematography of human urination. *Invest. Urol.* 6:605, 1966.
54. Zinner, N. R., Ritter, R. C., Sterling, A. M., and Harding, D. C.: Drop spectrometer: a non-obstructive, non-interfering instrument for analyzing hydrodynamic properties of human urination. *J. Urol.* 101:914, 1966.
55. Drake, W. M.: The uroflowmeter: an aid to the study of lower urinary tract. *J. Urol.* 59:650, 1948.
56. Rollema, H. J., Griffiths, W. A., VanDuyl, W. A., Vandenberg, J., and deHaan, R.: Flow rate versus bladder volume. *Urol. Int.* 32:401, 1977.
57. Siroky, M.B., Olsson, C. A., and Krane, R. J.: The flow rate nomogram. I. Development. *J. Urol.* 122:65, 1979.
58. Von Garrelts, B.: Intravesical pressure and urinary flow during micturition in normal subjects. *Acta Chir. Scand.* 114:49, 1957.
59. Drach, G. W., Layton, T., and Bottaccini, M. R.: A method of adjustment of male peak urinary flow rate for varying age and volume voided. *J. Urol.* 128:960, 1982.
60. Shoukry, I., Susset, J. G., Elhilali, M. M., and Dutartre, D.: Role of uroflowmetry in the assessment of lower urinary tract obstruction in adult males. *Br. J. Urol.* 47:559, 1975.
61. Siroky, M. B., Olsson, C. A., and Krane, R. J.: The flow rate nomogram. II. Clinical correlation. *J. Urol.* 123:208, 1980.
62. Sussett, J. G., and Dutarte, D.: Evolution of urinary flow rate with prostatectomy. *Urology* 5:763, 1975.
63. Kondo, A., Mitsuya, H., and Torii, H.: Computer analysis of micturition parameters and accuracy of uroflow. *Urol. Int.* 33:337, 1978.
64. Rollema, H. J.: Uroflowmetry in males: reference values and clinical application. In *Benign Prostatic Hypertrophy*. Dinkkerij van Denderen, Groninjen, B. V., 1981.
65. Strauss, B. S., and Blaufox, M. D.: Estimation of residual urine and urine flow rates without urethral catheterization. *J. Nucl. Med.* 11:81, 1970.
66. Platenkamp, G. J. J. M., Kramer, G., Hermans, Sterling, A., van Ness, J., Quverkerk, T. and Bout, C.: Voiding characteristics of normal man. In *Proceedings of the Sixth Annual Meeting of the International Continence Society*, Antwerp, 1976.
67. Spencer, R. P., and Treves, S.: Bladder empyting flow rate as a function of bladder volume. *Yale J. Biol. Med.* 44:401, 1971.
68. Layton, T., and Drach, G. W.: Selectivity of peak versus average male urinary flow rates. *J. Urol.* 125:839, 1981.
69. Gleason, D. M., and Lattimer, J. K.: The pressure flow study: a method for measuring bladder neck resistance. *J. Urol.* 87:844, 1962.
70. Frimødt-Moller, C., and Hald, T.: Clinical urodynamics, methods and results. *Scand. J. Urol. Nephrol.* 6:143, 1972.
71. Susset, J. G.: Resistance to flow in the lower urinary tract: clinical application. In Hinman, F., Jr. (ed.), *Hydrodynamics of Micturition*. Charles C Thomas. Springfield, IL, 1971, pp. 232–237, 249.
72. Bruskewitz, R., Jensen, K. M. E., Iversen, P., and Madsen, P. O.: Relevance of minimum urethral resistance in prostatism. *J. Urol.* 129:769, 1983.
73. Griffiths. D. J.: Mechanics of the urethra in micturition. *Br. J. Urol.* 45:497, 1973.
74. Griffiths, D. J.: The mechanical functions of the

bladder and urethra in micturition. *Int. Urol. Nephrol.* 6:177, 1974.
75. Griffiths, D. J.: Urodynamic assessment of bladder function. *Brt. J. Urol.* 49:29, 1977.
76. Griffiths, D. J., and Scholtmeijer, R. J., Precise urodynamic assessment of meatal and distal urethral stenosis in girls. *Neurourol. Urodyn.* 1:89, 1982.
77. Griffiths, D. J., and Scholtmeijer, R. J.: Precise urodynamic assessment of anatomic urethral obstruction in boys. *Neurourol. Urodyn.* 1:97, 1982.
78. Griffiths, D. J., and Scholtmeijer, R. J.: Detrusor/sphincter dyssynergia in neurologically normal children, *Neurourol. Urodyn.* 2:127, 1983.
79. Schäfer, W.: The contribution of the bladder outlet to the relationship between pressure and flow during micturition. In Hinman, F. (ed.), *Benign Prostatic Hypertrophy.* Springer-Verlag, New York, 1983.
80. Ryall, R. L., and Marshall, V. R.: The effect of a urethral catheter on the measurement of maximum urinary flow rate. *J. Urol.* 128:429, 1982.
81. Blaivas, J. G., Labib, B., Bauer, S. B., and Retik, A. B.: A new approach to elecromyography of the exteneral urethral sphincter. *J. Urol.* 117:773, 1977.
82. Chantraine, A.: EMG examination of anal and urethral sphincter. In Desmedt, J. E. (ed.), *New Developments in Electromyography and Clinical Neurophysiology,* Vol. 2. Karger, Basel, 1973, pp. 421–432.
83. DiBenedetto, M., and Yalla, S. V.: Electrodiagnosis of striated urethral sphincter dysfunction. *J. Urol.* 122:361, 1979.
84. Diokno, A. C., Koff, S. A., and Anderson, W.: Combined cystometry and perineal electromyography in the diagnosis and treatment of neurogenic urinary incontinence. *J. Urol.* 115:161, 1976.
85. Aminoff, M. J.: Electromyography, In *Electrodiagnosis in Clinical Neurology.* Churchill Livingstone, New York, 1973, pp. 197–228.
86. Goodgold, S., and Eberstein, A.: *Electrodiagnosis of Neuromuscular Disease,* 2nd ed. Williams & Wilkins, Baltimore, 1977, pp. 146–168.
87. Lanman, J. A. R., and Ritchie, E. E.: *Clinical Electromyography.* Lippincott, Philadelphia, 1977, pp. 119–151.
88. Diokno, A. C., Koff, S. A., and Bender, L. F.: Periurethral striated muscle activity in neurogenic bladder dysfunction. *J. Urol.* 122:361, 1977.
89. Siroky, M. B., Sax, D. S., and Krane, R. J.: Sacral signal tracing: the electrophysiology of the bulbocavernosus reflex. *J. Urol.* 122:661, 1979.
90. Sundin, T., and Petersen, I.: Cystometry and simultaneous electromyography from the striated urethral and anal sphincters and from levator ani. *Invest. Urol.* 13:40, 1975.
91. Butler, W. J.: Pseudomyotonia of the periurethral striated muscle in women with stress urinary incontinence. *J. Urol.* 122:838–840, 1979.
92. Dyro, F. M., Bauer, S. B., Hallett, M., and Koshbin, S.: Complex repetitive discharges in the external urethral sphincter in a pediatric population. *Neurourol. Urodyn.* 2:39, 1983.
93. Guld, C., Rosenfalck, A., and Willsion, R. G.: Report of the Committee on EMG Instrumentation, technical factors in recording electrical activity of muscle and nerve in man. *Electroencephalogr. Clin. Neurophysiol.* 28:399, 1970.
94. Anderson, R. S.: Increased motor unit fibre density in the external anal sphincter in genuine stress incontinence: a single fibre EMG study. *Neurourol. Urodyn.* 2:45, 1983.
95. Neill, M. E., and Swash, M.: Increased motor unit fiber density in the external anal sphincter in anorectal incontinence: a single fibre EMG study. *J. Neurol. Neurosurg. Psychiat-* 43:343, 1980.
96. Blaivas, J. G., Sinha, H. P., Zayed, A. A. H., and Labib, K.: Detrusor-external sphincter dyssynergia: a detailed EMG study. *J. Urol.* 545, 1981.
97. Blaivas, J. G., and Fisher, D. M.: Combined radiographic and urodynamic monitoring: advances in technique. *J. Urol.* 125:693, 1981.
98. Blaivas, J. G., Zayed, A. A. H., and Labib, K. B.: The bulbocavernosus reflex in urology: a prospective study of 299 patients. *J. Urol.* 126:197, 1981.
99. McGuire, E. J., and Brady, S.: Detrusor–sphincter dyssynergia *J. Urol.* 121:774, 1979.
100. Siroky, M. D., and Krane, R. J.: Neurologic aspects of detrusor–sphincter dyssynergia with references to the guarding reflex. *J. Urol.* 127:953, 1982.
101. Yalla, S. V., and Gittes, R. F.: Detrusor–urethral sphincter dyssynergia. *J. Urol.* 118:1026, 1977.
102. Kaplan, W. E., Firlit, C. F., and Schoenberg, H. W.: Female urethral syndrome: external sphincter spasm as etiology. *J. Urol.* 124:48, 1980.
103. Raz, S., and Smith, R. B.: External sphincter spasticity syndrome in female patients. *J. Urol.* 115:443, 1976.
104. Firlit, C. F., and Cook, W. A.: Voiding pattern abnormalities in children. *Urology* 10:25, 1977.
105. Maizels, M., King, L. R., and Firlit, C. F.: Urodynamic biofeedback: a new approach to treatment of vesical sphincter dyssynergia. *J. Urol.* 122:205, 1979.
106. Andersen, J. T., and Bradley, W. E.: Cystometric, sphincter and electromyelographic abnormalities in Parkinson's disease. *J. Urol.* 116:75, 1976.
107. Blaivas, J. G., O'Donnell, T. F., Gottleib, P., and Labib, K. G.: Measurment of bulbocavernosus reflex latency time as part of a comprehensive evaluation of impotence. In Zorgniotti, A. W., and Rossi, O. (eds.), *Vasculogenic Impotence.* Charles C Thomas, Springfield, IL, 1980.
108. Nordling, J., Andersen, J., Walter, H., et al.: Evoked response of the bulbocavernosus reflex. *Eur. Urol.* 5:36, 1979.
109. Ertekin, C., and Reel, F.: Bulbocavernosus reflex in normal men and in patients with neurogenic bladder and/or impotence. *J. Neurol. Sci.* 28:1, 1976.
110. Chantraine, A., de Leval, J., and Onkelinx, A.: Motor conduction velocity in the internal pudendal nerves. In Desmedt, J. E. (ed.), *New Developments in Electromyography and Clinical Neurophysiology,* Vol. 2. Karger, Basel, 1973, pp. 434–438
111. Bradley, W. E.: Urethral electromyelography. *J. Urol.* 108:563, 1972.
112. Bates, P., Bradley, W. E., Glen, E., Griffiths, D., Melchior, H., Rowan, D., Sterling, A., Zinner, N.,

and Hald, T.: The standardization of terminology of lower urinary tract function. *J. Urol.* 121:551, 1979.
113. Colstrup, H., Mortensen, S. O., and Kristensen, J. K.: A new method for the investigation of the closure function of the resting female urethra. *J. Urol.* 130:507, 1983.
114. Bors, E., and Comarr, A. E.: *Neurologic Urology.* University Park Press, Baltimore, 1971, p. 148.
115. Simons, I.: Studies on bladder function: the sphincterometer. *J. Urol.* 35:96,1936.
116. Hodgkinson, C.P.: Direct urethrocystometry. *Am. J. Obstet. Gynecol.* 79:664, 1960.
117. Enhörning, G.: Simultaneous recording of intravesical and intraurethral pressure. *Acta Chir. Scand.* [*Suppl*]. 276:1, 1961.
118. Donker, P. J., Ivanovici, F., and Noach, E. L.: Analysis of the urethral pressure profile by means of electromyography and administration of drugs. *Br. J. Urol.* 44:180, 1972.
119. Lapides, J., Ajemian, E. P., Stewart, B. H., Breskey, B. A., and Lichtwart, J. R.: Further observations on the kinetics of the urethrovesical sphincter. *J. Urol.* 84:86, 1960.
120. Tanagho, E. A., Miller, E. R., Myers, E. H., and Corbett, R. K.: Observations on the dynamics of the bladder neck. *Br. J. Urol.* 38:72, 1966.
121. Tanagho, E. A., Myers, E. H., and Smith, D. R.: Urethral resistance, its components and implications. 1. Smooth muscle components. *Invest. Urol.* 7:136, 1969.
122. Brown, M., and Wickham, J. E. A.: The urethral pressure profile. *Br. J. Urol.* 41:211, 1969.
123. Harrison, N. W., and Constable, A. R.: Urethral pressure measurement: a modified technique. *Br. J. Urol.* 42:229,1970.
124. Gleason, D. M., Reilly, R. J., Bottaccini, M. R., and Pierce, M. J.: The urethral continence zone and its relation to stress incontinence. *J. Urol.* 112:81, 1974.
125. Bradley, W. E., Scott, F. B., and Timm, G. W.: Sphincter electromyography. *Urol. Clin. North Am.* 1:69, 1974.
126. Robertson, J. R.: Gas cystometrogram with urethral pressure profile. *Obstet. Gynecol.* 44:72,1974.
127. Raz, S., and Kaufman, J. J.: Carbon dioxide urethral pressure profile. *J. Urol.* 115:439, 1976.
128. Edwards, L., and Malvern, J.: The urethral pressure profile: theoretical consideration and clinical applications. *Br. J. Urol.* 46:325, 1974.
129. Harrison, N. W.: The urethral pressure profile. *Urol. Res.* 4:95, 1976.
130. Brown, M.: In-vivo determination of error in the measurement of urethral pressure by the method of Brown and Wickham. *Br. J. Urol.* 47:445, 1975.
131. Abrams, P. H., Martin, S., and Griffiths, D. J.: The measurement and interpretation of urethral pressures obtained by the method of Brown and Wickham, *Br. J. Urol.* 50:33, 1983.
132. Anderson, R. S., Shepherd, A. M., and Feneley, R. C. L.: Microtip transducer urethral profile methodology: variations caused by transducer orientation. *J. Urol.* 130:727, 1983.
133. Van Geelen, J. M.: *The Urethral Pressure Profile in Continent Women.* Thesis. Schriks' Drukkerij, Asten, 1983.
134. Henriksson, L., Anderson, K. E., and Ulmsten, U.: The urethral pressure profiles in continent and stress incontinent women. *Scand. J. Urol. Nephrol.* 13:5, 1979.
135. Obrink, A., Bunne, G., and Ulmsten, U.: Intraurethral and intravesical pressures in continent women. *Acta Obstet. Gynecal. Scand.* 56:525, 1977.
136. Rud, T.: Urethral pressure profile in continent women from childhood to old age. *Acta Obstet. Gynecol. Scand.* 59:331, 1980.
137. Plante, P., and Susset, J.: Studies of female urethral pressure profile. I. The normal urethral pressure profile. *J. Urol.* 123:64, 1980.
138. Toguri, A. G., Bee, D. E.., and Bunce, H.: Variability of water urethral closure pressure profiles. *J. Urol.* 124:407, 1980.
139. Wein, A. J., Malloy, T. R., Hanno, P. M., and Raezer, D. M.: The reproducibility and signficance of carbon dioxide urethral profilometry. *J. Urol.* 122:651, 1979.
140. Blaivas, J. G.: Classification of stress urinary incontinence, *Neurourol. Urodyn.* 2:103, 1983.
141. Bates, C. P., and Corney, L. E.: Synchronous cine/pressure/flow cystography: a method of routine urodynamic investigation. *Br. J. Radiol.* 44:44, 1971.
142. Blaivas, J. G., Sinha, H. P., Zayed, A. A. H., and Labib, K. B.: Detrusor-external sphincter dyssynergia. *J. Urol.* 125:542, 1981.
143. McGuire, E. J.: Combined radiographic and manometric assessment of urethral sphincter function. *J. Urol.* 118:632, 1977.
144. Miller, E. R.: Combined monitoring for the study of continence and voiding. In Hinman, F. J., Jr. (ed.), *Hydrodynamics of Micturition.* Charles C Thomas, Springfield, IL, 1971, pp. 5-17.
145. Yalla, S. V., Rossier, A. B., and Fam, B.: Synchronous cystosphincterometry in patients with spinal cord injury. *Urology* 6:777, 1975.
146. Yalla, S. V., Sharma, G. V. R. K., and Barsamian, E. M.: Micturitional urethral pressure profile during voiding and the implications. *J. Urol.* 124:649, 1980.
147. Blaivas, J. G., and Salinas, J.: Type III stress urinary incontinence: the importance of proper diagnosis and treatment. *Surg. Forum,* 35:473, 1984.
148. McGuire, E. M.: Urodynamic findings in patients after failure of stress incontinence operations, In Zinner, N. R., and Sterling, A. M. (eds.), *Female Incontinence.* Alan R. Liss, New York, 1980.
149. McGuire, E. J., Woodside, J. R., Borden, T. A., and Weiss, R. M.: Prognostic value of urodynamic testing in myelodysplastic patients. *J. Urol.* 124:205, 1981.

Clinical Evaluation of Outlet Obstruction 11

SUBBARAO V. YALLA, M.D.

How strong or weak is your urinary stream? How often do you urinate? Do you empty your bladder completely? How long does it take you to initiate urination? Do you have to rush to urinate? Do you dribble at the end of urination? These and many other questions related to a patient's ability to urinate are usually asked during the clinical assessment of bladder outlet obstruction. A probing history of the patient's voiding habits and characteristics of his urination as well as a thorough physical and neurologic examination often yield useful information. On many occasions, however, the patient's history is inadequate, ambiguous, or unreliable. Objective clinical assessment is therefore critical for identifying the factors responsible for poor urination by any patient and for confirming the site and degree of any outlet obstruction that is present before therapy can be contemplated or recommended.

The traditional methods of urologic assessment of patients with urinary obstruction are radiologic and cystourethroscopic evaluations. Most bladder outlet problems can be recognized by these time-honored methods of examination, and therefore many experienced urologists are not convinced that urodynamic assessment is necessary unless a rare complex disorder associated with a neurologic problem is involved. Urodynamic studies may also be needed in situations in which failure of management has occurred and further therapy becomes a dilemma and requires a rational approach. Under these conditions, detailed urodynamic studies may be useful for guiding the urologist when planning judicious therapy and follow-up of the patient. The information obtained may also help to explain the problem to the patient in a rational and logical manner. It is for these reasons and to gain a better understanding of the pathophysiology of outlet obstruction that urodynamic and neurourologic evaluations have been recommended for its clinical evaluation. To develop a standardized nomenclature, previously ambiguous urodynamic terms are being redefined. Furthermore, attempts are being made to understand what precisely constitutes outlet obstruction in a particular age group and what testing methods are sufficiently sensitive to recognize not only the location but also the degree of obstruction. Several refined and innovative urodynamic methods are being introduced and evaluated for their merits and limitations; most, however, are invasive and have associated technical artifacts. Therefore efforts are being made to simplify and develop noninvasive urodynamic methods of clinical investigation of the obstructed patient. Despite current limitations of urodynamic techniques, their appropriate application with clinically oriented analysis may indeed lead to a better understanding of patient's problems and ultimately to their rational management.

Urodynamic testing techniques can be categorized as relatively simple, and complex electrourodynamic procedures. Hinman (*1*) held the view that several voiding problems can be studied successfully with simple urodynamic testing techniques such as obtaining a detailed history of voiding habits, stopwatch determination of urinary flow rate, measurement of residual urine volume, voiding cystourethrography, conventional cystometry, and neurologic evaluation. He believed that detailed electrourodynamic testing should be restricted to clinical problems that cannot be solved by standard clinical urodynamic tests and to medical centers that have the time and expertise to conduct them and thereby provide reliable answers. We, however, stress the necessity for early and accurate diagnosis by whatever means is available to properly manage the patient with suspected outlet obstruction.

Vesical outlet obstruction usually leads to variable degrees of change in the urinary stream as well as detrusor contractility. When left untreated, outlet obstruction can culminate in large residual urine volumes, chronic urinary retention, upper urinary tract stasis, urinary infection, and renal failure. Although the stage at which treatment of asymptomatic patients is required is not yet known precisely, we believe that urologists must diagnose and treat gross vesical outlet obstructions in order to prevent their deleterious consequences.

Most outlet obstructions can be recognized early by characteristics of the urinary stream and detrusor contractility. Objective assessment of outlet function includes recording urinary flow rates (uroflowmetry), recording intravesical pressures during filling and voiding (micturitional cystometry), and radiographically assessing changes in the configuration of the bladder and its outlet during voiding (*2,3*). Several workers add electromyography (EMG) of the periurethral musculature, perineal muscles, abdominal wall, or anal musculature (*4,5*) for assessing outlet function. The goal of any clinical method(s) of study is to accurately assess the voiding act and analyze the factor(s) responsible for any voiding dysfunction. Often more than one factor that mimics or complicates outlet obstruction is involved.

Nonneurogenic bladder outlet obstruction is rarely seen in women. In men, however, it is common in all age groups. Congenital valves, bladder neck obstruction, urethral strictures, and prostatic enlargement are known to cause bladder outlet obstruction. Neurogenic disorders also can produce outlet obstruction in both sexes and in all age groups. In this chapter, the advantages and disadvantages of each urodynamic testing technique are outlined, and my preferred methods of clinical evaluation of vesical outlet are presented in detail.

VOIDING CYSTOURETHROGRAPHY

Radiologic evaluation of the bladder and its outlet can provide useful information on their anatomic disposition and functional characteristics.The investigator can recognize the onset of a bladder contraction by carefully watching the bladder fill with radiocontrast solution. During such examination, cystometry to record intravesical pressure can be performed simultaneously. Additional fluoroscopy can provide details of the nature of bladder contraction, bladder base descent, vesicourethral funneling, urethral compliance, and the status of bulbous urethral filling. In the hands of an experienced urodynamicist, fluoroscopic study using videotaping alone may furnish adequate details of functional anatomy of the system, and further studies may not be required. When uroflowmetry and surface EMG of perineal muscles are combined with voiding cystourethrography, the value of clinical outlet assessment is greatly enhanced. It should be remembered, however, that the correct interpretation of functional aspects of any voiding cystourethrogram or urodynamic test depends on the experience of the interpreter.

In young male subjects with normal urinnary flow rates, the bladder contour is smooth and symmetrical with no evidence of thickening or trabeculation. The horizontal base of the resting bladder is usually above the upper border of the symphysis pubis. During voiding the bladder base descends into the pelvis and acquires a semilunar shape; the base merges smoothly into the well-funneled bladder neck, which together with the prostatic urethra appears well opacified. The narrow membranous urethra also shows caudal descent, and the adjacent bulbous urethra is well filled and distended (Fig. 11–1). With an obstructed outlet, the transition between the bladder base and the bladder neck is not smooth and gradual (Fig. 11–2). The bladder neck entrance may be the square or the reentrant type; it may open after undue delay; it may be stenotic with poor opacification of the posterior urethra; and some-

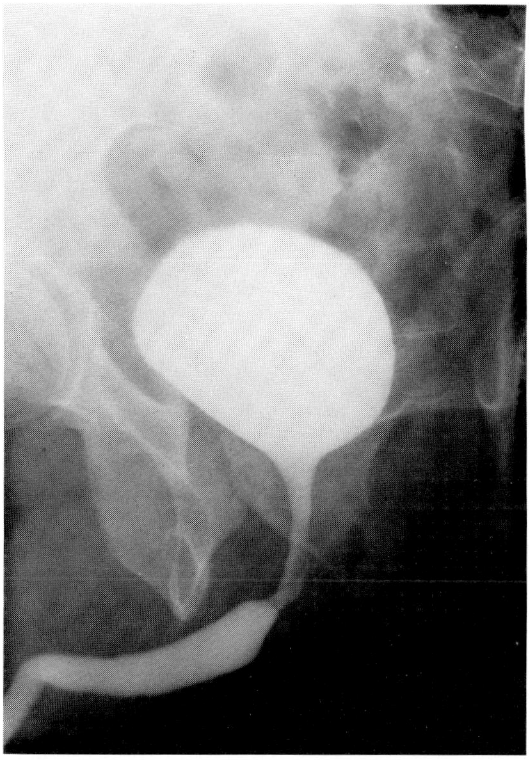

Figure 11–1. Normal voiding cystourethrogram showing a bladder of smooth contour, a well-funneled bladder neck, and a well-distended bulbous urethra. (From Yalla, S. V., *et al.*: *J. Urol.* 124:649, 1980. Copyright © 1980, The Williams & Wilkins Co., Baltimore.)

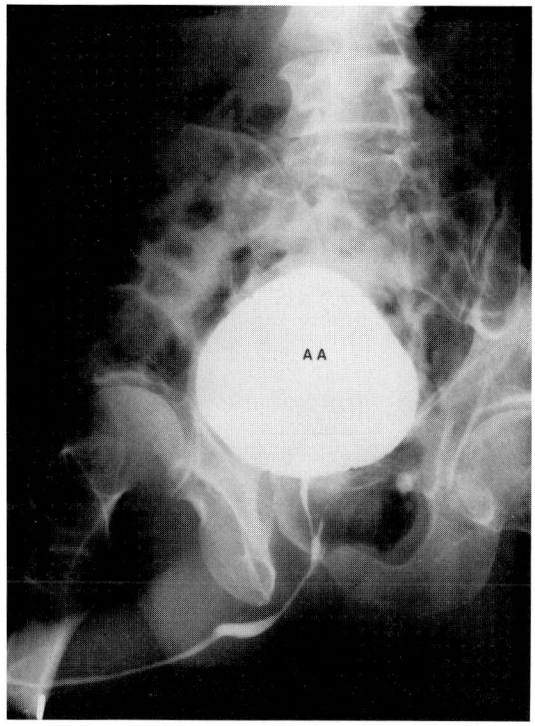

Figure 11–2. Patient with prostatic obstruction, a narrow, irregular prostatic urethra, and poor filling of the bulb; peak flow rates were 6 to 8 ml/s. (From Yalla, S. V., and Resnick, N. M.: *World J. Urol.* 2:196, 1984.)

times it is concealed by the lower segment of the bladder. For adequate visualization of the bladder neck region, radiographic exposures with the patient in the head-down (Trendelenburg) position or cephalad projections are recommended (Figs. 11–3 and 11–4). With posterior urethral obstructions, the bulbous urethra may not be filled in its proximal portion, creating the erroneous impression of a long, membranous urethra. After relief of proximal obstruction, the posterior urethra appears distended and well opacified (Figs. 11–5 and 11–6); the entire proximal portion of the bulbous urethra is filled and distended, and the membranous urethra appears shorter. With distal urethral obstructions, the proximal urethral region appears overdistended and sometimes masks a posterior urethral obstruction. Our recent urodynamic and radiologic studies in both male patients and canines suggested that a phenomenon called "Elastic Jump" may occur downstream of the membranous urethra, especially when associated with bladder neck or prostatic obstruction. Its appearance and location, however, seem to vary with obstruction or constrictions in both upstream and downstream of the narrow membranous urethra (*5a*). Further studies are certainly needed to understand this phenomenon of elastic jump.

UROFLOWMETRY

The final result of the summated events of micturition is urinary flow. Historically, the urologist has attempted to estimate urinary flow characteristics by either observing the urinary stream or obtaining details from the patient's own assessment of cast distance and force of the stream.

Urinary flow rate is expressed in millilters per second. The introduction of objective

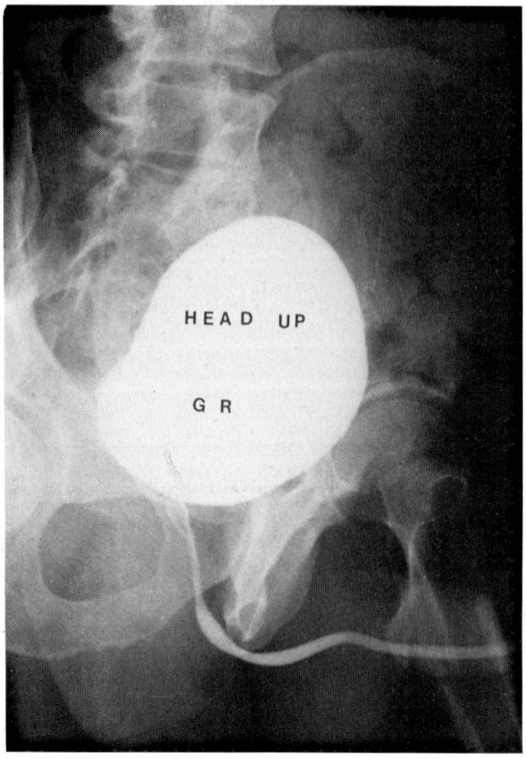

Figure 11–3. Forty-year-old man with bladder neck obstruction (x-ray film obtained in the oblique position). Note concealment of the bladder neck region by the bladder base; the filling defect represents verumontanum.

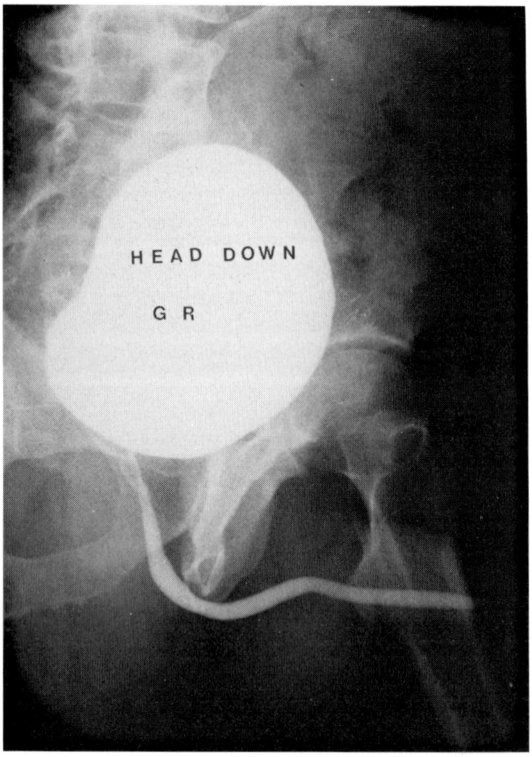

Figure 11–4. The patient voided in a head-down position, thereby showing the region of the narrow bladder neck; note better filling of the bulb and membranous urethra as the patient voided against gravity. (From Yalla, S. V., and Resnick, N. M.: *World J. Urol.* 2:196, 1984.)

techniques has allowed detailed analysis of the entire process of flow during an act of urination, including delay time, maximum flow rate, average flow rate, flow time, voiding time and volume, flow curve pattern, and exit force of the stream (*2,6*). Study of urinary flow is noninvasive and can be used as an initial screening procedure before any detailed urodynamic studies are undertaken. It is essential to have the patient's cooperation, and with privacy voiding acts representative of the patient's habitual patterns can be obtained.

Several commercial uroflowmeters that record urinary flow curves on paper charts are available. Some automatically record the volume voided, peak flow rate, average flow rate, and flow time. The patient is given privacy and advised to void in his usual manner, directing the stream at the bottom of the funnel, which leads to the flowmeter. At the end of voiding the patient is interrogated to determine if that voiding represented his usual voiding process, if he had to strain during voiding, and if he voluntarily or involuntarily interrupted the act. Repeat uroflowmetry is conducted whenever abnormal voiding patterns are noted. If the flow curves appear to be abnormal, further evaluation is recommended.

FLOW PATTERNS

Flow is initiated within 5 to 10 seconds after efforts to commence urination have begun. Delay of initiation usually results from nonrelaxation of urethral sphincters or from delay of the onset of detrusor contraction; it may also occur in patients with a hypoactive detrusor associated with delay of complete urethral sphincter relaxation.

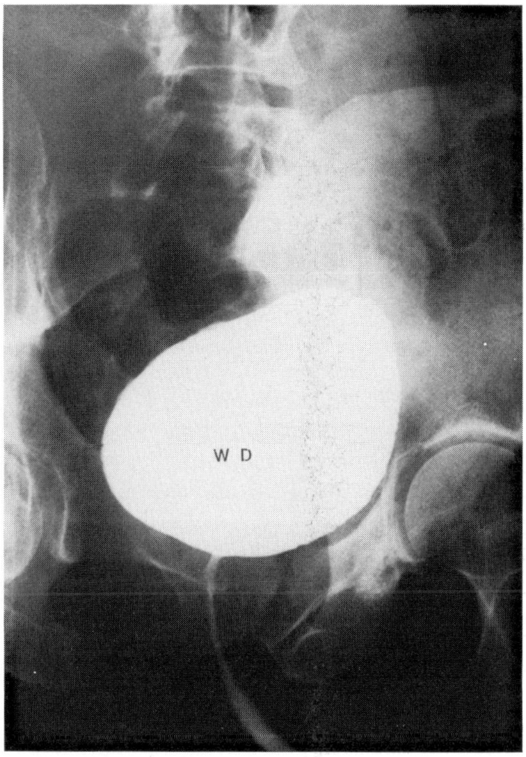

Figure 11–5. Prostatic obstruction with an inadequately filled bulbous urethra.

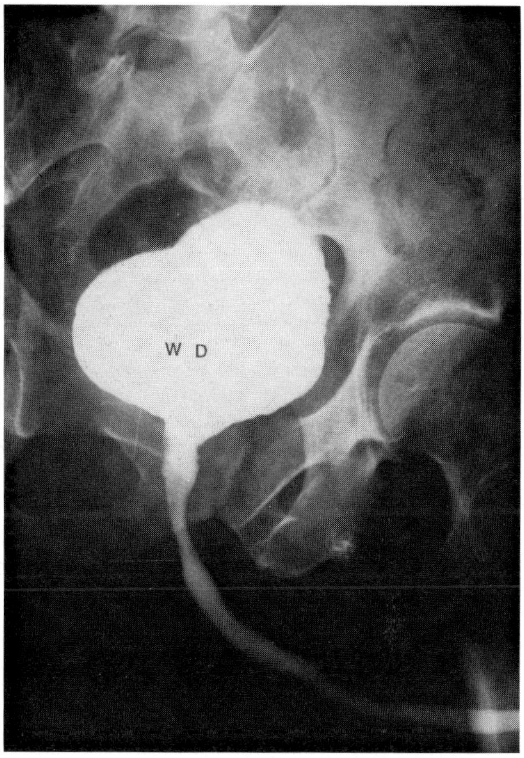

Figure 11–6. After transurethral resection (TUR) of the prostate, the bulb was better filled and well opacified.

Urinary flow rate depends on age, sex, and the volume voided, and can be expressed as either the maximum or average rate. Several nomograms have been devised to help interpret the flow rate values. Usually a flow rate exceeding 15 ml/s in men indicates normal lower urinary tract function. Normal (Fig. 11–7) or high flow rates may also be seen in outlet obstructions associated with high voiding pressures. Flow rates of less than 10 ml/s are suggestive of outlet obstruction. Such low flow rates may also be seen in conditions with a hypoactive detrusor. In conditions of intermittent flow, the actual flow time is less than the voiding time; intervals of voiding interruptions are not included in calculation of the flow time. Finally, it is important to study the flow curve pattern, as it gives more valuable information on outlet obstruction than some

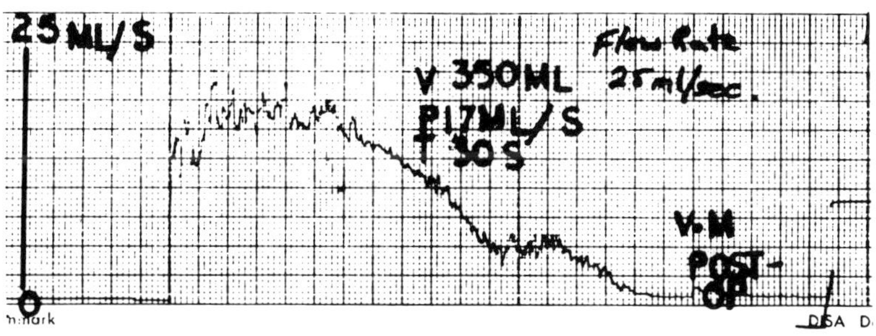

Figure 11–7. Uroflow curve showing an unobstructed pattern.

numerical values gathered from the flow curve.

Although the results of a urinary flow study may unmask an outlet obstruction, one cannot be certain whether they are attributed to detrusor hypoactivity, the obstruction, or both. Such results also cannot determine either the site or the degree of an obstruction. To accurately assess the latter, further studies combining uroflowmetry with radiologic evaluation and intravesical pressure measurements may be done.

FLOW AND VELOCITY DETERMINATIONS

Gleason and associates have studied "flow and velocity" properties of the urinary stream and concluded that combined measurements of the flow rate and exit-stream velocity could be used to distinguish clearly normal and obstructed subjects from those with a critical overlap (*6*). These authors compared patients with prostatism to normal subjects by instructing all to void against a light paddlewheel connected to a small generator; they then calculated the velocity of the urinary stream from the rotation velocity of that wheel; the peak flow rate was recorded simultaneously using a flowmeter. These authors believed that mere flow rate determination is not enough to distinguish a normal subject from a mildly obstructed patient; they suggested that flow rates of 12 to 18 ml/s can be indicative of obstruction if corresponding velocities stay lower than 100 cm/s, and that normalcy is indicated if the latter are higher than 200 cm/s.

We believe that the above observations and further studies of the same authors on the interrelations of stream velocity and other parameters such as voided volume and age are important contributions toward understanding the urodynamics of outlet obstruction. Such studies are not invasive and can easily be applied clinically.

SYNCHRONOUS PRESSURE/FLOW STUDIES

Synchronous pressure–flow voiding studies are designed to estimate bladder outlet resistance (*7*). By combining EMG of the perineal, anal, or periurethral muscles with radiographic monitoring, the accuracy of pressure–flow (P/F) tests is enhanced. It has been suggested that mathematic calculation of outlet resistance (P/F^2 or P/F) may help to accurately diagnose outlet obstruction; however, caution against using such mathematic formulas has been expressed (*8*). Nevertheless, pressure–flow studies are helpful in the diagnosis of more than two-thirds of cases of obstruction by monitoring intravesical voiding pressure, synchronous pressure–flow study, and radiologic study of outlet configuration. The remaining one-third of cases of obstruction are borderline and can be recognized by additional means of evaluation.

The patient is kept in the supine position, and intravesical pressure recordings are obtained by either an intraurethral 4F (ureteral) catheter or a percutaneous suprapubic cannula. The latter is ideal if the patient is cooperative. Intrarectal pressures are monitored through a rectal catheter in order to detect abdominal straining. Rectal pressure changes presumably represent paravesical intraabdominal pressure changes that might occur during a Valsalva maneuver or cough efforts. If additional monitoring of periurethral EMG is required, a transperineal, coaxial needle electrode is inserted under audiovisual control.

After obtaining residual urine, dilute radiocontrast solution is instilled into the bladder at a known rate. Cystometry is then performed, noting the following features: resting bladder pressure, proprioception, volume at which first desire to void occurs, cystometric bladder capacity, vesical compliance, ability to initiate and suppress detrusor contraction, and detrusor hyper- or hypoactivity. When voiding commences, simultaneous urinary flow rates are registered. In some urodynamic centers the entire study is videomonitored, superimposing pressure tracings on the radiographic images. A high detrusor pressure with a low flow rate indicates an obstruction. High voiding pressures with normal or high flow rates can also be observed in some obstructions. On the other hand, low pressure–low flow rate conditions may or may not be suggestive of outlet obstruction. In situations of ambiguity, static or total urethral pressure profile measurements (during voiding) may be helpful in defining the site of obstruction.

STATIC URETHRAL PRESSURE MEASUREMENTS DURING VOIDING

Several workers in the past have recognized that pressure, flow rate, fluid velocity, and diameter of the tube are interdependent (*8–10*). In the lower urinary tract the bladder pressure represents the total energy that is directed toward the transport system, i.e., the outlet. It has been postulated that the energy generated by the detrusor is dissipated within the urethra as the urine is expelled through the meatus. The frictional losses depend on the dynamic and static geometry of the outlet, as well as the fluid velocity. To recognize the sites of frictional losses of energy, techniques have been devised to measure pressures within the urethra by means of end-hole and side-hole catheters (*11,12*). The end-hole catheter (*13*), or end-on microtransducer (*12*), measures the total pressure, which is considered to be a measurement related to the velocity. It is also viewed as the sum of dynamic and static components of the pressure in the fluid system. The catheter with the side hole or lateral microtransducer measures the static pressure in the fluid system, which is less than the total pressure (or end-pressure) by an amount presumed to be equivalent to the kinetic energy of the flow. The static pressure therefore has an inverse relation with the velocity of the fluid.

Experiments designed by other workers to study the characteristics of dynamic and flexible models resembling the urethra have shown that some minor gradients were caused by acceleration and friction, which were flow rate-dependent (*12*). When an external pressure was applied on this model, the static pressure profile showed a gradient: a sudden fall of static pressure at the downstream side of the compression. It was suggested from these experiments that the static pressure profile measurement during flow could be a satisfactory method of direct measurement of extrinsic pressures. Zinner and colleagues applied these physical principles to clinical conditions and diagnosed minute degrees of outlet obstruction by measuring total urethral pressure along the length of the urethra with a small end-hole catheter (*11*). Similarly, Cass and Hinman studied static pressures in the female canine urethra that was subjected to vesical neck and meatal contrictions under varying flow rate (*14*). Constriction of the vesical neck of more than one-half of its cross-sectional area could produce a pronounced drop of static pressure across the constricted bladder neck even at low flow rates. Such a significant pressure drop was not seen when the vesical neck was constricted to only one-third of its cross-sectional area under low flow rate conditions. With higher flow rates, the pressure drop occurred at the site where the bladder neck was moderately constricted. Meatal constriction in these dogs produced an increase in the static pressure in the proximal urethral segments. Also, it has been shown that the intraluminal pressure-sensing probe (7F) could itself induce some degree of energy loss in a channel of 0.45 to 0.71 cm internal diameter (*15*). The aforementioned experiments indicate to us that these techniques of pressure measurement could be useful in clinical studies. Whe have realized, however, that they could be artifactual; recognition of such artifacts is important in clinical evaluations.

We have studied static pressure configurations of the urethra in male patients with proved outlet obstruction (*16–19*). We recognized that a significant drop in static pressure occurs at the site of an obstruction (Figs. 11–8 to 11–12). This drop occurs only when there is a detrusor contraction (there is some amount of urinary flow along the intraluminal catheter); a drop of pressure at the site of obstruction is not usually seen if an appreciable urinary stream is not expelled around the catheter. Moreover, proximal obstruction may be masked if the subject has significant additional obstruction distally. Factors such as detrusor contraction, concomitant urinary flow rate, and distal contrictions must always be considered in the interpretation of recordings of the static urethral pressure profiles.

Ideally, one should use end-hole catheters for precise estimation of energy losses (or frictional loss) at various regions of a conduit such as the bladder outlet. Evaluations with end-hole catheters, however, require synchronous suprapubic vesical pressure monitoring for proper interpretation. On the other hand, this additonal invasive procedure is not required in studies performed with urethral catheters that record intravesical and urethral static pressures simultaneously. For that purpose we use a 10F trilumen

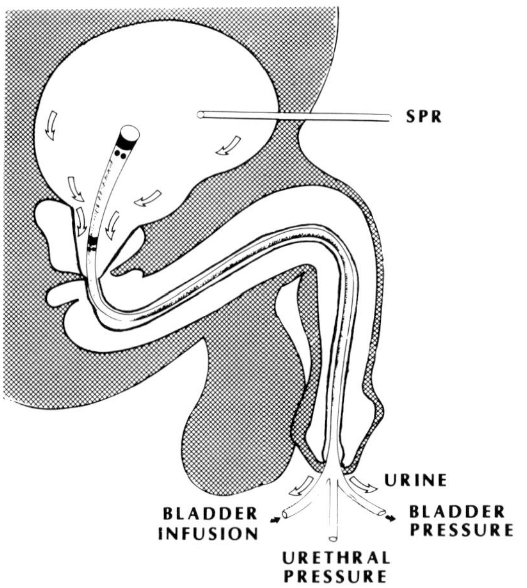

Figure 11–8. Voiding pressure profile recording. A 10F trilumen catheter was used to record vesical and urethral static (lateral) pressures simultaneously. SPR = Suprapubic route (From Yalla, S. V., *et al.*: *J. Urol.* 124:649, 1980. Copyright © 1980. The Williams & Wilkins Co., Baltimore.)

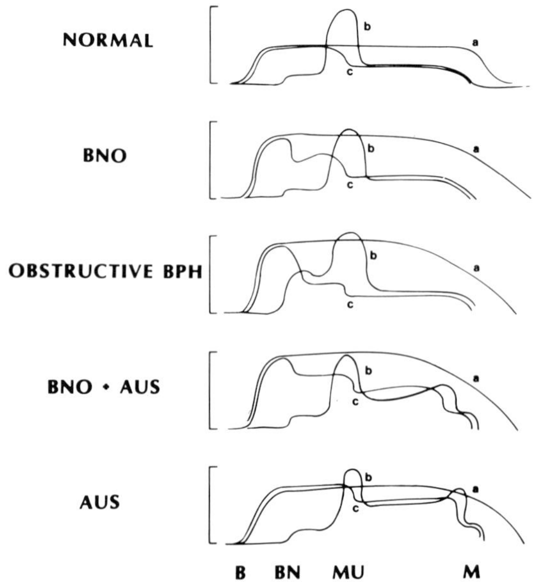

Figure 11–10. Normal and abnormal configurations of UCPP, voiding (static) pressure profiles, and detrusor contraction pressures. *a* = detrusor contraction pressure. *b* = UCPP configuration. *c* = static pressure (during voiding). *b* = bladder. *BN* = bladder neck. *MU* = membranous urethra. *M* = meatus.

catheter that has the capability of bladder filling and simultaneous vesical and urethral pressure recordings. We have also been using catheters with microtip transducers.

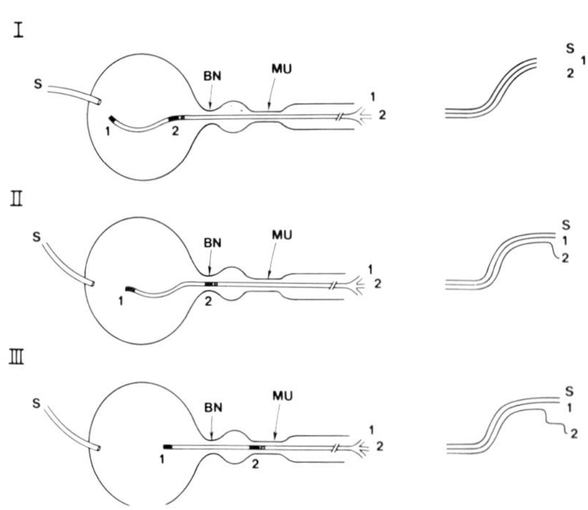

Figure 11–9. Stages of catheter withdrawal and respective pressure configurations during voiding. *S* = suprapubic cannula. *BN* = bladder neck (narrow). *MU* = membranous urethra. Lateral (static) pressure recorded through the two lateral holes (*2*) of the catheter drop at the BN and MU regions. (From Yalla, S. V., and Resnick, N. M.: *World J. Urol.* 2:196, 1984.

Our comparative studies performed with end-hole and side-hole catheters have shown almost identical clinical urodynamic information (Fig. 11–13). Therefore we seldom use end-hole urethral catheters or percutaneous suprapubic vesical pressure monitoring in our urodynamic evaluation of outlet obstruction.

ENDOURODYNAMIC EVALUATION

By combining endoscopic study with pressure recordings, outlet assessment can be carried out by adding visual impressions. We have evaluated this combined technique using a 10F to 11F Olympus fiberoptic scope. The terminal irrigating channel has been found to be ideal for measuring total urethral pressure during the voiding phase. Another advantage is that with the tiny flexible scope patients can stand up and void while endoscopic visualization and simultaneous intraurethral pressure monitoring are being carried out (*20*).

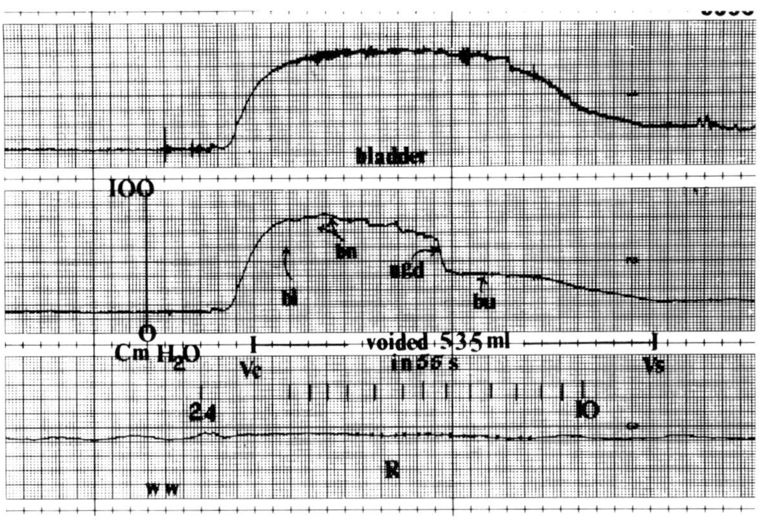

Figure 11–11. W.W., 62-year-old man with an almost normal static pressure profile configuration; a small (10 cm) pressure drop occurred along the bladder neck (bn) and prostatic urethra; a major pressure drop of 25 cm occurred in the region of the urogenital diaphragm (ugd). (From Hinman, F., Jr. [ed.]: *Benign Prostatic Hypertrophy*. Springer-Verlag, New York, 1983.)

URODYNAMIC TECHNIQUE

At our medical center the patient is first asked to void in a uroflowmeter in their usual manner. The residual urine is measured, and the patient is then subjected to a pressure-monitored voiding cystourethrogram (radiology monitored cystometry). The entire voiding process is thereby observed fluoroscopically. This part of the examination furnishes preliminary information on cystometry, the nature of detrusor reflex activity, the geometry of the bladder and its outlet, and the residual urine. Further detailed

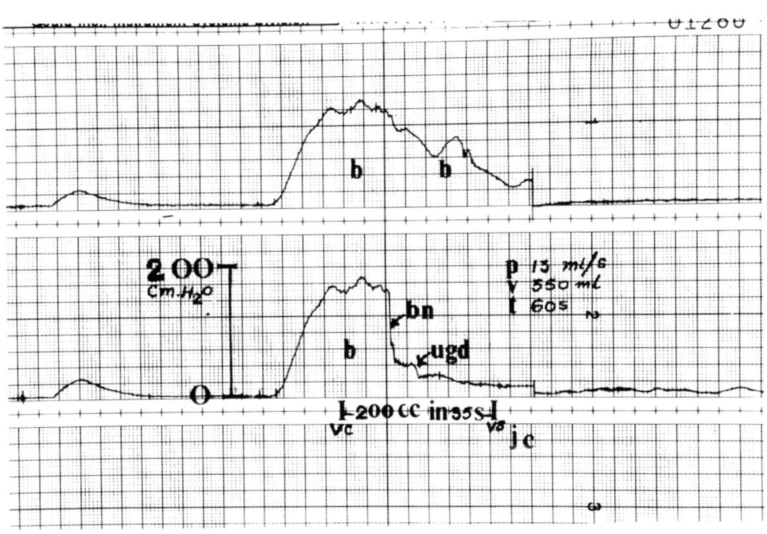

Figure 11–12. A 42-year-old man with bladder neck obstruction has markedly elevated detrusor contraction pressure (180 cm) and a precipitous pressure drop of 110 cm across the bladder neck (*bn*) region. *ugd* = region of the urogenital diaphragm. *b* = bladder. *VC* = voiding commenced. *vs* = voiding stopped.

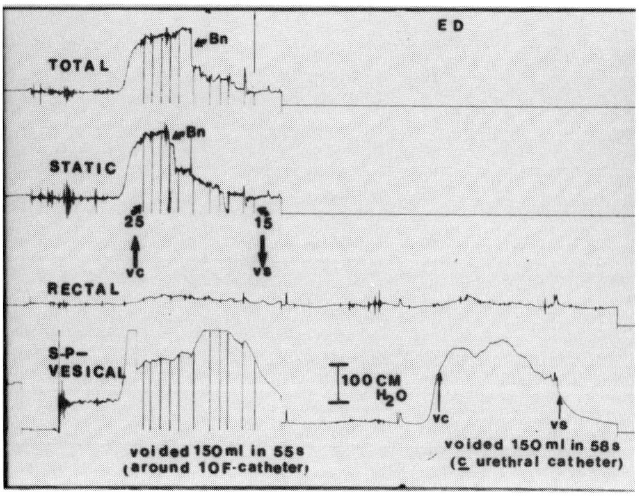

Figure 11–13. Simultaneous recording of total (end) and static (lateral) pressures in the urethra. Note the pressure drop across the bladder neck region in both recordings. Vesical pressure was recorded simultaneously through a separate cannula via the suprapubic route. In the lowermost tracings on the right, note the bladder pressure configuration and its high pressure without a catheter in the urethra.

urodynamic examination is undertaken only if the uroflowmetry and the pressure-monitored cystourethrography reveal abnormalities that require further amplification. In our current practice patients with normal uroflowmetry and normal pressure-monitored voiding cystourethrography are seldom subjected to routine micturitional vesicourethral pressure profile studies.

All studies are performed with fluoroscopic guidance. Videotaping and 100-mm spot films are used whenever necessary, and the entire study is performed in the supine position. The standing position is used only when the patient cannot void in the supine position. A rectal catheter (fluid-filled catheter with attached fingercot of a rubber glove) is inserted into the rectum to record rectal pressure changes (which reflect paravesical intraabdominal pressure changes). In several subjects we have seen spontaneous rectal pressure activity representing local activity rather than changes due to the Valsalva maneuver. Blind electronic subtraction can therefore lead to inaccurate analyses. In selected patients anal pressures are obtained as well. Xylocaine jelly is instilled into the urethra prior to introduction of an intraurethral pressure-sensing catheter, as the jelly minimizes the urethral discomfort that may occur with repeated catheter movements. Our observations in earlier studies have suggested that such instillation does not compromise the clinical value of the urodynamic study; no significant changes in the urethral closure or micturitional pressure profiles result from xyocaine instillation.

A 10F trilumen catheter designed to record intravesical and lateral urethral pressures simultaneously is used in the study; a smaller catheter would be ideal. The tip of the catheter and the site of the side hole (10 or 15 cm away from the catheter tip) are radiopaque so that their exact locations in the bladder and its outlet can be identified radiologically during the study. Dilute radiocontrast solution is used for bladder filling, and the bladder is filled until the subject experiences a desire to void. Under resting conditions and before the patient develops a desire to void, a urethral closure pressure profile (UCPP) is usually obtained using slow infusion through the catheter channel that leads to the two lateral holes. During this procedure the withdrawal of the catheter is observed fluoroscopically so as to recognize the anatomic and functional landmarks of the bladder outlet in relation to the graduation marks of the trilumen catheter. We also occasionally use a microtip transducer catheter for simultaneous recording of vesical and urethral pressures. Several microtransducers can be fixed in the catheter to record pressures at multiple sites in the urethra. By carefully designing such type of catheter, one can simultaneously record various regions of bladder outlet during an entire micturition cycle without moving the catheter.

The first rise in pressure in the UCPP

curve represents the beginning of the functional bladder neck. The maximum closure pressure in the pressure profile occurs in the vicinity of the pubic arch, which usually represents the peak pressure zone of the membranous urethra. When the patient develops a strong desire to void, he is instructed to relax his perineal muscles and allow urination to occur (in the supine position) around the 10F intraurethral catheter. The patient is also instructed not to apply any Valsalva maneuver unless it is a characteristic of the voiding habit. When voiding occurs at a steady rate, the catheter is gently withdrawn, and each centimeter of catheter withdrawal is noted on the strip chart of the recording with an event marker. Thus synchronous measurement of vesical pressure is obtained while pressures in the posterior and bulbous urethra are recorded. Simultaneous radiologic assessment of the posterior urethra during voiding can also be performed. At regions where abnormal pressure drops occur, spot films with a 100-mm camera are taken for further confirmation of their sites. Because of limitations in the design of the trilumen catheter, the vesical pressure cannot be synchronously recorded when the catheter is withdrawn toward the distal part of the anterior urethra. The tip of the catheter usually enters the bladder neck and the prostatic urethra when the lateral pressure recording site of the catheter enters the anterior urethra. A catheter with a different design is recommended to avoid these problems. The segment interposed between the catheter tip and the far site of the lateral hole should be as long as the entire male urethra. The other alternative is to monitor intravesical pressure via the suprapubic route. Several micturitional studies are attempted in each patient after repeated filling of the bladder to find out if pressure configurations during repeated micturitions are reproducible. Some patients are unable to void with the catheter positioned in the urethra. In these subjects suprapubic monitoring of vesical pressure is performed. Under fluoroscopic guidance a synchronous pressure/flow/EMG study may be attempted. In this type of study, surface EMG monitoring is all that is required, as we are attempting to study the behavior of the entire periurethral muscle mass, rather than the precise motor unit activity. Artifacts related to perineal surface EMG can be a problem when patients void with the Valsalva maneuver, and this situation must be taken into consideration when interpreting the study.

In conclusion, the clinical assessment of outlet obstruction can be carried out using several direct and indirect urodynamic techniques. A good understanding of the principles governing all techniques is mandatory for proper interpretation of the information they provide. With the emergence of newer technologies, further clinically relevant urodynamic methods will be introduced. Transrectal ultrasonography of micturition is such an example (*21,22*), and with further refinements in its imaging, it will attain an important role in clinical urodynamics.

REFERENCES

1. Hinman, F.: Residual urine—measurement and influence on management of obstruction. In Hinman, F. Jr., (ed.), *Benign Prostatic Hypertrophy* Springer-Verlag, New York 1983, pp. 589–596.
2. Siroky, M. B., Olsson, C. A., and Krane, R. J.: The flow rate nomogram. I. Development. *J. Urol.* 122:665, 1979.
3. Bates, C. P., Whiteside, C. G., and Turner Warwick, R.: Synchronous ciné/pressure/flow cystourethrography. *Br. J. Urol.* 42:714, 1970.
4. Webster, G. D., Lockhart, J. L., and Older, R. A.: The evaluation of bladder neck dysfunction. *J. Urol.* 123:196, 1980.
5. McGuire, E. J.: Combined radiographic and manometric assessment of urethral sphincter function. *J. Urol.* 118:632, 1977.

5a. Yalla, S. V., Cravalho, E., Resnick, N., Chiang, R., and Brown, K.: Elastic jump in male urethra during voiding: clinical observations in male subjects and experimental studies in dogs. *J. Urol.* 134:907, 1985.

6. Gleason, D. M., Bottaccini, M. R., Drach, G. W., and Layton, T. N.: Urinary velocity in prostatism. In Hinman, F., Jr. (ed.), *Benign Prostatic Hypertrophy.* Springer-Verlag, New York, 1983, pp. 539:544.
7. Abrams, P. H., and Griffiths, D. J.: The assessment of prostatic obstruction from urodynamic measurements and from residual urine. *Br. J. Urol.* 51:129, 1979.
8. Schäfer, W.: The contribution of the bladder outlet to the relation between pressure and flow rate during micturition. In *Benign Prostatic Hypertrophy*, Hinman, F., Jr. (ed.), Springer-Verlag, New York, 1983, pp. 470–496.
9. Elliott, E. A., and Dawson, S. V.: Fluid velocity greater than wave speed and the transition from supercritical to subcritical flow in elastic tubes. *Med. Biol. Eng. Comput.* 17:192, 1978.
10. Kamm, R. D., and Shapiro, A. H.: Unsteady flow in

a collapsible tube subjected to external pressure or body forces. *J. Fluid Mech.* 95:1, 1979.
11. Zinner, N. R., Ritter, R. C., Arbuckle, L. D., and Paquin, A. J.: Clincial urodynamics. III. Pressure profiles of the female urethra. *Surg. Forum* 14:481, 1963.
12. Scott, J. E. S., Clayton, C. B., Dee, P. M., and Simpson, W.: Dynamic and flexible models of the urethra. In Hinman, F., Jr., (ed.), *Hydrodynamics of Micturition.* Charles C Thomas, Springfield, IL, 1977, pp. 124—132.
13. Yalla, S. V., and Fraser, L.: Total and static pressure measurements in the male lower urinary tract. *Neurourol. Urodyn.* 1:159, 1982.
14. Cass, A. S., and Hinman, F., Jr.: Constant urethral flow in female dog model. In Hinman, F., Jr. (ed.), *Hydrodynamics of micturition.* Charles C Thomas, Springfield, IL, 1977, pp. 136:145.
15. Siroky, M. B., Willischer, M. K., and Krane, R. J.: The measurement of fluid energy loss during flow. *Invest. Urol.,* 17:514, 1980.
16. Yalla, S. V., Sharma, G. V. R. K., and Barsamian, E. M.: Micturitional static urethral pressure profile. *J. Urol.* 124:649, 1980.
17. Yalla, S. V., Blute, R. D., Snyder, H., Yap, W., Fraser, L., and Friedman, E.: Isolated bladder neck obstruction of undetermined etiology (primary) in adult male. *Urology* 17:99, 1981.
18. Yalla, S. V., Blute, R., Waters, W. B., Snyder, H., and Fraser, L.: Urodynamic evaluation of prostatic enlargements with micturitional vesicourethral static pressure profiles. *J. Urol.* 125:685, 1981.
19. Yalla, S. V., and Loughlin, K.: Urodynamic assessment of anterior urethral constrictions. *Urology* 19:106, 1982.
20. Loughlin, K., and Yalla, S. V.: Endo-urodynamics—another dimension in clinical urodynamics. *Neurourol. Urodyn.* 5:291, 1986.
21. Perkash, I., and Friedland, G. W.: Transrectal ultrasonography of the lower urinary tract: Evaluation of bladder neck problems. *Neuro. urol. Urodyn.,* 5:299, 1986.
22. Fellows, G. J., Cannell, L. B., and Ravichandran, G.: Transrectal ultrasonography compared with voiding cystourethrography after spinal cord injury. *Br. J. Urol.* 59:218, 1987.

12

Evaluation of Urinary Incontinence

EDWARD J. McGUIRE, M.D.

Most patients complaining of incontinence can be treated satisfactorily if the precise cause of involuntary loss can be identified. Although there are some shortcuts, a systematic approach is usually the best, keeping in mind the three broad categories of etiology: detrusor abnormalities, urethral abnormalities, and other factors including fistulae, diverticula, and even a psychogenic etiology.

CLINICAL HISTORY

Children

Bladder-Related Incontinence. The most common cause of incontinence in children is detrusor instability, which tends to occur suddenly and without any warning (*1*). The child is often characterized as inattentive or lazy, when in fact he/she has no idea when his or her bladder may contract. Parents should be thoroughly questioned about daytime urgency as well as nocturnal enuresis of their child. In females recurrent urinary tract infections frequently are associated with detrusor instability (or vice versa). In males detrusor instability may be related to obstruction but usually is not. Operations on the bladder or trigone can result in a poorly compliant bladder with urgency and urgency incontinence. A history of vesical or ureteral surgery is thus particularly important to identify; furthermore, previous surgery for imperforate anus, vaginal atresia, or hypospadias may be the cause of detrusor storage abnormalities.

Combined Vesical and Urethral Abnormalities. Myelodysplasia and lipomeningocele can be associated with overt neurogenic vesical dysfunction (*2*). Neither the extent of the associated neural deficit nor the area of bony involvement can be related to either the presence or the absence of vesical dysfunction. The most common clinical expressions of neurogenic vesical dysfunction in children with myelodysplasia are urinary infection, incontinence, and residual urine. This triad of clinical features in any child is sufficient reason for full radiographic and urodynamic evaluations.

Patients with myelodysplasia and or sacral agenesis frequently manifest a poor compliance areflexic vesical dysfunction in conjunction with a nonfunctional "internal sphincter" (the "wide bladder neck syndrome").

Ectopic Ureteral Insertion. Congenital abnormalities of ureteral insertion (Fig. 12–1) can easily be diagnosed if they are kept in mind. Typically, the resultant incontinence is not gross but is steady and in small amounts. There may be no other symptoms.

Adult Males

Detrusor Instability. Sudden reflex bladder contraction may be related to obstructive prostatism or cerebrovascular disease; it also may occur in Parkinson's disease or Par-

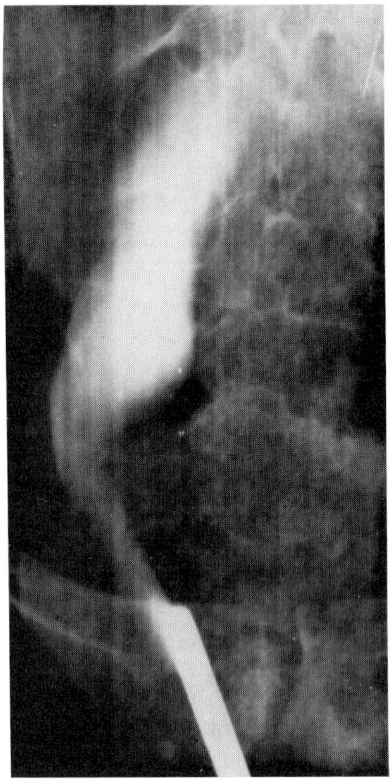

Figure 12–1. Retrograde ureterogram of a dilated ectopic ureter with an intraurethral orifice.

kinson-like syndromes, demyelinating diseases, spinal cord injury, infarction or tumor, dementia, and infrequently diabetes mellitus. Careful patient questioning should enable the examiner to suspect detrusor instability and to plan an appropriate evaluation of its probable underlying etiology. The crucial feature in the history is the occurrence of sudden and unanticipated detrusor activity.

Urethral Dysfunction. Urethral dysfunction causing incontinence in males is generally related to loss of internal sphincter activity and usually is worse in the upright position. Often it can be relieved transiently by volitional striated sphincter contraction. Urgency and urge incontinence are frequently associated with severe urethral dysfunction. A history of prostatectomy related temporally to the onset of the incontinence, a major pelvic trauma, or an intrapelvic operative procedure, e.g., an abdominoperineal rectal resection, may be related to the urethral dysfunction and can help to suggest the direction of subsequent evaluation.

Neurogenic Vesical Dysfunction. Neurogenic vesical dysfunction in adult males may be related to diabetes, spinal cord injury or disease, and peripheral neural injury or neuropathy; it may also follow extirpative surgery on the rectum, prostate, or adjacent organs.

Adult Females

Detrusor Instability. Historically, sudden urgency and incontinence with poor warning are reliable indicators of detrusor instability in adult females. There may be no other identifiable disease process, or the syndrome may be associated with stress incontinence, urinary infection, or a neuropathic condition. Persistent detrusor instability in adult females may occur following an operation for stress incontinence and occasionally is seen in patients with lumbar disk disease.

Urethral Dysfunction. Urinary loss coincident with an increase in intrabdominal pressure is usually associated with poor urethral support and clinically recognizable urethral hypermobility. It can occur in patients with well-supported urethral sphincteric mechansims, in which case inherent weakness of the urethral smooth muscle sphincter may be the underlying problem. Although incontinence in the latter group tends to be worse, there is no historical method to distinguish it from the former, unless the patient has had a previous transurethral resection (TUR) of the internal sphincter or a YV-plasty.

Fistulas. Incontinence due to fistulas often follows some operative procedure or radiation therapy and usually is not associated with urgency or a feeling of urethral urinary loss. Vesicovaginal fistulas can develop years after radiation therapy to pelvic organs.

Neurogenic Vesical Dysfunction. Frank neurogenic vesical dysfunction may follow pelvic surgery and frequently occurs in female patients with diabetes or multiple sclerosis. The patient's description of her incontinence generally is not sufficiently clear to enable a tentative diagnosis to be made without urodynamic testing.

PHYSICAL EXAMINATION

Children

Physical examination does not usually help make the definitive diagnosis of an unstable detrusor, but if combined with cystoscopy it usually enables the urologist to diagnose an ectopic ureter or vaginal atresia. Normal perineal sensation is diagnostically useful, as most patients with neurogenic vesical dysfunction secondary to myelodysplasia or sacral agenesis do not have it. Easy expression of bladder contents by the Credé maneuver in an infant or child usually indicates a urethral dysfunction, often in combination with bladder "denervation."

Adult Males

Dribbling incontinence in the upright position, which the patient can voluntarily stop by contraction of the striated sphincter, is sufficient to suggest urethral smooth sphincter dysfunction. Obstructive uropathy cannot be diagnosed reliably on physical examination unless gross urinary retention is present; even in that instance obstruction should not be considered as the exclusive etiology of such retention. Normal perineal sensation does not rule out peripheral neural pathology, particularly following pelvic extirpative surgery. A poor perineal sensation or anal sphincter tone, however, makes the diagnosis of benign prostatic hypertrophy unlikely. In adult males with known or suspected neurogenic vesical dysfunction, endoscopy is not the most reliable method to diagnose benign prostatic hypertrophy or any other obstructive process.

Adult Females

Classic stress urinary incontinence is associated with posterior rotational descent of the urethra and visible leakage during that movement. Associated conditions include cystocele, rectocele, uterine prolapse, and occasionally enterocele. Although these conditions are not directly related etiologically to stress incontinence, they cannot be ignored for any good reason when surgical repair of the stress incontinence is contemplated. Moreover, full radiographic evaluation is performed prior to surgical repair of a large cystocele to obviate the *de novo* appearance of severe stress incontinence during the postoperative period. That circumstance exists when a large cystocele is protective; acting as a sort of runoff for intravesical urine, it ceases to be protective after surgical repair. If hypermobility of the urethra is also present, it should be corrected at the time of operation on the cystocele.

Total Urethral Failure

Total urethral failure is usually associated with severe stress incontinence, urgency and frequency, and minimal findings on pelvic examination. Thus there is often a discrepancy between the symptom of urinary loss and the findings on vaginal examination that are commonly associated with stress incontinence, i.e., urethral hypomobility and poor pelvic support. Although poor coaptation of the proximal urethra can be diagnosed endoscopically (*3*), radiographic evaluation is easier and much more accurate, particularly if combined with urethral closing pressure profilometry (*4*).

Fistulas

Vesicovaginal and urethrovaginal fistulas are not difficult to find if the examiner is looking for them. Careful physical examination with a good light complemented by endoscopy is an accurate method of diagnosis and localization. Ureterovaginal fistulas are more difficult to identify; vaginal urine is often cloudy, and bladder urine is clear. Occasionally, a vesicovaginal fistula occurs in conjunction with a ureterovaginal fistula; full radiographic evaluation of both upper and lower urinary tracts is thus essential in any patient with a fistula.

URODYNAMIC EVALUATION

Primary assessment of urethral sphincter function is helpful in adult women and men with symptoms of incontinence and physical findings suggesting that a urethral lesion is present. If the urethral sphincter is found to function normally, other causes of incontinence can then be sought.

Method

Upright cystourethrography with pressure measurements probably provides the best single method of assessment of urethral sphincteric function. If a urethral striated sphincter electromyogram (EMG) is also recorded, a clear idea of such function is attainable (5). The EMG needles are placed under audible and oscilloscopic control within the urethral striated sphincter itself.

A 10F Bard urodynamic catheter with a triple lumen suitably marked for radiographic localization can be used. This catheter is inserted into the bladder. The urethral and bladder pressure channels are perfused at 1 ml/min with a Harvard syringe pump and the filling channel opened to a large reservoir with an inflow rate of 50 to 100 ml/min. The fluoroscopic table is placed in the upright position and the urethral pressure lumen advanced to just above the vesical outlet. The two pressure-sensing lumens should record almost equal pressures at this time except for the 6-cm separation between the two lumens. (The maximum pressure difference with a full bladder and a perfectly vertical table and recording tube is 6 cm H_2O). In practice, the tube bends and the mean difference is about 3 cm H_2O, which is not enough to make any difference. Under fluoroscopic control, the visible urethral pressure-sensing lumen is advanced slowly into the active urethral sphincter (Fig. 12–2). Normally, positive urethral closing pressure begins precisely as the lumen enters the vesical neck and rises until the peak pressure zone is reached. Just distal to the peak zone the pressure falls precipitously. Localization of sphincter components using EMG, fluoroscopy, and manometry is precise and reproducible. Volitional and reflex striated sphincter activities influence a well-defined area of the urethra that corresponds to the high-pressure of compressive zone (Fig. 12–3). This high-pressure zone and the EMG activity are lost in this segment after sacral rhizotomy.

Sphincter closure from the bladder neck to the area influenced by striated sphincter activity is about 2.8 to 4.0 cm in men, depending on the prostatic length, and about 1.2 to 1.8 cm in women. After sacral rhizotomy the

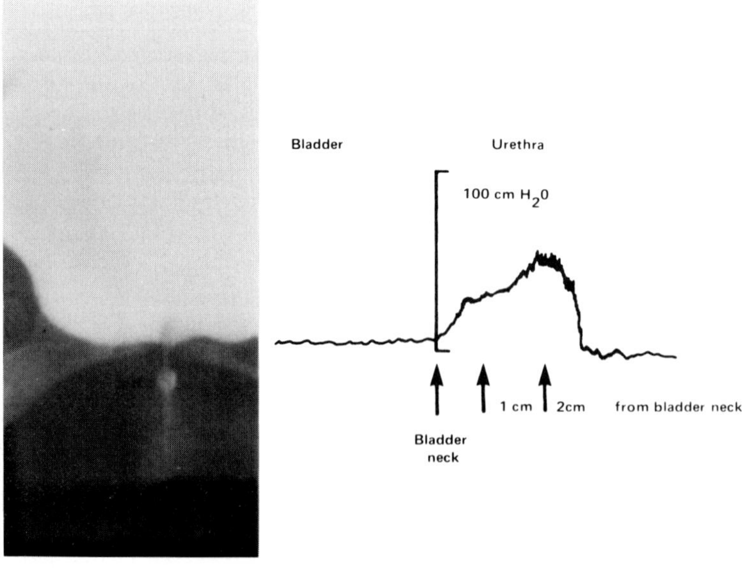

Figure 12–2. Urethral pressure profile using a Bard triple-lumen catheter. Note the disk marker entering the proximal urethra. The metal area indicates the position of the urethral pressure-sensing aperture. The manometric data show a normal female urethral pressure profile with onset at the bladder neck and peak pressure at 2 cm distal to the bladder neck.

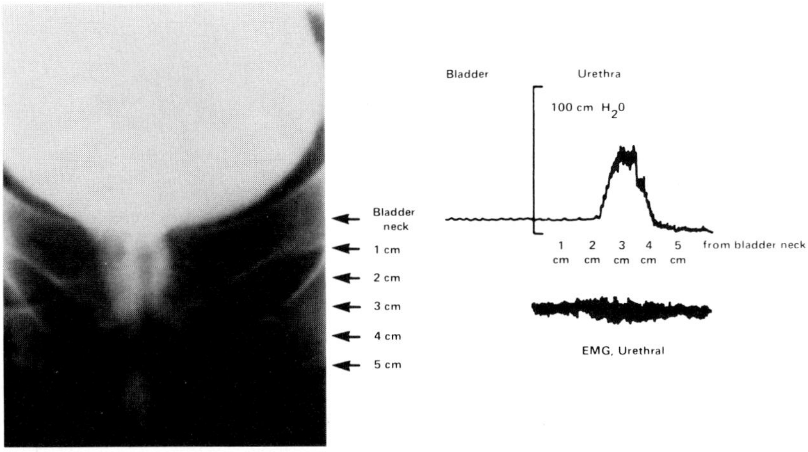

Figure 12–3. Combined manometric and radiographic assessment of urethral sphincter function. Note the absence of pressure measured in the first 2 cm of the urethra and no radiographic closure. Note the good peak pressure, with some EMG activity, and radiographic closure of the distal "volitional" sphincter area.

functional profile length remains unchanged, but peak pressures can no longer be recorded from the distal sphincter zone. With the bladder moderately full (200–400 cc volume) the continence mechanism is stressed by any increase in intraabdominal pressure. Leakage into the urethra distal to the active sphincter is easily recognized fluoroscopically and can be related to motion of the urethra in women with stress incontinence. It can be semiquantitated into the three basic types (Fig. 12–4). Provided that both smooth and striated urethral sphincter functions are normal and that the urethra does not move or leak with stress, both, sphincter areas are closed radiographically and manometrically.

DYSFUNCTION OF PROXIMAL URETHRAL MECHANISM

Dysfunction of the proximal urethral mechanism may be due to tissue loss after prostatectomy or YV-plasty, or it may result from sympathetic neural injury or a congenital neural deficit, as in myelodysplasia or sacral agenesis. The relation between loss of function of the proximal urethral continence mechanism and incontinence depends on the extent of the deficit and the length of urethra affected. After prostatectomy, continent individuals maintain urethral closure in an area from the distal verumontanum to the recognizable zone of volitionally controllable sphincter closure (Fig. 12–5). Postprostatectomy incontinence is associated with loss of radiographic coaptation of the urethra from the distal verumontarum to the area of volitional sphincter activity. The latter area is often normal, exhibiting a normal pressure that varies rapidly with coughing, straining, assumption of the upright position, and attempts to volitionally close the urethra (Fig. 12–6).

Neurologic lesions affecting the thoracolumbar sympathetic cell mass or more distal neural lesions in pelvic fracture, pelvic extirpative surgery, or prolonged alpha-adrenergic blockade in younger men without prostatic hypertrophy, result in loss of radiographic coaptation of the proximal mechanism, including the bladder neck, prostatic urethra, and urethra from the verumontanum to the volitional sphincteric zone. In this respect, urodynamic findings in men with postprostatectomy incontinence are similar to those in patients with a sympathetic neural deficit.

There is considerable debate over the type and innnervation of the muscle involved in closure of the male urethra from the verumontanum to the zone of the volitional sphincter. Such debate arose in part from anatomic studies indicating that this segment is closed principally by skeletal muscle, but the skeletal muscle that is referred to in this

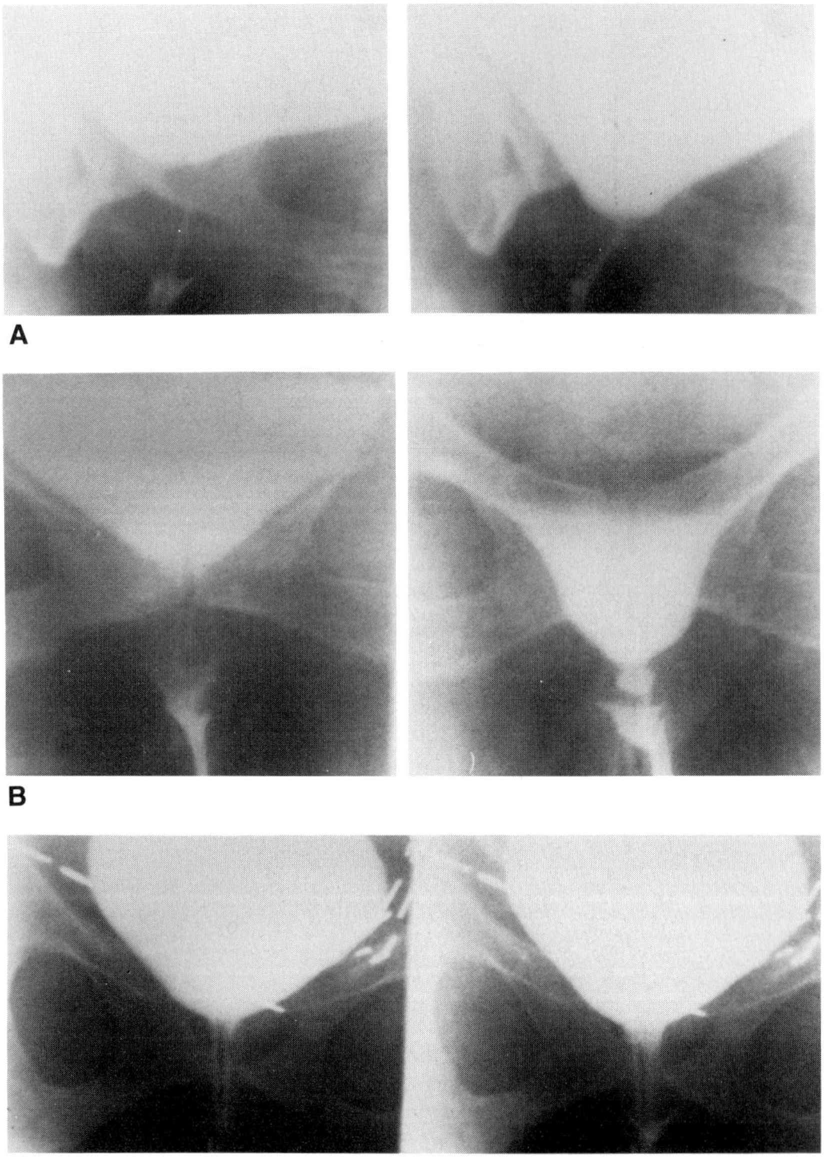

A

B

C

Figure 12–4. **A.** Type I stress urinary incontinence associated with minimal motion of the urethra and bladder base with an increased intraabdominal pressure. **B.** Type II stress urinary incontinence associated with marked hypermobility of the bladder base and urethra with severe urethral urinary loss. **C.** Type III stress incontinence. There is little motion with straining and an open bladder neck in the resting (*left*) and straining (*right*) films.

context is intrinsic to the urethra (*6*). That muscle is composed principally of slow tonic fibers (*7*). The extrinsic striated sphincter, which presumably is a part of the pelvic floor, is innervated by the pudendal nerves and is composed principally of fast-twitch fibers. Elbadawi and Schenk were the first to suggest that the intrinsic urethral striated musculature has autonomic innervation (*8*). Donker could not find pudendal neural fibers that directly innervate the intrinsic striated urethral sphincter and suggested that its in-

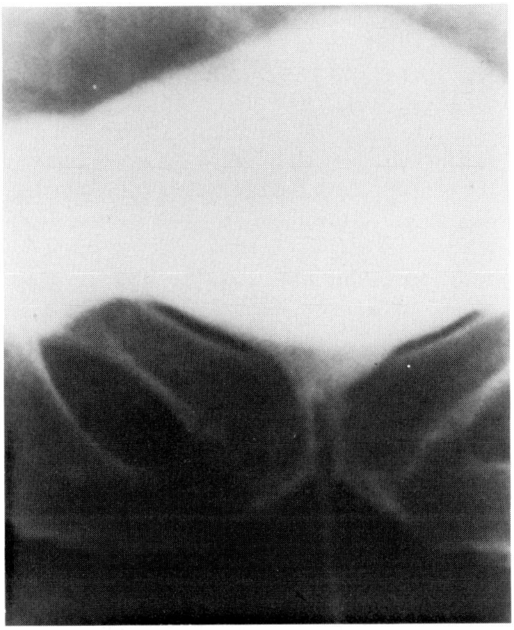

Figure 12–5. A continent 56-year-old man after prostatectomy. Note the open bladder neck and proximal urethra but no leakage.

nervation is derived from the pelvic nerves (P. Donker, personal communication, 1976). There must be some way to correlate the available anatomic and functional data; perhaps, we will be able at some time in the future to arrive at a common terminology and method of description of the urethral sphincter that has an acceptable meaning to urologists, engineers, and anatomists alike. Until that time the issue will remain an area of controversy that at present has limited clinical relevance. That part of the urethra lying distal to the verumontanum and proximal to the volitional controllable striated sphincter (which by inference but not proof is functionally fast twitch) is a crucial area in continence function. Whether it is a sympathetically innervated striated muscle composed of slow tonic fibers, a smooth muscle with sympathetic innervation, or both smooth and striated muscle provided with sympathetic innervation is in reality not important. My personal impression is that the area in question is a sympathetically innervated smooth muscle. The evidence for this impression seems clear; however, other workers hold opposing views.

URETHRAL DYSFUNCTION ASSOCIATED WITH ABNORMALITIES OF REFLEX VESICAL ACTIVITY

Normally, with and usually just before the onset of reflex bladder contractility, the en-

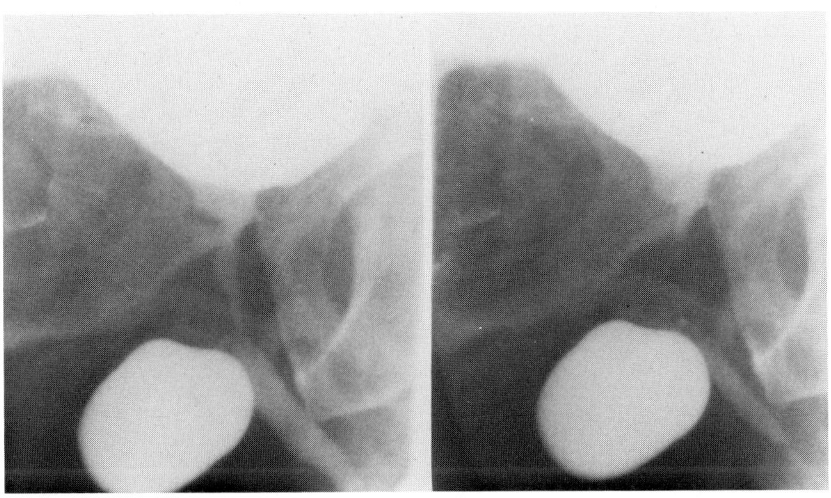

Figure 12–6. Postprostatectomy incontinence despite a Kaufman prosthesis. **Left.** Note at rest a column of contrast from the bladder neck across the entire sphincter, the prosthesis, and into the bulbous urethra. **Right.** The patient contracts the volitional sphincter on command and closes the area just proximal to the prosthesis. Note the narrow column of contrast just above the volitional sphincter that fills the 0.9-cm urethral segment distal to the verumontanum and proximal to the volitional mechanism.

tire urethral sphincter including its proximal and distal mechanisms visibly opens radiographically, and positive urethral pressure throughout the entire area is lost. With a rise in detrusor pressure, intraurethral pressure also rises, as the two areas are at that time a common hydraulic chamber.

For a number of technical reasons a forward-looking urethral pressure aperture should be superior to a lateral aperture in determining pressure relations between the bladder and urethra at midflow (during voiding). It so happens that it does not make any difference, and a lateral aperture is better to use because insertion and withdrawal is easier.

A sequence of sudden urethral pressure loss accompanied by a sharp fall in EMG activity with a fluoroscopically visible opening of the entire sphincter mechanism from the vesical neck to and including the distal mechanism has been termed "urethral instability" (*9*). These events also occur at the time of reflex bladder contractility when both proximal and distal sphincter elements open just prior to an increase in bladder pressure. The events in urethral instability are identical to those that occur with detrusor contraction and may be associated with urgency. Isolated loss of EMG activity, without opening of the vesical outlet and proximal urethral mechanism, can also occur volitionally or apparently for a number of other reasons. In that circumstance and in other cases where volitional sphincter contractility is lost as the result of a neural lesion, the primary (proximal) mechanism stays closed. While the detrusor is "storing" urine, certain changes may occur in the proximal urethra that result in a pressure loss and consequent opening of the proximal urethra. They do not occur in patients who have had prolonged administration of alpha-adrenergic blocking agents, sympathetic neural lesions, or TUR of the bladder neck. Opening of the internal mechanism is clearly linked to detrusor contraction or, rather, to the neural events that initiate reflex detrusor contraction (*10*). If the pelvic nerve is stimulated, the proximal mechanism opens and loses intrinsic pressure even with the detrusor excised. The usual neural event that opens the proximal mechanism is parasympathetic discharge. If the urethral sphincter opens fully during bladder filling it may be due to a reflex sacral neural response to that filling, i.e., a bladder contraction, which the patient can inhibit; or it may occur when the bladder, because of muscular injury, cannot respond to the parasympathetic neural discharge. Patients with unstable detrusor dysfunction frequently show what has been termed uninhibited urethral relaxation, or a drop in EMG activity and a sense of urgency associated with a drop in urethral relaxation, or a drop in EMG activity and a sense of urgency associated with a drop in urethral closing pressure and the sensation of "imminent micturition" (W.E. Bradley, personal communication, 1984). Most patients in such a circumstance can inhibit the detrusor response by vigorous striated sphincter contraction (Fig. 12–7). Observation of a sudden decrease in EMG activity during bladder filling, without volitional participation by the subject studied but with a fall in urethral closing pressure, is acceptable evidence of detrusor instability, even if the subject can inhibit the actual detrusor contractile response and prevent urinary loss.

Loss of EMG activity with bladder filling and reversal of the normal guarding reflex (a gradual increase in EMG activity and distal sphincter pressure during filling) are abnormal findings. There is considerable evidence that cortical control of reflex detrusor activity may be exerted through volitional striated sphincter contraction via pyramidal corticospinal pathways. Nonvolitional urinary loss, which on urodynamic evaluation is associated with striated sphincter instability, tends to respond to anticholinergic agents. Experimentally, administration of large doses of alpha-adrenergic agents does not influence pressure loss in the internal (smooth) sphincter with sacral root stimulation, whereas administration of a ganglionic blocking agent does.

Disorders of Detrusor Function Associated with Incontinence

Fixed disorders of urethral sphincter function related to tissue loss or neural injury are relatively easy to identify and should be ruled out early. Most individuals with severe sphincter lesions also show some degree of

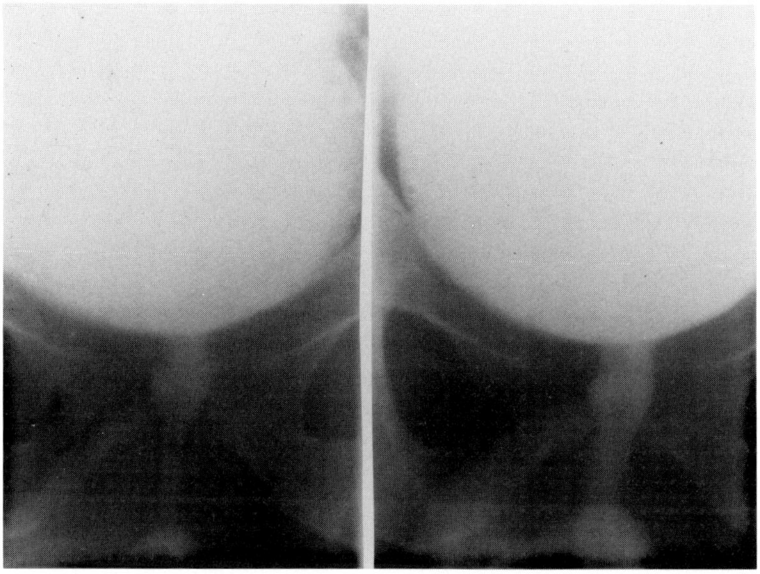

Figure 12–7. Uninhibited bladder contractility elicited by filling. The patient tries to "stop" voiding (**left**) but fails (**right**) and loses urine in the bulbous urethra. Note (**left**) the open "internal mechanism," which is linked to detrusor contractile activity. The area closed by a volitional attempt to stop voiding is clearly visible as the "distal mechanism."

bladder instability. Because detrusor instability often remits spontaneously after resolution of sphincteric incompetence, it is the sphincteric lesions that are approached first, diagnostically and therapeutically. If the sphincter is normal and the lesion is characterized, study of the detrusor response to bladder filling is the next step in urodynamic evaluation of the patient.

Disorders of Detrusor Compliance or Accommodation

Abnormal vesical storage of urine related to mural fibrosis or myogenic hypertonicity is characterized by a steep pressure–volume curve on the cystometrogram. The curve may rise with each volume increment, or there may be an initial flat curve followed by a slow but steady upward deflection. Relatively slow-fill cystometry seems to be the most accurate, as rapid filling, particularly with carbon dioxide, can induce an abnormally steep pressure–volume curve that is not elicited with slow fill rates (below 50 ml/min).

Poor vesical compliance may be related to defunctionalization, fibrosis, or neuromuscular-related hypertonicity. Some differential information can be obtained by subcutaneous injection of urecholine, which markedly increases the pressure response after preganglionic vesical decentralization, or intravenous injection of an anticholinergic agent, which flattens the pressure–volume curve of hypertonicity. Because these agents influence neuromuscular vesical activity, a pronounced effect of either agent indicates hypertonicity, usually secondary to "denervation."

The only method that *may* allow differentiation of vesical defunctionalization from actual fibrosis (which is not influenced by drug administration) is cyclic filling. This method may improve compliance, even in a fibrotic bladder, and thus is not an absolute test. The usual rationale for cyclic filling is to gain low-pressure reservoir capacity, rather than to investigate any underlying etiology. If the test fails, operative intervention to augment vesical capacity is the usual next step. Susset et al. used rapid-fill cystometry to investigate disorders of vesical compliance with good results (*11*).

DISORDERS OF REFLEX VESICAL ACTIVITY CONTROL

A normal bladder does not contract without its owner's permission. Volitional voiding is initiated by relaxation, and volitional constraint of micturition is associated with willful contraction of pelvic floor musculature. Despite considerable argument about the precise makeup and innervation of the distal urethral sphincter mechanism, volitional overriding of reflex bladder activity is first notable in the membranous urethra in males and the midurethral high-pressure zone in females (Fig. 12–7). Although uninhibited bladder contractions can often be diagnosed with a provocative cystometrogram, it is not universally the case, as many individuals with detrusor instability do not have detrusor contractions during urodynamic testing. In this respect, the history is often better at suggesting the diagnosis than a standard cystometrogram. James used continuous monitoring as an even better method of diagnosing detrusor instability (*12*). The technique involves continuous and simultaneous monitoring of intravesical pressure activity and urinary losses that occur while the patient performs everyday tasks. The results of such testing indicate that substantial false negative results could be seen in provocative cystometry. Therefore, a patient with a history suggestive of detrusor instability probably has it even if provocative cystometry does not help to provide the diagnosis unequivocally.

REFERENCES

1. Koff, S. A, Lapides, J., and Piazza, D. H.: Association of urinary tract infection and reflux with uninhibited bladder contractions and voluntary sphincteric obstruction. *J. Urol.* 122:373, 1979.
2. McGuire, E. J., Woodside, J. R., Borden, T. A., and Weiss, R. A.: Prognostic value of urodynamic testing in myelodysplasia. *J. Urol.* 126:205, 1981.
3. Robertson, J. A.: Gas endoscopy. In Raz, S. (ed.), *Female Urology*. Saunders, Philadelphia, 1983, pp. 68–78.
4. McGuire, E. J., Lytton, B., Kohorn, E. I., and Pepe, V.: The value of urodynamic testing in stress urinary incontinence. *J. Urol.* 124:256, 1980.
5. McGuire, E. J.: Combined radiographic and manometric assessment of urethral sphincter function. *J. Urol.* 118:632, 1977.
6. Gosling, J.: The structure of the bladder and urethra in relation to function. *Urol. Clin. North Am.* 6:31, 1979.
7. Gosling, J. A., Dixon, J. S., Critchley, H. O. D., and Thompson, S. A.: A comparative study of the human external sphincter and periurethral levator ani muscles. *Br. J. Urol.* 53:35, 1981.
8. Elbadawi, A., and Schenk, E. A.: A new theory of the innervation of bladder musculature. 4. Innervation of the vesicoureteral junction and external urethral sphincter. *J. Urol.* 111:613, 1974.
9. McGuire, E. J.: Reflex urethral instability. *Br. J. Urol.* 50:200, 1978.
10. McGuire, E. J., and Herlihy, E.: Bladder and urethral responses to isolated sacral motor root stimulation. *Invest. Urol.* 16:219, 1978.
11. Susset, J. G., Peters, N., Cohen, S., and Ghoniem, G. M.: Early detection of neurogenic bladder dysfunction caused by protruded lumbar disc. *Urology* 70:461, 1983.
12. James, D.: Continuous monitoring. *Urol. Clin. North Am.* 6:125, 1979.

Evaluation of the Upper Urinary Tract

13

BO COOLSAET, M.D., Ph.D.

Classification, investigation, and treatment of the wide upper urinary tract have been confusing. Such terms as obstruction, functional stenosis, and atonic distal ureter have been used as a basis for classifications that may appear to be mere scientific exercises but may become important when therapeutic measures are considered. Useful classifications by any international standardization group (*1*) have been simplified by others (*2*). There is general agreement on the distinction between a refluxing and a nonrefluxing wide upper urinary tract. Disagreement and confusion emerge, however, when distinction between an obstructed and a nonobstructed upper tract and a primary or secondary etiology is considered. The major misconception of the past has been the belief that the wide upper tract is not due to obstruction when reflux is present, but that it is when reflux is absent. Studies by Backlund and Reuterskiold (*3*), Struthers (*4*), Hanna and Edwards (*5*), Whitaker (*2*), and Whitfield *et al.* (*6*) have proved the fallacy of this clinical attitude. Other investigations (*7,8*) have shown, however, that although conceptual simplification is attractive it can be misleading. The more progress is made in both clinical and scientific research in the problem of upper urinary tract dilation, the more it becomes obvious that no clear-cut definition of obstruction or of primary and secondary pathogenetic mechanisms can easily be provided. For the time being, however, the urologist is faced with major problems in clinical management, including actual clinical questions related to: screening for wide upper tracts and the sequence and reliability of methods of their assessment; early detection of renal parenchymal dysfunction; the relation between outflow characteristics and parenchymal function as well as complications; the recoverability of upper tract and parenchymal functions; the distinction between refluxing systems with impaired and those with normal outflow; and methods of treatment, e.g., the choice between long-term conservative and operative treatment in cases of infection, the necessity of tailoring the wide system and indications for operative correction of vesicorenal reflux.

The ultimate goal of any clinical approach is the prevention of renal damage or, if already present, the prevention of further damage, prevention or treatment of complications, and control of symptoms. The clinical examination therefore must deal with the functional characteristics of both the transport system and the renal parenchyma.

Regardless of whether the ureterovesical junction (UVJ) is incompetent, routine clinical and urine analyses are followed by excretory urography, which by far is the most frequently used diagnostic procedure. Its major goal is to obtain information on renal morphology, urinary tract morphology, and urinary tract dynamics. It should be remembered, however, that it is of limited value in the assessment of renal parenchymal function; wide upper tracts that other methods indicate drain nearly normally functioning parenchyma may convey the false impression of impaired parenchymal function.

Determination of the morphology and dimensions of the renal parenchyma by excretory urography appears to be particularly important when correlated with the refluxing versus the nonrefluxing status of the upper tract. Nevertheless, the procedure cannot determine the causal relation between morphologic abnormalities of the upper tract and the kidney it drains. A wide upper tract system may be associated with a morphologically normal kidney, and an abnormal kidney may be drained by a morphologically normal upper tract. Morphologic parenchymal abnormalities therefore must be interpreted with great care, at least to rule out the possibility of being developmental in nature. Reliance on morphologic features of the parenchyma to determine indications for operative correction of morphologic upper tract abnormalities is thus not justified. Although an increase of parenchymal size after surgical correction may be a justification *a posteriori* for the operation, it must be remembered that accurate determination of total parenchymal volume is difficult or impossible in routine urologic practice.

When performed properly, excretory urography is indispensable for screening the anatomic morphology of the wide upper tract; it determines whether the involved part of the tract is a calyx, renal pelvis, or ureter, unilaterally or bilaterally (Fig. 13–1). Abdominal compression during the procedure is to be condemned, as it interferes considerably with natural filling and emptying of a wide system and with the accurate assessment of its natural dynamic behavior. Furthermore, abdominal compression can cause calyceal rupture. Better imaging of wide calyces is considered irrelevant when seeking a refined clinical diagnosis, particularly in any case where obstruction of the upper tract is clinically suspected.

The diagnostic value of excretory urography depends on the interest and compe-

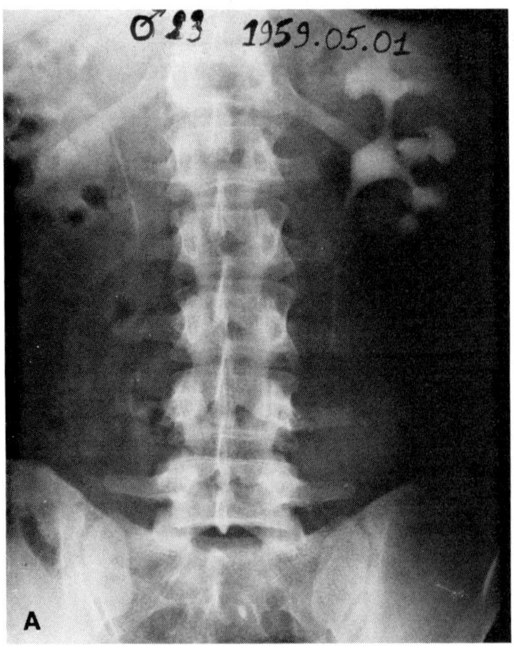

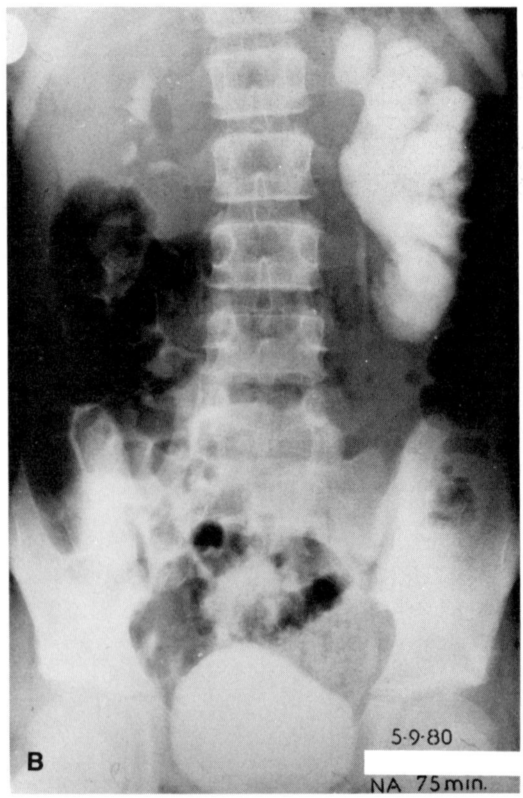

Figure 13–1. Dilation of the upper urinary tract is mostly localized by excretory urography, which is still the first screening test. Different parts of the upper tract may be involved: calices (**A**); renal pelvis and calices (**B**); unilateral calices pelvis and ureter (**C**); bilateral pelvis and ureter (**D**).

tence of the radiologist and the facilities available. The principal aim of the procedure is the qualitative assessment of outflow capabilities of the wide upper urinary tract in different bodily positions and under changing conditions of the bladder. Upper urinary tract dynamics can be evaluated satisfactorily by excretory urography. A "dynamic excretory urogram" can easily be obtained cinematographically when sufficient contrast medium is excreted in a wide system. From the moment the upper tract is visualized, important characteristics of upper tract dynamics can be recorded on static film or videotape. Characteristics of antegrade urine transport can subsequently be studied in both supine and erect positions. Drainage of urine from wide upper tracts into the bladder is sometimes achieved by passive antegrade flow. It should be remembered, however, that such antegrade urine transport, whether active or passive, must be determined by the contractile status of the detrusor. Data (*9*) have shown that the resistance to antegrade flow through the UVJ is determined mainly by intravesical pressure and detrusor stretch. The status of the upper urinary tract is investigated when the bladder is empty and subsequently when it is filled. Occurrence of ureteral wall coaptation at propulsive contraction sites and of retrograde peristaltic waves are interesting features to evaluate during such assessment. It is impossible, however, to clearly relate retrograde peristalsis, ureteral reflux, and impaired upper tract outflow with upper tract stasis to the presence or threat of renal parenchymal injury. A noncoapting system with ureteral reflux and stasis sometimes drains a normal renal parenchyma and vice versa. Data obtained from excretory urography therefore is analyzed in correlation with data obtained by other investigations, especially specialized tests of renal nephron function. Obviously, neither the ordinary nor the dynamic excre-

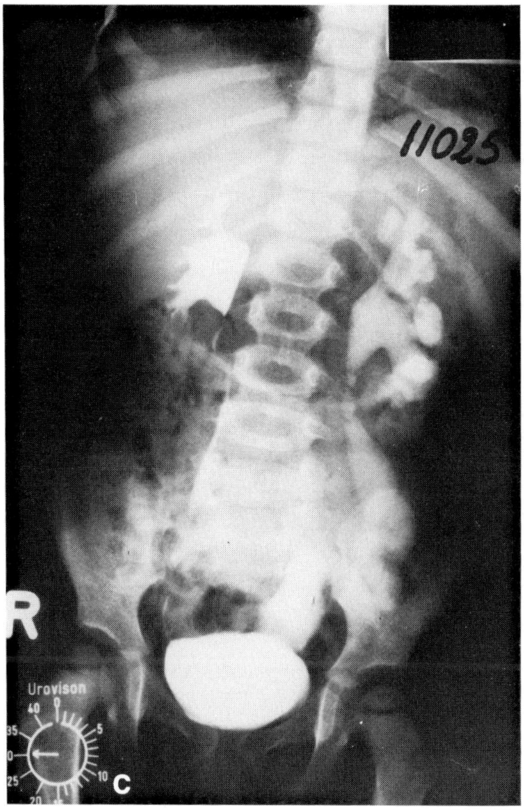

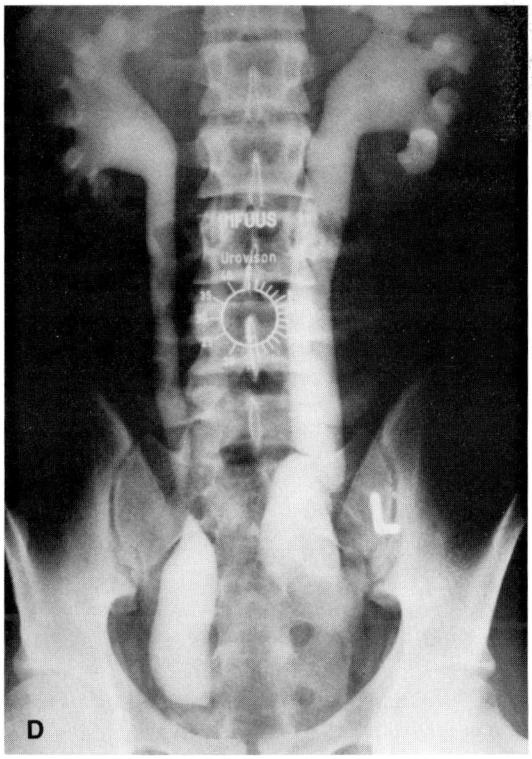

Figure 13–1 *(cont.)*

tory urogram is of value alone in the evaluation of an upper tract system in which contrast material is insufficiently visualized for one reason or another. Although it has previously been stated that the clinical diagnosis of ureteral disease depends almost entirely on radiologic examination, it would be unrealistic to diagnose "obstruction" or "nonobstruction" on the basis of data obtained even by a carefully performed and evaluated dynamic excretory urogram.

The application of excretory urography can be extended by studying the opacified upper tract 20 minutes after a diuretic injection of agent in order to study the influence of hyper-diuresis on visualized renal pelvic dimensions. When upper urinary tract outflow is impaired, the renal pelvis is unable to evacuate the amount of the urine excreted under diuretic conditions, resulting in a greater volume of the pelvis. Such an increase in volume can be estimated by measuring diameters of the renal pelves on the excretory urogram. When the pelvic diameter is increased more than 22 percent beyond the norm, a severely impaired upper tract outflow is likely (*10*). Although this method provides some necessary information, spurious findings may result from extensibility characteristics of the upper urinary tract, including the anatomic location of the renal pelves.

Methods other than radiographic techniques have been developed for quantitation of renal function and imaging of the renal parenchyma. ^{99m}Tc-DMSA (dimercaptosuccinic acid) is a cortical labeling agent that is largely bound to plasma proteins. Its early excretion is minimal, half of its administered dose is bound to the tubular cell mass (*11*), and the percentage of its renal parenchymal distribution appears to be directly related to tubular function (*12*) and differential renal blood flow (*13*). The major advantages of the technique are that it can be repeated with minimal risk, it can assess differential tubular function, and it is practically independent of urinary flow rate as well as anatomic urinary tract morphology. The test is particularly easy to perform when a gamma camera and a data processor are available and is especially useful because it can allow expression of relative tubular cell mass and function in terms of total tubular function (Fig. 13–2). Specific evaluation of tubular function is particularly important in the assessment of renal parenchymal function in cases with wide urinary tracts. There is clinical and experimental evidence that the distal tubular function is threatened before other parts of the nephron in patients with impaired tract outflow (*14,15*). Although the potential causal relation between nephron function and a wide upper urinary tract may be difficult to determine, the assessment of distal tubular function remains a valuable test when operative intervention is considered. It is particularly true when nontubular parts of the nephron are determined to function normally and when during follow-up tubular function is observed to decrease. At present, the potential of recovery of nephron function is not fully known; what is known is that tubular cell mass and function can recover considerably, even when its estimated relative function is less than 10 percent, particularly in children.

Both nephron and upper tract evacuation functions can best be screened and evaluated further by diuresis renography (*16,17*), especially using the same computerized gamma camera as in the above-described procedure. Whitefield *et al.*, using radioisotope transit times, were able to distinguish nephropathy from obstructive uropathy (*18*). It is known that renal parenchymal function is not influenced by the diuretic furosemide. With the patient sitting, a furosemide dose of 0.5 mg/kg body weight is administered intravenously, and 10 minutes later a radionuclide is administered. ^{99m}Tc-DTPA (diethylenetriaminepentaacetic acid) can be used to determine relative glomerular functions and ^{123}I- or ^{131}I-hippuran to assess proximal tubular function; the latter is determined 2 minutes after injection of about 10 mCi of the radionuclide (Figs. 13–3 and 13–4). Computerized data collection is continued from 20 to 30 minutes. Each kidney, ureteral segment, or bladder can be analyzed separately by selecting regions of interest at retrospective examination of the records (Fig. 13–5).

Three types of time–activity curves can be recognized by diuresis renography (Fig. 13–6). The first type represents a group of wide upper tracts that excrete the radionuclide rapidly during high diuresis, resembling the pattern obtained in normal systems. There is evidence that such wide tracts are innocuous to the renal parenchyma, and that

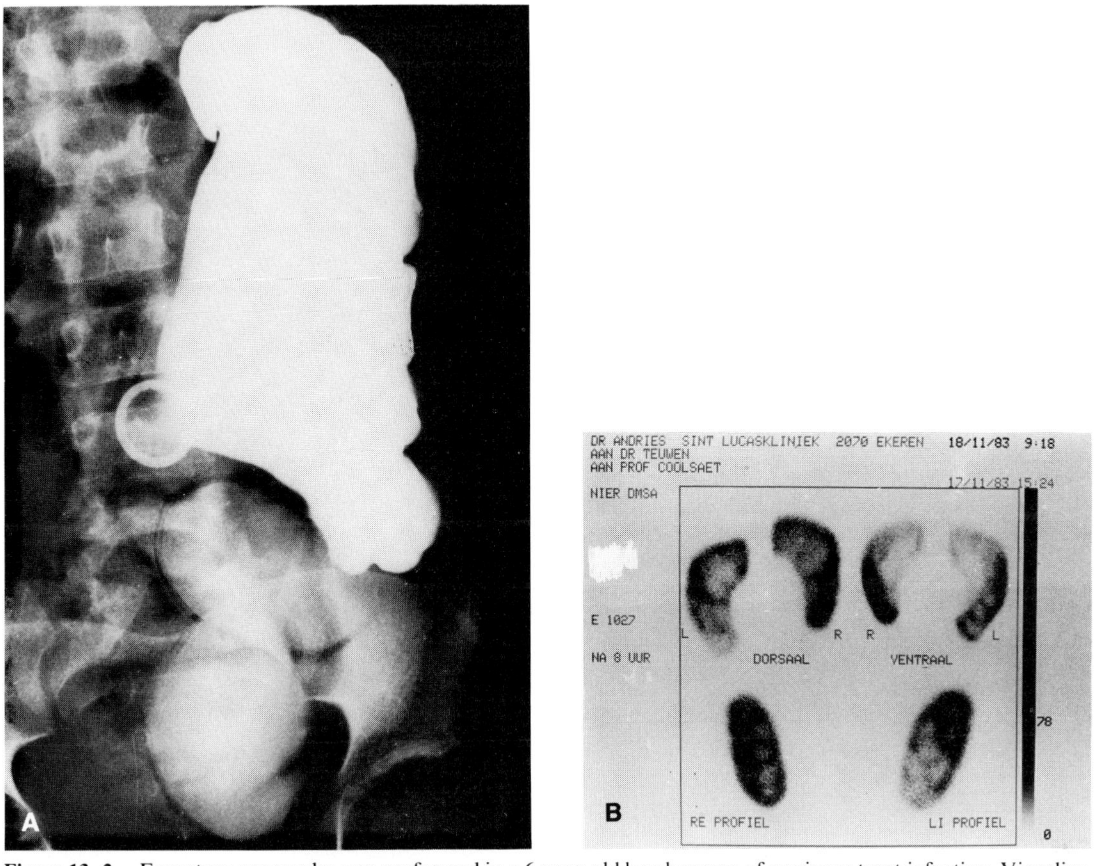

Figure 13–2. Excretory urography was performed in a 6-year-old boy because of a urinary tract infection. Visualization of the upper tract was nearly impossible. A 90-minute exposure showed bilateral highly dilated upper tract systems. Percutaneous puncture on the left side and an antegrade x-ray film show extensive dilation. **A.** A ^{99m}Tc-DMSA scan was performed. **B.** Tubular function determination was performed 8 and 234 hours after injection. Tracer captation was, respectively, 71.7 and 63.8 percent of the injected dose. After 24 hours relative tubular function was (left/right): 48.0/52.0. Results are within the normal limits. Maximal concentration ability (Minirin-Test), however, was decreased to 439, 409, and 405 on the left side and to 421, 442, and 243 on the right side. Diuresis renography (^{99m}Tc-DTPA) revealed a severely impaired outflow, and relative glomerular function was (left/right) 50.1/49.9 at 2 minutes. Creatinine clearance was 86.9 ml/min. Pressure studies revealed no significant pressure rise in the left renal pelvis at maximal diuretic stimulation.

their surgical correction may be unnecessary. Using standard renography, the radionuclide appears to be accumulated in most cases with such systems, suggesting that stasis does occur under normal diuretic conditions. At present, however, it is not known if this normal pattern of evacuation of some wide

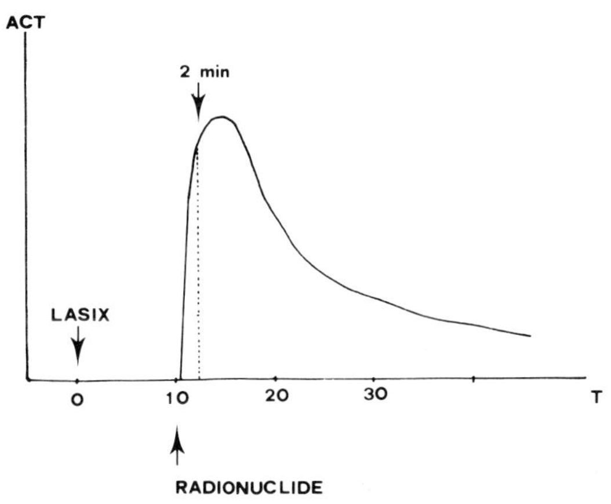

Figure 13-3. Relative nephron function is determined 2 minutes after injection of about 10 mCi radionuclide.

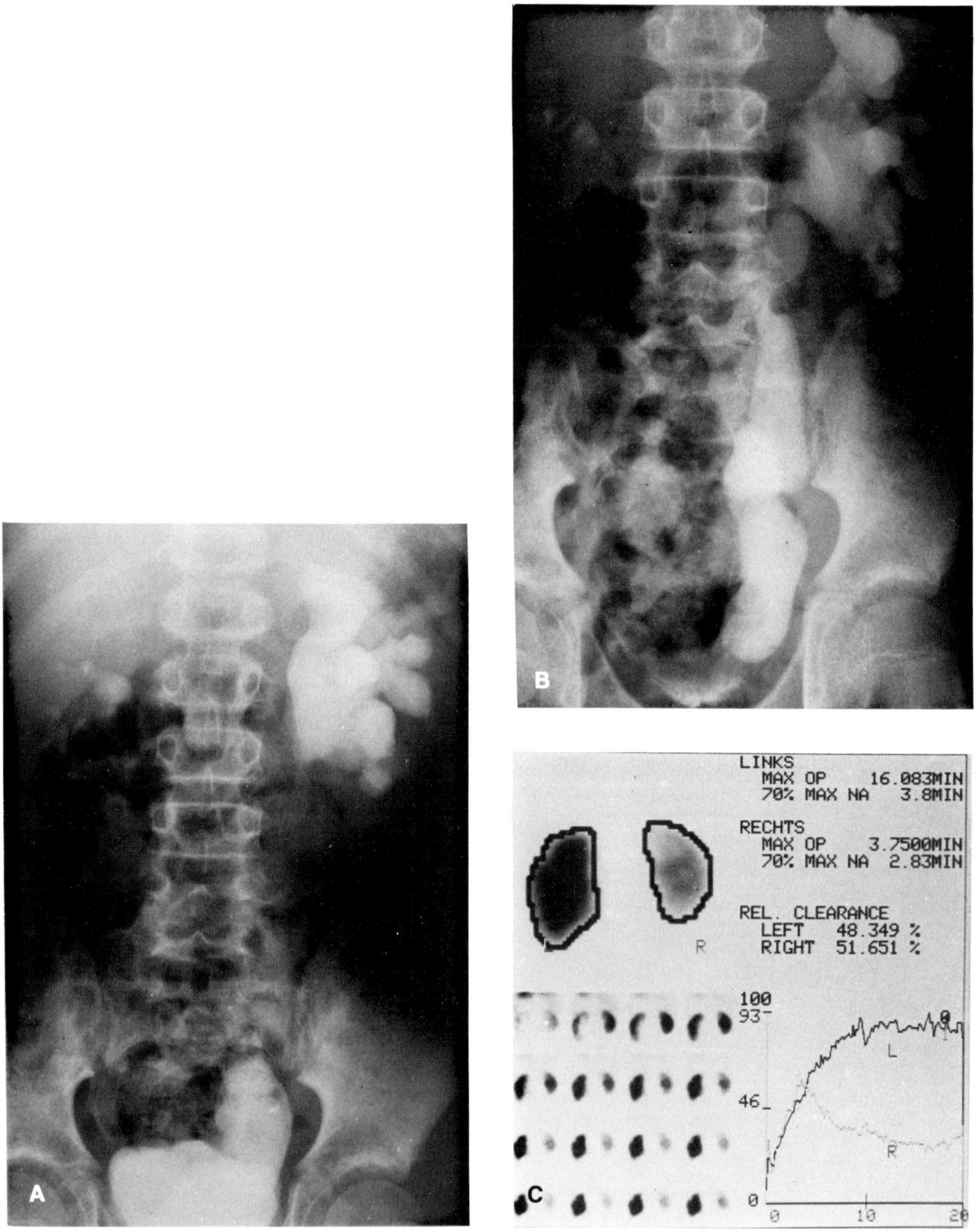

Figure 13–4. **A.** Intravenous urography (IVU) in a 6-year-old boy showing a wide left system. Diuresis renography was performed and demonstrated similar function in both kidneys and normal evacuation capabilities. No treatment was undertaken. **B.** IVU 4 years later showed similar morphology although the left ureter might appear more dilated in its proximal part. **C.** ^{99m}TcDPTA diuresis renography at the time of the last IVU, however, still demonstrated nearly identical function of both parenchymas, and evacuation is now severely disturbed.

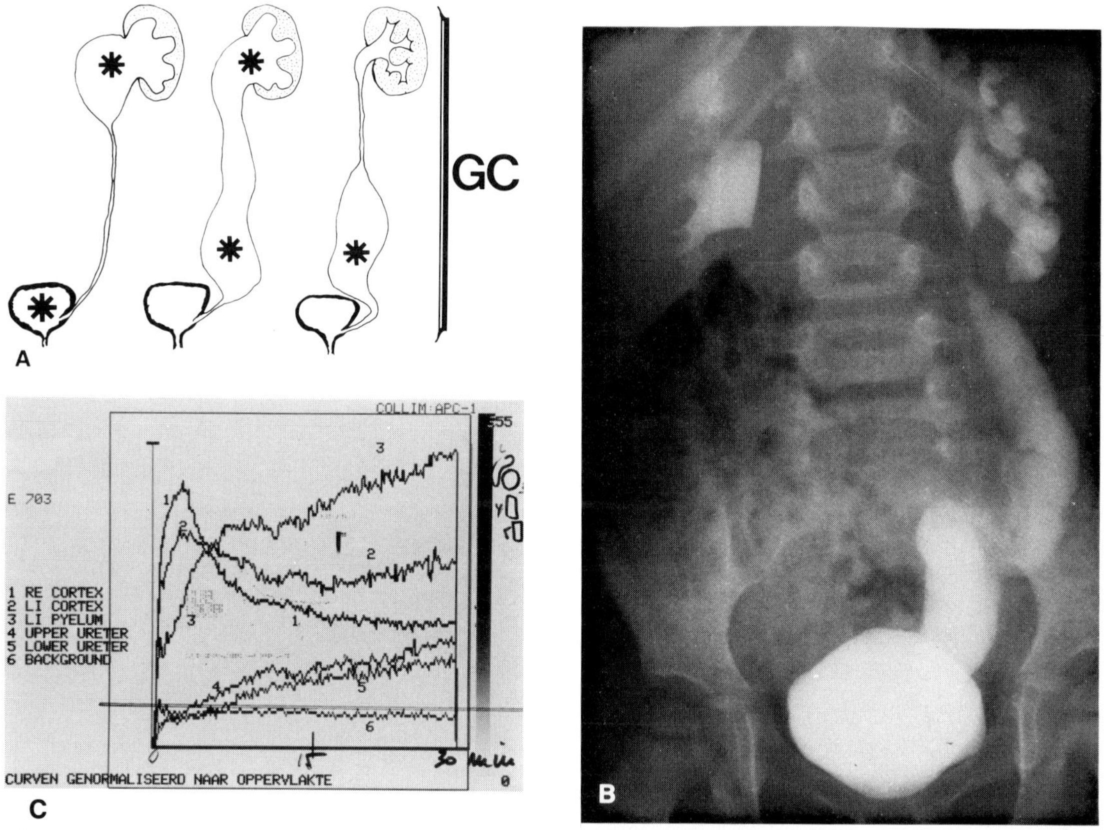

Figure 13–5. **A.** By selecting regions of interest, each parenchyma, renal pelvis, and ureter as well as the bladder can be analyzed separately. GC = Gamma camera. **B.** IVU on a 7-year-old girl with a wide left ureter. The left renal pelvis has nearly normal dimensions. **C.** Diuresis renography. Different regions of interest have been selected: (*1*) right renal cortex, (*2*) left renal cortex, (*3*), left renal pelvis (*4*) left proximal ureter, and (*5*) left distal ureter.

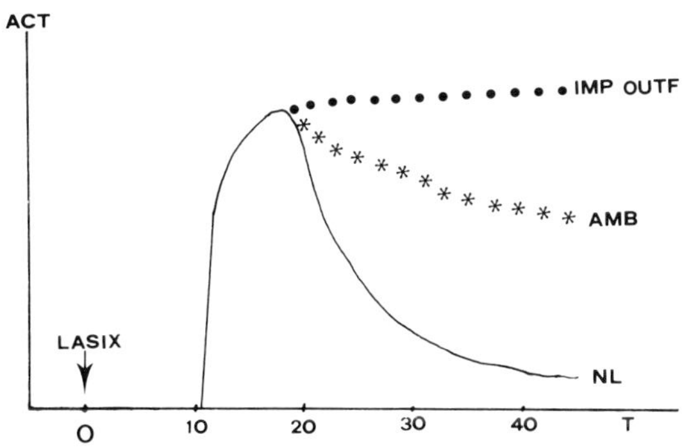

Figure 13–6. The shape of the time-activity curve obtained at diuresis renography can be grossly divided into three groups: *IMP OUTF*–a group of systems probably with a severely impaired outflow. *NL*–a group of systems most likely with a normal outflow. *AMB*–an ambiguous group where outflow is moderately delayed.

upper tracts is related to complications such as infection and lithiasis. Although renal parenchymal function can be maintained for years only to deteriorate with the onset of complications, a conservative attitude in therapeutic management of such cases can be fully justified.

The second type of observed curves represents a group of wide upper tracts in which the excreted radionuclide is accumulated in the kidney over a 20 to 30-minute period, even under high diuresis. Such tracts have a markedly impaired capability to evacuate urine and, with or without reflux, may be associated with normal parenchymal function (Fig. 13–5), impaired distal tubular function (Fig. 13–7), or a more severe renal parenchy-

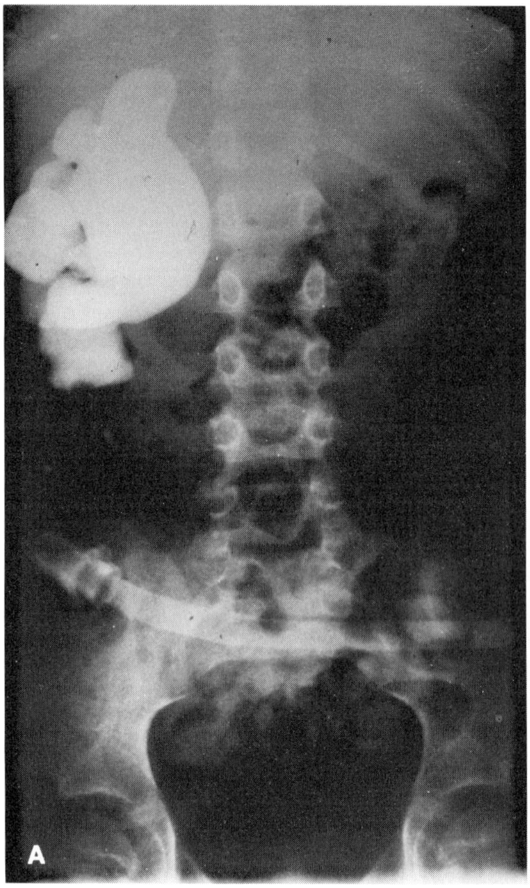

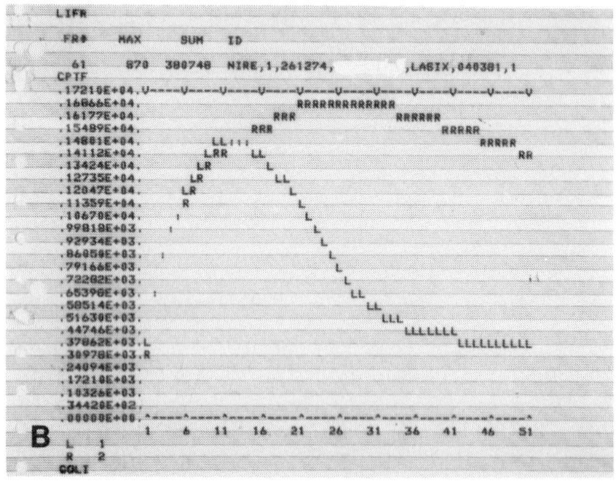

Figure 13–7. **A.** IVU in a 10-year-old boy showing hydronephrosis of the right system (^{131}I-hippuran). **B.** Diuresis renography revealed normal nephron function, although evacuation was severely disturbed. Maximum concentration function was severely disturbed (maximal osmolarity < 500 mosm).

mal dysfunction. An observed partial failure of radionuclide washout thus does not necesarily mean that nephron function is impaired. Some wide upper tracts show impairment of outflow (the "obstructive pattern") by diuresis renography in the presence of normal renal parenchymal function. The fact that insufficiently draining upper tracts associated with urinary stasis do not necessarily have adverse effects on nephron function will arouse even more controversy than it already has. Careful and repeated follow-up examinations, however, can obviate any irrational discussions on 'he clinical definittion of obstruction in these particular cases.

The third, relatively frequent pattern of curves represents an ambiguous type of wide upper urinary tract with moderately delayed urine evacuation. So far, the scope of this ambiguity has not been clearly defined. Some have tried to express numerically the fraction of tract evacuation after 10 or 20 minutes. As a result of this approach, many urologists became confident that they have at their disposal a method of clinical assessment that is reliable simply because of its quantitative implications. It is doubtful, however, that this approach can solve the fundamental problem in question.

When interpreting the results of diuresis renography, the following additional limitations must be considered: (a) The shape of the evacuation curve can be falsely positive for the existence of obstruction depending on the assessed degree of parenchymal functional impairment; the more the parenchymal function is impaired, the less reliably diagnostic is the evacuation curve. (b) In cases of severely impaired parenchymal function with creatinine clearance less than 25 ml/min (adjusted for body weight), the procedure is unreliable and should not be performed. (c) The procedure can yield falsely positive results in upper tracts with high capacity, as

well as in the presence of increased parenchymal transit times, e.g., with polycystic kidneys (Fig. 13–8). (d) False-negative results are obtained, although seldom, in small-capacity but high-pressure upper tracts.

Diuresis renography also has been proposed as a means for evaluating the function of the distal segment of the ureter (Fig. 13–9) on the basis of the idea that although the renal pelvis may have good drainage urine can be transported only to accumulate in a wide distal ureteral segment. It was expected that by tracing the accumulation of urine in, and its evacuation by, the distal ureteral segment, its normal and abnormal function can be distinguished. This idea, however, is illogical; it is impossible for the renal pelvis to continue draining urine into a wide distal ureteral segment that does not evacuate its contents to the bladder at the same flow rate. Accumulation of urine in that segment, certainly occurring with high diuresis, would necessarily be reflected on the evacuation curve of the upper urinary tract.

Despite the above limitations, diuresis renography remains a valuable, noninvasive clinical method for investigating nephron function and upper tract evacuation of urine, especially when combined with DMSA renal scanning. This method appears to be reasonable and justified, at least for following conservatively the important groups of patients who have wide upper tracts but normal urinary washout at high levels of diuresis and those with abnormal urinary washout but normal parenchymal function. The problem continues to exist because diuresis renography is not the gold standard and correlation between washout pattern and intrapelvic pressure is poor.

Based on current knowledge, urologists should be aware of the fact that a clear-cut clinical distinction between an obstructed and a nonobstructed upper urinary tract is impossible and probably unrealistic, and that whatever means we currently have at our disposal can provide data only on some parameters, the value of which will, hopefully, become clear as clinical trials proceed and become reported. On the other hand, it has been shown that normal renal parenchymal function can remain stable over time in the presence of a wide upper tract but no complications, e.g., infections or lithiasis (*19*). In view of this finding, it probably is justified to continue follow-up of those patients with a wide upper tract that drains a normally functioning kidney but has impaired washout on diuresis renography.

Diuresis renography also has introduced the possibility of evaluating patients with both vesicoureteral reflux and impairment of upper tract outflow (*20*). Such a case is illustrated in Figure 13–10. Further studies,

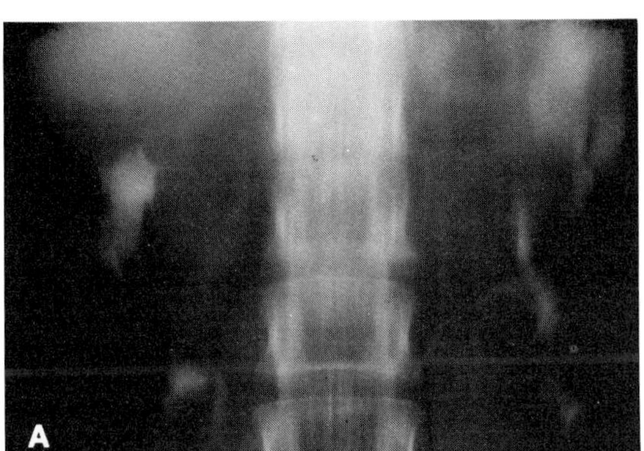

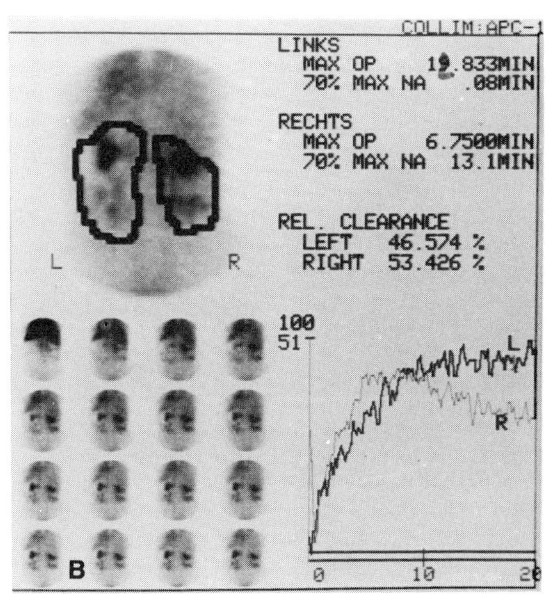

Figure 13–8. **A.** IVU of polycystic kidneys. **B.** Diuresis renography shows falsely impaired outflow due to increased parenchymal transit times.

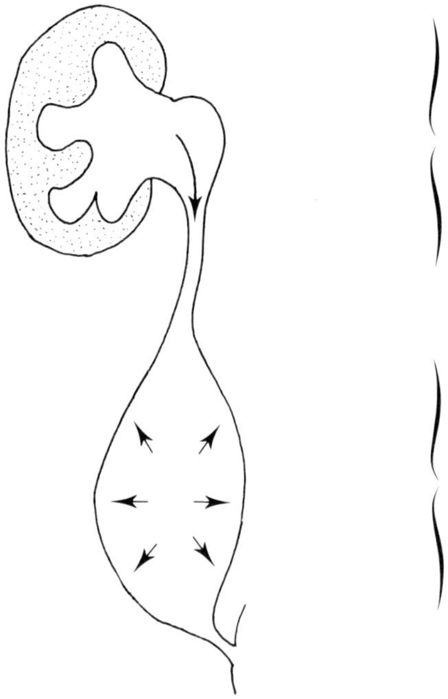

Figure 13–9. Evaluation of the evacuation capabilities at the distal ureter is used in systems where the pelvis and the ureter, or only the ureter, is dilated.

however, are necessary to accurately define the clinical indications based on such testing for reimplanting a refluxing ureter.

When more sophisticated clinical study of a wide upper tract than so far indicated is required, more invasive techniques are available. Percutaneous puncture of the wide system allows quantitative determination of divided renal function, pressures, and pressure–flow measurements. From the practical standpoint, puncture of a wide renal pelvis should not be a problem, as it can be performed routinely after localization of the system by palpation, fluoroscopy, or ultrasound imaging. Retrograde puncture techniques may be necessary for adequate catheter positioning in moderately distended systems (*21*). Complications, particularly infection, do occur but can be avoided by sterile techniques. Two catheters can be placed in a wide system.

Investigation of nephron function is started 1 day after positioning the catheter(s) and focuses on assessment of distal tubular function. The maximum ability of urine concentration is evaluated by the Minirin-Test, performed on the morning after 12 hours of fluid restriction; it is done by measuring the osmolarity of urine samples taken 1, 2, and 4 hours after intranasal administration of 40 μg of desmopressin (or less, depending on body weight) (*15*). A urine osmolarity of 800 mosm/kg water indicates normal concentrating ability, 500 to 800 mosm moderately decreased ability, and 500 mosm or less severely decreased concentrating ability. In some wide systems impairment of distal tubular function may be the only abnormal parameter that indicates a possible threat to renal parenchymal function. It is possible to predict the capability of recovery of impaired renal parenchymal function by short-term evaluation of maximal distal tubular concentrating ability following 2 to 3 weeks of free upper tract outflow.

Pyelostomy tubes allow further information to be obtained concerning the effect of changing urinary inflow rates and bladder volumes on the dynamics of a wide upper urinary tract. The main advantages of such an approach are that no general anesthesia (which may alter upper tract dynamics) is required and that the resistance of the UVJ can be studied without a catheter passing through it. Moreover, fluoroscopic or video techniques allow detailed study of peristalsis and urine evacuation by the tract.

In the past, the idea had been generated that renal parenchymal function can be impaired by continuous or intermittent back-pressure in a wide upper tract system. Investigative techniques have therefore been developed to measure baseline pressures in a wide system and to provoke diuretic inflow rates (*22*). These studies indicate that baseline pressures may not be increased in the presence of a wide system. Apparently a delicate balance exists between urine excretion, back-flow, and evacuation. Urine evacuation in a partially "obstructed" upper system is not achieved by elevation of its baseline pressure. If it becomes clear in a wide system with slightly impaired outflow that the renal parenchyma is in danger, however, other pathogenetic mechanisms for such danger must be investigated.

It also has been advocated that a wide upper tract can be further evaluated by measuring its maximal pressure at the maximal diuresis the kidney can produce. Such maximal diuresis can be provoked by in-

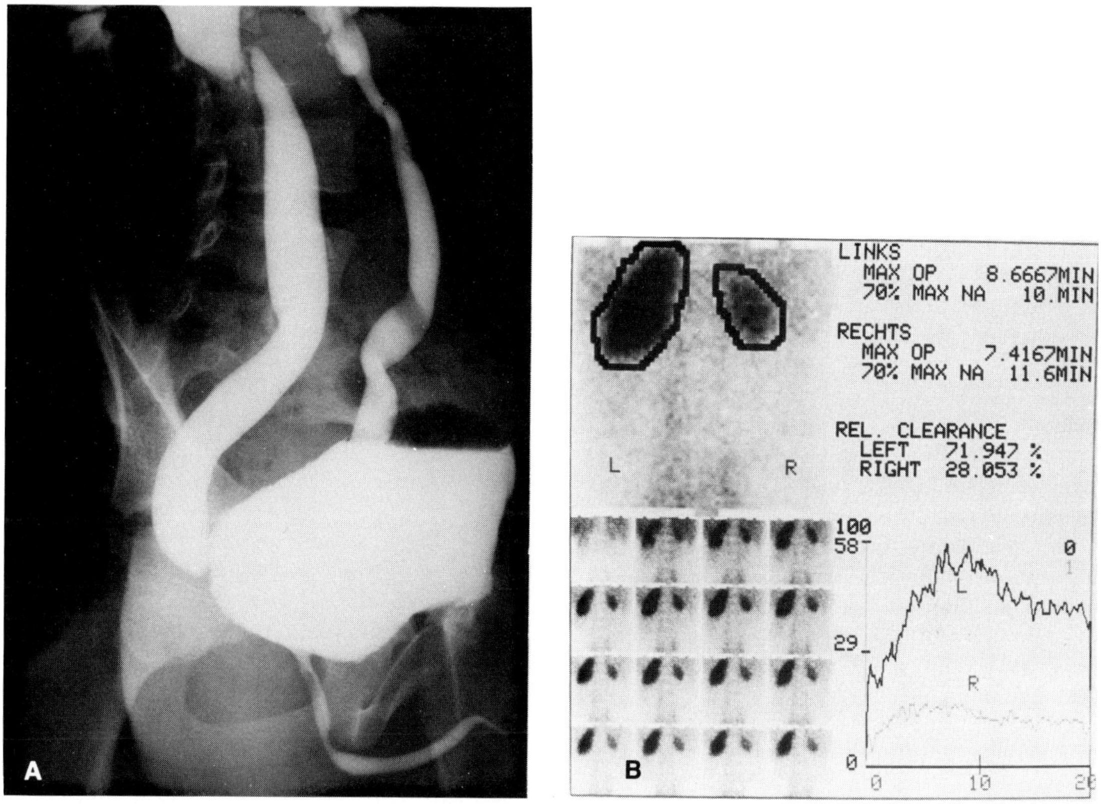

Figure 13–10. A. Cystography in a 16-year-old girl showing bilateral refluxing systems. **B.** Diuresis renogrpahy has made with an open bladder catheter. Relative parenchymal function (left/right) is 72/28. Evacuation toward the bladder of the good functioning left system is severely disturbed.

travenous administration of a 5 percent glucose solution plus furosemide 0.5 mg/kg body weight. Short-term pressure peaks during the test may indicate the nephron functional changes have been induced or that the renal parenchymal function is further decreased. Moreover, during osmotic diuresis the pressure increases in both the normal and the wide upper tracts. Because some researchers did not find these differences, large series and long follow-up studies need to be done.

In our ongoing studies, pressure in the renal pelvis and bladder are continuously recorded (Fig. 13–11) in combination with diuresis renography. The bladder is allowed to fill and empty two or three times during the examination, and the patient is changed from the supine to the sitting position. The pressures measured under these circum-

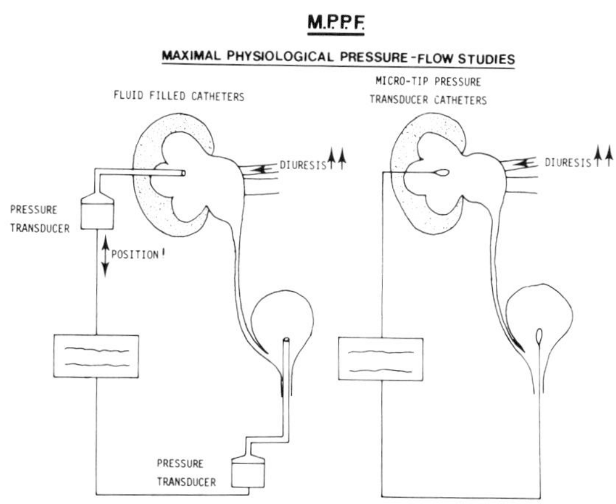

Figure 13–11. Graphic representation of the method used for MPPF measurements.

stances depend on the intraluminal volume, the passive mural properties of the wide system, and the active properties of its muscularis (*7*). The intraluminal volume depends on nephron function and outflow capabilities; urine production by nephrons usually varies between 7 and 10 ml/min. Viscoelastic properties have been investigated extensively in the detrusor (*23,24*) and the upper tract wall (*25*). They implicate time and rate dependence on the pressure-volume relation. A slowly increasing volume provokes only a minimal increase of pressure, as is also seen in the bladder during cystometry. Stretch of the tissue induces changes in its initial length; the tissue thus becomes longer by stretching, and still unknown metabolic processes are required to reestablish its original architectural characteristics. Smooth muscle contractility is not decreased in a large group of wide systems. The force that is generated by the smooth muscle, however, is not reflected in the intraluminal pressure. This concept can be understood by applying Laplace's equation. In some systems, however, tissue contractility is lowered because of excessive stretching beyond the optimal limit. Infection and probably the duration of dilation also seriously interfere with contractility.

Compliance, which denotes the volume–pressure relation ($\Delta V/\Delta P$), is determined by all the above factors; neglect of compliance may result in oversimplified and misleading statements. Pressures measured under different conditions do not allow clear distinction between the "obstructed" and "nonobstructed" systems; even completely closed systems sometimes do not show a pressure increase (*7*). Some investigators have demonstrated that infected systems appear to be incapable of building up high pressures.

The major disadvantages of the maximal physiologic pressure–flow test are that it is time-consuming and requires complicated equipment. Moreover, problems may arise in severely malfunctioning kidneys that are unable to produce large amounts of urine but that can recover, especially in children. All that can be asked of the test under these conditions is to reveal the maximal pressure that can be developed by the malfunctioning kidney. We do not know what that parameter might indicate in regard, to outflow characteristics and recoverability. In these circumstances a perfusion technique can be applied (*2*); an arbitrary perfusion rate of 10 ml/min is used to test some aspects of outflow capability.

Aside from the discussion of the clinical significance of the test, some basic biologic (*7*) and nonbiologic (*26*) sources of error must be known and considered. All pressure measurements are performed so that there is a minimal possibility of error. Pressures in the renal pelvis and bladder can be measured using microtip transducers or fluid-filled tubes that are connected to external transducers. The major advantage of the former is that pressure measurement is independent of the position of the renal pelvis or bladder. When fluid-filled tubes are used, it is necessary to fluoroscopically control and equalize the end of the tube and the external transducer for the renal pelvis and the bladder. Simplified techniques (*2*), in which only one transducer is used to measure pressures in both renal pelvis and bladder, are a possible source of error. Results obtained by such methods must be interpreted with caution. Aside from the influence of needle type, flow rate, and perfusate, pressure depends on the height of the fluid column in the wide system above the level of the external transducer. Changes of several centimeters of water are therefore to be taken into account.

Nonbiologic factors (*26*) can cause pressure changes of up to 55 cm H_2O, which would seriously interfere with the proposed criteria. It has been proposed that relative pressures (pressure in the renal pelvis minus detrusor pressure) of up to 15 cm H_2O indicate normal outflow, those between 15 and 22 cm H_2O are equivocal, and those more than 22 cm H_2O indicate obstruction.

Biologic variables of the system also introduce other problems related to its geometry, viscoelasticity, and contractility, as well as in relation to bladder physiology. The results of carefully performed and technically reliable investigations must be compared to results of refined parenchymal function tests and other evacuation parameters such as those obtained by diuresis renography and dynamic excretory urography. There is evidence that high pressures obtained during perfusion with 10 ml/min indicate a severely impaired outflow although these elevated pressures can be related to a "nonobstructed" diuresis renography pattern. Nevertheless, negative and ambiguous pressures may be found in wide systems that evacuate poorly or even not at all. Although useful additive information might be obtained in some limited indications, the pressure–flow technique by no means allows characterization of a wide system definitively as "obstructed" or "nonobstructed."

In addition to the above-mentioned limitations, the bladder influences outflow from the ureter into the lower tract (*9*). Increased detrusor pressure, bladder wall stretch, and detrusor contractions severely interfere with the resistance at the ureterovesical junction. Although simplicity is attractive, the present state of knowledge does not allow us to make simple and practical classifications of the wide upper tract. For this reason and because none of the above-mentioned techniques can provide parameters on the basis of which clear-cut distinction between "obstructed" and "nonobstructed" systems can be made, the term "obstruction" is better put to rest until long-term follow-up studies on carefully investigated wide upper tracts become available. As upper tract symptoms can occur in all wide systems (with and without abnormal outflow parameters), the surgical indication should be based on alterations in parenchymal function associated with impaired outflow. Currently, there is no single parameter than can be used as a gold standard for obstruction.

REFERENCES

1. Smith, E., Cussen, L., Glenn, J., Hendren, W., Jeff, R., Tanagho, E., Whitaker, R., and Woodard, J.: International nomenclature for the large ureter. In *International Pediatric Urology*. Alan R. Liss, New York, 1977.
2. Whitaker, R.: Some observations and theories on the wide ureter and hydronephrosis. *Br. J. Urol.* 47:377, 1975.
3. Backlund, L., and Reuterskiold, A. G.: The abnormal ureter in children. I. Perfusion studies on the wide non-refluxing ureter. *Scand. J. Urol. Nephrol.* 3:219, 1969.
4. Struthers, N. W.: The role of manometry in the investigation of pelvi-ureteral junction. *Br. J. Urol.* 41:129, 1969.
5. Hanna, M. K., and Edwards, L.: Pressure perfusion studies of the abnormal uretero-vesical junction. *Br. J. Urol.* 44:331, 1972.
6. Whitfield, H. N., Harrison, N. W., Sherwood, T., and Williams, D. I.: Upper urinary tract obstruction: pressure flow studies in children. *Br. J. Urol.* 48:427, 1976.
7. Coolsaet, B. L. R. A., Griffiths, D. J., Van Mastrigt, R., and van Duyl, W. A.: Urodynamic investigation of the wide ureter. *J. Urol.* 124:290, 1980.
8. Coolsaet, B. L. R. A., Urodynamic approach of the upper urinary tract by percutaneous puncture nephrostomy. *Acta Urol. Belg.* 51:458, 1983.
9. Coolsaet, B. L. R. A., van Venrooij, G. E. P. M., and Blok, C.: Detrusor pressure versus wall stress in relation to ureterovesical resistance. *Neurourol. Urodynam.* 1:105, 1982.
10. Whitfield, H. N., Britton, K. E., Hendry, W. F., and Wickham, J. E. A.: Furosemide intravenous urography in the diagnosis of pelvi-ureteric junction obstruction. *Br. J. Urol.* 51:445, 1979.
11. Enlander, D., Weber, P. M., and dos Remedios, L. V.: Renal cortical imaging in 35 patients: superior quality with ^{99m}Tc-DSMA. *J. Nucl. Med.* 15:743, 1979.
12. Daly, M. J., Jones, W., and Rudd, T. G., Differential renal function using technetium^{99m} dimercaptosuccinic acid (DMSA): in vitro correlation. *J. Nucl. Med.* 20:63, 1979.
13. Kawamura, J., Hosokawa, S., Yoshiba, O., Fujita, T., Ishii, Y., and Torizuka, K.: Validity of ^{99m}Tc DMSA renal uptake for an assessment of individual kidney function. *J. Urol.* 119:305, 1978.
14. Kinn, A.: *Urodynamics and renal function in hydronephrosis*. Thesis, Stockholm, 1982.
15. Nilsson, S., Aurell, M., and Bratt, C.G.: Maximum urinary concentration ability in patients with idiopathic hydronephrosis. *Br. J. Urol.* 51:432, 1979.
16. O'Reilly, P. H., Testa, H. J., Lawson, R. S., Farrar, D. J., and Charlton Edwards, E.: Diuresis renography in equivocal urinary tract obstruction. *Br. J. Urol.* 50:76, 1978.
17. Koff, S. A., Thrall, J. H., and Keyes, J. W.: Diuretic radionuclide urography: a non-invasive method for evaluating nephroureteral dilation. *J. Urol.* 122:451, 1979.
18. Whitfield, H. N., Britton, K. E., Hendry, W. F., Nimmon, C. C., and Wickham, J. E. A.: The distinction between obstructive uropathy and nephropathy by radioisotope transit times. *Br. J. Uro.* 50:433, 1978.
19. Bratt, C. G., Aurell, M., and Nilsson, S.: Renal function in patients with hydronephrosis. *Br. J. Urol.* 49:249, 1977.
20. Kesavam, P., and Fowler, R.: Vesicoureteric reflux and ureterovesical obstruction. *Urology* 10:105, 1977.
21. Hunter, P. T., Hawkins, I. F., Finlayson, B., Nanni, G., and Senior, D.: Hawkins-Hunter retrograde transcutaneous nephrostomy: a new technique. *Urology* 6:583, 1983.
22. Djurhuus, J. C., and Stage, P.: Percutaneous intrapelvic pressure registration in hydronephrosis during diuresis. *Acta Chir. Scand.* 147:43, 1976.
23. Coolsaet, B. L. R. A., Van Duyl, W. A., Van Mas-

trigt, R., and van der Zwart, A.: Viscoelastic properties of the bladder wall. *Urol. Int.* 30:16, 1975.
24. Coolsaet, B. L. R. A.: *Stepwise cystometry*. Thesis, Rotterdam, 1975.
25. Weiss, R. M., Bassett, A. L., and Hoffman, B. F.: Dynamic length-tension curves of cat ureter. *Am. J. Physiol.* 222:388, 1971.
26. Toguri, A., and Fourmier, G.: Factors influencing the pressure flow perfusion system. *J. Urol.* 127:1021, 1982.

Section Three
Urodynamic and Neurourologic Disorders

14

Voiding Dysfunctions in Children: Diagnosis and Management

DAVID M. BARRETT, M.D., AND JEFFREY R. WOODSIDE, M.D.

A wide spectrum of voiding abnormalities is seen in pediatric patients (*1*). Urologists, pediatricians, and primary care clinicians are charged with the responsibility of defining the characteristics of voiding problems in children early so as to prevent subtle but potentially significant deterioration of the bladder and upper urinary tract. Certain congenital defects that are obvious at birth, e.g., myelodysplasia and urogenital sinus anomalies, signal the potential for an underlying voiding dysfunction (*2*). In such instances it has been shown that early assessment of the neurourologic status allows placement of the patient into either a therapeutic or a regular surveillance group (*3,4*). Such a program greatly decreases the likelihood of insidious vesical deterioration and upper tract disease as the child matures. (*5*).

Unfortunately, not all children with a potential voiding problem can be identified early. Many patients have no apparent problem with urination. Thus parents and physicians are unable to note subtle changes in voiding function until retention, marked incontinence, or urosepsis develops. Children are typically poor historians and are unlikely to communicate a subtle voiding problem to their parents or physicians. Moreover, because they may not perceive changes in voiding as abnormal, significant micturitional abnormalities may remain undetected for some time. This situation does not mean that all children with mundane alterations in urination require extensive neurourologic evaluation. Awareness of the potential for serious urinary tract disease, however, does mandate the need for a thorough understanding of the peculiarities of voiding dysfunction in children. Knowledge of their normal and abnormal physiology of micturition, the indications and reliability of diagnostic testing modalities, and current concepts of therapeutic alternatives is necessary for all practitioners caring for children with a voiding dysfunction. The symptoms and conditions indicating further investigations of a child's neurourologic status are listed below. However, clinical experience and intuition must also be included as important ingredients in the decision-making process as to which child should undergo further investigation of vesicourethral function (Table 14–1).

It is the goal of this chapter to outline a practical approach to the problem of vesicourethral dysfunction in children (Table 14–1). Diagnostic modalities are presented with references to their relative importance and usefulness in the pediatric age group. Certain conditions common to vesicourethral dysfunction in children are discussed and the nuances relative to their diagnosis and management presented.

NORMAL VESICOURETHRAL MATURATION

In the newborn urination is regulated by a relatively simple spinal reflex mechanism (*6*). When the bladder becomes distended by urine, stretch receptors in the detrusor evoke

Table 14–1. Indications for Pediatric Neurourologic Investigation

Urosepsis
Retention
Hematuria
Dripping incontinence
Overt neurologic disease (including trauma)
Painful urination
Straining or squatting during urination
Secondary enuresis
Frequency and urgency incontinence
Encopresis
Polydipsia
Urogenital sinus abnormality

sensory impulses that are conducted by autonomic afferent fibers to the spinal cord where they evoke autonomic efferent stimuli that cause contraction of the detrusor. This spinal reflex mechanism is coordinated with simultaneous relaxation of the urethral striated sphincter, which probably requires an intact brainstem (*7–12*). In young children the spinal reflex mechanism lacks the inhibitory influence of cephalic areas above the brainstem. Although there is little volitional control of voiding, the functions of urine storage and continence are maintained, and it is the relative state of bladder fullness and bladder wall distension that triggers detrusor contraction and subsequent bladder emptying.

Goellner *et al.* (*13*) studied the various aspects of micturition during the first 3 years of life. They pointed out that most children sleep approximately two-thirds of the day, and that almost half of the voidings occur during the sleep period. During the first 12 months the number of voidings averages 20 per day. As the child matures the frequency of voiding decreases but the volume increases to approximately four times that of the newborn. It has been suggested that the increase in voided volume and the decrease in voiding frequency are a function of a subtle assumption by central areas above the brainstem of neurologic control of urination (*14*). Physiologic studies, however, indicate that a change in the relation between voided volume and frequency during the first 3 years of life is related more to the fluid volume ingested and the changing functional volume of the child's bladder.

It seems reasonable to conclude that both factors influence enhanced urinary control. By the end of the third year most children are able to have some conscious control over urination. Nonetheless, enuresis and daytime accidents do occur. Bladder volume is adequate and central urinary control is complete in most individuals at age 4 years. The degree of neuromuscular maturation that occurs is most dramatic in the assumption of voluntary control of the urethral striated sphincter and detrusor contractility. Both of these functions are related to neurologic organization of centers in the midbrain and cerebral cortex. As in adults, the brainstem must be intact for normal coordinated voiding to occur. There is no question that there are some neurologically normal children who have a temporary delay in the maturation of these functions and may well exhibit significant voiding dysfunction at the ages of 4, 5, or 6 years but eventually "outgrow" their problem. If one aspect of maturation lags behind the others, discoordinated voiding patterns may occur.

PEDIATRIC NEUROUROLOGIC EVALUATION

History and Physical Examination

For all practical purposes, no neurourologic tests are ordered for a child with suspected vesicourethral dysfunction without first obtaining a complete history and performing a physical examination. A history suggestive of subtle disease of the central nervous system, e.g., a traumatic birth, neonatal anoxia, a convulsive disorder, and head or back trauma, may explain many voiding abnormalities despite the absence of overt neurologic disease.

Neurourologic Evaluation. The neurourologic evaluation includes the history, physical examination, neurologic examination, urine studies, renal function studies (including isotopes), ultrasonography, voiding cystourethrography, excretory urography, cystoscopy, and urodynamic evaluation.

During the initial interview with the child and parents, an assessment is made of the fluid ingested during a 24-hour period. Historical approximations of this volume may be misleading, however; and when it is clinically related to a voiding problem such as diabetes insipidus, the child or parents are asked to bring a documented list of the volumes ingested and voided.

The voiding history itself may well hold the clue as to which of the various available tests offer the best opportunity for an accurate and cost-effective diagnosis. Parents of infants are questioned about their observations of diaper wetness, number of diapers used, diaper rash, dripping loss of urine, leakage while crying, stream characteristics, straining during urination, and apparent pain or discomfort when voiding. The older child may be asked questions about painful urination, urgency, frequency, and unusual voiding positions, although corroboration from parents is often necessary for information related to enuresis, soiling, and the problem of malodor.

Aside from the potential damage to the bladder and upper tracts, vesicourethral dysfunction in children, especially incontinence, may have a dramatic impact on the psychological and sociologic adjustment of the child or the family as a unit. During the initial interview, an assessment is made about the impact of the "voiding problem" on the child and parents. This information is important not only diagnostically, because psychogenic voiding dysfunction must be excluded, but also therapeutically, because the eventual selection of therapeutic alternatives depends greatly on the psychosocial status of the patient and the family.

The physical examination is directed to those conditions that may foretell underlying neurologic disease or suggest the more immediate problem of bladder overdistension and hydronephrosis. In the absence of overt neurologic problems, the examination is first directed toward the integrity of the spinal column by looking for clues to vertebral dysrhaphism. Hairy patches, depressions, or dimples over the spine or sacral area may indicate underlying dysrhaphism or sacral agenesis. A rough estimate of intact reflex arc activity can be evaluated by evoking deep tendon reflexes in the lower extremities. The sensory neurologic integrity of the abdomen, perineum, and lower extremities can also be roughly estimated. Further neurologic assessment is left to the pediatric neurologist.

After the initial history and physical examination have been completed and urinalysis obtained, the severity of the "voiding problem" must be determined. Does it require further evaluation, or can the child and parents be reassured that the symptoms are normal variants and there is no threat to the unseen portions of the urinary tract? Clinical judgment becomes the most important indicator at this time. Children with the conditions listed earlier are evaluated further. However, for those children who cannot be placed in a particular category, one must weigh the relative costs and degree of invasiveness involved in additional tests against the risk of failing to diagnose a potentially serious vesicourethral abnormality.

Urodynamics

In many children a satisfactory evaluation for the cause of a voiding abnormality can be made with various combinations of uroradiographic studies and cystoscopy. The voiding cystourethrogram is most efficient for evaluating the detrusor and bladder outlet. Vesicoureteral reflux, ureterocele, impaired urethral valves, ureteral ectopy, and fistula may be related to voiding difficulties and must be excluded before an abnormality of intrinsic vesicourethral function can be implicated as the cause of a particular voiding problem. It is not unusual to have a combination of abnormalities (e.g., vesicoureteral reflux and detrusor hyperreflexia) that simultaneously produce an abnormal voiding symptom (*15*).

Once structural abnormalities have been excluded, a urodynamic evaluation is considered to more accurately define voiding dynamics (*16*) (Table 14–2). The goals of urodynamic testing in children are to define the nature and cause of voiding symptoms, help determine the best mode of therapy, and provide a means to assess therapeutic progress (*17*). The urodynamic parameters available to most urologists (Table 14–3) include uroflowmetry, cystometry, pelvic floor skeletal muscle electromyography (EMG), urethral pressure profilometry, and combined studies (i.e., simultaneous measurement of various combinations of the aforementioned studies with or without abdominal pressure recordings). For all practical purposes, videourodynamics, in which

Table 14–2. Classification of Voiding Dysfunction: Urodynamic Findings

Failure to store
Detrusor abnormality
Hyperreflexia
Decreased compliance
Sphincter abnormality
Areflexia: internal, external, both
Increased compliance: patulous
Decreased compliance: rigid, scarred
Combined detrusor and sphincteric abnormality
Failure to empty
Detrusor abnormality
Areflexia
Increased compliance
Sphincter abnormality
Dyssynergia: smooth, striated, both
Decreased compliance: mechanical obstruction
Combined detrusor and sphincter abnormality

multiple voiding parameters are recorded in sequence with voiding cystourethrography, are only occasionally indicated in children. Because the necessary equipment is rarely available outside the medical center environment (*18*), only the most complex voiding disorders in children require true videourodynamic assessment (Table 14–3).

The more complex a urodynamic test is, the more its degree of invasiveness tends to become. Invasiveness increases the possibility of alienating children, thus introducing an unacceptable degree of artifact into the study. Therefore it is generally best to begin the urodynamic testing sequence with a minimally invasive examination, yet one that produces reliable data relative to the abnormal voiding symptom. At the beginning, the examiner asks two basic questions: "What do we want to know?" Do the symptoms suggest a detrusor or an outlet abnormality, or could they be the result of both?

Table 14–3. Urodynamic Tests

Detrusor function
Cystometry
Uroflowmetry
Combined studies
Videourodynamics
Outlet function
Uroflow
Electromyography (EMG)
Urethral profilometry
Combined studies
Videourodynamics.

Sedation, e.g., by intramuscular meperidine 1 mg/kg, has been proposed to decrease discomfort and anxiety during urodynamic testing of some patients (*19*). Others reported reliable results in children using nitrous oxide anesthesia (*20*).

Uroflowmetry. Regardless of the methodology used, which depends on the preferences of the urologist and the particulars of the case, uroflowmetry remains a cost-effective means for evaluating vesicourethral dysfunction in children. Furthermore, no other urodynamic test allows assessment of the lower urinary tract during the natural act of voiding with the accuracy, reproducibility, and lack of invasiveness of the uroflowmetric study. Modern urodynamic methods can provide for conversion of the dynamics of the voided stream into an electrical signal that can be plotted on a strip chart recorder (*21*). This technique produces a permanent record of voiding that can be used to evaluate stream characteristics, measure voided volume, and calculate mean and peak flow rates in milliliters per second. Many of the new uroflow recording devices calculate as well as plot the data (Fig. 14–1.)

When dealing with children, patient cooperation is essential for recording any urodynamic parameter; because uroflowmetry is the least invasive of all urodynamic tests, many urologists prefer to use it as the initial screening tool. It of course requires that the child be old enough to follow instructions and void in a typical manner. This prerequisite practically eliminates children younger than 4 to 5 years of age. If the recorded uroflow is normal, subsequent, more invasive urodynamic testing may not be necessary. On the other hand, when it is abnormal, additional tests may be chosen to focus on the specific voiding abnormality (Table 14–3).

It is not infrequent that the volume voided by a child under study is insufficient for accurate assessment of rate and pattern of urinary flow. Despite some degree of invasiveness, an accurate test may be obtained in such cases by filling the bladder to the point of comfortable fullness with body-temperature sterile water through a small catheter (*22*); the catheter is then removed, and the child is instructed to void. An accurate estimate of

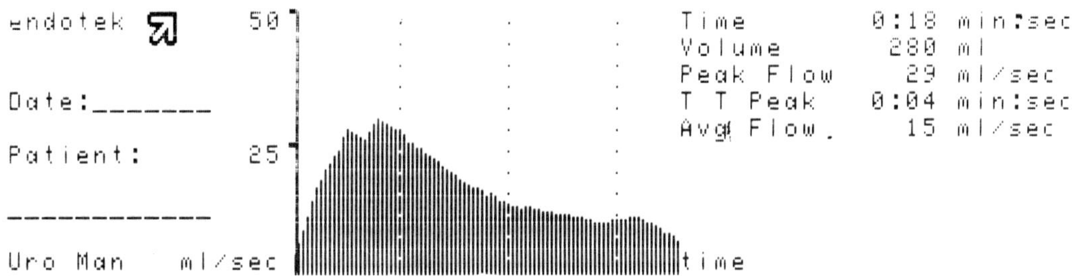

Figure 14–1. Sample record from a uroflow device.

residual volume can also be obtained by subtracting the voided volume from the volume instilled in the bladder.

Many urologists prefer to record pelvic floor or abdominal striated muscle activitity by EMG during uroflowmetry. This method requires placing electrodes on or in muscles of the perineum and abdominal wall (*26*). Normal micturition in the absence of pelvic floor EMG activity confirms relaxation of the urethral striated sphincter during detrusor contraction (Fig. 14–2). A lack of coordination of detrusor contraction and urethral striated sphincter relaxation is manifested by an interrupted flow pattern, with corresponding burst of EMG activity (Fig. 14–3). Straining to void produces concomitant contractions in abdominal and perineal skeletal muscles that may or may not produce significant outflow obstruction; when obstruction occurs, the flow rate is decreased and the EMG activity increases.

Cystometry. Although moderately invasive and dependent on the child's cooperation, cystometry can provide enlightening information on detrusor contractility and compliance (*27*). Each investigator has preferences regarding the age of the child to be investigated, the size of the catheter, the infusion medium, the rate of filling, and the

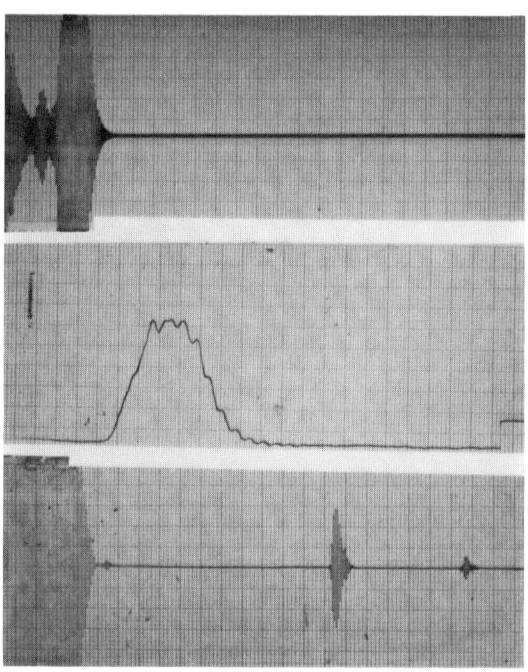

Figure 14–2. Uroflow rate with abdominal wall EMG (*top*) and urethral sphincter EMG (*bottom*). Flow rate is normal, with a peak rate of 30 ml/s; scale is 0 to 50 ml/s. Abdominal wall and striated urethral sphincter appropriately relax during voiding.

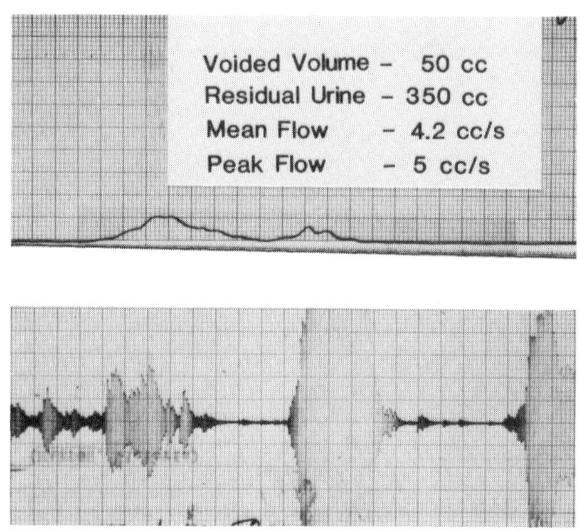

Figure 14–3. Uroflow rate with urethral sphincter EMG. Interrupted flow pattern with EMG activity during voiding indicates intermittent urethral sphincter closure; the result is incomplete voiding with excessive residual volume.

need for simultaneous EMG recording (*28*). The amount of information obtained from childhood cystometry is directly related to the degree of interest and care directed to the test by the clinician. More so than with adults, childhood cystometry requires a gentle hand and the ability to abate the fears of the child during the testing sequence. Extremely young children who undergo cystometry may be surprisingly cooperative, especially if there are associated neurologic deficits; however, others may require sedation or even light general anesthesia (Fig. 14–4).

Many younger children, especially boys, require the use of small intraurethral catheters (5–8F) to infuse the bladder during cystometry. When water is used as a testing medium, larger tubes are preferred so as to decrease the erroneous pressure increases that occur during moderate infusion rates (5–100 ml water/min). Alternatively, carbon dioxide may be used conveniently without fear of false pressure increases, even at high infusion rates. However, one should be aware of the alteration in detrusor compliance as the infusion rate is increased (Fig. 14–5). Infusion rates higher than 100 ml of water or carbon dioxide per minute are unphysiologic and produce a recording that may reflect a significant decrease in detrusor compliance. When testing for the possibility of detrusor instability, higher infusion rates may be used advantageously to provoke what may otherwise be an undetected hyperreflexic detrusor contraction (Fig. 14–6). On the other hand, infusion rates that are too high and extremely unphysiologic may induce a detrusor contraction that ordinarily would not be seen during the child's normal voiding sequence. It is especially true in children less than 4 years of age, when the inhibitory mechanism of micturition has not completely matured. Therefore the interpre-

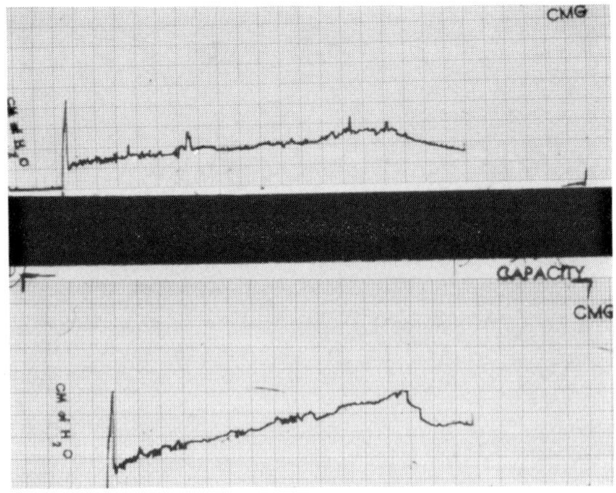

Figure 14–5. CMG demonstrating artifactual changes in detrusor compliance by varying the infusion rate: 100 ml/min (*top*) and 200 ml/min (*bottom*).

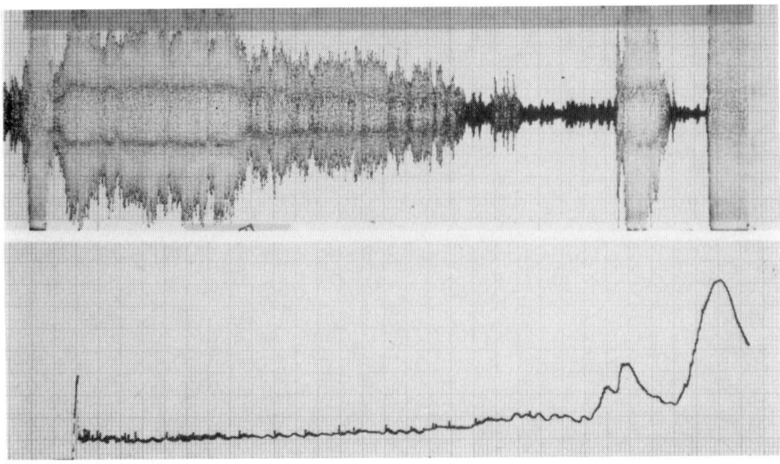

Figure 14–4. Normal cystometrogram (CMG)–EMG in a 12-year-old girl. The tonus limb reflects normal compliance, and EMG activity is noted to decrease during detrusor contractions that are under voluntary control. ECG patch electrodes were used to record EMG activity.

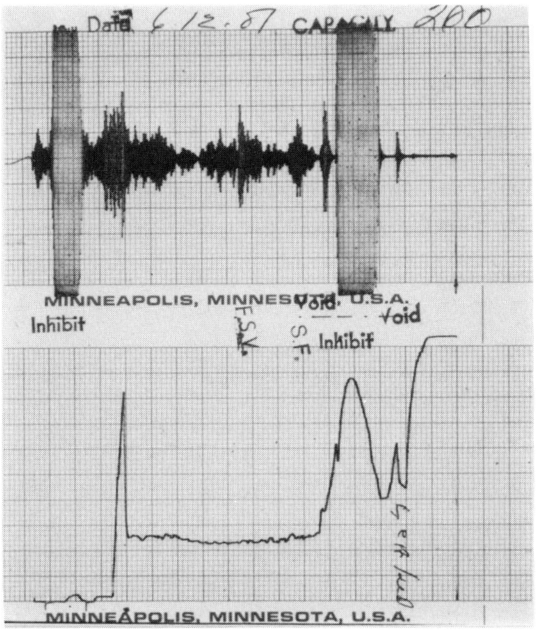

Figure 14–6. CMG–EMG in a 9-year-old girl who complained of urgency and urgency incontinence. A strong detrusor contraction is seen during carbon dioxide infusion at 100 ml/min. She had decreased ability to suppress this contraction, although the external sphincter contracted appropriately in an attempt to block it.

tation of cystometry data must take into account all such variables, and care must be taken not to produce the extreme unphysiologic conditions that may produce data that are overinterpreted and thus lead to erroneous conclusions regarding vesicourethral dysfunction (*29*).

At times during cystometry it may be unclear as to whether an increase in intravesical pressure is related to a "true" detrusor contraction or transmitted from increases in intraabdominal pressure during straining. Measurement of the intraabdominal pressure through a closed catheter system placed in the rectum may clarify this source of artifact. Again, more invasiveness is required, and additional pressure recording equipment is necessary. However, most modern urodynamic recording devices provide the capability of simultaneously measuring rectal pressure, bladder pressure, and subtracted detrusor pressure (bladder pressure minus rectal pressure).

Urethral Pressure Profile. Static urethral pressure profilometry has only limited use in pediatric urodynamic testing. It was devised to assess the status of the bladder outlet and offer information relative to the inherent resistance of the continence mechanism. Its drawback centers on evaluation of tissues when they are static and equating this information to their function during the dynamics of voiding. In most situations, information relative to the continence mechanism (combined smooth and skeletal muscle sphincters) can be obtained more accurately from other urodynamic tests or combinations thereof.

Urethral pressure profile measurement has occasionally been useful for following the function of artificial sphincter occlusive cuff pressures; however, radiographic studies are usually more diagnostic when there is a sphincter malfunction.

Sphincter Electromyography. The term "electromyography" has been used loosely relative to urodynamic testing. The electrical activity in striated muscles of the pelvic floor can be measured in two forms. The raw form is known as classic EMG and is basically a study of the action potentials of skeletal muscle. The other form of EMG is a result of a counted or integrated electrical signal derived from several muscle bundles and is best classified as a kinesiologic measurement (*30*). Raw EMG requires the introduction of fine needles or wire electrodes directly into the muscle of the external sphincter. With the proper recording equipment, action potentials from the muscle may be converted to an auditory or a visual signal. Variations in the action potentials allow accurate determination of the denervation characteristics within the muscle. In addition, the presence or absence of electrical activity in the sphincter muscle during a detrusor contraction can be assessed. In essence, it is the latter characteristic of EMG that is most useful to urodynamic testing. The absence of EMG activity during voiding implies neurologic coordination, but EMG activity noted during voiding is typical or uncoordination between the detrusor muscle and the sphincter muscle and is classically known as sphincter–detrusor dyssynergia. In most urodynamic settings, only the presence or absence of EMG activity is important to exclude the possibility of sphincter–detrusor dyssynergia. In pediatric urodynamics, accurate recording of EMG activity in pelvic floor skeletal muscles has been reliably produced using surface electrodes such as the patch electrocardiogram (ECG) electrodes that may be pasted on the skin overlying the perineal skeletal muscles (Fig. 14–7). Not only is invasiveness reduced, but the reliability of recording electrical activity in the muscles has been shown to be accurate. This type of electrical activity measurement can easily be recorded on a strip chart recorder and combined with other urodynamic testing modalities such as cystometry or uroflowmetry.

Combined Studies. During the initial screening urodynamic investigation, it may not be clear whether an obvious voiding defect is the result of a detrusor contractility abnormality or an outlet abnormality. A combination study of simultaneous cystometry (with or without rectal pressure measurement), uroflowmetry, and EMG is ideally suited to better define the voiding abnormality (*31*). Children who are candidates for this relatively invasive test are those who fail to completely empty or those with interrupted voiding thought to be related to sphincter–detrusor dyssynergia. From the information gained from this study, a rough calculation of outflow resistance can be made when voiding pressure is compared to peak flow rate (Fig. 14–8).

Cooperation from the child is necessary during combined studies, as considerable manipulation is necessary to set up for such testing (*32*); EMG electrodes must be placed on the perineum or abdominal musculature, rectal pressure catheters must be inserted, and one or two urethral catheters must be placed for the infusion of fluid and the recording of pressure. For a combined study, one has the option of inserting one catheter through which the water medium is infused and intravesical pressure is recorded. However, experience has shown that it is convenient to insert into the bladder a small 4F or 5F polyethylene feeding tube through which pressure is measured, followed by an 8F catheter through which the water medium is instilled into the bladder. Prior to recording the voiding pressures, the 8F catheter is removed, allowing easy voiding around the

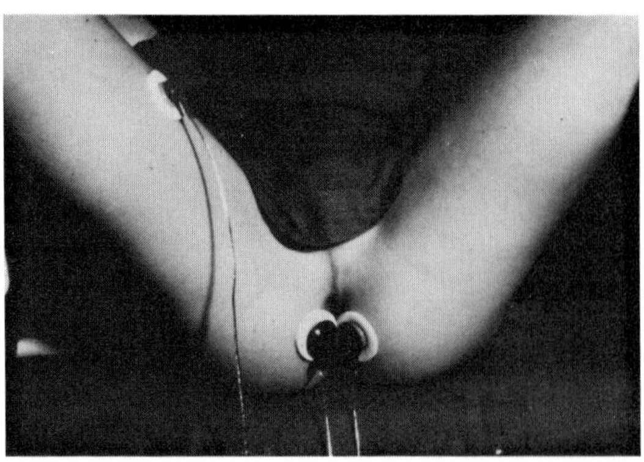

Figure 14–7. Placement of perineal ECG electrodes used to record electrical activity in pelvic floor skeletal muscles during urodynamic testing. Electrode on the thigh serves as a ground. (From Barrett, D. M.: Electromyography: the practical approach. In Barrett, D.M., and Wein, A. J. [eds.], *Controversies in Neuro-urology.* Churchill Livingstone, New York, 1984.)

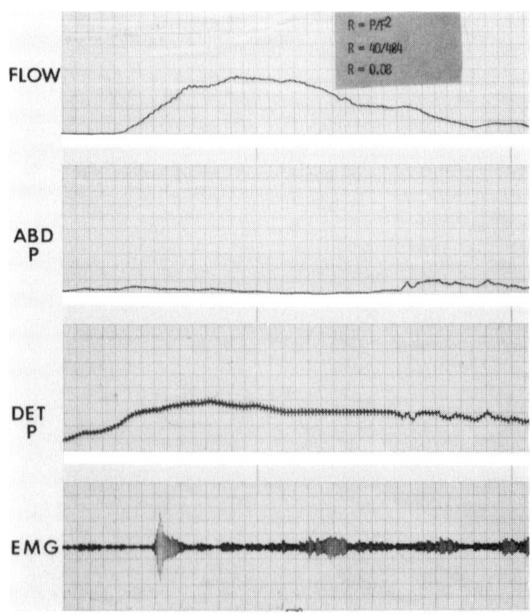

Figure 14–8. Combined study comparing uroflow rate, peak 22 ml/s (scale 0–50 ml/s) (*first line*); abdominal pressure, 0 ml H_2O (scale 0–100 ml H_2O) (*second line*); detrusor pressure, 40 ml H_2O (scale 0–100 ml H_2O) at the point of peak flow rate (*third line*); and pelvic floor EMG activity (*fourth line*). A rough estimate of resistance can be calculated and has a normal value of 0.08.

small catheter. There is no question that the catheter, especially in young children with small-diameter urethras, introduces some element of outflow obstruction and thereby decreases the peak flow rate. However, this problem appears to be negligible in most clinical settings.

Children with high voiding pressures and low flow rates may have outflow obstruction. When there is increased EMG activity during the voiding sequence, one may suspect an uncoordinated striated sphincter giving rise to this degree of obstruction. On the other hand, if EMG activity is coordinated, other causes of outflow obstruction must be excluded. When both voiding pressures and flow rates are low, it is reasonable to conclude that detrusor contractility is lacking. This abnormality may be the result of neurologic impairment to the detrusor or myogenic detrusor decompensation. One must also take into account the possibility of poor patient cooperation during the testing sequence. In such a situation, a patient may volitionally fail to initiate a detrusor contraction and augment voiding by straining or subtle increases in intravesical pressure, which generally results in low detrusor pressures and low flow rates.

In most instances an experienced urodynamic technician can define the degree of patient compliance during urodynamic testing and thereby guard against misinterpretation of this type of study.

Video urodynamics. The true essence of pediatric urodynamics is achieved when the parameters of the combined study are coupled with voiding cystourethrography. The bladder is filled with contrast medium, and the voiding parameters are recorded while fluoroscopic monitoring of the sequence is carried out. Limited use of the fluoroscope during bladder filling keeps the radiation exposure to a minimum (*33*).

The main benefit of this technique is visualization of the bladder neck and proximal urethra of the child with a voiding abnormality due to outflow obstruction. A true detrusor contraction is a prerequisite for adequate interpretation of the study when outflow obstruction is suspected. When a normal bladder contraction occurs, the bladder neck (smooth muscle) is pulled upward and outward, assuming a funnel configuration. There is concomitant relaxation of the striated sphincter that allows free passage of urine through the urethra. In clinical situations where sphincter dyssynergia is suspected as the cause of outflow obstruction, the origin may be at the bladder neck and proximal urethra (internal sphincter–smooth muscle), the striated sphincter, or a combination of both sphincteric areas (Fig. 14–9).

Webster *et al* (*34*) have defined other categories of micturitional abnormalities in neurologically normal children that may be observed with videourodynamics. In general, those conditions that fail to result in a detrusor contraction, e.g., detrusor areflexia and increased detrusor compliance, can be evaluated with tests that are less expensive and invasive. As before, patient cooperation is extremely important during this testing sequence, as actual voiding must occur for an adequate study to be obtained.

ENURESIS

Enuresis may be defined as the nocturnal or diurnal incontinence of urine in a child

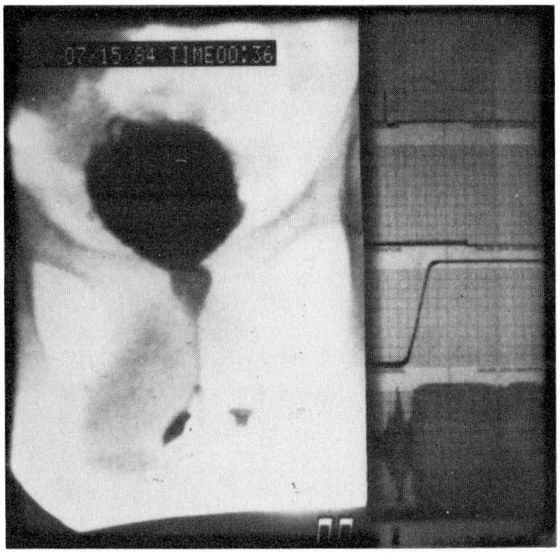

Figure 14–9. Videourodynamic study in a 15-year-old paraplegic (T5) boy who had high residuals and recurrent urinary infection. Intravesical pressures exceeded 100 ml H_2O (scale 0–100 ml H_2O), and EMG activity was excessive during the detrusor contraction. Although the bladder neck opened, the prostatic urethra was dilated to the level of the striated sphincter. There was no urinary flow (*top*) or increase in abdominal pressure (*second from top*). This picture is a classic for detrusor–external sphincter dyssynergia.

more than 4 years of age. Primary enuresis is present from birth, and secondary enuresis is preceded by a dry interval of 6 to 12 months. The incidence of enuresis has been estimated at 12 percent of children of age 4 to 5 years (*35*), and it is known to have a familial predisposition (*36*). Theories regarding the cause of enuresis include such factors as delayed level of central nervous system maturation, psychogenic and behavioral components, environmental influences, deep sleep, allergies, small bladder capacity, uninhibited neurogenic bladder, and structural abnormalities of the urinary tract (*31,37–39*). The incidence of underlying organic problems is higher in the older patient population. This discussion emphasizes those children with enuresis who have no overt neurologic or urologic disorder.

The extent of the urologic evaluation of enuretic children has undergone reevaluation. In the past, most children underwent intravenous urography (IVP), voiding cystourethrography (VCUG), and endoscopy. However, many investigators currently recommend a much more selective evaluation that is tailored to the individual child and family. The importance of the history, physical examination, and results of urinalysis and urine culture in this evaluation are stressed. One determines the pattern of incontinence, whether nocturnal, diurnal, or both; associated urinary frequency or urgency; fecal soiling or constipation; and if there is a history of urinary tract infection and obstructive voiding symptoms. Careful examination of the spine, abdomen, genitalia, and sacral spinal cord segments is necessary, and the voided stream is observed. Urinalysis and urine culture, if indicated, are performed. A history or laboratory findings suggestive of urinary tract infection or evidence suggestive of a hyperactive striated urethral sphincter, urinary tract obstruction, or a neurologic problem mandates further evaluation. Determination of the uroflow rate, possibly combined with surface perineal EMG, may be indicated (*24*). If a screening IVP is indicated, additional information can be obtained from voiding urethral and postvoiding bladder films.

Many investigators have performed urodynamic evaluations of enuretic children in an attempt to identify any specific abnormality of vesicourethral function responsible for their incontinence. Whiteside and Arnold (*36*) studied 50 patients who had normal urinary flow rates and complete bladder emptying. Among 13 patients with nocturnal enuresis only, 15 percent had detrusor instability. In constrast, 97 percent of 37 patients with both diurnal and nocturnal enuresis had detrusor instability. Blaivas *et al* (*15*) evaluated 13 children with diurnal and nocturnal enuresis and found two with neurogenic bladder dysfunction. Seven of the remaining 11 patients had decreased bladder capacity. Firlit *et al.* (*31*) performed pressure, flow, and EMG urodynamic studies on 34 children with diurnal and nocturnal enuresis and found 13 patients with uninhibited bladders, 17 with hyperactive striated sphincters, and 4 with normal results. Kass *et al.* (*37*) urodynamically evaluated 65 children with primary enuresis. Forty-two of these patients had either a history or evidence of urinary tract infection. Among the 42, there were 30 with uninhibited detrusor contractions, 10 patients were normal, and 2 had mixed types of neurogenic bladder dysfunction. Of the remaining 23 patients, 5 had uninhibited detrusor contractions and 18 were normal. Smey *et al.* (*40*) reported a subgroup of enuretic children who had hyperactive striated urethral sphincters as a factor contributing to incontinence. Diurnal enuresis, urinary frequency and urgency, urinary tract infection, and fecal soiling or constipation appear to correlate with the presence of uninhibited detrusor contractions, hyperactive striated urethral sphincters, or both.

The role of radiographic studies of enuretic children has also undergone reevaluation. Redman and Seibert (*41*) obtained an IVP, VCUG, or both in 138 enuretic children. Twenty-one children had abnormal results, and each had a history of urinary tract infection, signs and symptoms of lower urinary tract obstruction, or both. No significant radiographic abnormalities were found in children with diurnal enuresis unless accompanied by symptoms or findings suggestive of urinary tract infection or obstruction. Kass *et al.* (*37*) similarly reported that an IVP revealed a significant abnormality only in children with a history of urinary tract infection.

Various treatment modalities have been used for the enuretic child, including reassurance, psychotherapy, behavior modification techniques, hypnotherapy, pharmacologic manipulation, and various surgical techniques. The preponderance of evidence currently suggests that the history, physical examination, and basic laboratory findings indicate the appropriate extent of evaluation and initial management of most enuretic children. Children with past or present urinary tract infection, evidence of lower urinary tract obstruction, or abnormalities on physical or neurologic examination should undergo thorough urologic evaluation followed by appropriate treatment. Meatotomy may be helpful in the male child with documented meatal stenosis, but it may be associated with a high relapse rate. The routine use of meatotomy or urethral dilation is to be condemned. Children with none of the above findings or those who have had a negative urologic evaluation may be managed in a more conservative manner.

When deciding whether to initiate therapy it is important to assess the effect of the problem on the patient and the family as a whole. When some parents and children are informed that no significant organic or psychological problem is causing enuresis, reassurance and fluid restriction before bedtime may be the only treatment required. Many are quite willing to wait for the spontaneous resolution of enuresis, which occurs at a rate of 15 percent per year in patients 5 to 19 years of age (*35*). Should treatment be desired, a conditioning device such as a pad and bell bed alarm is successful in as many as 60 percent of patients, and behavior modification therapy aimed at making the patient responsible for changing his behavior, complemented by positive reinforcement, is helpful in as many as 70 percent of patients (*39*).

For patients who are unable to accept or who fail these approaches, pharmacologic therapy may be effective. The results of the thorough study by Kass *et al.* (*37*) suggest that successful empiric pharmacologic treatment of these patients can be instituted on the basis of historical information, physical examination, and urinalysis. Eighty-five percent of patients with nocturnal enuresis and daytime urgency and frequency respond well to anticholinergic medication. Seventy percent of patients with nocturnal enuresis only are successfully treated with imipramine hydrochloride. It is the authors' experience that nortriptyline hydrochloride may be efficacious in those patients who do not respond to imipramine hydrochloride. The former drug has the additional benefit of a more rapid onset of action and a shortened half-life should undesirable side effects be encountered. Some of those who fail imipramine hydrochloride therapy respond to an anticholinergic drug. A high relapse rate can be expected if drug therapy is withdrawn early, particularly in young children. Pharmacologic therapy is more effective if it is suggested in a positive manner and combined with a program of behavior modification and positive reinforcement techniques. Patients with hyperactive striated urethral sphincters may be successfully treated with diazepam (*40*) or biofeedback training (*42,43*). Further urologic and radiologic evaluation of these patients is frequently indicated if they fail pharmacologic therapy, particularly the older child.

MYELODYSPLASIA

Myelodysplasia (spinal dysraphism) is a serious congenital anomaly that occurs in 1 to 2/1000 births in the United States. Multifactorial genetic and environmental influences are thought to be responsible for the unfused neural arches and the associated spinal cord defects (*44*). Although early neurosurgical intervention has decreased the incidence of meningitis and hydrocephalus during infancy (*45*), urologic complications resulting from neurogenic vesical dysfunction (NVD) remain the leading cause of morbidity and mortality in the survivors (*46*). For most, urinary incontinence is a formidable social handicap, and in some vesicoureteral reflux, hydroureteronephrosis, chronic pyelonephritis, and urolithiasis ultimately result in renal failure (*47*). In recent years, sophisticated urodynamic evaluation of these children has permitted more precise and rational treatment. Pharmacologic therapy, often in conjunction with intermittent catheterization, and the application of new surgical techniques have rendered many of these patients continent and promoted the preservation of renal function.

The term "spinal dysraphism" encompasses a spectrum of anomalies—from the more occult dermal sinus, lipoma of the spinal cord, aberrant roots or fibrous traction bands, and abnormal filum terminale to the more apparent and generally more serious lesions of meningocele and myelomeningocele (*48*). Although the occult forms may be associated with significant NVD, this discussion is primarily concerned with the more common form encountered by the urologist: myelomeningocele. Myelomeningoceles are most frequently lumbosacral (42%), thoracolumbar (27%), and sacral (21%); only 10 percent are thoracic or cervical (*49*). Some investigators maintain that the level of the vertebral defect largely determines the degree of neurologic damage (*50*), but most studies suggest no correlation between the level and NVD (*51,52*). Indeed, significant NVD can be associated with minimal body defects (*48*). These disparities can be explained by the various possible neuropathologic lesions of the spinal cord, which include hydromyelia, syringomyelia, failure of upward migration or tethering of the cord, and dysplasia of the cord itself. Furthermore, these changes may extend several segments above and below the actual site of the myelomeningocele. The importance of urodynamic evaluation to determine the precise vesicourethral dysfunction present in an individual patient is thus apparent.

Clinical Presentation

Nearly all forms of spinal dysraphism are associated with a cutaneous abnormality of the back such as hypertrichosis, skin pigmentation, lipoma, skin dimple, or the more obvious meningocele (*48*). Many patients have lower extremity othopedic deformities, paresis, or paralysis. Inability to void, urinary incontinence, and fecal incontinence unfortunately are common problems.

Urologic Evaluation

As soon as is practical after repair of the myelomeningocele and shunting of the cerebrospinal fluid, several urologic studies are done if necessary. They include IVP, VCUG, urine culture, and serum blood urea nitrogen and creatinine determinations. These tests are performed for the purpose of identifying those patients who require immediate treatment and as a baseline in others. Approximately 20 percent of patients have an abnormal IVP demonstrating hydroureteronephrosis, caliectasis, or hydroureter (*53*). It is of particular importance that nearly two-thirds of patients with a normal IVP have an abnormal VCUG showing vesicoureteral reflux, a thickened bladder wall, diverticula, or abnormalities of the bladder shape and outlet (*53*). Thus these radiographic examinations are complementary, and we believe that a VCUG should be obtained even when the IVP is normal. Urodynamic evaluation of neonates has been performed infrequently, but Bauer *et al.* (4) have obtained important data suggesting that neonates should routinely undergo urodynamic investigation.

Urodynamic Evaluation

Sophisticated urodynamic evaluation of children with myelodysplasia is essential in order to render rational therapy for urinary incontinence and to preserve renal function. The optimum urodynamic techniques to identify specific abnormalities of vesicourethral function include liquid cystometry, urethral closure pressure profilometry, simultaneous determination of intravesical and urethral pressures during bladder filling and voiding, and determination of EMG activity of the striated urethral or anal sphincter, all in conjunction with fluoroscopic monitoring. It is important to ascertain several urodynamic parameters, including bladder capacity, intravesical filling pressure, intravesical pressure at the moment of urethral urinary loss, the presence or absence of reflex detrusor activity and the competence of the smooth and striated muscular sphincteric mechanisms. The degree of coordination of the detrusor and sphincter mechanisms and the postvoid residual urine volume should also be determined.

Several investigators have reported similar results of urodynamic studies in myelodysplastic children (*3,52,54*). Reflex detrusor activity in response to bladder filling is present in 17 to 40 percent of patients. The reported incidence of detrusor–sphincter dyssynergia depends on its definition. If it is defined as an actual increase in EMG activity and urethral pressure at the area of the striated sphincter during a reflex detrusor contraction, the incidence is 7 percent (*3*). If it is defined as failure of sustained sphincter relaxation during reflex detrusor contraction or voiding maneuvers such as Valsalva or Credé, the incidence is 50 percent (*52*). Between 60 and 80 percent of patients have detrusor areflexia. In many it is the result of neural injury, but in others it may represent myogenic failure resulting from chronic distension or recurrent urinary tract infection with bladder wall fibrosis. Detrusor hypertonia (decreased detrusor compliance) during bladder filling occurs in as many as 85 percent of patients with detrusor areflexia and manifests as a progressive increase in intravesical pressure with increasing volume, culminating in urethral urinary loss when the intravesical and intraurethral pressures are equal. A striking relation exists between intravesical pressure at the time of urethral urinary loss and the incidence of ureteral complications. In one report, if urethral urinary loss occurred at an intravesical pressure of less than 40 cm H_2O, no patient had vesicoureteral reflux and only 10 percent had ureteral dilation (*3*). On the other hand, if urethral urinary loss occurred at an intravesical pressure of more than 40 cm H_2O, 68 percent of patients had vesicoureteral reflux and 81 percent had ureteral dilation. Most patients have open bladder necks (determined radiographically), and these patients tend to have a lower maximum urethral closure pressure than patients with closed bladder necks. The major clinical problem in these patients tends to be urinary incontinence. In those with higher urethral closure pressures, upper urinary tract deterioration and vesicoureteral reflux tend to occur.

The results of these investigations have important prognostic and therapeutic implications for children with myelodysplasia. McGuire *et al.* (*55*) described six patients with detrusor hypertonia on initial urodynamic evaluation but no upper tract complications. Subsequently, upper urinary tract deterioration or vesicoureteral reflux developed in all patients, and persisting detrusor hypertonia was demonstrated on follow-up urodynamic testing (Fig. 14–10). This upper tract deterioration may occur after many years of normalcy and as late as the midteenage years. Similar urodynamic abnormalities have been demonstrated in neonates, including upper tract deterioration developing in patients who initially had detrusor–sphincter dyssynergia and normal upper tracts (*4*).

Bladder wall fibrosis causes detrusor hypertonia in some patients. However, the fact that bilateral surgical transection of all sacral roots often results in a hypertonic, areflexic detrusor response to bladder filling suggests that this response is usually intrinsic to the vesical musculature freed from central neural regulation (*56*). Experimental data indicate that an increase in adrenergic innervation and alpha-receptor activity occurs in the bladder after parasympathetic decentralization (*57*). Histochemical fluorescent studies of excised detrusor muscle from normal and parasympathetically decentralized human bladders show that the adrenergic nerve terminals of the denervated detrusors are thicker, more strongly fluorescent, and more densely distributed than in normal detrusors (*58*). Interestingly, the patients with decentralized bladders had filling curves typical of hypertonia on cystometry. Although the precise mechanism responsible for increased adrenergic activity is unknown, unmasking of already exisitng alpha-receptors or an induction of alpha-receptors by parasympathetic denervation seems probable (*58*).

Treatment

Urologic disorders requiring treatment in children with myelodysplasia include recurrent urinary tract infection, vesicoureteral reflux, urinary incontinence, inadequate bladder emptying, discoordinate voiding, and detrusor hypertonia with resultant upper tract changes. The same treatment modality or combination of modalities may be appropriate for several urodynamic abnormalities in an individual patient. The type of treatment or the necessity of treatment may differ depending on the age of the child.

Until recently, if the traditional urologic evaluation of the neonate revealed no significant abnormalities, routine surveillance with IVP or ultrasonography, VCUG, urine culture, and tests of renal function was fairly standardized. However, the data reported by Bauer *et al.* (*4*) suggested a reappraisal. Their experience indicated that neonatal urodynamic evaluation is important, and that the results should dictate the type and

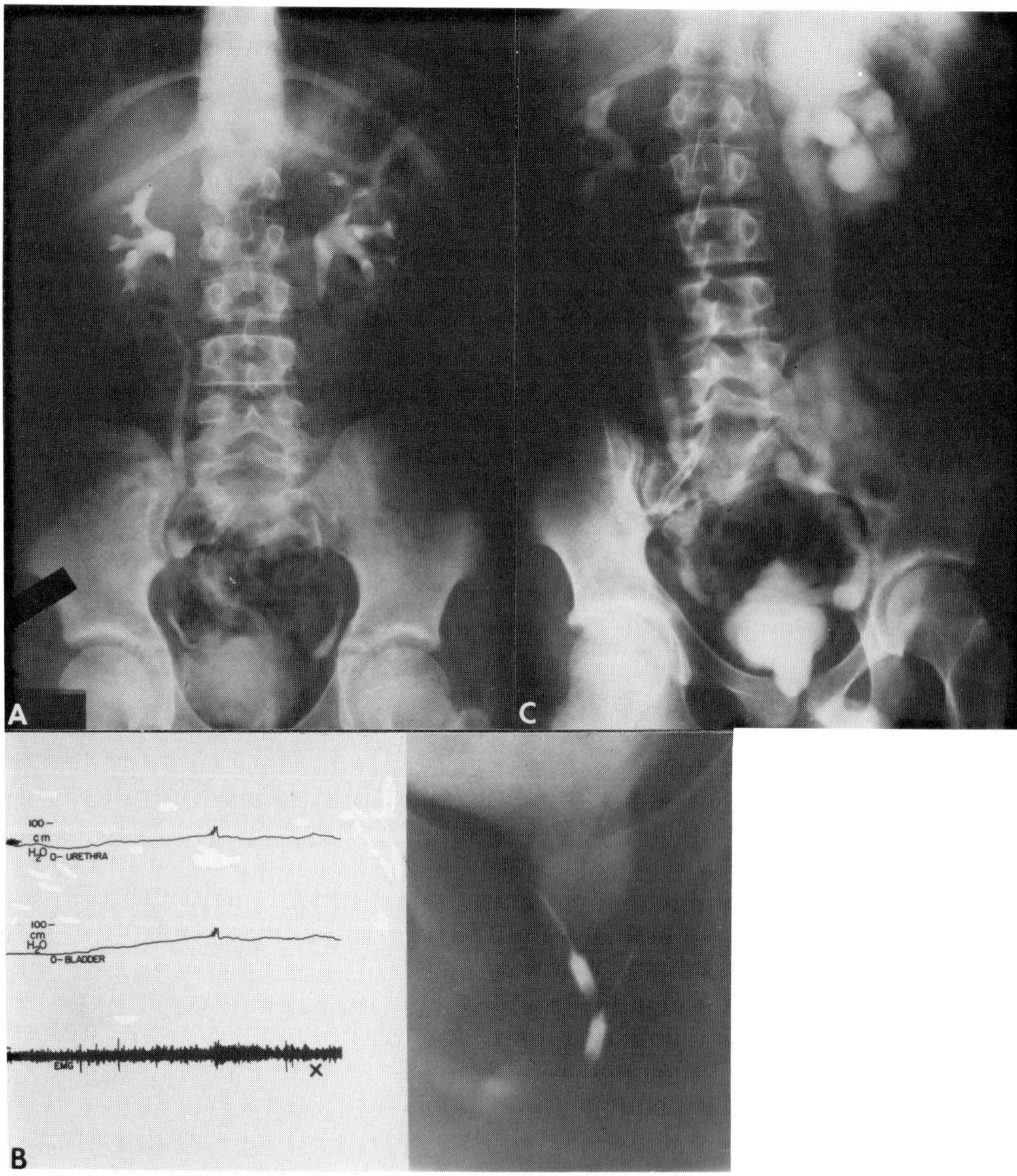

Figure 14–10 **A.** Normal intravenous urogram from a 12-year-old boy with myelodysplasia. **B.** *Left.* Urodynamic recordings show detrusor areflexia and a hypertonic filling curve with an intravesical pressure of 56 cm H_2O at 100 ml bladder volume. *Right.* Radiograph (exposed at X, left) shows open vesical neck and urethral urinary loss. **C.** Intravenous urogram 2.5 years later shows early right caliectasis and moderate left hydroureteronephrosis. Repeat urodynamic evaluation showed persisting detrusor hypertonia. (From McGuire, E. J., *et al. J. Urol.* 121:458–461, 1979. Copyright © 1979, The Williams & Wilkins Co., Baltimore.)

frequency of periodic evaluation. Those infants with complete denervation of the striated urethral sphincter and normal intravesical filling pressure require only a yearly renal ultrasonogram or IVP. Infants with synergic sphincter activity require a yearly renal ultrasonogram or IVP and a urodynamic study in order to detect the development of dyssynergia. In infants with dyssynergic sphincter activity, the frequency of evaluation with renal ultrasonography or IVP, VCUG, and urodynamic study is increased to every 6 months during the first 2 years of life and yearly thereafter until the age of 5 years.

Treatment must be initiated in patients who develop detrusor hypertonia, increased voiding pressure, increased postvoiding residual urine volume, recurrent urinary tract infection, or vesicoureteral reflux. Anticholinergic medication can suppress reflex detrusor activity and lower intravesical pressure; it may be used in conjunction with intermittent catheterization to ensure adequate bladder emptying. Intermittent catheterization is feasible in neonates, and children as young as age 2 to 3 years may learn self-catheterization. For infants in whom intermittent catheterization is not technically feasible or acceptable to the family or who do not improve with this form of treatment, cutaneous vesicostomy may be performed. Cutaneous vesicostomy, an acceptable means of urinary diversion in children still in diapers, may be reversed when the child is desirous of being dry and has been taught self-catheterization, and generally is not associated with loss of bladder volume (*59*).

The use of the Credé maneuver for bladder emptying is controversial. Most investigators think it is contraindicated in the presence of vesicoureteral reflux, and others think it should not be used at all (*60*). It probably should not be used in a patient with a bladder neck that radiographically appears closed because of the high probability of developing detrimental intravesical pressures. If one considers its use in a patient with a bladder neck that appears to be open radiographically, the intravesical pressure produced during the Credé maneuver can be determined at the time of urodynamic evaluation.

The application of intermittent catheterization, with or without concomitant pharmacologic therapy, represents a significant advance in the treatment of myelodysplastic children. If detrusor hypertonia exists, with or without hydroureteronephrosis, catheterization is useful to ensure bladder emptying prior to attaining the volume at which detrimental pressure occurs. This situation frequently requires treatment with either an anticholinergic or an alpha-adrenolytic drug to decrease intravesical filling pressure (*55*). Upper urinary tract changes have resolved or improved in up to 80 percent of patients so treated (*61*). Experience suggests that renal preservation is better accomplished by this regimen than with ileal conduit urinary diversion (*62*). If detrusor hypertonia associated with upper tract changes persists despite treatment, bladder augmentation or superselective sacral 2, 3, and 4 dorsal root rhizotomy is considered (*63*).

Urinary continence depends on the balance between intravesical filling pressure, bladder capacity, urethral sphincteric function, and the presence or absence of reflex detrusor activity. To optimize the opportunity for continence, specific therapy may be required for one or several of these parameters. Intermittent catheterization is an integral component of the treatment for incontinence in nearly all myelodysplastic children. It ensures periodic complete bladder emptying and is performed at a frequency adequate to prevent reaching the bladder volume at which incontinence occurs. An anticholinergic drug may be necessary to increase bladder capacity enough to allow a reasonable frequency of catheterization (*61,64–66*). Complete or nearly complete continence may be attained in 50 to 60 percent of patients so treated. The highest continence rate occurs in patients who have vesical necks that appear closed radiographically (*3,67*). Treatment with an alpha-adrenergic agonist to increase proximal urethral resistance and establish continence seems attractive, but results have been disappointing (*3, 64*).

Some patients remain unacceptably incontinent despite treatment with intermittent catheterization and pharmacotherapy. They are potential candidates for surgical procedures designed to establish continence by augmenting urethral resistance. Surgical techniques that have had varying degrees of success include the Young-Dees, the Marshall-Marchetti-Krantz, and the pubovaginal sling procedures (*59,68*). We have also used suprapubic endoscopic vesical neck suspension (Stamey procedure) successfully in three pubertal girls, but the follow-up is short (*69*). The artificial urinary sphincter offers an attractive surgical option and has been used successfully in myelodysplastic patients, even in conjunction with intermittent catheterization (*70,71*). Caution must be exercised when selecting patients for any procedure that augments urethral resistance. If detrusor hypertonia coexists with urethral sphincteric incompetence, the urethra may act as a "pressure relief valve" for the hypertonic detrusor. If urethral resistance is then surgically augmented, detrimental intravesical pressure can occur and result in upper tract deterioration (*72*). Cystometry performed with the bladder outlet occluded by an inflated Foley catheter balloon can detect this occult detrusor hypertonia (*73*). If hypertonia cannot be eliminated or controlled by pharmacologic therapy, bladder hydrodilation, or possibly bladder augmentation, surgical elevation of urethral resistance is contraindicated.

Until recently, vesicoureteral reflux in the myelodysplastic child was treated by urinary diversion. As experience with intermittent catheterization increased, it became apparent that reflux was cured or improved in many patients. If urinary infection can be prevented, intermittent catheterization results in either cessation, downgrading or stabilization of reflux in as many as 75 percent of patients (*2,74*). Ureteroneocystostomy may be necessary in children who continue to have significant reflux, with or without recurrent urinary tract infection. Surgical success rates of 76 to 100 percent have been reported in patients with grade 2B or greater reflux when they were operated on with the Politano-Leadbetter, Cohen cross-trigonal, or Paquin techniques (*2,74,75*). Ureteral dilatation requiring tapering or a severely trabeculated bladder are significant factors in operative failure. It may be particularly important to treat the patient with a severely trabeculated bladder with an anticholinergic drug after ureteroneocystostomy.

Regardless of the initial favorable status of the urinary tract or favorable responses to various treatment modalities, silent deterioration of upper tract function can occur. Therefore these patients require life-long urologic surveillance. Nash (*76*) has graphically described the myelomeningocele victim as a "paraplegic incontinent cripple, who may be snatched from the jaws of death in the neonatal months, only to be delivered over to the tragedy of an expanding head or, in the past, to a life of social exclusion amid the fumes and filth of double incontinence and trophic ulcers." With the evolution in surgical and nonsurgical therapeutic modalities, the child with myelodysplasia is usually spared from these terrible consequences.

CAUDAL REGRESSION SYNDROME

The syndrome of caudal regression was described by Duhamel (*77*); in its most severe form it results in sacral agenesis, imperforate anus, fusion of the lower extremities, and absence of the genitourinary tract except for the gonads. The disordered embryogenesis appears to occur at the fourth to fifth week of fetal life when the lumbosacral spine and nephrogenic masses are forming and the cloacal septum is separating the genitourinary sinus from the rectum. Fortunately, the most severe form is rare, but imperforate anus and sacral agenesis are relatively common, as separate and combined congenital anomalies.

Imperforate Anus

Several classifications of imperforate anus have been proposed, and that of Santulli *et al.* (*78*) is widely used. These authors classified imperforate anus into four major groups based on the level of the imperforation in relation to the puborectalis muscle or the pelvic floor: low or translevator lesions, intermediate lesions (uncommon), high or supralevator lesions, and miscellaneous lesions. In nearly all male patients with supralevator lesions, a fistulous communication exists between the prostatic urethra and the blind end of the rectal pouch; in female patients a rectovaginal fistula is common. Patients with translevator lesions do not have fistulas between the intestinal and urinary tracts; rather, the rectal fistula opens near the posterior scrotal raphe in men and the distal vagina or posterior fourchette in women.

Patients with supralevator lesions are managed with a diverting colostomy shortly after birth, with the definitive rectal pull-through and repair of the rectourethral fistula performed when the child has grown to approximately 25 pounds. Those who have infralevator lesions are treated with a primary anoplasty. All patients undergo uroradiographic studies to detect associated genitourinary anomalies. Patients with supralevator lesions have a 52 to 67 percent incidence of genitourinary anomalies, but those with infralevator lesions have an incidence of 16 to 18 percent (*79,80*).

Imperforate anus may be associated with many urologic problems, including a broad spectrum of congenital upper tract anomalies. Additionally, complications may result from the definitive surgical correction of the lesion. Excessive surgical dissection of the fistula has resulted in urethral stricture or sphincteric damage and urinary incontinence (*81,82*); failure to adequately excise the fistula has resulted in pseudodiverticulum formation (*81*).

Although it is difficult to ascertain the precise cause, neurogenic vesical dysfunction is also common among patients with imperforate anus. Approximately 25 percent of patients have abnormalities of the lumbosacral spine, and most are supralevator lesions, which alone could be responsible for voiding dysfunction (see Sacral Agenesis, below) (*83*). In addition, the pelvic plexuses can be injured by surgical dissection of the rectal pull-through procedure. These plexuses lie deep in the pelvis on either side of the rectum and contain pre- and postganglionic parasympathetic and sympathetic neurons. Thus abnormalities of innervation of the bladder, urethra, or both may occur, including partial or complete denervation of the bladder manifested as poor detrusor contractility, detrusor areflexia, or decreased detrusor compliance with increased intravesical filling pressure. Varying degrees of urethral denervation may also result in a low maximum urethral closure pressure and urinary incontinence. A similar clinical situation exists in patients who have undergone radical or Wertheim hysterectomy or abdominoperineal resection of the rectum (*84,85*). Because of the spectrum of potential abnormalities in patients with imperforate anus, urodynamic investigation is important to precisely identify the disordered vesicourethral function and thus direct specific treatment. We have most commonly encountered poor detrusor function, usually detrusor areflexia, as the cause of incomplete bladder emptying and as a factor contributing to urinary incontinence. Some patients have also had sphincteric insufficiency, with a bladder neck that appears open radiographically, and severe urinary incontinence (Fig. 14–11).

Sacral Agenesis

Sacral agenesis results from failure of ossification of the sacral segments early in fetal development. It manifests as a complete or partial absence of one or more scaral vertebral segments. Several authors have noted an increased incidence of sacral agenensis in the offspring of mothers with diabetes mellitus (*86–88*). The neuropathologic abnormalities of the spinal cord, spinal roots, and spinal canal have been ascertained from postmortem anatomic dissections and from the findings encountered at neurosurgical procedures. In some patients the sacral roots caudad to the lowest formed vertebral segment fail to develop, whereas in others sacral roots are present despite the absence of the corresponding vertebral bodies (*89*). There may be dense fibrous tissue within the spinal canal as well as an intradural lipoma, a dermoid cyst, or tethering of the cord (*90*). Sacral agenesis may also coexist with forms of spinal dysraphism such as myelomeningocele and diastematomyelia (*88*). The resulting neurologic deficits may result from

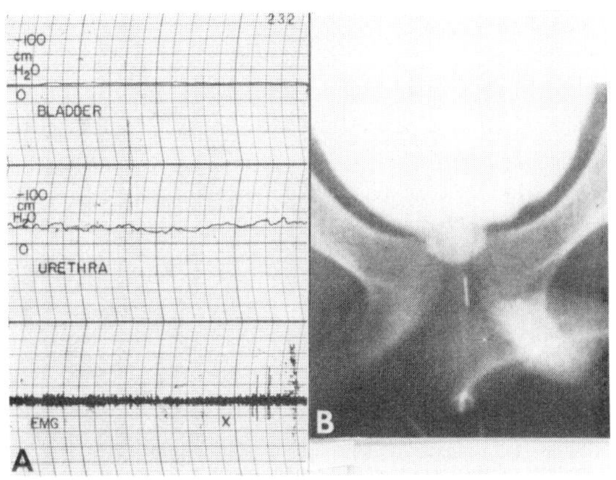

Figure 14–11. A 6-year-old boy with an imperforate anus, status post rectal pullthrough procedure, with urinary incontinence. **A.** Urodynamic recordings show detrusor areflexia and low urethral pressure. **B.** Radiograph (exposed at X, left) illustrates an open vesical neck.

an absence of spinal roots, compression or entrapment of the spinal cord or spinal roots, and traction on the spinal cord during growth of the vertebral column due to tethering.

Many patients wth sacral agenesis have either no apparent or only subtle neurologic symptoms, and the condition may thus elude diagnosis for many years (*91*). Unfortunately, some patients with NVD have undergone multiple urologic surgical procedures before the underlying condition was diagnosed (*90,92*). The condition may be misdiagnosed if only anteroposterior radiographs of the lower spine are obtained because the sacrum may be poorly visualized if an exaggerated lumbosacral angle exists. Therefore it is important to obtain lateral sacral radiographs (*87*). Patients with neurogenic vesical dysfunction may initially present with hydronephrosis, urinary tract infection, vesicoureteral reflux, difficulty of voiding, urinary incontinence, or bladder trabeculation (*90*). Several investigators have determined that NVD occurs in patients with agenesis of one of two sacral segments (*87,93*). The findings on physical examination may include a palpable defect in the sacrum, a sacral dimple, a flattened gluteal region, foot deformities, decreased perineal sensation and resting external anal sphincter tone, and flaccid paralysis of the muscles innervated by sacral roots 2 through 5 (*88,90*). Motor deficits are generally more pronounced than sensory deficits (*87,94*), and in many patients these deficits do not correlate with those expected from the bony deficiency (*86,89*).

Similarly, the type of NVD does not correlate with the bony lesion (*86,93*). Because the clinical neurologic evaluation is also not helpful in identifying the specific type of NVD in a given patient, urodynamic evaluation is extremely important. Koff and Deridder (*86*) performed sophisticated urodynamic evaluations in 11 patients with sacral agenesis. Three patients had uninhibited detrusor dysfunction, four had detrusor areflexia, and four had a mixed type of detrusor dysfunction. Perineal EMG was performed in 12 patients, seven of whom showed evidence of denervation, although some had normal external anal sphincter activity in the presence of detrusor dysfunction. The pattern of NVD may change with time, probably because of traction of the spinal cord due to tethering.

An example of a patient with sacral agenesis and late presentation of urologic disease is the 22-year-old woman who had been completely asymptomatic until she developed several episodes of urinary retention requiring catheterization. An abdominal plain film revealed partial right sacral agenesis (Fig. 14–12A), and an IVP showed bilateral hydroureteronephrosis (Fig. 14–12B). A complete neurologic evaluation performed by a neurosurgeon failed to detect any neurologic deficit of the sacral spinal cord segments or lower extremities. Urodynamic evaluation demonstrated detrusor –sphincter dyssynergia, with an intravesical voiding pressure as high as 90 cm H_2O and poor urinary flow (Fig. 14–12C). A myelogram showed tethering of the spinal cord and an intradural filling defect (Fig. 14–12D). She underwent excision of an intradural lipoma and release of tethering. Urodynamic studies repeated 3 and 6 months after operation showed detrusor areflexia that was presumably secondary to the surgical dissection.

The consequences of vesicourethral dysfunction that required treatment in these patients were urinary incontinence, incomplete bladder evacuation, or both. Urinary incontinence may result from urethral sphincteric incompetence or detrusor hyperreflexia, alone or in combination. Detrusor hyperreflexia is treated with an anticholinergic medication, but some patients may then be unable to void and require intermittent catheterization. In some patients alpha-adrenergic agonists may increase proximal urethral resistance and alleviate the incontinence resulting from sphincteric insufficiency. In those patients with sphincteric insufficiency who do not respond to pharmacologic treatment, proximal urethral resistance may be augmented by various surgical procedures. In carefully selected patients a pubovaginal sling, Stamey urethral suspension, or artificial urinary sphincter may be an excellent form of treatment. Coexisting detrusor hypertonia must be treated pharmacologically in patients undergoing these procedures (see Myelodysplasia, above). Patients with detrusor areflexia or impaired detrusor contractility who cannot adequately

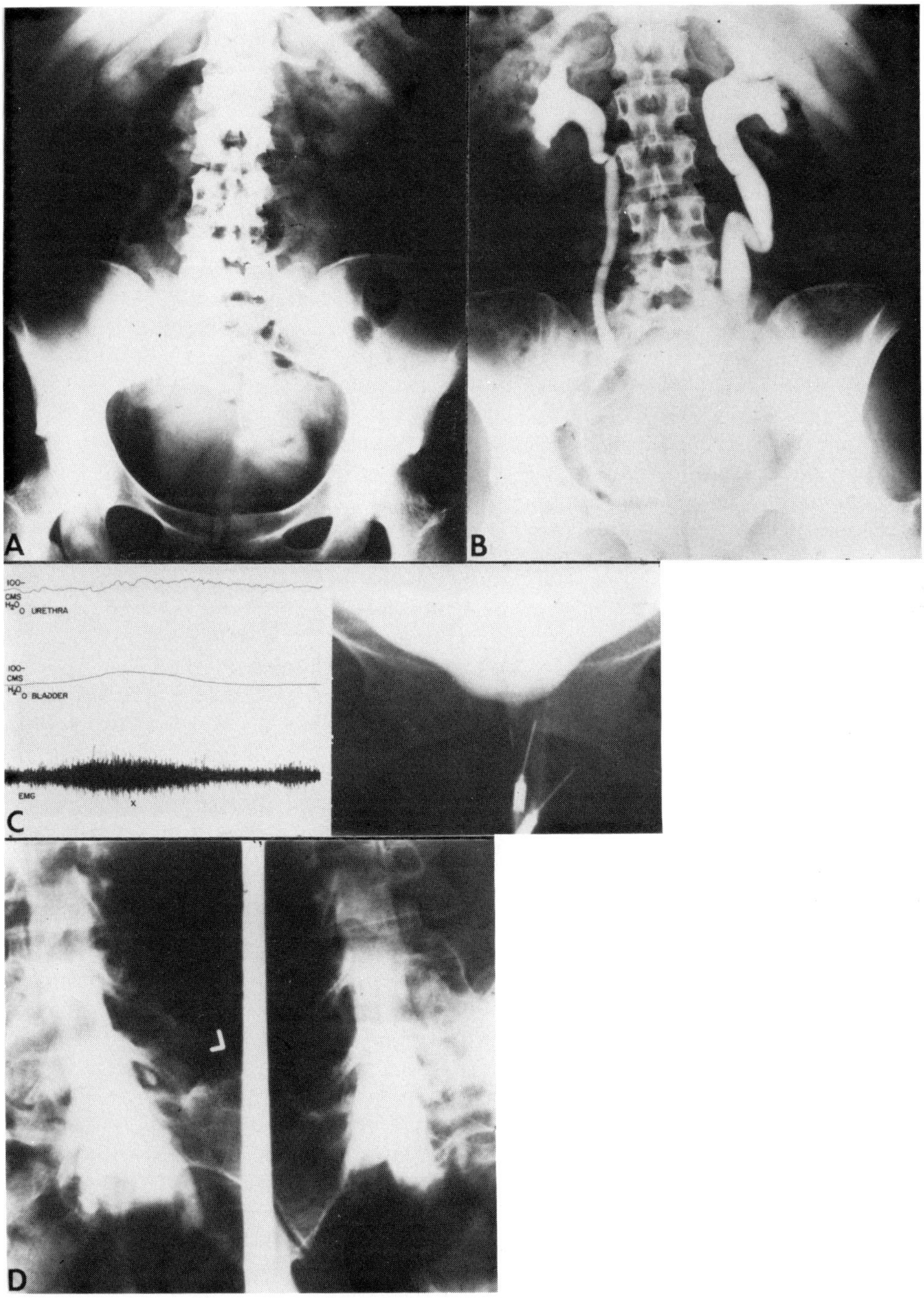

Figure 14–12. **A.** Abdominal plain film demonstrates partial right sacral agenesis. **B.** Intravenous urogram shows bilateral hydroureteronephrosis. **C.** *Left.* Urodynamic recordings show detrusor-sphincter dyssynergia and a voiding pressure of 90 cm H_2O. *Right.* Radiograph (exposed at X, left) shows open vesical neck and poor urinary flow despite the high voiding pressure. **D.** Myelogram shows an intradural filling defect and tethering of the spinal cord.

empty the bladder are managed with intermittent catheterization.

NONNEUROGENIC VOIDING DYSFUNCTION

The true challenge to the pediatric neurourologist is the definition of vesicourethral dysfunction in the child who has no overt neurologic deficits. These children present to the clinician only after voiding difficulties have led to either urinary tract infection or significant social disability. The spectrum of voiding abnormalities seen is not unlike that of patients with true neurologic disease (*95*). Thus to label this type of vesicourethral dysfunction as nonneurogenic speaks only to the general neurologic state of the child, not to the problem of vesicourethral dysfunction. Because this group of patients has no outward indicators for the potential of underlying vesicourethral problems, it becomes important for all clinicians to assess carefully the subtle changes in voiding mentioned by the child or his parents. When in doubt as to the significance of a particular symptom, a simple noninvasive test such as uroflowmetry may better define its importance.

When voiding dysfunction is identified without overt neurologic disease or evidence of spinal dysraphism, confusion abounds as to its cause. Some investigators have suggested an underlying psychological defect, and other emphasize an occult neuropathy (*96–100*). Regardless of their origin, many of the voiding abnormalities are thought to be related to a disorder of coordination between the detrusor contraction and striated sphincter relaxation. Support for a nonneurologic acquired abnormality comes from Bauer *et al.* (*101*), who failed to show denervation potentials on raw EMG data obtained from the sphincter in such children. In addition, many such voiding abnormalities are associated with acquired bowel defects such as encopresis. Also supporting an acquired cause is the fact that many such voiding abnormalities can be corrected by a period of bladder retraining that may include biofeedback methods. The full spectrum of voiding dysfunction may be seen, and the diagnostic characteristics are the same as those seen with true neurologic disease (*102*). Many such patients have subtly sustained irreversible damage to the detrusor, resulting in myogenic decompensation (Fig. 14–13). In others, vesicoureteral reflux may have developed, and surgical repair is necessary to ensure adequate bladder emptying (*103*). In all such patients, therapy is designed to promote adequate bladder emptying and an acceptably low voiding pressure in order to protect the upper urinary tract.

Patients with urgency, frequency, and wetting related to vesicourethral incoordination are ideally suited for bladder retraining with biofeedback methods. However, those with significant failure-to-empty defects may be better managed with conventional techniques of intermittent catheterization with or without the use of adjunctive pharmacologic agents. The length of therapy in both categories of patients depends on the degree of detrusor decompensation, upper tract disease, and the likelihood of relapse into a state of vesicourethral incoordination. Regular follow-up is necessary in these patients to ensure that relapse has not occurred and that the upper tracts are in fact being protected.

URINARY UNDIVERSION

Until recently many children with NVD and urinary incontinence, upper tract deterioration, or both underwent supravesical urinary diversion. However, improved urodynamic technology, a better understanding of the neurophysiology and pharmacology of the lower urinary tract, the introduction of intermittent catheterization, and the development of a workable prosthetic sphincter device have permitted satisfactory management of most of these patients without the need for supravesical urinary diversion. It is not surprising, therefore, that some of these early patients are now being considered for undiversion. The pioneering work of Hendren (*104*) demonstrated the efficacy of this treatment in selected patients. The various reconstructive surgical techniques are beyond the scope of this discussion; instead, the evaluation of potential candidates is discussed, with emphasis on evaluation of the defunctionalized vesicourethral unit. The suggested protocol represents the consensus of several investigators from various institutions (*105*).

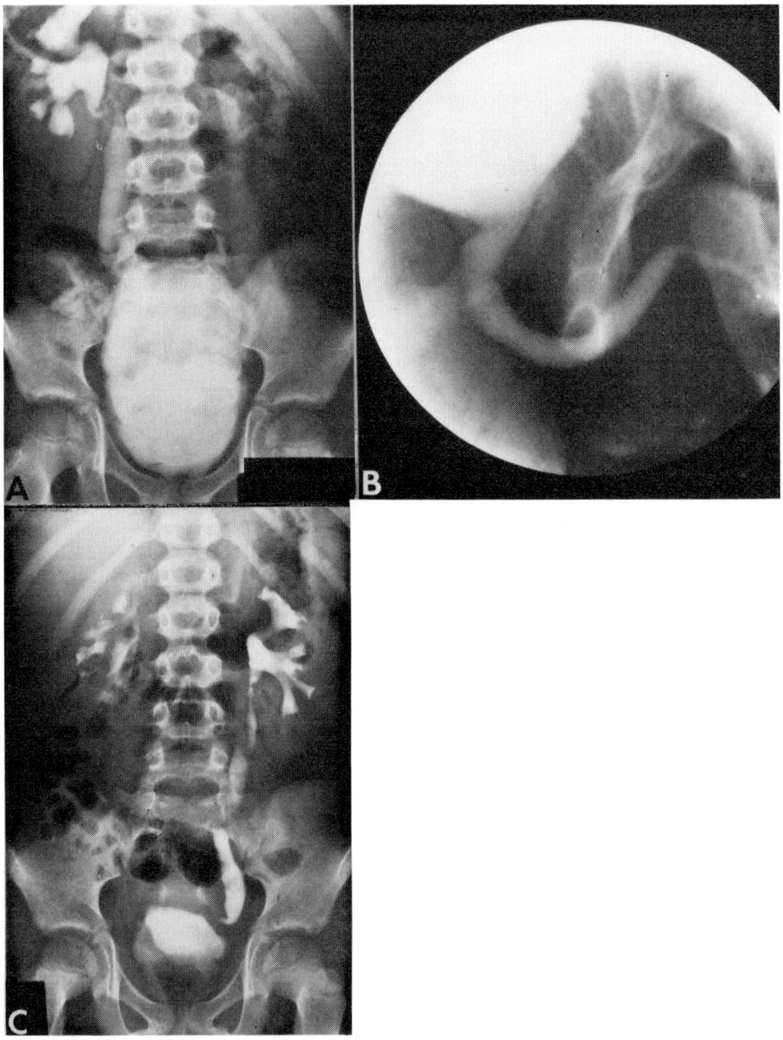

Figure 14–13. **A.** Excretory urogram in a 10-year-old boy with wetting. Neurologic examination reflected no neurologic disease. **B.** Voiding cystourethrogram is normal with the exception of excessive postvoided residual volume. **C.** Excretory urogram after a 6-month interval following combined bladder retraining and intermittent self-catheterization.

The most frequent reason for assessment for undiversion is poor psychological adjustment to the diversion. Patient selection is extremely important, and a candidate should be reliable, compliant, and highly motivated. In addition, the patient should be receptive to and capable of managing adjunctive techniques, e.g., intermittent catheterization, if necessitated by the undiversion. In general, renal function should be stable, and the corrected creatinine clearance should exceed 30 ml/min. Radiographic evaluation of the upper and lower urinary tracts is mandatory. Although many patients have an abnormal IVP, it is thought by most investigators that they are still acceptable candidates if the IVP is stable. A simultaneous cystogram and conduitogram may be helpful in deciding if reconstruction is technically feasible. Finally, the complications and the risk of failure of the procedure, including rediversion, must be stressed to both patient and family.

The anatomy and function of the lower urinary tract are assessed (Fig. 14–14). Ana-

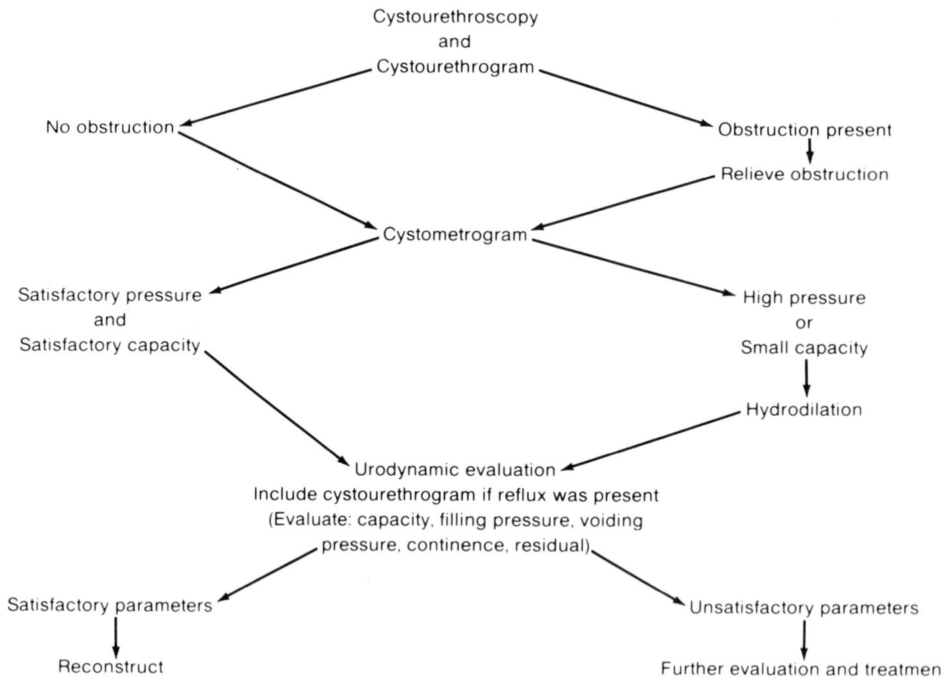

Figure 14–14. Algorithm for the initial evaluation of lower urinary tract anatomy and function in patients considered for undiversion. (From Borden, T. A. *et al. Urology* 18:223, 1981.)

tomic obstruction due to posterior urethral valves, bladder neck contracture, and urethral stricture are sought with cystourethroscopy and cystourethrography and generally are relieved prior to undiversion. Contrary to some reports (*106,107*), many investigators think that meaningful physiologic evaluation of the defunctionalized bladder and urethra is feasible. Detrusor function is first assessed with cystometrography to determine the bladder capacity, intravesical filling pressure, voiding pressure, presence or absence of reflex detrusor activity, and efficiency of bladder emptying. Poor detrusor compliance, manifesting as detrusor hypertonia at a small bladder volume, may result solely from defunctionalization, vesical wall fibrosis, or peripheral or suprasacral denervation (*108*). Patients with diminished bladder capacity or poor detrusor compliance undergo cyclical bladder filling, which may be done in either the inpatient or outpatient setting (*109*). Several weeks of cycling may be required to attain the patient's maximum bladder capacity. If a patient probably is to be managed by intermittent self-catheterization after undiversion, a trial of cyclic dilation with self-catheterization is essential for determining if the patient is capable and accepting of the procedure. If the patient can void, the volume voided and the postvoid residual are recorded.

In addition to assessment of bladder capacity and voiding function, continence can be ascertained by the patient performing the activities of daily living with a full bladder. The parameters of vesical function most favorable for successful undiversion include a capacity sufficient to allow interval continence (approximately 300 ml) with an intravesical pressure of less than 40 cm H_2O. Detrusor areflexia can be managed by intermittent catheterization after undiversion so long as continence is ensured. If a patient satisfies all these criteria, he is a candidate for reconstruction. If not, further evaluation is necessary (Figure 14–15).

Continued cyclic bladder hydrodilation may ultimately result in satisfactory detrusor parameters. When they are attained, it is important to determine the function of the bladder and urethra as a unit. It is best done by

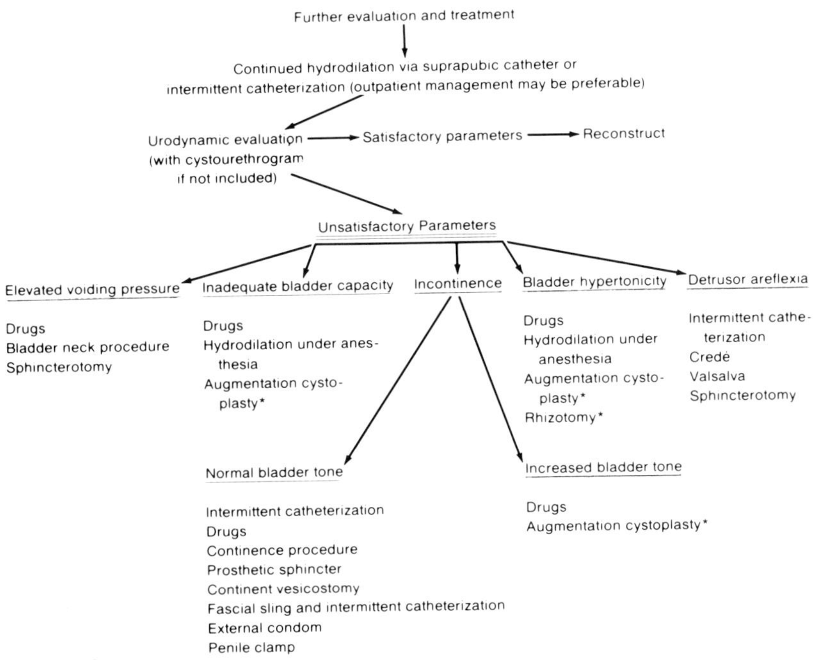

*Potential value is currently unknown.

Figure 14–15. Algorithm describing the further evaluation and treatment of the defunctionalized bladder in patients who do not initially satisfy all criteria for undiversion. (From Borden, T. A., *et al. Urology* 18:223, 1981.)

formal urodynamic study incorporating the simultaneous determination of intravesical and intraurethral pressures during both filling and voiding, in conjunction with striated anal or urethral sphincter EMG recordings and fluoroscopic monitoring (*110*).

If urethral dysfunction results in urinary incontinence and the intravesical filling pressure is normal, treatment with an alpha-adrenergic agonist may achieve continence. However, intermittent catheterization may be required for adequate bladder emptying. If incontinence persists, treatment options include various bladder neck sling procedures, continent vesicostomy, prosthetic sphincter, and in male patients a penile clamp or condom catheter. If a continence device or precedure is deemed necessary, careful evaluation of the intravesical filling pressure is of the utmost importance because a poorly functioning urethra may provide a pressure relief valve for excessive intravesical pressure. Elimination of this safety mechanism by augmentation of urethral resistance could result in increased intravesical pressures and detrimental effects on the upper urinary tract. The true intravesical filling pressure may be determined in a patient with sphincteric incompetence by performing cystometrography with the bladder neck occluded by an inflated Foley catheter balloon (*84*). A vesical capacity of approximately 300 ml is adequate, and the intravesical pressure should not exceed 40 cm H_2O. If urinary incontinence and increased intravesical filling pressure coexist, an attempt is made to lower the filling pressure pharmacologically. If this measure is unsuccessful, augmentation cystoplasty can be considered.

Similarly, a patient with an inadequate bladder capacity can be treated pharmacologically, with hydrodilation under anesthesia, or by augmentation cystoplasty. Detrusor hypertonicity may be managed pharmacologically, with hydrodilation under anesthesia. with augmentation cystoplasty, with rhizotomy in selected patients with neural lesions. Patients who void with a significantly increased voiding pressure may be treated with drugs that decrease outlet resistance; and in some instances they require surgical ablation of the bladder neck or striated urethral sphincter. This step, of course, may result in urinary incontinence that would also require management.

Many patients with NVD have detrusor areflexia and require intermittent catheterization, Credé or Valsalva maneuvers or external sphincterotomy to ensure bladder emptying. Some patients have persistent overt detrusor hyperreflexia that cannot be satisfactorily suppressed pharmacologically or with bladder hydrodilation. This problem probably contraindicates undiversion in female patients because no satisfactory external collecting device exists. However, this condition does not contraindicate undiversion in a male patient if he is willing to use an external condom catheter.

The gravity of the decision and the complexity of the evaluation that must be undertaken prior to urinary undiversion must be emphasized. Undiversion is a reasonable surgical treatment in select patients with NVD, but the decision to remove a satisfactorily functioning conduit must not be undertaken lightly. The patient is selected only after a thorough, detailed, and properly conducted evaluation.

REFERENCES

1. Allen, T. D., and Bright, T. C., III: Urodynamic patterns in children with dysfunctional voiding problems. *J. Urol.* 119:247, 1978.
2. Bauer, S. B., Colodny, A. H., and Retik, A. B.: The management of vesicoureteral reflux in children with myelodysplasia. *J. Urol.* 128:102, 1982.
3. McGuire, E. J., Woodside, J. R., Borden, T. A., and Weiss, R. M.: The prognostic value of urodynamic testing in myelodysplastic patients. *J. Urol.* 126:205, 1981.
4. Bauer, S. B., Hallett, M., Khoshbin, S.: Predictive value of urodynamic evaluation in newborns with myelodysplasia. *JAMA* 252:650, 1984.
5. Raezer, D. M., Benson, G. S., Wein, A. J., and Duckett, J. W., Jr.: The functional approach to the management of the pediatric neuropathic bladder: a clinical study. *J. Urol.* 117:649, 1977.
6. Bradley, W. E., Timm, G. W., and Scott, F. B.: Innervation of the detrusor muscle and urethra. *Urol. Clin. North Am.* 1:3, 1974.
7. De Groat, W. C.: Nervous control of the urinary bladder of the cat. *Brain Res.* 87:201, 1975.
8. De Groat, W. C., and Saum, W. R.: Adrenergic inhibition in mammalian parasympathetic ganglia. *Nature* 231:188, 1971.
9. De Groat, W. C., and Theobald, R. J.: Reflex activation of sympathetic pathways to vesical smooth muscle and parasympathetic ganglia by electrical stimulation of vesical afferents. *J. Physiol (Lond.)* 259:223, 1976.
10. Elbadawi, A., and Schenk, E. A.: A new theory of the innervation of the bladder musculature. I. Morphology of the intrinsic vesical innervation apparatus. *J. Urol.* 99:585, 1968.
11. Elbadawi, A., and Schenk, E. A.: A new theory of the innervation of bladder musculature. 2. The innervation apparatus of the ureterovesical junction. *J. Urol.* 105:368, 1971.
12. Elbadawi, A., and Schenk, E. A.: A new theory of the innervation of bladder musculature. 4. Innervation of the vesicourethral junction and external urethral sphincter. *J. Urol.* 111:613, 1974.
13. Goellner, M.H., Ziegler, E. E., and Fomon, S. J.: Urination during the first three years of life. *Nephron* 28: 174, 1981.
14. Yeates, W. K.: Bladder function in normal micturition. *Clin. Dev. Med.* 48/49: 28, 1973.
15. Blaivas, J. G., Labib, K. L., Bauer, S. B., and Retik, A. B.: Changing concepts in the urodynamic evaluation of children. *J. Urol.* 117:778, 1977.
16. Bauer, S. B.: Urodynamics in children: indications and methods. In Barrett, D. M., and Wein, A. J. (eds.), *Controversies in Neuro-urology*. Chruchill Livingstone, New York, 1984, pp. 193–202.
17. Gierup, J.: Micturition studies in infants and children: intravesical pressure, urinary flow and urethral resistance in boys without infravesical obstruction. *Scand. J. Urol.* 4:217, 1970.
18. Mundy, A. R., Borzyskowski, M., and Saxton, H. M.: Videourodynamic evaluation of neuropathic vesicourethral dysfunction in children. *Br. J. Urol.* 54:645, 1982.
19. Evans, A. T., Felker, J. R., Shank, R. A., III, and Sugarman, S. R.: Pitfalls of urodynamics. *J. Urol.* 122:220, 1979.
20. Koff, S. A., Solomon, M. H., Lane, G. A., and Lieding, K. G.: Urodynamic studies in anesthetized children. *J. Urol.* 123:61, 1980.
21. Backman, K.-A., and von Garrelts, B.: Apparatus for recording micturition. *Acta Chir. Scand.* 126:167, 1963.
22. Barrett, D. M.: Urinary flow rate: theory and methods. In Barrett, D. M., and Wein, A. J., (eds.), *Controversies in Neuro-urology*. Churchill Livingstone, New York, 1984, pp. 133–143.
23. Barrett, D. M., and Wein, A. J.: Flow evaluation and simultaneous external sphincter electromyography in clinical urodynamics. *J. Urol.* 125:538, 1981.
24. Barrett, D. M.: Disposable (infant) surface electrocardiogram electrodes in urodynamics: a simultaneous comparative study of electrodes. *J. Urol.* 124:663, 1980.
25. Maizels, M., and Firlit, C. F.: Pediatric urodynamics: a clinical comparison of surface versus needle pelvic floor/external sphincter electromyography. *J. Urol.* 122:518, 1979.
26. Koff, S. A., and Kass, E. J.: Abdominal wall elec-

tromyography: a noninvasive technique to improve pediatric urodynamic accuracy. *J. Urol.* 127:736, 1982.
27. Merrill, D. C., Bradley, W. E., and Markland, C.: Air cystometry. II. A clinical evaluation of normal adults. *J. Urol.* 108:85, 1972.
28. Gleason, D. M., Bottaccini, M. R., and Reilly, R. J.: Comparison of cystometrograms and urethral profiles with gas and water media. *Urology* 9:155, 1977.
29. Grossman, H. B., Koff, S. A., and Diokno, A. C.: Cystometry in children. *J. Urol.* 117:646, 1977.
30. Barrett, D. M.: Electromyography: the practical approach. In Barrett, D. M., and Wein, A. J. (eds.), *Controversies in Neuro-urology*. Churchill Livingstone, New York, 1984, pp. 85–92.
31. Firlit, C. F., Smey, P., and King, L. R.: Micturition urodynamic flow studies in children. *J. Urol.* 119:250, 1978.
32. Cook, W. A., Firlit, C. F., Stephens, F. D., and King, L. R.: Techniques and results of urodynamic evaluation of children. *J. Urol.* 117:346, 1977.
33. Webster, G. D., and Older, R. A.: Video urodynamics. *Urology* 16:106, 1980.
34. Webster, G. D., Koefoot, R. B., Jr., and Sihelnik, S.: Urodynamic abnormalities in neurologically normal children with micturition dysfunction. *J. Urol.* 132:74, 1984.
35. Forsythe, W. I., and Redmond, A.: Enuresis and spontaneous cure rate: study of 1129 enuretics. *Arch. Dis. Child.* 49:259, 1974.
36. Whiteside, C. G., and Arnold, E. P.: Persistent primary enuresis: a urodynamic assessment. *Br. Med. J.* 1:364, 1975.
37. Kass, E. J., Diokno, A. C., and Montealegre, A.: Enuresis: principles of management and results of treatment. *J. Urol.* 121:794, 1979.
38. Lennert, J. B., and Mowad, J. J.: Enuresis: evaluation of perplexing symptoms. *Urology* 13:27, 1979.
39. Marshall, S., Marshall, H. H., and Lyon, R. P.: Enuresis: an analysis of various therapeutic approaches. *Pediatrics* 52:813, 1973.
40. Smey, P., Firlit, C. F., and King, L. R.: Voiding pattern abnormalities in normal children: results of pharmacologic manipulation. *J. Urol.* 120:574, 1978.
41. Redman, J. F., and Seibert, J. J.: The uroradiographic evaluation of the enuretic child. *J. Urol.* 122:799, 1979.
42. Libo, L. M., Arnold, G. E., Woodside, J. R., Borden, T. A., and Hardy, T. L.: EMG biofeedback for functional bladder-sphincter dyssynergia: a case study. *Biofeedback Self. Regul.* 8:243, 1983.
43. Sugar, E. C., and Firlit, C. F.: Urodynamic biofeedback: a new therapeutic approach for childhood incontinence/infection (vesical voluntary sphincter dyssynergia). *J. Urol.* 128:1253, 1982.
44. Emery, J. L., and Lendon, R. G.: The local cord lesion in neurospinal dysraphism (meningomyelocele). *J. Pathol.* 110:83, 1973.
45. Laurence, K. M.: The natural history of spina bifida cystica: detailed analysis of 407 cases. *Arch. Dis. Child.* 39:41, 1964.
46. Smith, E. D.: *Spina Bifida and The Total Care of Spinal Myelomeningocele*. Charles C. Thomas, Springfield, IL: 1965, pp. 92–123.
47. Light, K., and Van Blerk, P. J. P.: Causes of renal deterioration in patients with meningomyeloceles. *Br. J. Urol.* 49:257, 1977.
48. Anderson, F. M.: Occult spinal dysraphism: a series of 73 cases. *Pediatrics* 55:826, 1975.
49. Kaplan, G. W.: Myelomeningocele and related disorders. *J. Contin. Educ. Urol.*, October:15, 1978.
50. Barson, A. J.: Spina bifida: the significance of the level and extent of the defect to the morphogenesis. *Dev. Med. Child. Neurol.* 12:129, 1970.
51. Thomas, G. G., Zachary, R. B., and Lister, J.: Serial follow-up studies of bladder pressure in spina bifida infants. *J. Pediatr. Surg.* 9:471, 1974.
52. Bauer, S. B., Labib, K. B., Dieppa, R. A., and Retik, A. B.: Urodynamic evaluation of boy with myelodysplasia and incontinence. *Urology* 10:354, 1977.
53. Gaum, L. D., Wese, F. X., Alton, D. J., Hardy, B. E., and Churchill, B. M.: Radiologic investigation of the urinary tract in the neonate with myelomeningocele. *J. Urol.* 127:510, 1982.
54. Mayo, M. E., Chapman, W. H., and Shurtleff, D. B.: Bladder function in children with meningomyelocele: comparison of cine-fluoroscopy and urodynamics. *J. Urol.* 121:458, 1979.
55. McGuire, E. J., Woodside, J. R., and Borden, T. A.: Upper urinary tract deterioration in patients with myelodysplasia and detrusor hypertonia: a follow-up study. *J. Urol.* 129:823, 1983.
56. McGuire, E. J., and Wagner, F. C., Jr.: The effects of sacral denervation on bladder and urethral function. *Surg. Gynecol. Obstet.* 144:343, 1977.
57. Sundin, T., and Dahlström, A.: The sympathetic innervation of the urinary bladder and urethra in the normal state and after parasympathetic denervation at the spinal root level: an experimental study in cats. *Scand. J. Urol. Nephrol.* 7:131, 1973.
58. Sundin, T., Dahlström, A., Norlén, L., and Svedmyr, N.: The sympathetic innervation and adrenoreceptor function of the human lower urinary tract in the normal state and after parasympathetic denervation. *Invest. Urol.* 14:322, 1977.
59. Snyder, H. McC., III, Kalichman, M. A., Charney, E., and Duckett, J. W.: Vesicostomy for neurogenic bladder with spina bifida: follow-up. *J. Urol.* 130:724, 1983.
60. Stafford, S. J., Fried, F. A., Sackett, C. K., Woosley, R. E., Herrington, R. T., and Mandell, J.: Hydronephrosis in the asymptomatic neonate with myelodysplasia. *J. Urol.* 129:340, 1983.
61. Perez-Marrero, R., Dimmock, W., Churchill, B. M., and Hardy, B. E.: Clean intermittent catheterization in myelomeningocele children less than 3 years old. *J. Urol.* 128:779, 1982.
62. Kyker, J., Gregory, J. G., Shah, J., and Schoenberg, H. W.: Comparison of intermittent catheterization and supravesical diversion in children with meningomyelocele. *J. Urol.* 118:90, 1977.
63. McGuire, E. J., and Savastano, J. A.: Urodynamic findings and clinical status following vesical denervation procedures for control of incontinence. *J. Urol.* 132:87, 1984.

64. Drago, J. R., Wellner, L., Sanford, E. J., and Rohner, T. J., Jr.: The role of intermittent catheterization in the management of children with myelomeningocele. *J. Urol.* 118:92, 1977.
65. Schoenberg, H. W., and Meador, M.: Analysis of 48 children with myelodysplasia. *J. Urol.* 127:749, 1982.
66. Mulcahy, J. J., James, H. E., and McRoberts, J. W.: Oxybutynin chloride combined with intermittent clean catheterization in the treatment of myelomeningocele patients. *J. Urol.* 118:95, 1977.
67. Rabinovitch, H. H., and Kendall, A. R.: Management of the failures of intermittent catheterization in children with myelomeningocele. *Soc. Pediatr. Urol. Newslett.* March:20, 1979.
68. Woodside, J. R., and Borden, T. A.: Pubovaginal sling procedure for the management of urinary incontinence in a myelodysplastic girl. *J. Urol.* 127:744, 1982.
69. Stamey, T. A.: Endoscopic suspension of the vesical neck for urinary incontinence. *Surg. Gynecol. Obstet.* 136:547, 1973.
70. Barrett, D. M., and Furlow, W. L.: The management of severe urinary incontinence in patients with myelodysplasia by implantation of the AS 791/792 urinary sphincter device. *J. Urol.* 128:484, 1982.
71. Scott, F. B., Bradley, W. E., Timm, G. W., and Kothari, D.: Treatment of incontinence secondary to myelodysplasia by an implantable prosthetic urinary sphincter. *South. Med. J.* 66:987, 1973.
72. Gonzalez, R., and DeWolf, W. C.: The artificial bladder sphincter AS-721 for the treatment of incontinence in patients with neurogenic bladder. *J. Urol.* 121:71, 1979.
73. Woodside, J. R., and McGuire, E. J.: Technique for detection of detrusor hypertonia in the presence of urethral sphincteric incompetence. *J. Urol.* 127:740, 1982.
74. Kaplan, W. E., and Firlit, C. F.: Management of reflux in the myelodysplastic child. *J. Urol.* 129:1195, 1983.
75. Woodward, J. R., Anderson, A. M., III, and Parrott, T. S.: Ureteral reimplantation in myelodysplasia children. *J. Urol.* 126:387, 1981.
76. Nash, D. F. E.: Congenital spinal palsy. *Br. Med. J.* 2:1333, 1956.
77. Duhamel, B.: From the mermaid to anal imperforation: the syndrome of caudal regression. *Arch. Dis. Child.* 36:152, 1961.
78. Santulli, T. V., Kiesewetter, W. B., and Bill, A. H., Jr.: Anorectal anomalies: a suggested international classification. *J. Pediatr. Surg.* 5:281, 1970.
79. Belman, A. B., and King, L. R.: Urinary tract abnormalities associated with imperforate anus. *J. Urol.* 108:823, 1972.
80. Wiener, E. S., and Kiesewetter, W. B.: Urologic abnormalities associated with imperforate anus. *J. Pediatr. Surg.* 8:151, 1973.
81. Persky, L., Tucker, A., and Izant, R. J., Jr.: Urological complications of correction of imperforate anus. *J. Urol.* 111:415, 1974.
82. Resnick, M. I., and King, L. R.: Use of the Leadbetter anti-incontinence procedure in children. *J. Urol.* 116:366, 1976.
83. Tank, E. S.: The urologic complications of imperforate anus and cloacal dysgenesis. In Harrison, J. H., Gittes, R. F., Perlmutter, A. D., Stamey, T. A., and Walsh, P. C. (eds.), *Campbell's Urology*, 4th ed., Vol. 2. Saunders, Philadelphia, 1979, pp. 1889–1900.
84. Woodside, J. R., and McGuire, E. J.: Detrusor hypertonicity as a late complication of a Wertheim hysterectomy. *J. Urol.* 127:1143, 1982.
85. McGuire, E. J.: Urodynamic evaluation after abdominal-perineal resection and lumbar intervertebral disk herniation. *Urology* 6:63, 1975.
86. Koff, S. A., and Deridder, P. A.: Patterns of neurogenic bladder dysfunction in sacral agenesis. *J. Urol.* 118:87, 1977.
87. Mariani, A. J., Stern, J., Khan, A. U., and Cass, A. S.: Sacral agenesis: an analysis of 11 cases and review of the literature. *J. Urol.* 122:684, 1979.
88. White, R. I., and Klauber, G. T.: Sacral agenesis: analysis of 22 cases. *Urology* 8:521, 1976.
89. Smith, E. D.: Congenital sacral anomalies in children. *Aust. N.Z. J. Surg.* 29:165, 1959.
90. Cumes, D.: Sacral dysgenesis associated with occult spinal dysraphism causing neurogenic bladder dysfunction. *J. Urol.* 117:127, 1977.
91. Braren, V., and Jones, W. B.: Sacral agenesis: diagnosis, treatment and followup of urological complications. *J. Urol.* 121:543, 1979.
92. Koontz, W. W., Jr., and Prout, G. R., Jr.: Agenesis of the sacrum and the neurogenic bladder. *JAMA* 203:481, 1968.
93. Williams, D. I., and Nixon, H. H.: Agenesis of the sacrum. *Surg. Gynecol. Obstet.* 105:84, 1957.
94. Sarnat, H. B., Case, M. E., and Graviss, R.: Sacral agenesis: neurologic and neuropathologic features. *Neurology* 26:1124, 1976.
95. Allen, T. D.: The non-neurogenic neurogenic bladder. *J. Urol.* 117:232, 1977.
96. Hinman, F.: Urinary tract damage in children who wet. *Pediatrics* 54:142, 1974.
97. Dorfman, L. E., Bailey, J., and Smith, J. P.: Subclinical neurogenic bladder in children. *J. Urol.* 101:48, 1969.
98. Johnston, J. H., and Farkas, A.: Congenital neuropathic bladder: practicalities and possibilities of conservational management. *Urology* 5:719, 1975.
99. Martin, D.C., Datta, N. S., and Schweitz, B.: The occult neurological bladder. *J. Urol.* 105:733 1971.
100. Williams, D. I., Hirst, G., and Doyle, D.: The occult neuropathic bladder. *J. Pediatr. Surg.* 9:35 1974.
101. Bauer, S. B., Retik, A. B., Colodny, A. H., Hallett, M., Khoshbin, S., and Dyro. F. M.: The unstable bladder of childhood. *Urol. Clin. North Am.* 7:321, 1980.
102. Wein, A. J.: Classification of voiding dysfunction: a simple approach. In Barrett, D. M. and Wein, A. J. (eds.), *Controversies in Neuro-urology*. Churchill Livingstone, New York, 1984, pp. 239–250.
103. Snyder, H. M., Caldamone, A. A., Wein, A. J., and Duckett, J. W.: The Hinman syndrome—alternatives for treatment. Presented at the Annual Meeting of the American Urological Association, Kansas City, MO, 1982.
104. Hendren, W. H.: Reconstruction of previously diverted urinary tracts in children. *J. Pediatr. Surg.* 8:135, 1973.

105. Borden, T. A., McGuire, E. J., Woodside, J. R.: Urinary undiversion in patients with myelodysplasia and neurogenic bladder dysfunction: report of a workshop. *Urology* 18:223, 1981.
106. Hendren, W. H.: urinary diversion and undiversion in children. *Surg. Clin. North. Am.* 56:425, 1976.
107. Kogan, S. J., and Levitt, S. B.: Bladder evaluation in pediatric patients before undiversion in previously diverted urinary tracts. *J. Urol.* 118:443, 1977.
108. McGuire, E. J.: Neurogenic incontinence in males. *Urol. Clin. North Am.* 5:335, 1978.
109. Kogan, S. J., Kim, K., and Levitt, S. B.: Preoperative evaluation of bladder function prior to renal transplantation or urinary tract reconstruction in children: description of a method. *J. Pediatr. Surg.* 11:1007, 1976.
110. Woodside, J. R., and McGuire, E. J.: A simple inexpensive urodynamic catheter. *J. Urol.* 122:788,1979.

15

Adult Female Urology

EDWARD J. McGUIRE, M.D.

The most common urologic symptoms in women, as in men, are urgency and frequency. Peculiar to female urologic conditions is a relative lack of the obstructive voiding disorders so commonly encountered in men.The dramatic response of men with urethral strictures or benign prostatic hypertrophy to appropriate surgical procedures initially led to the application of procedures aiming at correcting urethral obstruction in women with irritative bladder symptoms. Unfortunately, the more common causes of such symptoms in women proved not to be obstructive, and the treatment usually failed or, in the case of transurethral resection (TUR) of the vesical outlet or YV-plasty, occasionally led to intractable urinary incontinence. The procedures that lead to incontinence have largely been abandoned; moreover, urethral dilatation is not commonly used today because in most patients it does not lead to relief of symptoms (*1*).

URINARY INFECTION

One of the most common causes of irritative bladder symptoms in women is recurrent urinary tract infection, which occurs in 7 to 15 percent of the female population. Although residual urine, poor voiding, and neuromuscular functional changes induced by pregnancy increase the risk of urinary tract infection, its incidence does not appear to be influenced by these ancillary problems. Women with neurogenic vesical dysfunction related to spinal cord injury or multiple sclerosis appear to have an increased risk of urinary tract infection, but exactly what that risk is has so far not been accurately defined. Overt neurogenic vesical dysfunctions that induce incontinence are frequently treated by Foley or suprapubic tube vesical drainage by a Foley catheter, or by a suprapubic catheter with predictably poor results over a 10 to 15-year period due to upper urinary tract deterioration, urolithiasis, or ultimately vesical fibrosis requiring augmentation cystoplasty or supravesical diversion. Patients without neurogenic dysfunction or recurrent urinary infections rarely show anatomic abnormalities. Radiographic, endoscopic, and urodynamic evaluation of young adult women with recurrent urinary tract infection are rarely indicated and rarely productive.

URGENCY AND FREQUENCY WITH INCONTINENCE

Urgency and frequency are protean irritative bladder symptoms; and when they are associated with urinary incontinence, detailed clinical and urodynamic evaluation is usually indicated. The most common etiology of such symptoms is probably detrusor instability, but occasionally that dysfunction can be difficult to confirm urodynamically. Under standard circumstances of urodynamic testing, in an alert patient, detrusor instability may not be disclosed even by painful overfilling of the bladder. Cerebral disinterest and lack of conscious appreciation of vesical functional events, especially vesical filling, are fairly consistent features of detrusor instability (*2,3*). Because urodynamic testing tends to obviate cerebral disinterest, it is often nondiagnostic in patients with detrusor instability due to poor appreciation of the degree of bladder filling or imminence of a detrusor contraction. Continuous intravesical pressure monitoring (*4–6*) may uncover detrusor instability.

The standard treatment of detrusor instability is anticholinergic agents; clinicians frequently prescribe them on the basis of the patient's history and cystoscopy that reveals no abnormality. Provided there is no residual urine, such treatment, though empiric, is reasonable and often effective.

A cystometrogram (CMG) combined with electromyography (EMG) and urethral pressure measurements can amplify the results of urodynamic testing. The normal bladder tolerates filling with a minimal increase in vesical pressure, slight striated sphincter (EMG) activity, and an increase in urethral closure pressure. The latter two events consititute the guarding reflex (*7*) and should remain active in the area associated with volitional sphincteric closure unless the subject studied volitionally relaxes the urethral sphincter to void. A sudden fall in EMG activity with a sharp drop in urethral closing pressure and gradual downward drift of both EMG and urethral closing pressure recordings are abnormal (*8*). Because sphincteric relaxation is an integral part of the reflex detrusor response, these findings are indicative of unrecognized sphincter relaxation (Fig. 15–1).

Sphincteric pressure falloff is a reasonable indicator of detrusor instability that the examiner can usually suspect from the history alone. It is sufficient evidence to initiate treatment, usually with anticholinergic agents and timed or prospective voiding. It is important to point out to the patient that sudden, unanticipated reflex detrusor contractile activity is part of the problem and that micturition on a timed prospective schedule before the need to void is apparent is an effective way of dealing with the problem. Anticholinergic agents only delay the reflex response; they do not necessarily cure the condition.

URGENCY AND FREQUENCY WITHOUT INCONTINENCE

Urgency and frequency as apparently isolated symptoms are fairly common in office urologic practice after urinary infection, bladder calculi, ureteral calculi, and carcinoma *in situ* have been eliminated as diagnostic possibilities by appropriate endoscopy, urine culture, and radiographic studies. It is this particular group of patients and the difficulty urologists have had in treating them

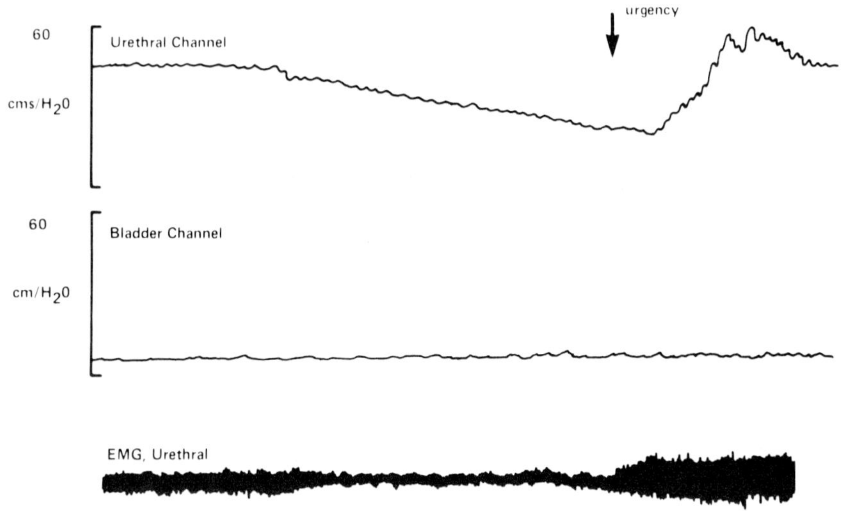

Figure 15–1. Urodynamic study shows a slow drift in urethral pressure with filling associated with diminished EMG activity, culminating in a sensation of urgency and brisk volitional sphincter response. This picture is reasonable urodynamic evidence of detrusor instability (see text).

effectively that led to interest in urodynamics as a method of assessment in the office. Unfortunately, urodynamic evaluation has neither improved our diagnostic ability in this patient group nor led to more effective treatment. It seems clear that relative volume intolerance resulting in urgency and frequency of urination in otherwise healthy women is not a single disease entity. Some of these women have "interstitial cystitis," some a syndrome similar to interstitial cystitis, some the "urethral syndrome," and many an idiopathic condition. It may be that there is an emotional component to the complaints, but it has not been demonstrated conclusively.

Urethral dilatation, internal urethrotomy, or fulguration of microabscesses in the urethra are certainly not universally effective methods, although in occasional cases they seem to be. The problem lies in patient selection, and it may be that measurement of urethral compliance will turn out to be a method to detect those patients who will improve with urethral dilatation (J. J. Susset, personal communication, 1983).

Anticholinergic agents are ineffective for pure sensory urgency and probably should not be used. Treatment of volume intolerance with bladder overdistension under anesthesia and administration of dimethylsulfoxide (DMSO) can be effective, but there is no accurate method to determine that preoperatively, either endoscopically or urodynamically.

URINARY INCONTINENCE

Stress urinary incontinence is defined as involuntary urinary loss, with an increase in intraabdominal pressure and without any evidence of detrusor contraction. This condition is relatively common, and accurate diagnosis rests on the history and physical examination, with appropriate urodynamic evaluation when indicated.

PATHOPHYSIOLOGY OF STRESS URINARY INCONTINENCE AND ASSOCIATED ABNORMALITIES

About 30 percent of women with stress urinary incontinence have associated detrusor instability or a bladder that contracts without its owner's permission (*9*). Although there is no real agreement among experts in the field regarding the precise relation between the two conditions, there is good evidence in a substantial number of patients with both conditions that cure of the stress incontinence relieves detrusor instability.

Stress incontinence appears to be the result of urethral sphincter inefficiency in the face of increased intraabdominal pressure. Because in women the proximal urethra from the bladder neck to the high-pressure zone is intraabdominal, it normally is exposed to the same abdominal pressure excursion as the bladder. Both structures normally maintain their resting pressure relations or a higher urethral than bladder pressure despite changes in intraabdominal pressure. In women with stress incontinence this relation is imperfectly maintained. It appears to be due to loss of integrity of urethral supporting structures so that an increase in intraabdominal pressure actually results in posterior and inferior rotational descent of the urethra and anterior vaginal wall, with shortening and telescoping of the sphincter active area. With urethral motion, intraabdominal pressure is less effectively transmitted to the moving urethra, which is forced into an extraabdominal position, and the bladder, compresssed by the intraabdominal pressure change, briefly registers a pressure higher than the urethra, resulting in a brief spurt of urine. The fact that there is an association between urethral mobility and stress incontinence has been exhaustively documented (a) radiographically using catheters, bead chains, and mercury-filled balloons; (b) utlrasonically; (c) by physical examination; and (d) endoscopically (*10*) (Fig. 15–2).

The problem is that not all women with urethral hypermobility have stress incontinence, whereas some women with no urethral hypermobility are incontinent, some clearly with stress incontinence. A particular illustration involves women with pronounced cystocele formation and urethral hypermobility who rarely complain of stress urinary incontinence and indeed may show evidence of fairly high-grade urethral obstruction. These findings suggest that static radiography is not the best method to clearly diagnose stress incontinence; probably the single most accurate method requires fluoroscopy to document urethral and bladder mo-

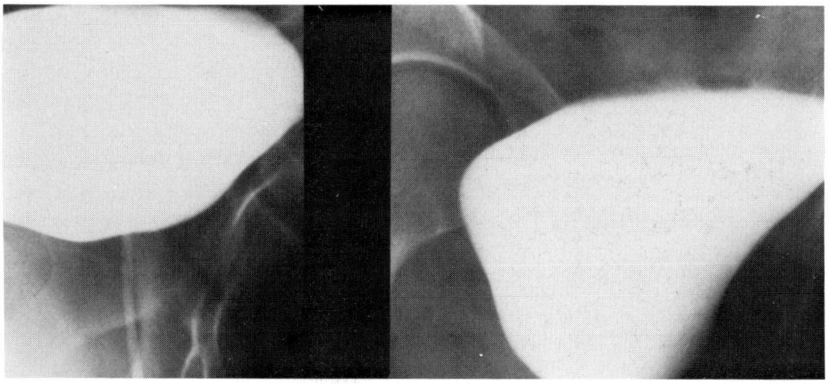

Figure 15–2. Radiographic findings in a 54-year-old woman with stress incontinence. Note the bladder prolapse with straining (*right*), hiding the urethra; at rest (*left*) the bladder is in normal position.

bility as well as any associated urinary loss, which is quite easy to visualize. That method, particularly if combined with intravesical pressure monitoring, provides information on anatomic distortion of the organs; this information helps when planning repair and allows fairly accurate characterization of internal sphincter competence, as well as documentation of the presence of urethral leakage in conjunction with posterior and inferior rotational descent of the urethra and bladder base. It is particularly valuable to use that method in women with large symptomatic cystoceles, as urinary incontinence, although potentially present, is not usually symptomatic. If urethral hypermobility is present, that abnormality should be repaired at the time of repair of the cystocele to prevent the *de novo* appearance of stress urinary incontinence as a result of replacement of the bladder within the abdominal cavity.

Although genital prolapse, rectocele, cystocele, and even enterocele formation are not causally related to stress incontinence, they are associated with that condition in 16 to 20 percent of the patients. These problems cannot realistically be ignored when the stress incontinence is being corrected with an operative procedure.

HISTORY

The examiner must inquire about the characteristics of the incontinence. Typical stress urinary incontinence is brief, related to coughing, jogging, or exertion, and worse in the upright position. Urinary loss while sleeping, on the way to the toilet, in large amounts suddenly, or when water is run in the sink or bath usually indicates bladder instability.

Urinary loss at odd intervals without sensation, or coughing, or exertion, e.g., while walking about, is an indeterminant symptom that should prompt further investigation. Prior operations have an important bearing on the usual evaluation. A prior operation for stress incontinence that resulted in no change in symptoms or made the symptoms worse is often associated with poor urethral sphincter function and not classic urethral motion-related stress incontinence. A prior operation(s) that effectively "cured" stress incontinence for a time is usually associated with recurrent urethral hypermobility. Multiple prior operative procedures for stress incontinence are often associated with poor or no urethral sphincter function, as is the incontinence that began after surgery for a urethral diverticulum or major pelvic extirpative procedures. Incontinence after both of the latter, however, may be related to fistula formation as well. Concurrent medication can influence vesical and urethral function adversely, especially pharmacologic agents, including the phenothiazines, which have anticholinergic and alpha-adrenergic blocking properties, and antihypertensive agents with alpha-adrenergic blocking properties. Chronic disease, e.g., diabetes, can result in both urethral failure and detrusor atony and areflexia, as can prior pelvic irradiation or surgery.

PHYSICAL EXAMINATION

Motion of the urethra and bladder base palpable through the anterior vaginal wall with an increase in intraabdominal pressure, if associated with a brief spurt of urine from the urethra, is diagnostic of stress incontinence. Lack of motion with leakage suggests a severely impaired urethral sphincter or sometimes a fistula. The characteristics of the urethra and surrounding tissues as well as fixation of the urethra due to prior operations are determined. If the urethra is firmly fixed to the surrounding tissue and immobile, a standard retropubic suspension is sometimes difficult. Contractility of the pelvic floor and striated sphincter is determined if any associated cystocele, rectocele, or uterine prolapse is noted.

ANCILLARY TESTING

Radiography, as mentioned above, particularly combined with urodynamic evaluation, provides the best overall method of assessment. We use a 10F Bard triple-lumen urodynamic catheter with a radiographic marker to identify the bladder and urethral perfusion apertures on fluoroscopy. The three channels are perfused with a radiopaque medium (20% Hypaque). The catheter is inserted into the bladder and the patient placed in the upright oblique position on the fluoroscopy table. The urethral perfusion aperture is withdrawn through the sphincter area to obtain a radiographic and manometric assessment of urethral resting sphincter activity. The urethral perfusion aperture is then replaced in the proximal 2 cm of urethra, and the bladder is filled to 300 ml, at which time the patient is asked to cough and perform the Valsalva maneuver. At such time the bladder and urethra are visualized fluoroscopically, the urethral and bladder motion is characterized, and urine leakage is visually detected. Bladder filling is then continued until capacity is reached or a bladder contraction occurs. If no bladder contraction occurs before bladder capacity is reached, the patient is asked to volitionally urinate. Once a bladder contraction is well in progress, the patient is asked to stop voiding.

The above method provides fairly precise information on the characteristics and extent of urethral hypermobility, the presence and relative severity of urinary incontinence, function of the resting voluntary and involuntary sphincter mechanism, and the presence of detrusor instability and detrusor contractile function. The patient's ability to volitionally override detrusor contractility can also be ascertained. Episodes of urethral instability during filling characterized by a fall in urethral closing pressure, with or without a detrusor contraction, are also detectable.

Using the above methodology led to recognition of several syndromes associated with incontinence, as well as some types of incontinence in women. Type I or II urinary incontinence is characterized by minor to major urethral hypermobility associated with visible urinary loss (Fig. 15–3). Such incontinence occurs in about 90 percent of patients referred for urodynamic testing who never had an operation for stress incontinence. It occurs in 70 percent of patients who have failed one operation but is less common in patients who have failed successive operations.

Type III stress incontinence is characterized by an open proximal urethra with an increase in intraabdominal pressure, with or without hypermobility of the urethra (Fig. 15–4). This type is usually seen in women who have failed successive vaginal and retropubic operative procedures, occasionally in young women or even adolescents, and fairly frequently in elderly women. The latter patients rarely show total proximal urethral nonfunction but, rather, have extremely low pressures in the first 1.5 to 1.8 cm of the urethra.

INCIDENCE OF VARIOUS TYPES OF INCONTINENCE AND ASSOCIATED DETRUSOR INSTABILITY

In a study of 603 women with radiographically and urodynamically determined stress incontinence, 169 (28%) had type I, 340 (56%) type II, and 94 (16%) type III stress incontinence. As reported in a previous study, the incidence of type III urinary in-

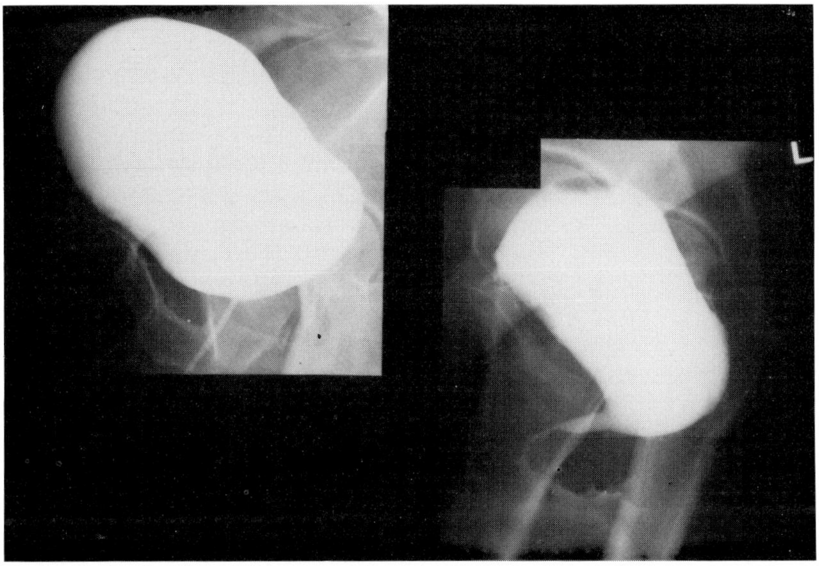

Figure 15–3. Resting (*left*) and straining (*right*) lateral cystourethrograms showing urethral and bladder base hypermobility with visible urethral urinary loss: type II stress incontinence.

continence in patients who never had an operation is 10 percent or less; the incidence of type III incontinence after a single operation increases to 25 to 30 percent in women and to 60 to 75 percent in those with multiple successive operative failures.

Ninety-nine patients with type I incontinence had a 7 percent failure rate after anterior colporrhaphy with recurrent urethral hypermobility and stress incontinence. In a 5-year follow-up study there were no failures due to recurrent urethral hypermobility in 51 patients with type I stress incontinence who had a retropubic operation. None of seven patients treated by a Raz needle suspension failed with recurrent hypermobility and stress incontinence over a 2-year period.

Of 283 patients with type II incontinence treated by retropubic suspension or the Raz procedure, there was failure with recurrent urethral hypermobility and stress incontinence in four (1.3%). There were no failures over a 3- to 4-year follow-up period as a result of recurrent urethral hypermobility and stress incontinence in 24 patients with type II incontinence treated by a pubovaginal sling. Anterior repair had a 60 percent failure rate due to recurrent urethral hypermobility in patients with type II and virtually a 100 percent rate in those with type III incontinence. Of 93 type III patients treated by a pubovaginal sling, four had recurrent stress

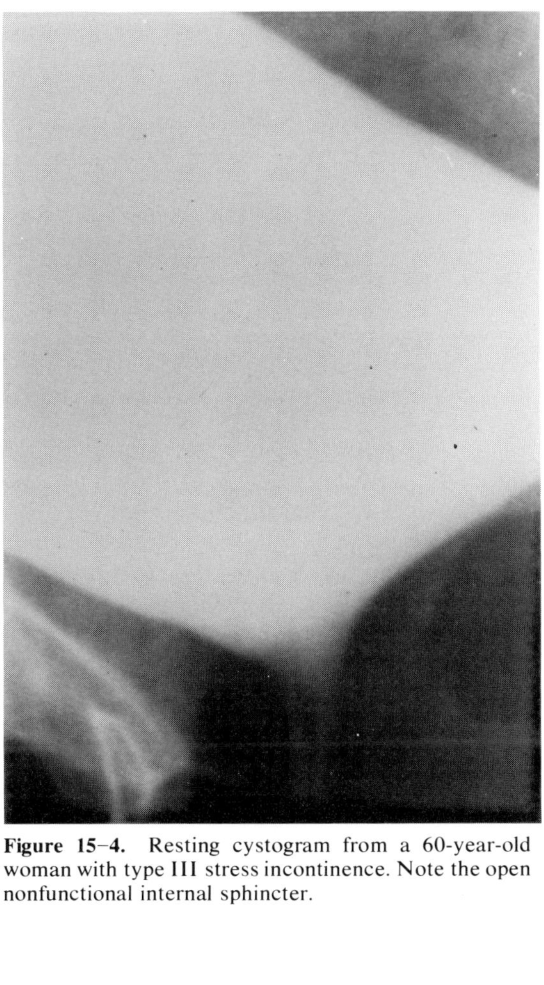

Figure 15–4. Resting cystogram from a 60-year-old woman with type III stress incontinence. Note the open nonfunctional internal sphincter.

incontinence over a 10-year period (a failure rate of 4.3%).

RELATION BETWEEN STRESS INCONTINENCE AND DETRUSOR INSTABILITY

In the above series of 603 patients, 180 (29.8%) had preoperative detrusor instability on cystometry or by history. Of this group of women, 56 (31%) still had detrusor instability postoperatively; that is, 31 percent of those with preoperatively determined detrusor instability still had the problem. In other words, it appears that detrusor instability was relieved by the operation in 69 percent of patients. Twenty-four patients (4 %) developed detrusor instability only postoperatively. The problem of instability thus persisted postoperatively in 80 patients and ultimately was the cause of an unsatisfactory operative result in 23, or about one-third of this group. Operative failure due solely to detrusor instability occurred in 4 percent of the entire group of patients.

The incidence of failure due to intractable detrusor instability was 2.2 percent after anterior repair, 5.1 percent after a Marshall-Marchetti-Krantz operation, 4.1 percent after a Burch retropubic suspension, 5.6 percent after the sling procedure, but 0 percent after Raz needle suspension. These data suggest that in some cases intractable detrusor instability may be related to the obstructive character of the operation. It should be remembered that in most patients detrusor instability appears to be causally related to stress incontinence and is often relieved by its operative treatment, but that there are no preoperative criteria that allow the examiner to predict the outcome of an operation with respect to detrusor instability. Indeed, most patients with overt and easily elicited detrusor instability at low volumes, particularly when associated with severe stress incontinence, had a good postoperative result.

SPINAL CORD INJURY AND DEMYELINATING DISEASES

Violent trauma resulting in spinal cord injury has become more common in women than in the past. Methods to manage the lower urinary tract that are applicable to men are often inappropriate in women.

During spinal shock, intermittent catheterization is the method of choice for management of the lower urinary tract. Bladder volumes greater than 500 ml should be avoided, and hospital-acquired urinary tract infections should be prevented or appropriately treated. Direct instillation of an antimicrobial agent into the bladder at the time of intermittent catheterization seems to be a reasonable and practical method (*11*). We instill 20 to 30 ml of gentamicin (240 mg/L of saline) into the bladder after each catheterization.

In patients with lesions above T_{12}, spontaneous reflex bladder activity is recovered, on the average, 1 to 3 months after injury. Suppression of reflex vesical activity with anticholinergic agents and continued intermittent catheterization is still the method of choice for bladder management at this stage. Although female patients with spinal cord injury can develop upper tract dilatation without incontinence due to detrusor sphincter dyssynergia, it is relatively unusual. This finding appears to be related to both detrusor power and the strength of the striated sphincter, which generates pressures that are considerably lower than those measured in men.

In female patients with transverse suprasacral spinal cord lesions managed by intermittent catheterization, a danger to upper urinary tract function is almost always associated with urinary incontinence. Initial urodynamic evaluation is performed when a patient who is expected to develop reflex bladder activity becomes intermittently incontinent between catheterizations. The purpose of the urodynamic evaluation is to ascertain the volume required to elicit a bladder contraction, the intravesical pressure required to drive urine across the sphincter, and the presence or absence of vesicoureteral reflux. A baseline intravenous urogram is also helpful at that time in determining the status of the upper urinary tracts.

Urodynamic testing is best done with a trilumen urodynamic catheter, which allows measurement of bladder and urethral pressures, and fluoroscopic monitoring to detect leakage in the presence of detrusor–sphincter dyssynergia as well as vesicoureteral reflux. A combination of anticholinergic agents (e.g., oxybutynin chloride plus imipramine hydrochloride) may help control incontinence and ameliorate intravesical pressure.

PATTERNS IN FEMALE PATIENTS WITH TRANSVERSE SUPRASACRAL SPINAL CORD INJURY: QUADRIPLEGICS

Women with high spinal cord lesions and limited hand function are usually unable to perform intermittent self-catheterization. These patients also have a 60 percent rate of developing autonomic dysreflexia and may require alpha-adrenergic blocking agents, sacral rhizotomy, or both to control this problem (*12*). Forty percent of these patients develop intractable incontinence due to uncontrollable detrusor contractility, which is frequently treated by Foley or suprapubic catheter drainage, particularly if the incontinence is associated with autonomic dysreflexia. It is important to remember, however, that autonomic dysreflexia may be related to bladder volume and not invariably to bladder contraction or increased vesical pressure. Quadriplegics occasionally develop severe autonomic dysreflexia after treatment with anticholinergic agents because of relatively high bladder volumes. Such patients are treated with alpha-adrenergic blocking agents (e.g., prazosin 1 mg. b.i.d. or thorazine 25 mg t.i.d.), but the anticholinergic agents are also continued (*12*). Urodynamic evaluation of these patients is helpful in determining whether the autonomic dysreflexia is related to high bladder volumes or is in fact related to detrusor contractile activity. If it is the former, an effort is made to control the dysreflexia and preserve continence.

Patients who escape anticholinergic medication and develop detrusor hyperreflexia with uncontrollable incontinence can be converted to areflexic bladder by S_{2-4} dorsal root ganglionectomy or intradural sacral rhizotomy. Alternatively, subtotal cystectomy with augmentation cecocystoplasty can be performed. These procedures may need to be combined with creation of a continent vesicostomy or an abdominal stoma to facilitate self-catheterization in women with limited hand function (*13,14*).

In practice, about 50 percent of quadraplegic women can be managed by intermittent catheterization with the help of anticholinergic agents, and alpha-adrenergic blocking agents as required. These patients continue to maintain normal upper urinary tracts by intravenous urography and are free from stones, sepsis, and urethral erosion, all of which are common in patients treated by catheter drainage on a chronic basis. Another 25 to 30 percent of patients require and accept one or two procedures to achieve an areflexic bladder and facilitate intermittent self-catheterization. The remainder of the patients choose management by catheter; these can expect a 40 percent rate of upper urinary tract deterioration and a 100 percent rate of bladder and urethral complications over time. Although these percentages are better than those in comparable male patients treated by catheter they are still dismal, and every effort should be made, once the lesion is stable at 2 years, to encourage patients to accept an appropriate procedure(s) that will protect them from upper urinary tract dysfunction and irreparable bladder injury. The latter, which culminates in a fibrotic end-stage bladder, often leads to unremitting autonomic dysreflexia, prolonged hospitalization, supravesical diversion, and often cystectomy, with early or delayed development of struvite calculi in the upper urinary tracts.

PARAPLEGICS WITH SUPRASACRAL TRANSVERSE SPINAL CORD LESIONS

Paraplegic patients with suprasacral transverse spinal cord lesions are not subject to the syndrome of autonomic dysreflexia but have problems with control of reflex detrusor activity of the same severity as in quadriplegics. Appoximately one-third of the patients, however, never develop effective high-pressure reflex activity and can be managed easily by intermittent catheterization, with or without anticholinergic agents. Another one-third require vigorous anticholinergic therapy to control hyperreflexic bladder activity and facilitate intermittent self-catheterization. These individuals can be expected to maintain normal upper urinary tracts and to remain free of serious bladder and urethral complications. In the remaining one-third, operative intervention is necessary to control reflex vesical activity by rhizotomy, ganglionectomy, or subtotal cystectomy with augmentation cystoplasty. Invariably, some patients choose catheter drainage; 30 to 40 percent of these patients can be expected to develop, with time, upper urinary tract dysfunction, upper urinary tract infection, or struvite stone formation; and all experience lower urinary tract complications.

LESIONS BELOW T_{12}–L_1

Lesions below T_{12}–L_1 are associated with detrusor areflexia and often preservation of some striated sphincter activity. Although early upper urinary tract problems are unusual, incontinence is often the major problem. Most such patients can be managed by intermittent self-catheterization with or without anticholinergic agents. These agents are required to decrease intrinsic detrusor tone, which is elevated following a sacral cord or root lesion. If incontinence is still a problem, urodynamic evaluation consisting in upright bladder pressure registration during filling under fluoroscopic control, can be useful. If vesical compliance is the underlying problem, cyclic filling or augmentation cystoplasty may be required. If maintenance of the internal sphincter is the underlying problem, a pubovaginal sling, or a Scott inflatable prosthesis, may be required.

DEMYELINATING DISEASES

The demyelinating diseases are more frequently encountered in women than in men. When uncomfortable lower urinary tract symptoms prompt urologic referral, three basic urodynamic patterns may be encountered. These patterns have similar clinical expressions and symptoms, including pressure sensation, incontinence, urgency, inability to initiate micturition, and nocturnal enuresis. As such, the symptoms have no differential value, being common to patients with urodynamic evidence of uninhibited detrusor activity, with or without detrusor–sphincter dyssynergia, and profound detrusor areflexia.

Measurement of residual urine volumes is helpful. Large volumes are usually associated with detrusor areflexia (which can be managed by intermittent self-catheterization), moderate volumes with detrusor hyperreflexia and discoordinate striated sphincter activity, and minimal to no residual volumes with simple detrusor instability with a coordinated striated sphincter.

On initial urodynamic testing, about 45 percent of patients with multiple sclerosis demonstrate unstable detrusor responses associated with discoordinated reflex striated sphincter activity and an inability to volitionally initiate micturition by conscious sphincteric relaxation. Although some of these patients respond to anticholinergic medication, most either develop urinary retention or continue to be incontinent as a result of detrusor reflex contractility. Only about one-half of the patients respond to treatment with anticholinergic agents, which usually must be coupled with intermittent self-catheterization as it is in spinal cord injury patients. Treatment of incontinence by Foley or suprapubic catheter drainage is usually unsuccessful over time and frequently results in permanent urethral injury, requiring ever larger catheters, or the development of vesical calculi and upper urinary tract deterioration.

Patients with multiple sclerosis satisfactorily treated by intermittent self-catheterization and anticholinergic agents for protracted periods of 1 to 3 years usually had stable disease with only slow and gradual deterioration in general function, whereas those who responded poorly often had progressive neurologic disease.

Patients with simple detrusor instability without sphincter discoordination respond reasonably well to anticholinergic medication. Ten percent of these patients gradually progress and develop sphincter discoordination in association with detrusor hyperreflexia and recurrent urinary incontinence. Most individuals with areflexic vesical dysfunction can be managed by intermittent self-catheterization over time, but 20 percent gradually develop intractable incontinence related to the development of detrusor–sphincter dyssynergia and detrusor hyperreflexia.

REFERENCES

1. Gleason, D., and Bottaccini, M. R.: In: McGuire, E. J. (ed.), *Urinary Incontinence*. Grune & Stratton, New York, 1981.
2. Yeates, W. K.: Disorders of bladder function. *Ann. R. Coll. Surg.* 50:335, 1972.
3. Torrens, M. J., and Collins, C. D.: The urodynamic assessment of adult enuresis. *Br. J. Urol.* 47:433, 1975.
4. James, D.: Continuous monitoring. *Urol. Clin. North Am.* 6:125, 1979.
5. Bradley, W. E., Bhatia, N., and Haldeman, S.: Twenty-four hour continuous urodynamic monitoring. In *Proceedings of the AUA*, abstract 113, 1982.
6. Frohneberg, D., Thüroff, J. W., Petri, E., and Jonas, U.: Telemetric urodynamic investigations in patients with intravesical obstruction. In *Proceedings of the AUA*, 1981.
7. Blaivas, J. G.: A critical appraisal of specific diagnostic techniques. In Krane, R., and Siroky, M. (eds.), *Clinical Neurourology*. Little, Brown, Boston, 1979.
8. McGuire, E. J.: Reflex urethral instability. *Br. J. Urol.* 50:200, 1978.
9. McGuire, E. J., Pepe, V., Kohorn, E., and Lytton, B.: The value of urodynamic testing in stress urinary incontinence. *J. Urol.* 124:256, 1980.
10. McGuire, E. J.: Causes of involuntary loss and ways to recognize it. In: McGuire, E. J. (ed.), *Urinary Incontinence*. Grune & Stratton, New York, 1980.
11. Rhame, F.S., and Perkash, I.: Urinary tract infections occurring in recent spinal cord injury patients on intermittent catheterization. *J. Urol.* 122:669, 1979.
12. McGuire, E. J., and Rossier, A. B.: Treatment of acute autonomic dysreflexia. *J. Urol.* 129:1185, 1983.
13. McGuire, E. J., and Wagner, F.: The effect of complete sacral rhizotomy on bladder and urethral function. *Surg. Gynecol. Obstet.* 144:343, 1977.
14. Green, D. H., Micheson, D., and McGuire, E. J.: Management of the bladder by augmentation ileocecocystoplasty. *J. Urol.* 130:133, 1983.

16

Prostatic Enlargement and Prostatism

SUBBARAO V. YALLA, M.D.

Enlargement of the prostate gland in men over 50 years of age has traditionally been held responsible for most of their lower urinary tract symptoms. Despite modern innovative technology, the urologist continues to depend for clinical evaluation on the patient's symptoms and the size of the prostatic gland as assessed by rectal and endoscopic examination. Often successful management of these patients can be accomplished using these conventional methods of assessment. In certain patients, however, these time-honored methods may not be helpful in determining the degree of outlet obstruction or predicting the outcome of prostatic surgery. In most instances the urologist, based on previous training, makes therapeutic decisions that may be debated by peers. A survey of second opinions on urologic surgical procedures showed that a significant number (26%) of patients who were advised to have transurethral resection of the prostate (TURP) were successfully managed by noninvasive therapy after a second opinion was sought (*1*). In other words, there is a wide difference of opinion among urologists in regard to the management of patients with prostatic enlargement. The reasons for this discrepancy are (a) the lack of precise objective criteria for clinical assessment of the problem and (b) the lack of specific information related to the outcome of surgical versus nonsurgical management.

Currently, obstructive symptoms secondary to prostatic enlargement can be evaluated with techniques that involve simple clinical observations as well as sophisticated electronic urodynamic testing. Despite modern innovative urodynamic techniques, there is no consensus with respect to the definition of the term "obstruction" (*2*). Nevertheless, it remains possible to clinically evaluate such patients with techniques that are mentioned in this and other chapters of this book.

Most urodynamic studies in the patient with prostatic enlargement have been designed to record urinary flow rates (*3*), exit velocities (*4*), urethral closure pressure profiles (to assess prostatic urethral length) (*5*), the degree of prostatic enlargement and the resultant urethral compression, pressure–flow relations to assess outlet resistance (*6*), and micturitional pressure profiles to localize the site and degree of outlet obstruction (*7*). Abrams studied patients with prostatism and suggested that symptoms such as a slow urinary stream and hesitancy can be attributed to the presence of outflow obstruction (*8*); the symptoms of frequency, nocturia, urgency, and incontinence have all been attributed to bladder overactivity. Their study involved an analysis of 318 male patients 45 to 85 years of age who had symptoms suggestive of outflow obstruction (*8*). Thirteen percent of these patients showed no urodynamic abnormalities with cystometry and urinary flow rate determinations. We suspect that more sensitive evaluations such as exit flow and energy determination (velocity and flow) as well as micturitional total or static urethral pressure profiles would reveal some element of obstruction in the "nonobstructed" group. Abrams (*8*) also reported that 107 of 318 patients were not surgically treated on clinical grounds, and on later review (after 5 years) 53 were shown to be obstructed by urodynamic criteria, and 10 of these patients required surgery because of deterioration of the obstructive problems.

Confusion about the components of obstructive and irritative symptoms in men over 50 years of age can be related to several factors. Patients in this age group may be taking medications that influence the function of the bladder and its outlet. The patient may also have a subclinical neurogenic condition, e.g., discogenic compression, diabetic autonomic neuropathy, or cerebrovascular disease. In addition, the effect of aging on the bladder wall about which little is known could influence the mechanics of the bladder and its outlet. When the patient has moderate or mild prostatic enlargement in association with disproportionate bladder wall changes the clinical picture can be more confusing.

METHODS OF EVALUATIONS

Rectal Evaluation of Prostatic Size

Digital examination of the prostate per rectum often does not indicate if the patient is obstructed. It has been suggested by several workers that a moderate degree of prostatic enlargement may not be associated with obstruction. A clear correlation between the size of the prostate and urodynamic findings of outlet obstruction is often lacking (*9*).

Cystourethroscopy

The studies of Andersen and Nordling have suggested that the cystourethroscopic findings and grading of prostatic lobe occlusion may be correlated with the degree of bladder outlet obstruction (*11*). They found that grade I and II lateral lobe occlusions were associated with a reduction in peak flow rates and suggested that estimation of bladder neck-to-verumontanum distance can be a good criterion for assessing outlet obstruction; they also noted that marked rigidity of the bladder neck can be associated with reduced flow rates.

Intravenous Urography

Studies have shown that the intravenous urogram has limited value in patients who have obstructive symptoms but no hematuria (*12*). Although certain features of the bladder observed on the intravenous urogram (trabeculation, diverticula, large amount of residual urine, thick wall, and defects at the base) have been considered to be indicative of outlet obstruction, their precise value when making decisions about treatment has not been established.

In his review Abrams mentioned that intravenous urography plays a minimal role in the assessment of patients with prostatic enlargement (*8*). He analyzed the urograms of a large group of patients who were subjected to urodynamic studies. Several features (trabeculation, diverticula, prostatic filling defect on the base of the bladder, residual urine, increased bladder wall thickness, and the presence of prostatic calculi) have been studied. Although he found a relation between trabeculation, diverticula, bladder instability, prostatic urethral configurations, and obstruction, he believed that the intravenous urogram provides only limited information to help make the diagnosis of outlet obstruction. Although Abrams' studies revealed upper tract dilation in 5 percent, renal cysts in 3 percent, renal calculi in 1 percent, pyelonephritis in 1 percent, and congenital renal anomalies in 1.5 percent of the cases, these abnormalities did not affect the ultimate management of outlet obstruction. Several other studies led to similar impressions on the value of the intravenous urogram in the management of prostatism and to the conclusion that routine urography is not necessary in the evaluation of the vesical outlet but is advisable if the patient has urinary infection or hematuria. Turner-Warwick *et al.* believed that positive urographic renal findings, despite their low incidence, are of great importance in clinical management of the patient with prostatic enlargement; they therefore advocated a modified urogram that they termed the "intravenous urodynamogram" (*12*). With this study a lower tract postvoiding film is obtained after an upper tract spot film series. It is suggested from this type of study that the modified upper urinary tract radiologic screening coupled with a more physiologic assessment of the lower urinary tract reduces the radiation exposure and the cost.

Voiding Cystourethrography

Functional and anatomic study of the lower urinary tract can be accomplished by well-performed voiding cystourethrography. Although this test is known to be a valuable radiographic procedure, the urologist does not routinely depend on it during clinical assessment of prostatic enlargement. We believe that voiding cystourethrography is underutilized in clinical evaluation of the lower urinary tract, and that when properly used it can yield valuable information that negates the need for urodynamic testing. These impressions are further supported by Manolin who conducted synchronous radiologic and urodynamic studies in several men and was able to predict outlet obstructions by Radiologically measuring the prostatic diameter (*12a*).

During bladder filling with radiocontrast solution, vesical adaptation can be assessed by visualizing the rate of flow of contrast material in the drip chamber. During initiation of voiding, bladder base descent into the pelvis and the extent of bladder neck opening and funneling also can be observed. During voiding the amount of opacification of the posterior urethra, any filling defect, and the location of the verumontanum (sometimes visualized) can provide information of the length of the urethra and the degree of prostatic encroachment on its lumen. By observing the patient's abdominal wall movements and radiologically assessing the descent of the bladder base during voiding, it is possible to recognize if the patient is applying a Valsalva maneuver. Observations on the degree of bulbous urethral filling with radiocontrast material can provide further information on the degree of outlet obstruction (*13*). We have noted that prostatic urethral, or bladder neck obstructions can produce inadequate filling of the proximal portion of the bulbous urethra, creating the appearance of a long membranous urethra (Figs. 16–1 and 16–2), and that with less severe obstruction the bulb may be filled but not adequately distended. Other features such as contour and wall thickness of the bladder, the presence or absence of trabeculation, cellules, and diverticula, prostatic calculi and reflux into the prostatic ducts and the seminal vesicles, and ureters can be studied by voiding cystourethrography. Upon completion of voiding, the amount of postvoid residual urine can be determined. Details of the functional and anatomic aspects of the voiding cystourethrogram can provide more reliable information on lower urinary tract dysfunction than any other test.

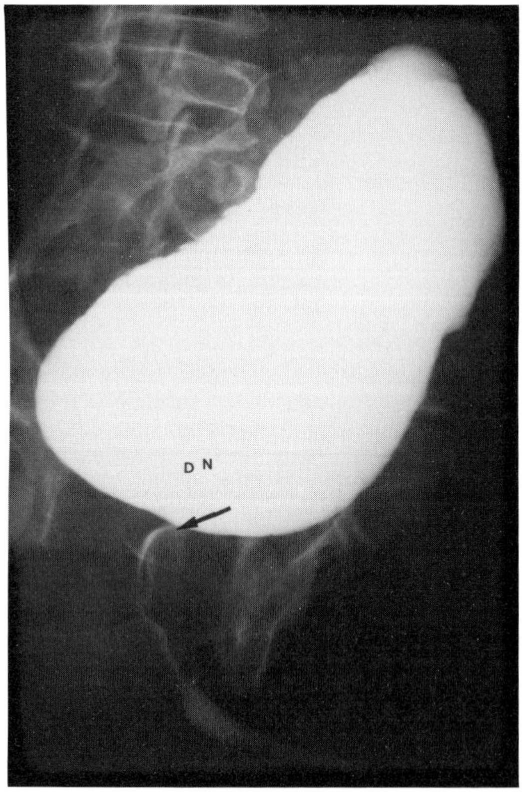

Figure 16-1. VCUG of a patient with prostate enlargement causing outlet obstruction. (From Hinman, F., Jr. [ed.]: *Benign Prostatic Hypertrophy*. Springer-Verlag, New York, 1983.)

Uroflowmetry

It has been suggested that uroflowmetry (Fig. 16–3) is the most accurate physiologic and noninvasive test for assessing bladder outlet obstruction. Among the several parameters that can be measured, the peak flow rate has been considered as the best correlate of outlet obstruction. Siroky *et al.* described several abnormal patterns of uri-

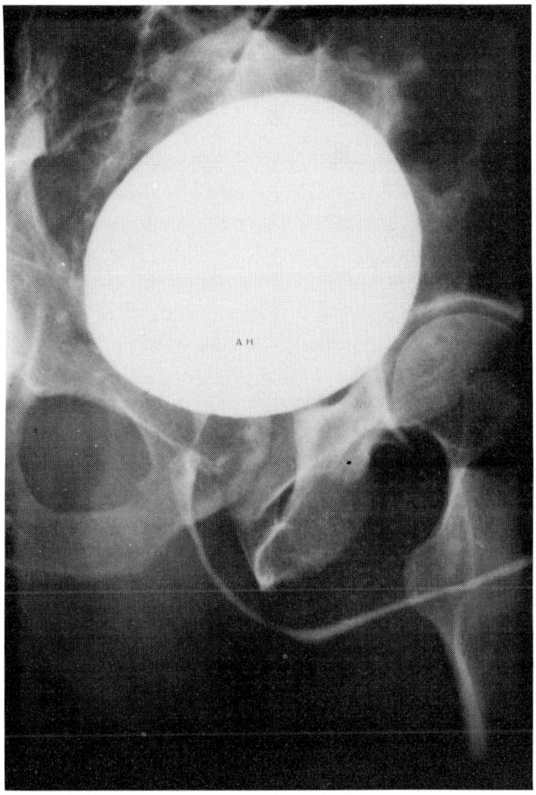

Figure 16-2. VCUG showing prostatic urethral obstruction. Rectal examination revealed minimal prostatic enlargement.

nary flow rate curves that are characteristic of obstructive voiding dysfunction (*14,15*).

It has been suggested that urinary flow rates may not be diminished in some patients with outlet obstruction (*16*). It is also believed that a high flow rate does not exclude the presence of infravesical obstruction. In one study 16 of 225 patients (7%) had a high-flow (>15 ml/s) infravesical obstruction diagnosed by simultaneous recording of the intravesical pressure and urinary flow rates (*16*).

Although it is recognized that urinary flow rate determination may not be sensitive enough to detect early obstruction, most investigators believe that it is a clinically adequate noninvasive test that can help make appropriate judgments in the management of prostatism. Further details of the techniques, rationale, and interpretation of uroflowmetry are described in other chapters of this book.

Urethral Closure Pressure Profile

The urethral closure pressure profile (UCPP) does not yield information on the functional status of the lower urinary tract in patients with prostatic enlargement. Kitada and Ishisawa showed no direct correlation between peak prostatic closure pressure and urethral length or size of the enlarged prostate (*17*). More specifically, not only patients

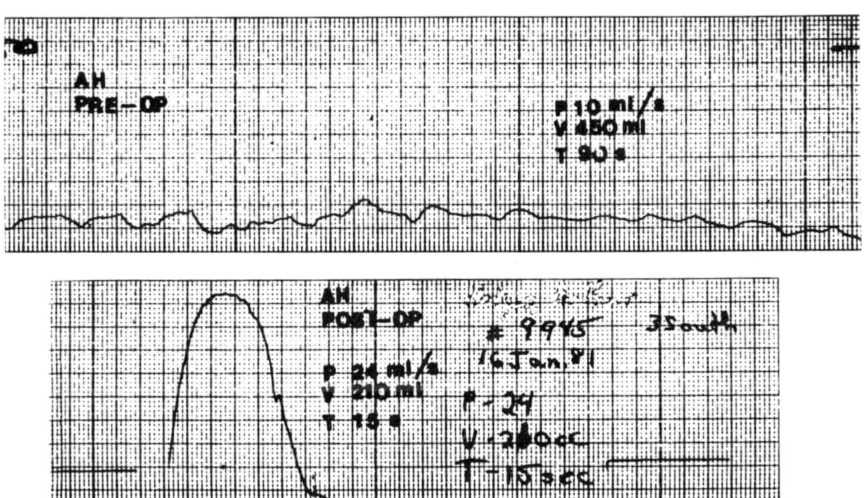

Figure 16-3. Pre- and postoperative urinary flow rate configurations.

with a large prostatic area but also those with small prostates and normal prostatic areas may have outlet obstruction. The closure pressure profiles obtained under resting conditions may not represent the nature and degree of obstruction when voiding commences (*18*).

Voiding Urodynamic Studies

Voiding urodynamic studies are recommended when simpler and less invasive procedures such as uroflowmetry and voiding cystourethrography are not conclusive. They can establish the degree of prostatic obstruction, evaluate the detrusor muscle mechanics, and rule out neurogenic dysfunction of urethral sphincters as the cause of obstruction.

Several combinations of voiding studies have been recommended: (a) pressure–flow study combined with periurethral electromyography (EMG); (b) synchronous cystosphincterometry with periurethral EMG; and (c) micturitional vesicourethral static or total urethral pressure profiles. Studies performed under fluoroscopy can be videotaped.

We rarely perform detailed voiding urodynamic studies in patients who are neurologically normal, have urinary flow rates that appear unequivocally to be obstructed, and complain of symptoms of severe obstruction. We prefer micturitional vesicourethral static pressure profilometry (*7*) when detailed urodynamic studies are indicated. EMG is rarely combined with such studies. Our experience with the voiding profile technique has convinced us that it is useful in patients who have obstructive symptoms but no rectally or endoscopically detected prostatic enlargement (*19*) (Figs. 16–4 and 16–5).

Static urethral pressure profilometry cannot be performed initially in patients with urinary retention, although it can be attempted in such patients after 1 to 2 weeks of catheter drainage. Micturitional static pressure profiles assisted by the Valsalva maneuver might help identify outlet obstruction in patients who have a hypoactive detrusor (*20*). The Valsalva maneuver is encouraged during the midvoiding phase with instructions to the patient to avoid voluntary contraction of pelvic floor muscles. The principle underlying this test is to impart additional energy or pressure to the bladder by the maneuver and to determine how the additional pressure is distributed along the posterior urethra. In patients with no prostatic obstruction, this additional pressure can be equally transmitted to the prostatic urethra

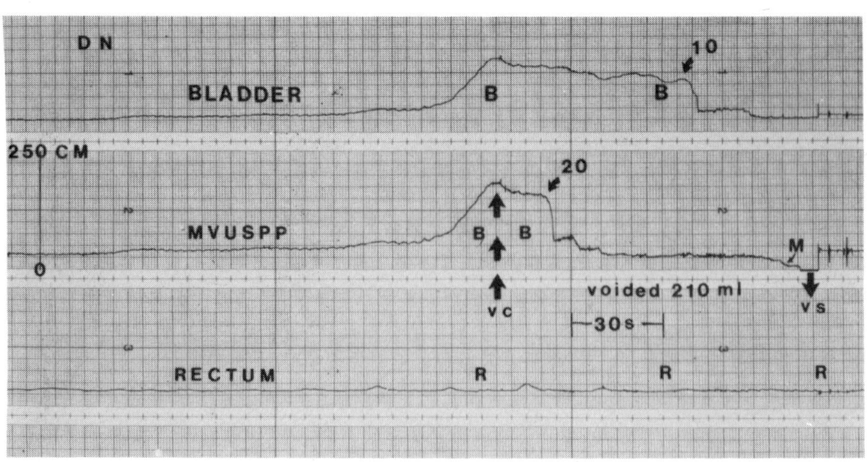

Figure 16-4. Voiding pressure profile of a patient whose VCUG is shown in Figure 16-1. Note abrupt drop of pressure of 100 cm H_2O in the vicinity of the vesicoprostatic junction 20 cm proximal to the meatus. *B*=bladder. *R*=rectal pressure tracing. Voiding pressure profile (MVUSPP) is shown in the middle tracing. *Arrows* at the *vc* = voiding commencement. As the catheter is withdrawn, the outlet pressures adjacent to the lower segment of the bladder are registered and then the anterior urethra. *M*=pressure at the meatal region. (From Hinman, F., Jr. [ed.]: *Benign Prostatic Hypertrophy*. Springer-Verlag, New York, 1983.)

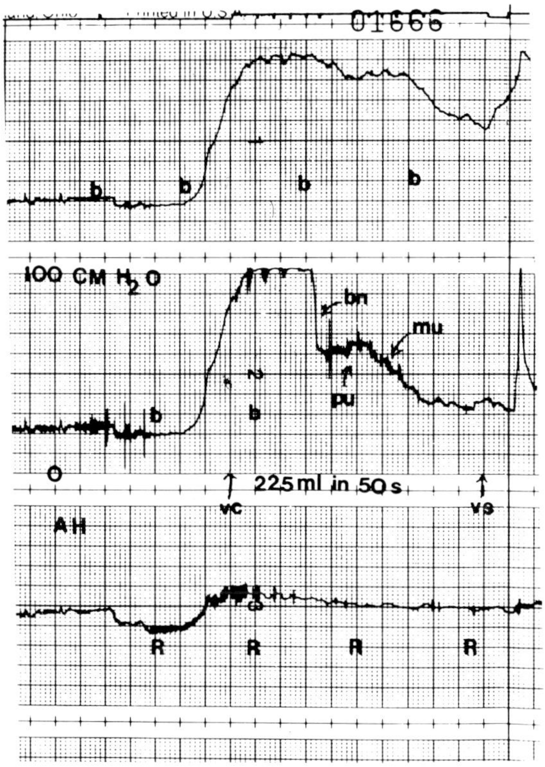

Figure 16-5. VCUG and urinary flow rates of this patient are shown in Figures 16-2 and 16-3. The voiding pressure profile is seen here. Note the abrupt drop of pressure at the bladder neck (*bn*) region. pu and mu = regions of prostatic and membranous urethral regions. *b* = bladder. *R* = rectum. *vc* = voiding commenced. *vs* = voiding stopped.

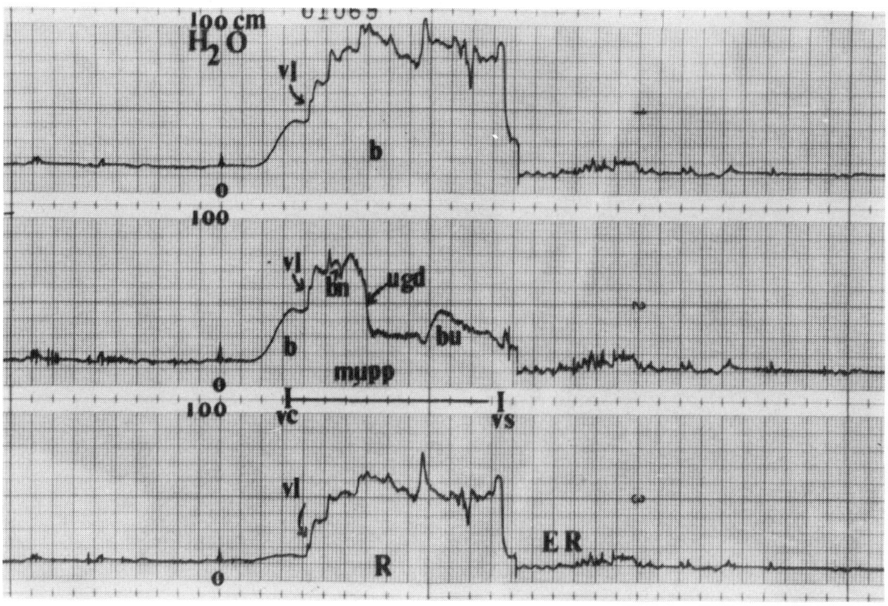

Figure 16-6. Voiding profile during voiding assisted with Valsalva (*vl*) in a 45-year-old man with symptoms of prostatism. It shows no evidence of a pressure drop in the bladder neck and prostatic urethral regions. *b* = bladder. *bn* = bladder neck. *ugd*=area of urogenital diaphragm or membranous urethra. *R* =rectum. *vc*=voiding commenced. *vs*= voiding stopped. *bu* = bulbous urethral region.

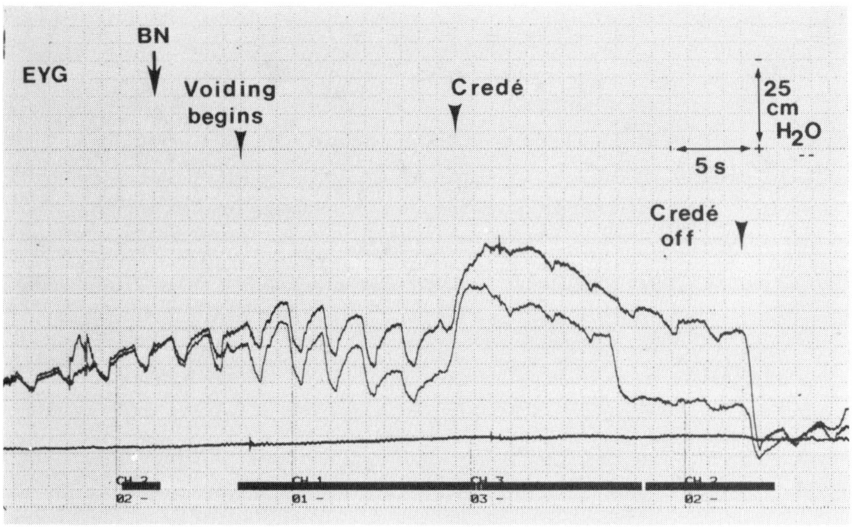

Figure 16–7. Voiding profile of an 80-year-old patient assisted with the Credé maneuver. The region of the bladder neck (*BN*) was isobaric; the midprostatic urethral region shows a drop of 5 to 10 cm H_2O. When the Credé maneuver was applied, the disparity in the midprostatic region becomes slightly accentuated by 10 cm H_2O. Note the difference in the pressure in the region distal to the membranous urethra, where a difference of 25 cm H_2O pressure was seen between the bladder and the membranobulbous urethral region. When the Credé pressure was off, no difference was noted.

(Fig. 16–6). On the other hand, obstruction in the posterior urethra can enhance the increase of the pressure drop across the bladder neck and prostatic urethra (Figs. 16–7 and 16–8). Studies utilizing the Valsalva maneuver are not helpful in patients with detrusor–striated sphincter dyssynergia or with severe pelvic floor descent and abnormal angulation at the prostatomembranous urethral junction. In the latter group of patients, when Valsalva is applied exaggeration of malalignment of the prostatomembranous urethral axis occurs and creates further mechanical obstruction.

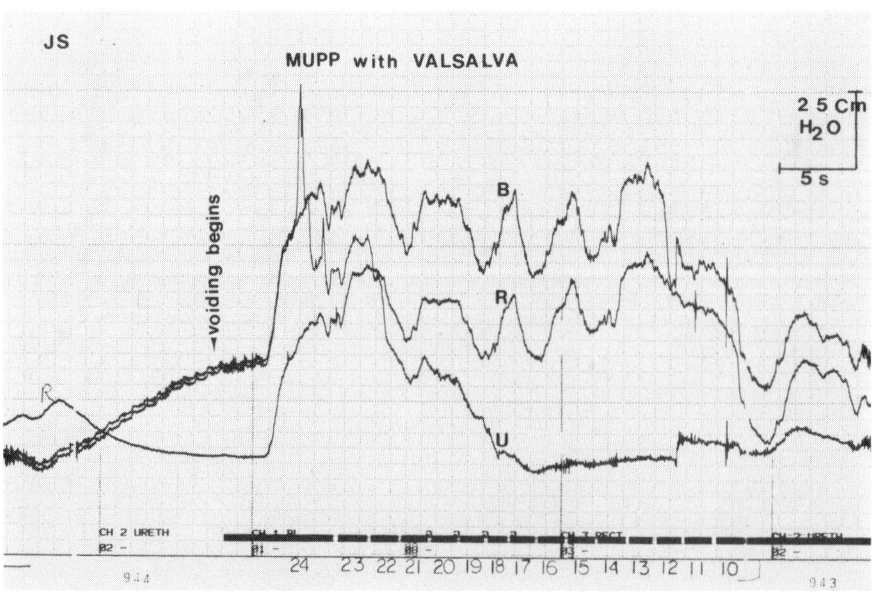

Figure 16–8. Voiding pressure profile during Valsalva-aided detrusor contraction shows the disparity of pressure between the bladder outlet and the bladder. A 45 cm H_2O pressure difference can be seen about 23 cm proximal (bladder neck) to the meatus.

REFERENCES

1. Schlossberg, S. M., Finkel, M. L., Vaughan, E. D., Jr., Jensen, D., Riehle, R. A., Jr., and McCarthy, E. G.: Second opinion for urologic surgery. *J. Urol.* 131:209, 1984.
2. Sterling, A. M., Ritter, R. C., and Zinner, N. R.: The physical basis of obstructive uropathy. In Hinman, F., Jr. (ed.), *Benign Prostatic Hypertrophy.* Springer-Verlag, New York, 1983, pp. 432–442.
3. Susset, J. G., Picker, P., Kretz, M., and Jorset, R.: Critical evaluation of uroflowmeters and analysis of normal curves. *J. Urol.* 109:874, 1973.
4. Gleason, D. M., Bottaccini, M. R., Reilly, R. J., and Byrne, J. C.: The residual stream energy is a diagnostic index of male urinary outflow obstruction. *Invest. Urol.* 10:72, 1972.
5. Abrams, P. H., and Torrens, M. J.: Urethral closure pressure profiles in the male. *Urol. Int.* 32:137, 1977.
6. Bates, C. P., Whiteside, C. G., and Turner Warwick, R.: Synchronous cine pressure-flow cystourethrography. *Br. J. Urol.* 42:714, 1970.
7. Yalla, S. V., Sharma, G. V. R. K., and Barsamian, E. M.: Micturitional static urethral pressure profile. *J. Urol.* 124:649, 1980.
8. Abrams, P.H.: Use of the intravenous urogram in diagnosis. In Hinman, F., Jr. (ed.), *Benign Prostatic Hypertrophy.* Springer-Verlag, New York, 1983, pp. 605–609.
9. Meyhoff, H. H., and Hald, T.: Are doctors able to assess prostatic size? *Scand. J. Urol. Nephrol.* 12:219, 1978.
10. Yalla, S.V., Blute, R., Waters, W. B., Snyder, H., and Fraser, L.: Urodynamic evaluation of prostatic enlargements with micturitional vesicourethral static pressure profiles. *J. Urol.* 125:685, 1981.
11. Andersen, J. T., and Nordling, J.: Relation of prostatic lobes to degree and rate of obstruction. In Hinman, F., Jr. (ed.), *Benign Prostatic Hypertrophy.* Springer-Verlag, New York, 1983, pp. 678–681.
12. Turner Warwick, R., Whiteside, C. G., Milroy, E. G. G., Pengelly, A. W., and Thompson, D. T.: The intravenous urodynamogram. *Br. J. Urol.* 51:15, 1979.

12a. Manolin, R. A.: Voiding cystourethrography with synchronous measurements of pressure and flow in the diagnosis of subvesical obstruction in men: A radiological view. *J. Urol.*, 137:1196, 1987.

13. Yalla, S. V., Cravalho, E., Resnick, N., Chiang, R., Gilliam, J., and Brown, K.: Elastic jump in the bulbous urethra during voiding. *J. Urol.*, 1987 134:907, 1985.
14. Siroky, M. B., Olsson, C. A., and Krane, R. J.: The flow rate nomogram. I. Development. *J. Urol.* 122:665, 1979.
15. Siroky, M. B., Olsson, C. A., and Krane, R. J.: The flow rate nomogram. II. Clinical correlation. *J. Urol.* 123:208, 1980.
16. Gerstenberg, T. C., Andersen, J. T., Klarskov, P., Ramirez, D., and Hald, T.: High flow infravesical obstruction. *J. Urol.* 127:343, 1982.
17. Kitada, S., and Ishisawa, N.: Urethral pressure profilometry in the preoperative assessment for prostatectomy. *J. Urol.* 126:89, 1981.
18. Gessner, F. B., and Zinner, N. R.: Urethral pressure profiles. In Hinman, F., Jr. (ed.), *Benign Prostatic Hypertrophy.* Springer-Verlag, New York, 1983, pp. 566–576.
19. Yalla, S. V.: Urethral static pressure profile. In Hinman, F., Jr. (ed.), *Benign Prostatic Hypertrophy.* Springer-Verlag, New York, 1983, pp. 577–588.
20. Yalla, S. V., Dyro, F. M., and Koyle, M.: Diagnosis of outlet obstruction with Valsalva assisted voiding studies in patients with hypoactive detrusor and low urinary flow rates. Presented at the American Urological Association Annual Meeting, 1984.

17

Bladder Neck Obstruction and Urethral Strictures

SUBBARAO V. YALLA, M.D., AND KEVIN LOUGHLIN, M.D.

PRIMARY BLADDER NECK OBSTRUCTION

Bladder neck obstruction of undetermined etiology is seen much more often in adult men than women. It is this disorder that Marion (*1*) in 1933 described as an "acquired type" of the "disease of bladder neck." He also believed that a congenital form occurs in infants and children. In both forms of the disease he found dysuric symptoms similar to those of prostatic hypertrophy but without evidence of that disease, no visible lesions in the bladder neck region, and no neurologic deficits.

A few decades ago the condition of bladder neck obstruction was a popular entity, and indiscriminate bladder neck resections and YV-plasties were often performed without objective evidence. Consequently several surgical failures occurred, as a result of which the diagnosis of bladder neck obstruction itself was questioned and the entity once again became a curiosity. Sporadic attempts, however, were made to recognize the site and degree of obstruction using urodynamic studies (*2,3*). These direct methods of evaluation have not been reliable for localization of outlet obstructions. It was not until the introduction of radiology-aided synchronous pressure–flow studies (*4–7*) that primary bladder neck obstruction has become a real entity. The essential features of this condition are elevated detrusor contraction pressures, poor urinary flow rates, a narrow bladder neck region, and poor opacification of the posterior urethra. In our studies on male outlet obstruction, inadequate bulbous urethral filling and downstream migration of elastic jump have also been observed (*8*). Voiding pressure profile techniques have been employed to precisely localize and estimate the degree of bladder neck obstruction (*9,10*). We have employed these techniques of recording voiding profiles in more than 25 patients (*11*). Based on these studies, it was recognized that the obstruction occurs at the level of the bladder neck region, and that the degree of obstruction can be graded as mild, moderate, or severe (*12*). The age distribution was between 30 and 58 years. Other reports suggested that bladder neck obstruction can also occur in women although it is extremely rare (*13,14*).

Patients usually have both obstructive and irritative lower urinary tract symptoms. Hesitancy and varying degrees of postvoiding dribbling are the usual complaints. Patients with longstanding obstruction of severe degree may develop marked vesical trabeculation, diverticula, reflux, or upper tract obstruction.

The urodynamic features depend on the degree and duration of obstruction. The spectrum of obstruction may vary from a mere delay of opening of the bladder neck during detrusor contraction to the most severe variety characterized by a marked pressure drop across the bladder neck, elevated detrusor pressure, and marked morphologic changes of the bladder wall (Figs. 17–1 to 17–3). We have also seen patients with long-standing lesions who exhibited

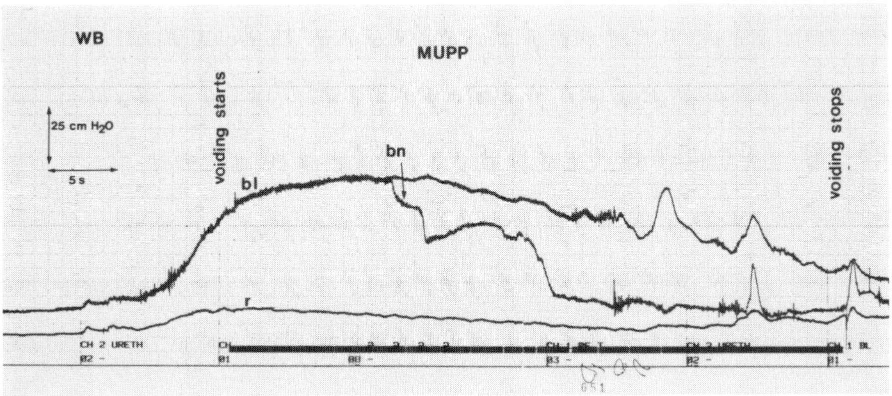

Figure 17–1. Mild degree of bladder neck obstruction showing about 68 cm H_2O of detrusor pressure and a drop of 22 cm H_2O across the bladder neck region. Note that both pressure-sensing sites of the 10F trilumen pressure recording catheter were recording the bladder pressure (*bl*) during the initial phase of voiding (pressures are superimposed). Upon catheter withdrawal the urethral pressure-sensing site of the catheter arrives at the stenotic bladder neck (*bn*) region and records the lower pressure. As the catheter was further withdrawn, more pressure drop occurred at the narrow membranous urethra.

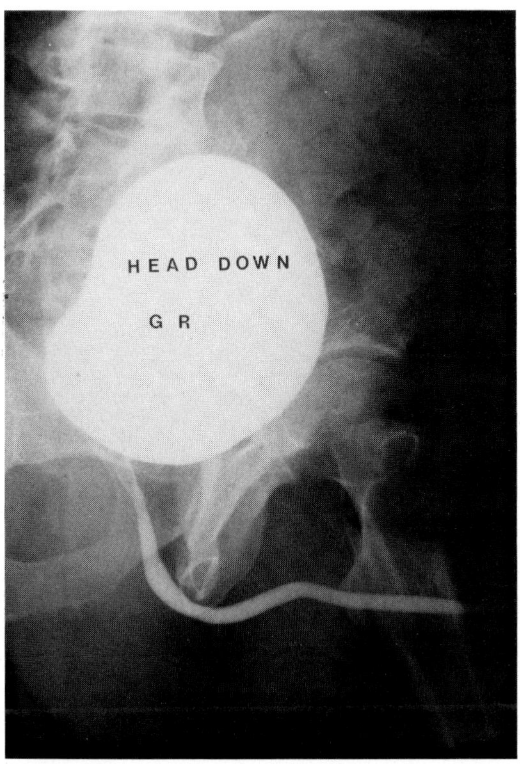

Figure 17–2. Severe stenosis of the bladder neck in a 42-year-old man. He voided in the head-down position to unmask the bladder neck from the bladder base. (From Yalla, S. V., and Resnick, N.: *World J. Urol.* 2:196, 1984.)

decompensated bladders that resulted in a large bladder capacity, lowered detrusor contraction pressures, increased residual urine volumes, and a drop of pressure across the bladder neck. This pressure drop can be magnified when patients apply the Valsalva maneuver during a detrusor contraction.

Our earlier report showed that the range of detrusor contraction pressure varied between 55 and 225 cm H_2O. The pressure drop across the bladder neck region was 20 to 110 cm H_2O. Postoperatively, flow rates improved, pressure drops disappeared or diminished, residual urine volumes decreased, and detrusor contraction pressures were lowered (Figs. 17–4 and 17–6). Other urodynamic studies involved assessment of maximum opening time (*7*) and X-Y recorder plots of pressure–flow data (*14*). Maximum opening time is defined as the time interval between the prevoiding rise of intravesical pressure and peak flow rates (*7*).

The etiology of primary bladder neck obstruction is uncertain. Turner-Warwick suggested that it is a form of intrinsic dyssynergia (*15*). Another view is that it may result from a fault in dissolution of mesenchyme at the bladder neck or inclusion of abnormal amounts of nonmuscular connective tissue (*16*).

Bladder neck obstruction can occur in both young adult and elderly men. The etiologic factors may vary depending on the age at which the manifestations begin to appear. In children and young adults the lesion

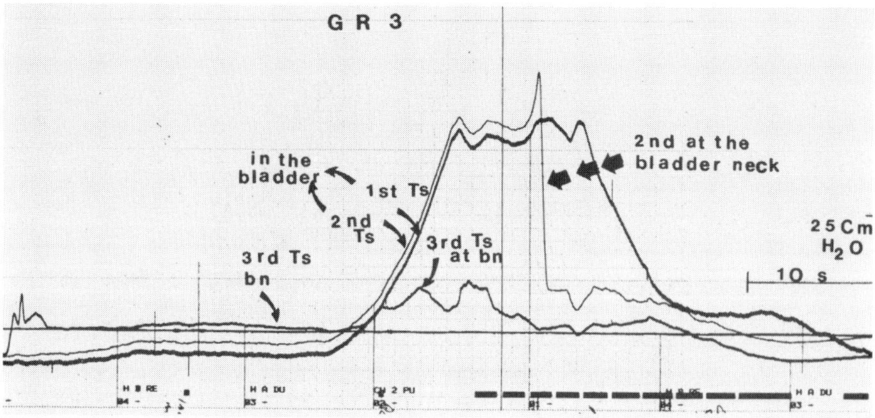

Figure 17-3. Note the pronounced drop of pressure (65 cm H_2O) at the bladder neck region in patient. Bladder pressure was 110 cm H_2O. This study was performed with a triple microtransducer catheter. Prior to voiding, the catheter was positioned with two transducers *(ts)* inside the bladder and the third at the bladder neck *(bn)* region. When voiding commenced, the catheter was withdrawn at the rate of 1 cm/2 s (shown as a heavy interrupted line at the baseline) (From Yalla, S. V., and Resnick, N.: *World J. Urol.* 2:196, 1984.)

probably is congenital in origin. In older age groups (40–60 years) the obstruction probably is caused by fibrosis and fibromuscular hyperplasia of prostatic enlargement. Studies at the Johns Hopkins Hospital Center suggested that the prostate may begin to enlarge during the fourth decade (*17*).

The management of bladder neck obstruction depends on the age of the patient and the severity of the condition. With mild conditions and those suspected to be nonfibrotic

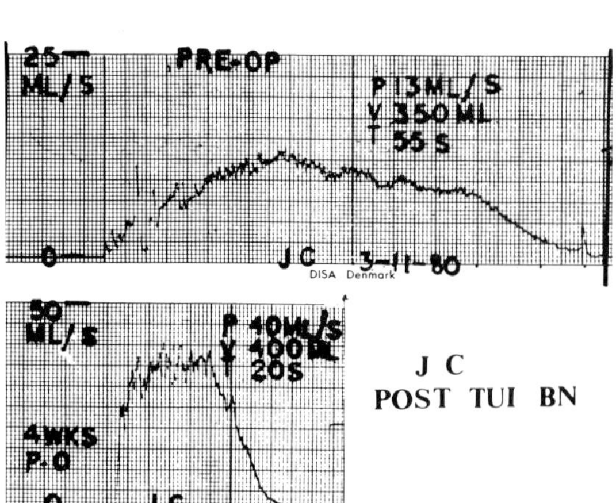

Figure 17-4. Preoperative obstructed flow pattern (*above*) and postoperative (bladder neck incision) flow pattern (*below*) in a 42-year-old man. (From Yalla, S. V., *et al.*: *J. Urol.* 125:677, 1981. Copyright © 1981, The Williams & Wilkins Co., Baltimore.)

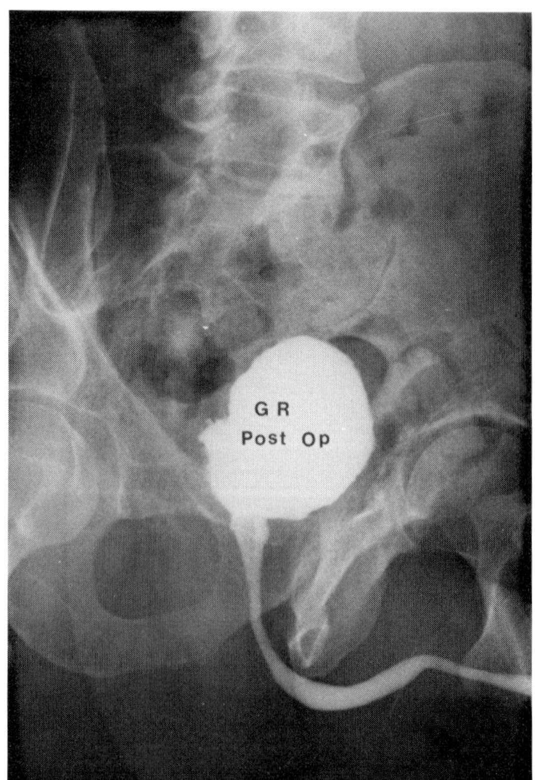

Figure 17-5. Postoperative voiding cystourethrogram in patient, showing the wide bladder neck region. (From Yalla, S. V., and Resnick, N.: *World J. Urol.* 2:196, 1984.)

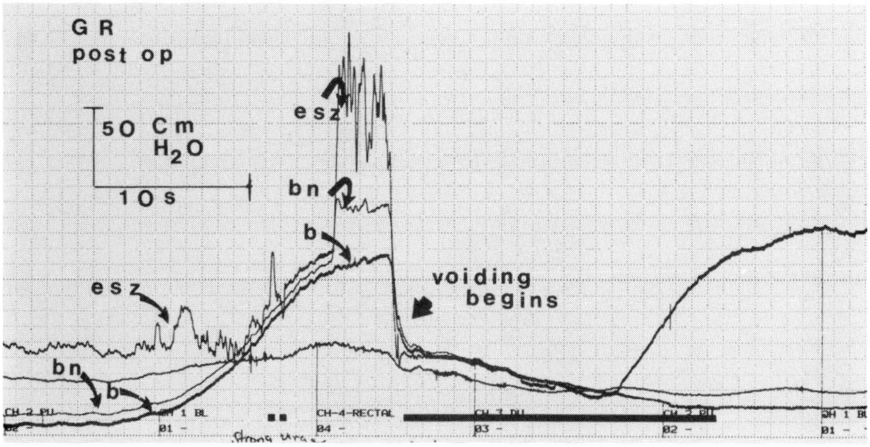

Figure 17-6. Postoperative urodynamic study in patient shows isobaric pressures in the bladder neck and distally after the patient commenced voiding by releasing his voluntary efforts of holding urine. During the hold maneuver, pressures at the external sphincter (*esz*) and bladder neck (*bn*) regions were higher than bladder (*b*) pressures. During voiding they all became isobaric at low pressures. (From Yalla, S. V., and Resnick, N.: *World J. Urol.* 2:196, 1984.)

obstructions, alpha-adrenergic blockade can yield good results. Long-standing severe lesions suspected to be fibrotic and in older age groups benefit more from surgical relief. We favor unilateral incisions of the bladder neck without encroaching on the verumontanum. The incision must extend into the bladder in order to ascertain that the entire bladder neck is incised.

ANTERIOR URETHRAL STRICTURES

Anterior urethral strictures can be diagnosed with the patient's history, urethrography, and endoscopic study (urethroscopy). Detailed urodynamic evaluations are rarely needed for the diagnosis.

Several urodynamic methods have been used to diagnose subtle urethral strictures and objectively document severe strictures (*18–20*). Studies have also been performed to determine the effect of strictures on bladder function and urinary flow rates (*21*). With severe strictures, low urinary flow rates and changes in their pattern are usually observed. With less severe strictures, such changes in flow rates may not be seen (*22*). Maintenance of normal flow rates has been attributed to detrusor compensatory hypertrophy secondary to increased outlet resistance. Hedenberg *et al.* (*21*), on the other hand, did not find evidence of detrusor compensation. Their studies showed that maximum voiding and peak flow pressures varied from normal to values of up to 300 cm. H_2O. The same distribution was found postoperatively. They found after-contraction in five of nine patients postoperatively but in none preoperatively. Other parameters that were studied were flow invariables ($Q_{1\,s}$, Q_{max}, and $Q_{max\ time}$), minimal urethral resistance, maximum exit velocity, and urethral energy losses. Preoperatively, $Q_{1\,s}$ was within normal limits; but the mean value was lower. The Q_{max} related to the square root of bladder volume was below normal in all preoperative studies; postoperatively, it was increased. Minimal urethral resistance was markedly decreased in most of the postoperative patients.

The preoperative maximum exit velocity varied between 0 (dribbling) and 140 cm/s (normal values 131–335 cm/s; mean 73 cm/s). Postoperatively, the mean values improved to 137 cm/s. The preoperative urethral energy losses were 85 to 100 percent (mean 96%), and postoperatively the loss was still high (mean 90%; normal values for boys 33–86%, mean 65%).

Pressure–flow studies may reveal several abnormalities. The intravesical pressure during voiding may show sustained elevated pressures. The pressure at which flow com-

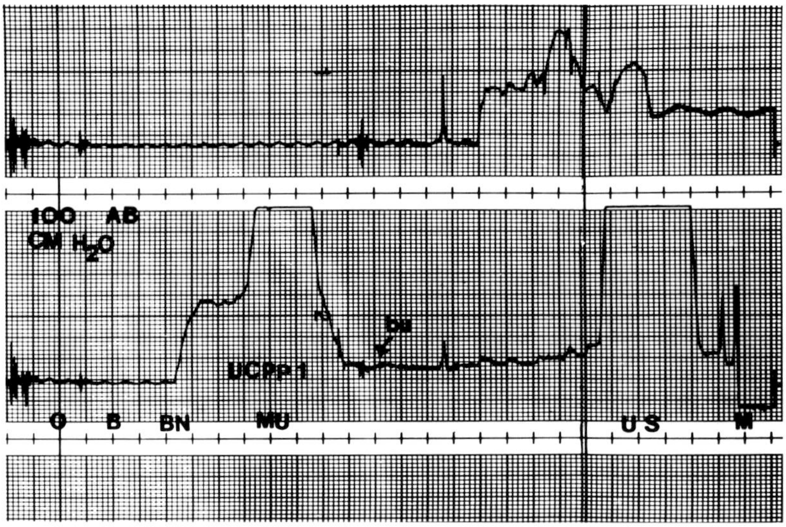

Figure 17–7. Patient A.B. First UCPP done with a 10F trilumen infusion catheter (2.2 ml/min). Note the high pressure zone in the distal urethra suggesting severe strictures (*VS*). (From Yalla, S. V., and Loughlin, K.: *Urology* 19:106, 1982.)

mences is usually higher than the values seen in normal people. Nyman's studies of intravesical pressure measurements showed that the pressures during voiding were considerably higher than in normal men (*23*). However, he discovered that the maximum detrusor pressure was lower in high than in low-volume voidings. He concluded that a patient with a low urinary flow rate, a high residual urine volume, and an increased intravesical pressure during voiding is obstructed.

Urethral closure pressure profiles (UCPP) have been described in patients with urethral strictures (*20*). Depending on the technique and the size of the catheter, the pressure configurations and the magnitude of the pressures may vary. The closure pressure depends on the severity of the obstruction caused by the stricture. The urethral closure pressure configuration of the severely stenotic anterior urethra may vary in the same patient when repeat studies are performed (Figs. 17–7 and 17–8). We believe that this pronounced variation can occur in patients with severe distal constrictions and whenever the pressure-sensing catheters that deal with fluid infusion are used with the slow withdrawal technique. The infusate used in this technique may be trapped in the segment between the competent membranous urethra and the stricture in the distal urethra. This "fluid entrapment effect" can result in artifactual pressure readings and can be minimized if the trapped infusate is milked from the urethra before a repeat study is started. A fluid entrapment effect may also be eliminated if studies are performed with catheters such as microtransducer catheters and membrane catheters that do not need constant fluid infusion.

Although urethral closure profiles may demonstrate the sites of anterior urethral constriction, they may not all represent the severity of the clinical obstruction. It appears that patients with severe constrictions of the anterior urethra experience significant clinical obstructive symptoms. Our previous studies confirm that a correlation usually exists between the diagnosis obtained from the UCPP and the findings of micturitional vesicourethral static pressure profiles (*24*). All patients who demonstrated anterior urethral strictures in the UCPP studies have shown abnormal urodynamic findings in micturitional studies (Figs. 17–9 and 17–10). All these urodynamic abnormalities can be reversed after dilation of the strictures (Figs. 17–11 and 17–12).

Our experience with the recordings of the static (lateral) pressure measurements during voiding suggests that this method is useful for identifying distal urethral strictures (*24*). A significant drop of static pressure occurs at

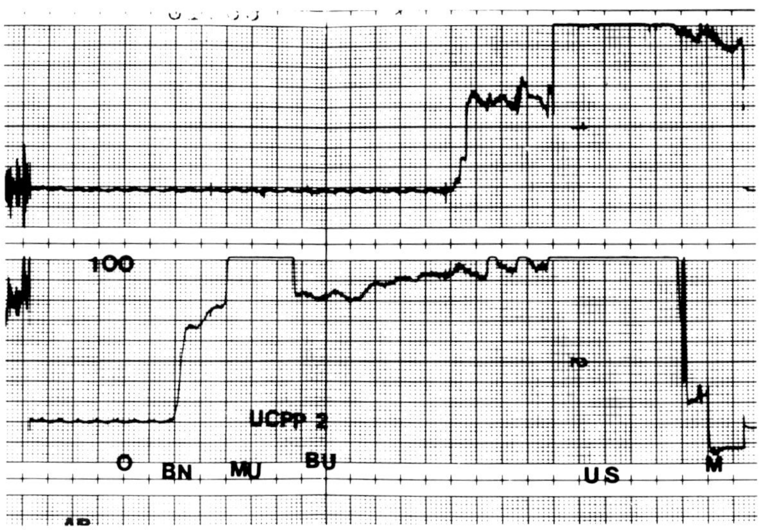

Figure 17-8. Patient A.B. Repeat UCPP (*2*) shows an entirely different configuration. The infusate is trapped between the competent membranous urethra and the stricture in the anterior urethra. This high closure pressure in the bulb does not mean stricture at this region. (From Yalla, S. V., and Loughlin, K.: *Urology* 19:106, 1982.)

the site of anterior urethral constriction (Fig. 17–13). With severe constrictions the urethral pressure-sensing probe can produce complete occlusion at the site of the stricture (Figs. 17–14 and 17–15). Consequently, the fluid in the bladder is in continuity (without motion) with the fluid in the proximal anterior urethra when the detrusor contracts and the bladder outlet sphincters relax. The fluid pressure proximal to the strictured segment becomes identical with the bladder pressure.

In conclusion, detailed urodynamic studies are rarely needed for identifying clinically significant anterior urethral strictures. However, recognition of these segments becomes important for understanding proximal obstructions in the region of the bladder outlet.

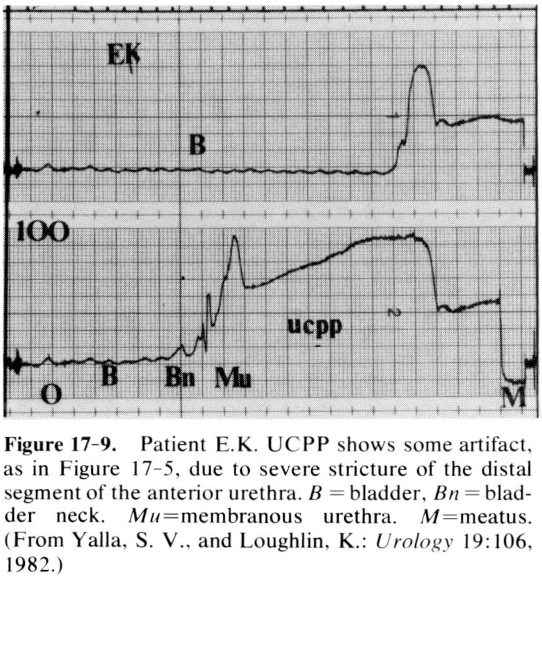

Figure 17-9. Patient E.K. UCPP shows some artifact, as in Figure 17-5, due to severe stricture of the distal segment of the anterior urethra. *B* = bladder, *Bn* = bladder neck. *Mu*=membranous urethra. *M*=meatus. (From Yalla, S. V., and Loughlin, K.: *Urology* 19:106, 1982.)

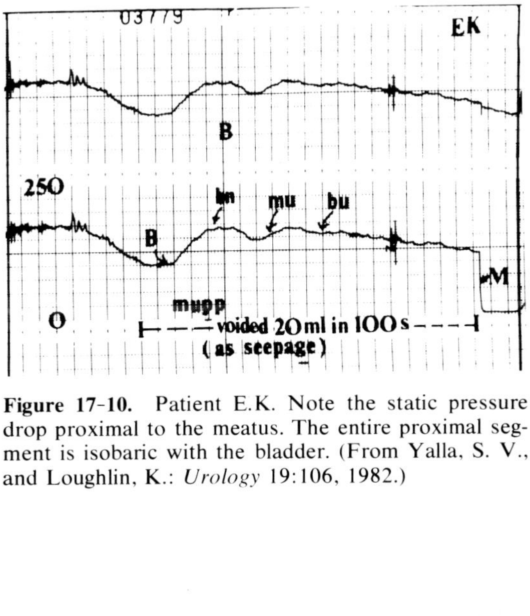

Figure 17-10. Patient E.K. Note the static pressure drop proximal to the meatus. The entire proximal segment is isobaric with the bladder. (From Yalla, S. V., and Loughlin, K.: *Urology* 19:106, 1982.)

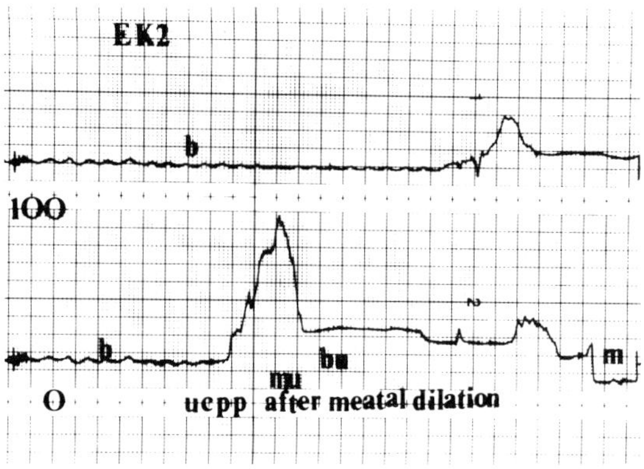

Figure 17-11. Patient E.K. after meatal dilation. The artifact of infusate entrapment is not seen. UCPP shows a normal configuration. (From Yalla, S.V., and Loughlin, K.: *Urology* 19:106, 1982.)

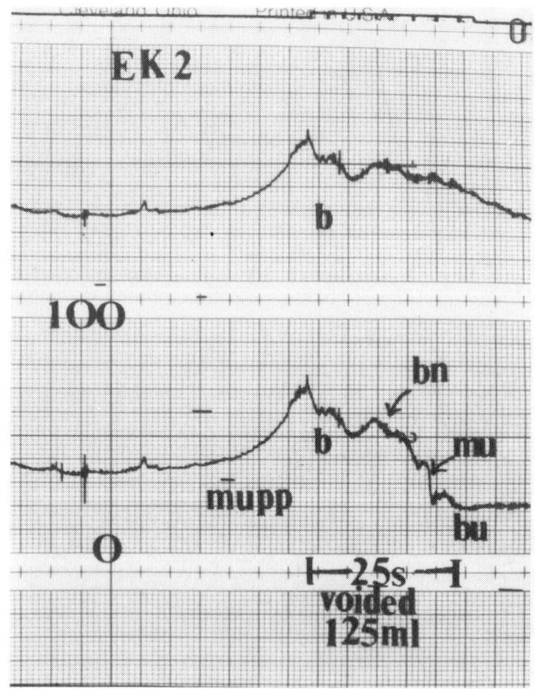

Figure 17-12. Patient E.K. Voiding study shows a normal configuration of the posterior urethra. The pressure drop at the membranous urethra (*mu*) is physiologic, which was not seen in the preoperative study. (From Yalla, S. V., and Loughlin, K.: *Urology* 19:106, 1982.)

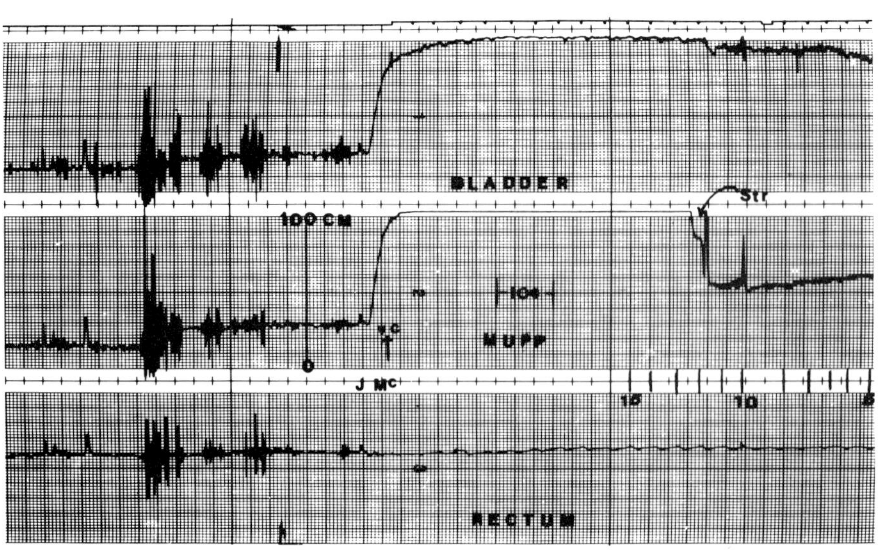

Figure 17-13. Patients with strictures in the anterior urethra showing decreased static pressure in the distal bulb (11 cm from the meatus). The stricture region (*STR*) is shown with an arrow in the middle tracing of vesicourethral static pressure during voiding.

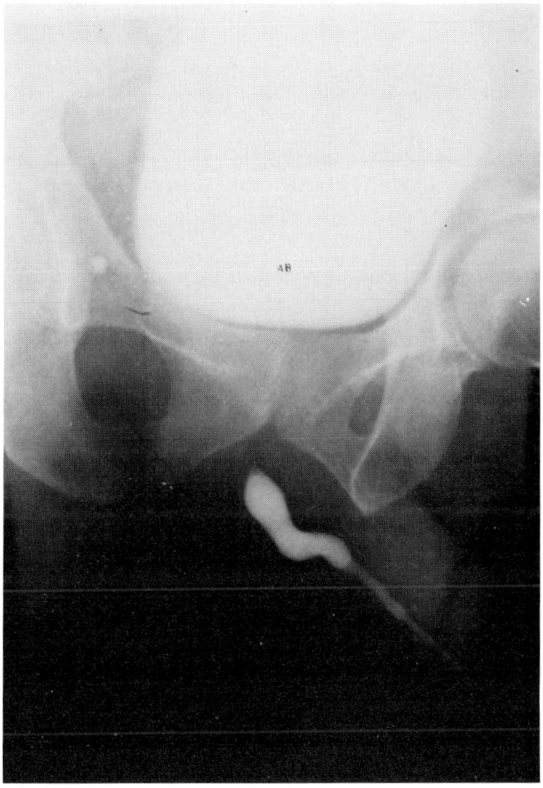

Figure 17-14. Patient A.B. Retrograde urethrogram showing a strictured segment of the distal anterior urethra. (From Yalla, S. V., and Loughlin, K.: *Urology* 19:106, 1982.)

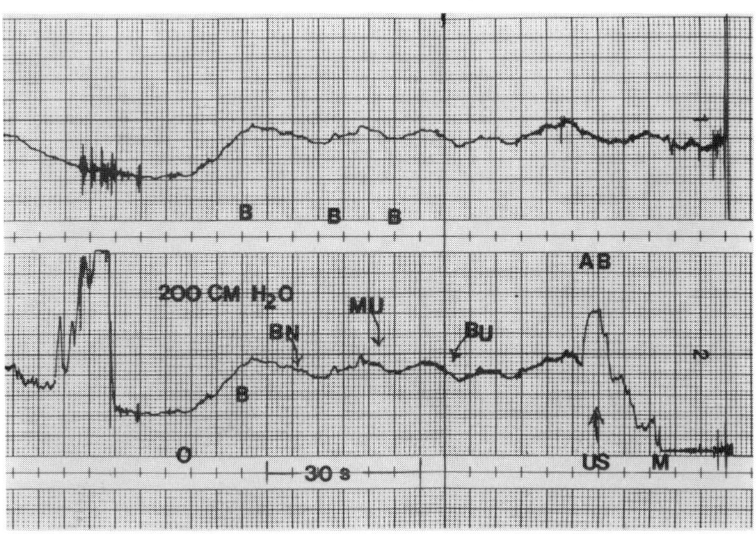

Figure 17-15. Patient A.B. The pressure is identical in the entire segment proximal to the stricture (*us*) area. Top tracing shows isobaric bladder pressure similar to that in the middle tracing. The strictured segment, however, shows higher pressure. *B* = bladder. *BN* = bladder neck. *MU* = membranous urethra. *BU* = bulbous urethra. *M* = meatus. The entire study was done under fluoroscopy. (From Yalla, S. V., and Loughlin, K.: *Urology* 19:106, 1982.)

REFERENCES

1. Marion, G.: Surgery of the neck of the bladder. *Br. J. Urol.* 5:351, 1933.
2. Nunn, I. N.: Bladder neck obstruction in children, *J. Urol.* 93:693, 1965.
3. King, L. R., Mellens, H. A., and White, H.: Measurement of the intravesical pressure during voiding. *Invest. Urol.* 2:303, 1965.
4. Turner-Warwick, R. T., Whiteside, C. G., Worth, P. H. L., Milroy, E. J. G., and Bates, C. P.: A urodynamic view of the clinical problems associated with bladder neck dysfunction and its treatment by endoscopic incision and transtrigonal posterior prostatectomy. *Br. J. Urol.* 45:44, 1973.
5. Andersen, J. T., Jacobsen, O., Gammelgard, R. A., and Hald, T.: Dysfunction of the bladder neck: a urodynamic study. *Urol. Int.* 31:78, 1976.
6. Gierup, J., Ericsson, N., and Von Hedenberg, C.: Urodynamic studies in boys with disorders of the lower urinary tract in congenital bladder neck obstruction. *Scand. J. Urol. Nephrol.* 12:195, 1978.
7. Webster, G.D., Lockhart, J.L., and Older, R.A.: The evaluation of bladder neck dysfunction. *J. Urol.* 123:196, 1980.
8. Yalla, S. V., Cravalho, E., Resnick, N., Chiang, R., Gilliam, J., and Brown, K.: Elastic jump in male urethra during voiding. *J. Urol.,* 134:907, 1985.
9. Yalla, S. V., Sharma, G. V. R. K., and Barsamian, E. M.: Micturitional static urethral pressure profile: a method of recording urethral pressure profile during voiding and implications. *J. Urol.* 124:649, 1980.
10. Yalla, S. V., Waters, W. B., Snyder, H., and Fraser, L.: Urodynamic localization of isolated bladder neck obstruction in the male: studies with micturitional vesicourethral static pressure profiles. *J. Urol.* 125:685, 1981.
11. Yalla, S. V., Blute, R. D., Snyder, H., Yap, W., Fraser, L., and Friedman, E.: Isolated bladder neck obstruction of undetermined etiology (primary) in adult male. *Urology* 17:99, 1981.
12. Yalla, S. V., Blute, R. D., Waters, W. B., Snyder, H., and Fraser, L.: Urodynamic evaluation of prostatic enlargements with micturitional vesicourethral static pressure profiles. *J. Urol.* 125:677, 1981.
13. Diokno, A. C., Hollander, J. B., and Bennett, C. J.: Vesical neck contracture in women: a real entity. In *Proceedings of AUA Meeting,* 1984, abstract 604.
14. Abrams, P. H., and Griffiths, D. J.: The assessment of prostatic obstruction from urodynamic measurements and from residual urine. *Br. J. Urol.* 51:129, 1979.
15. Turner-Warwick, R.: A urodynamic review of bladder outlet obstruction in the male and its clinical implications. *Urol. Clin. North Am.* 6:171, 1979.
16. Leadbetter, G. W., and Leadbetter, W. F.: Diagnosis and treatment of congenital bladder neck obstruction in children. *N. Engl. J. Med.* 260:633, 1959.
17. Berry, S. J., Coffey, D. S., Walsh, P. C., and Ewing, L. L.: Development of human benign prostatic hyperplasia with age. *J. Urol.* 132:474, 1984.
18. Von Garrelts, B.: Micturition in urethral stricture. *Acta Chir. Scand.* 114:466, 1958.
19. Gierup, H. J. W., and Ericsson, N. O.: Micturition studies in infants and children: urodynamics in boys with disorders of the lower urinary tract. *Scand. J. Urol.* 10:72, 1971.
20. Brown, M., and Wickham, J. E. A.: The urethral pressure profile. *Br. J. Urol.* 41:211, 1969.
21. Hedenberg, C. V., Ericsson, N. O., and Gierup, J.: Urodynamic studies in boys with disorders of the lower urinary tract. I. Urethral strictures: a pre and post-operative study. *Scand. J. Urol. Nephrol.* 11:111, 1977.
22. Beck, A. D., and Gaudin, H. J.: The measurement and significance of the urinary flow rate. *Aust. N.Z. Surg.* 39:99, 1969.
23. Nyman, C. R.: Urodynamics in urethral stricture. *Scand. J. Urol. Nephrol.* [*Suppl.*] 39:1, 1979.
24. Yalla, S. V., and Loughlin, K.: Urodynamic assessment of anterior urethral constrictions: studies with micturitional vesicourethral static profile. *Urology* 19:106, 1982.

18

Spinal Cord Injury

BUSHRA A. FAM, M.D., MEHDI SARKARATI, M.D., AND SUBBARAO V. YALLA, M.D.

In the United States 30 to 40 new spinal cord injury patients are seen yearly per one million population. Most acute injuries are caused by automobile accidents and are due to fractures or fracture-dislocations of the spine. Other causes are gunshot wounds and diving accidents. Vascular injuries related to the major blood supply of the spinal cord are less common (*1,2*). Epidural and subdural hematoma, disk prolapse, and rarely aortography are known to produce acute spinal cord lesions.

NEUROPATHOLOGY

Spinal injuries can lead to varying degrees and patterns of neurologic deficits, which depend on the level of the injury. Complete transection of the spinal cord is rare. The essential pathologic features in the spinal cord are edema, hemorrhage, and cord necrosis. Hemorrhagic necrosis is seen in grey matter of the cord, and the tissue damage may extend in cephalad as well as caudad directions (*3*). Consequently, the injury may be extensive and often does not confine itself to one cord segment. Other causes, such as local anoxia secondary to local circulatory arrest and production of toxic neurotransmitter agents, have been suggested as factors compounding the injury. Delayed features of cord injury include cystic degeneration of the cord, resulting in cystic gliosis or syringomyelia (*4*).

TYPES OF LESIONS

Cervical and thoracic vertebral injuries form the major group. Depending on the site of spinal injury, partial or complete lesions can result. Injury to the thoracic spine most often leads to a complete cord lesion because of its narrow vertebral canal (*1*). Injury at the T_{12} and L_1 vertebrae may not conform to either an upper or a lower motor neuron lesion; at this level, mixed (combined) lower and upper motor neuron lesions usually occur. Neurologic lesions proximal to the S_{2-4} sacral cord segments produce an upper motor neuron type of hyperreflexia of the bladder and striated sphincter (*5*).

Ischemic changes may occur distal to the thoracolumbar cord segments and may involve sacral cord nuclei; such a lesion may lead to a lower motor neuron type of bladder and sphincter behavior. Occasionally, the S_{2-4} segments of the cord are involved in injuries to the sacral roots and pelvic and pudendal nerves, leading to bizarre patterns of vesicourethral dysfunction. Extensive thoracolumbar lesions may also involve sympathetic neural pathways (*6–9*). When such lesions occur, various combinations of parasympathetic, sympathetic, and somatic dysfunctions may be seen.

EARLY PHASE OF SPINAL INJURY (SHOCK)

During the phase of acute trauma and the immediate posttraumatic state, all skeletal and visceral reflexes are suppressed below the level of the cord lesion. This condition is known as spinal shock (*10*) and was first described in 1843. Alternate terms such as posttransectional areflexia or hyporeflexia have been proposed. This stage of spinal shock may last a few weeks to a few months, although sometimes it is present only a few hours. During the recovery phase, anal and genital reflexes are the earliest somatic reflexes to reappear when the cord lesion is above the level of sacral cord centers (*11,12*).

URODYNAMIC MANIFESTATIONS

The urodynamic features of spinal cord injury depend on the level, duration, and completeness of the cord lesion. They can be classified into the following categories: (a) stage of spinal shock (b) stage of recovery, and (c) established patterns of voiding dysfunction.

Spinal Shock Phase

Although tendon reflexes have been considered to remain flaccid during the phase of spinal shock, it was observed that conus reflexes (superficial anal reflex, bulbocavernosus reflex) return within a few hours after the injury (*11,12*). The presence of any degree of spasticity immediately after injury indicates an incomplete lesion. The reflexes tend to return in a cephalad fashion. The conus reflexes recover before ankle reflexes, and the latter before knee reflexes. Plantar reflexes initially become flexor before they eventually become extensor in nature.

During the phase of spinal shock, the bladder is completely areflexic, resulting in urinary retention. The reflex activity of the detrusor usually returns within 6 to 8 weeks, although the deficit is prolonged in some cases (*13,14*). The precise causes of detrusor areflexia and the factors responsible for return of its activity are unclear. It has been suggested, however, that loss of facilitatory influences of suprasacral micturition centers may occur during the stage of spinal shock. It has been suggested that after spinal shock the central nervous system develops a form of central supersensitivity to neurotransmitters that accounts for the return of reflex activity. Neural sprouting has also been suggested as a cause of the return of spinal reflex activity and development of the mass reflex (*15*). Bradley *et al.* suggest that in experimental animals, the ascending and descending tracts involving motor neurons of pontine detrusor nucleus, are long routed (*16,17*). It is for this reason that permanent alteration in voiding takes place after spinal cord injury (*16,17*). The same authors also maintain that such a reflex provides a bladder contraction of adequate duration; interruption of spinal tracts in spinal cord injury thus leads to loss of the detrusor reflex during spinal shock. In their opinion, detrusor hyperreflexia occurs subsequently, on recovery, with short-circuit currents at the level of the spinal cord transection. Hyperreflexia indicates a bladder reflex with a low volume threshold (*16,17*).

The essential urodynamic features of the spinal shock phase are as follows. The cystometrogram (CMG) shows a shift to the right in the pressure–volume curve. The detrusor is areflexic and does not respond to any stimulation. Compliance of the bladder wall (absolute compliance) is unchanged; that of the entire organ (apparent compliance) appears to be increased owing to increased bladder capacity and the absence of the detrusor reflex. The bladder contour on x-ray films indicates a loss of its globular shape and seemingly reflects the shape of a flabby organ that changes by filling and position.

Various rehabilitative stimulatory bladder maneuvers are unsuccessful in producing reflex activity of the detrusor. The ice-water test may show an increase in tonicity and reduction of compliance, but it does not evoke contraction. The test is carried out by recording intravesical pressure while rapidly injecting 100 ml of solution to 4°C (*18*).

The urethral closure pressure profiles (UCPPs) are stunted in the early part of the spinal shock but later return to the normal pressure ranges (*11,12,19*). Although reflex activity of the external sphincter region may be sluggish in the earlier stages of recovery, it gradually returns to normal and often becomes exaggerated. Radiologically, the bladder base is within its normal confines, and the bladder has a smooth contour. There may not be any trabeculation during this phase. The bladder neck region is closed under resting conditions. Bladder filling is accompanied by increased pressure and resistance in both the internal and external sphincter zones without a corresponding increase in electromyographic (EMG) activity at the latter zone. One may therefore assume that the somatic muscular component is more suppressed than the smooth muscle component in spinal shock (*19*).

The treatment during spinal shock phase is to subject the patient to intermittent catheterizations (*13,14,20*). Frequent evaluations of the physiology of the bladder and its outlet during this phase can be performed at the bedside by cystometry and the ice-water tests. These tests can be useful for prognosticating the return of reflex detrusor activity (*18,21,22*).

Stage of Recovery

The recovery phase is characterized by a gradual return of reflex activity of the centers of undamaged spinal cord segments below the level of injury. The somatic superficial anal and bulbocavernosus reflexes recover initially, usually preceding recovery of the visceral reflexes. The detrusor reflex appears 6 to 8 weeks (or more) but is sometimes delayed for more than a year.

During the recovery phase the detrusor develops reflex contractions in response to visceral stimuli such as intravesical filling or manual suprapubic compression (*6*). These contractions may not be sustained or powerful and consequently may not result in voiding. During this minor detrusor activity the bladder neck may not open completely. The striated sphincter may not relax during detrusor activity during the recovery phase. Gradually, the detrusor contractions become more powerful and thus produce voiding in one or more spurts. However, the bladder is not emptied completely, as the striated musculature around the urethra may become dyssynergic (*23–26*). Ineffectual voiding may also be caused by the nonsustained nature of detrusor activity (*6*). It is well known that during normal micturition the striated sphincter relaxes in a sustained fashion during the detrusor contraction, which also is sustained. This coordination between the detrusor and the striated sphincter is not seen during the phase of recovery; it is especially true with complete suprasacral cord lesions. During such incomplete and incoordinated voiding the periurethral striated muscles are unusually sensitive to any external stimulation; contractions from such stimulations inhibit detrusor activity, causing cessation of voiding. Such unusual contractile responses of the periurethral striated muscle is not seen during normal voiding (*27*).

Established Patterns of Voiding Dysfunction

Following the recovery phase, voiding dysfunctions of specific patterns become established. All suprasacral complete cord injuries lead to abnormalities of voiding in relation to both detrusor activity and outlet function. Because the brainstem region is known to be responsible for maintenance of coordination between the detrusor and the striated sphincter, a complete cord lesion leads to detrusor–sphincteric incoordination of a minor or major degree in most such patients (*23–26*). On the other hand, detrusor contractions are not sustained, and the detrusor would relax inappropriately during voiding before the bladder is empty. Detrusor activity is inhibited when striated sphincter contraction or other pelvic floor muscle activity occurs. Moreover, decreased stimulation of bladder wall receptors may occur after voiding of small amounts of urine and before bladder emptying is completed. It may result from loss of facilitation of the sacral reflex arc due to disconnection from higher brainstem centers of micturition (*6*). Intermittent and unsustained detrusor activity leading to interrupted voiding with poor urinary flow rates and high residual volumes are thus seen.

Any one or more of a number of abnormal urodynamic findings may be present in upper motor neurogenic bladders.

1. There may be delayed opening of the bladder neck (Figs. 18–1 and 18–2); A mild degree of striated sphincter dyssynergia may coexist despite some voluntary control (Figs. 18–3 and 18–4).

2. Phasic or oscillatory, often prolonged contractions of the bladder may be present with alternating peaks and troughs of pres-

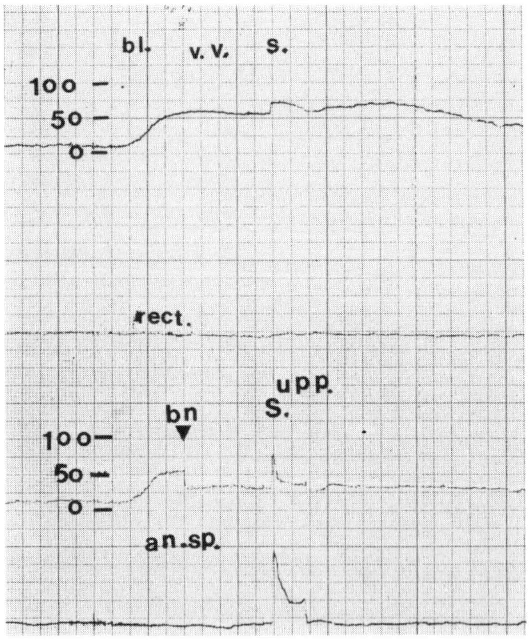

Figure 18-1. Urodynamic studies of a fully ambulatory 21-year-old man with grossly incomplete C_6 tetraplegia after injury. Urethral pressure profile (UPP) was performed during voiding to demonstrate delayed bladder neck opening and bladder neck obstruction. Note the marked drop in UPP at the bladder neck (*bn*). Stop voiding (*s*) was voluntary; note the isometric bladder contraction that occurs at the same time. Anal sphincter (*an sp*) contracts synchronously, but contraction is not sustained. *v*=voiding. Pressure is expressed in centimeters of water.

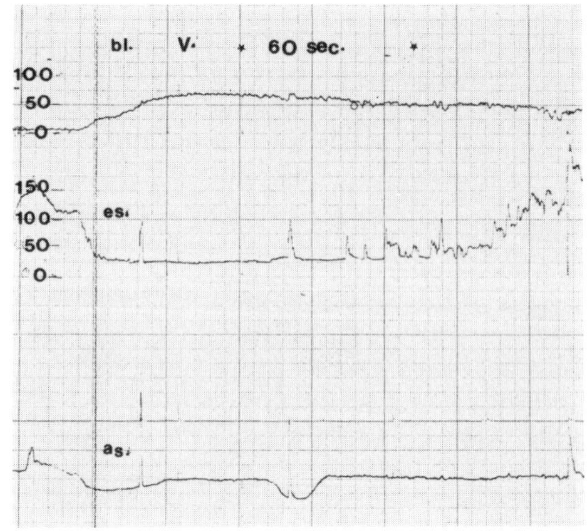

Figure 18-3. Urodynamic studies of the patient in Figure 18-1. Pressure is in centimeters of water. *bl* = bladder. *es* = external sphincter. *as* = anal sphincter. Note: (*1*) a small degree of detrusor-striated sphincter dyssynergia; and (*2*) a prolonged wave of bladder contraction due to delayed bladder neck opening.

sure; Such a pattern manifests mostly in patients with detrusor–sphincter dyssynergia (Figs. 18–5 and 18–6).

3. Intermittent small voidings with sudden interruptions beginning with closure at the external sphincter zone and continuing closure in a proximal milking fashion toward the bladder neck may be seen.

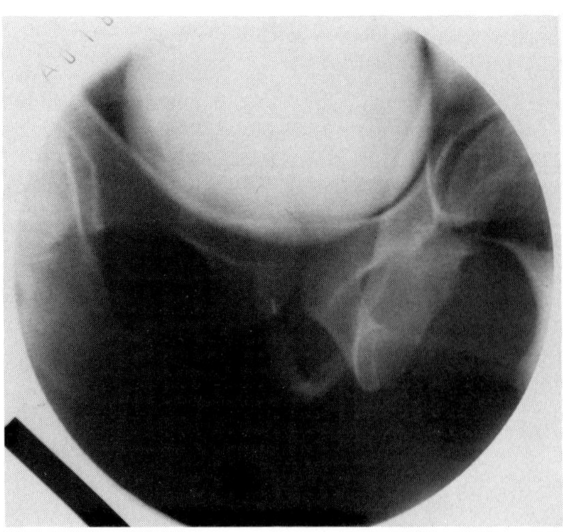

Figure 18-2. Radiograph of the same patient as in Figure 18-1, demonstrating radiopaque marker in the striated sphincter zone; radiograph was obtained before the stop voiding order (*s*).

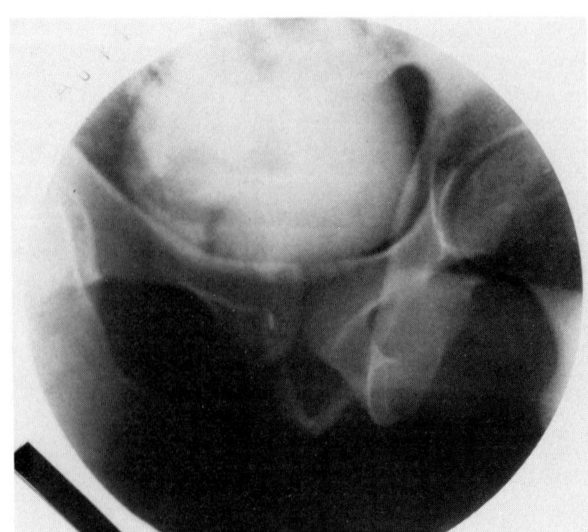

Figure 18-4. Radiograph of the patient in Figure 18-1, demonstrating a moderate voiding stream and a narrow bladder neck.

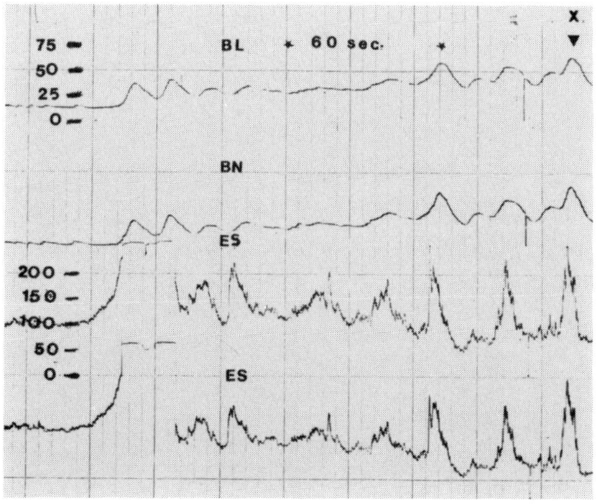

Figure 18-5. Urodynamic studies of an 18-year-old male tetraplegic, C_7 complete, 5 months after injury. Examination was performed with a five-microtransducer catheter. Not the marked degree of detrusor–sphincter dyssynergia with delayed bladder neck opening. Approximately 3 minutes after the start of bladder activity, the bladder neck opened slightly (see x-ray film); voiding never took place; and autonomic dysreflexia occurred during the examination.

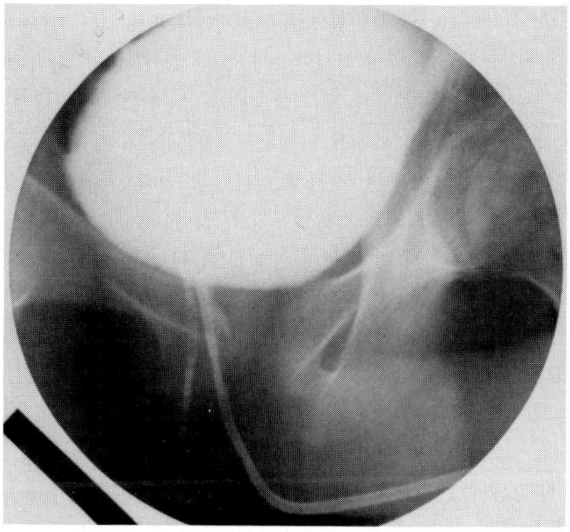

Figure 18-6. X-ray films of the patient in Figure 18-5. Note the five-microtransducer catheter in place with minimal bladder neck opening; note the three microtransducer catheter in the anal canal and rectum.

4. Despite an open bladder neck, delay in voiding occurs because of a lack of relaxation of the striated sphincter; sometimes complete obstruction at the striated sphincter zone is seen.

5. A rapid decrease of detrusor contraction occurs and residual vesical volume to a minimum is not seen (Figs. 18–7 and 18–8).

6. Although the basic voiding reflex of striated sphincter relaxation and bladder contraction may be present, it is much reduced in magnitude and is often interrupted by spasmodic sphincter contractions.

7. The bladder responds to repeated gentle percussions (tappings), with resultant detrusor contractions and voidings; urine expulsion occurs seconds after the end of each stimulus. This pattern may eventually achieve an acceptable degree of bladder emptying.

8. Uninhibited bladder contractions are sometimes opposed by a sudden rise in striated sphincter-generated pressure, followed by sphincter relaxation and adequate voiding.

9. Incomplete upper motor neuron lesions may leave patients with some bladder sensation and voluntary sphincteric control; yet careful urodynamic assessment of bladder function may unsuspectingly reveal one or more of the above findings (Figs. 18–9 and 18–10).

Although voiding dysfunctions appear to be established after injury, they occasionally change. The factors responsible for such a change are (a) changing interneuronal activity in isolated cord segments; (b) anatomic/structural changes in the bladder; (c) obstructive changes if the patient develops an enlarged prostate; and (d) changes due to urinary infection.

Spinal cord damage may extend distally when an injury occurs at the low lumbar segmental level, resulting in bizarre patterns of voiding dysfunction. Detrusor activity may be sluggish or absent, but reflex activity of the striated sphincter may persist. Reflex activity below the level of the lesion may not appear owing to complete damage to lower spinal cord segments secondary to extensive necrosis or infarction; in such cases a completely flaccid bladder with soft abdominopelvic musculature may result, and the pa-

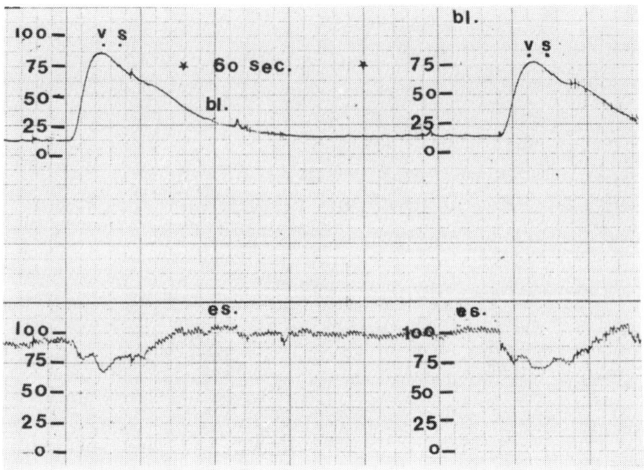

Figure 18–7. Urodynamic studies of a 22-year-old C_8-T_1 complete tetraplegic man. Pressure is in centimeters of water. *bl* = bladder. *v* = void. *es* = striated sphincter. *s* = stop void. Examination was done 1 hour after a bilateral pudendal block with marcaine to overcome dyssynergia. There is no evidence of detrusor-sphincter dyssynergia; the voiding contraction is not sustained, nor is the striated sphincter relaxation.

tient may be unable to void without the Valsalva maneuver ability.

CLASSIFICATION OF VOIDING DYSFUNCTION SECONDARY TO CORD DAMAGE

Simplifying an original proposal by Bors and Comarr (*5*), Thomas outlined the following classification based on the level and degree of cord damage above and below the site of maximum cord injury (*6*).

Vesicourethral dysfunction secondary to spinal cord injury can be classified as upper motor, lower motor, or mixed. Dysfunctions secondary to complete or incomplete upper motor neuron lesions are due to cord damage proximal to the sacral cord (S_2, S_3, S_4 segments), which remains intact. Lower motor neuron lesions of sacral cord segments or the cauda equina also can be complete or incomplete and produce dysfunctions. Mixed lesions leading to bizarre combinations of upper and lower motor neuron dysfunctions can result from partial damage to the lumbosacral cord region. In addition to the above dysfunctions, sympathetic neural damage may also occur when the lesions are extensive and involve thoracolumbar cord segments; passive bladder neck opening in such cases is often encountered (Fig. 18–11) (*7–9*). When upper motor detrusor dysfunc-

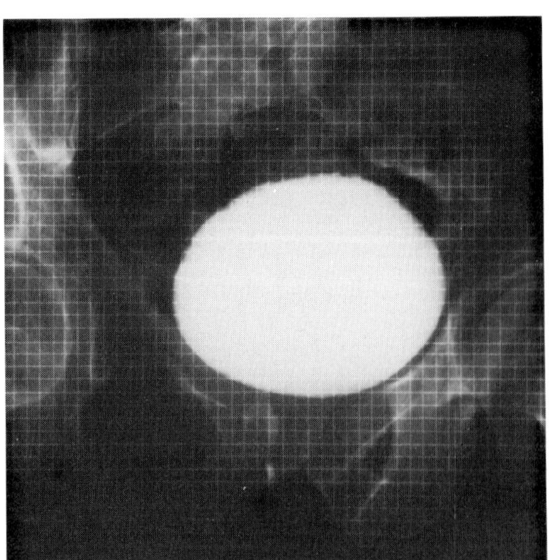

Figure 18-8. X-ray film of the same patient in Figure 18–7 during voiding. Note the minor bladder neck opening; only a small amount of urine emerged.

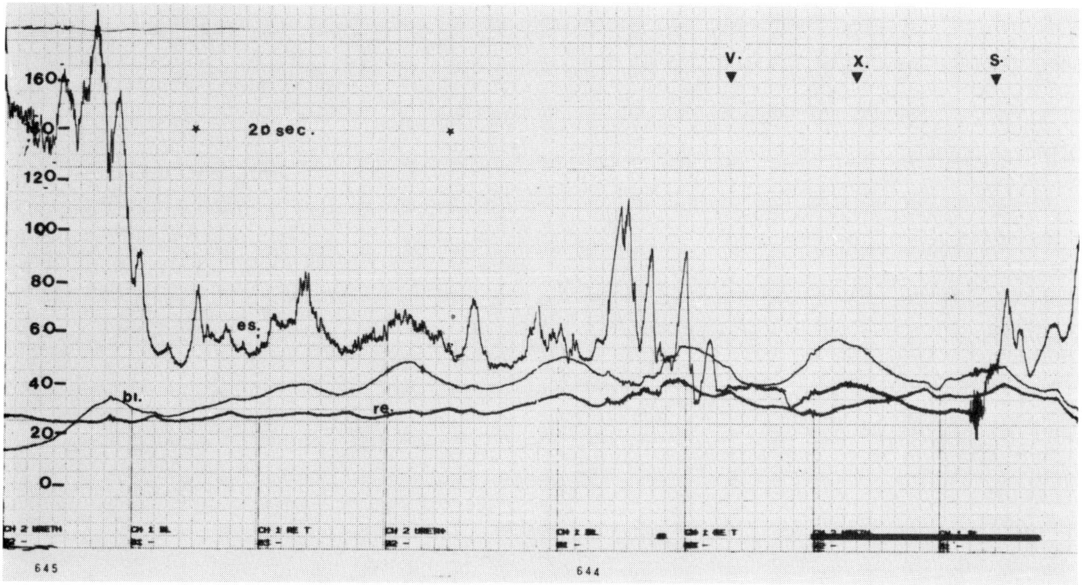

Figure 18-9. Urodynamic studies 6 months after injury in a 27-year-old, grossly incomplete C_8 tetraplegic man. The patient was able to ambulate with crutches; he had voluntary control over his striated sphincter, sensations of bladder fullness and of passage of urine, and good bladder emptying. The patient thought he had normal voiding. Pressure is given in centimeters of water. bl=bladder. v=void. *x*=X-ray films. *re*=rectum. *s*=stop void. *es*=external sphincter. Despite adequate sphincter relaxation, detrusor-sphincter dyssynergia is present with delayed bladder neck opening; the urinary stream is adequate.

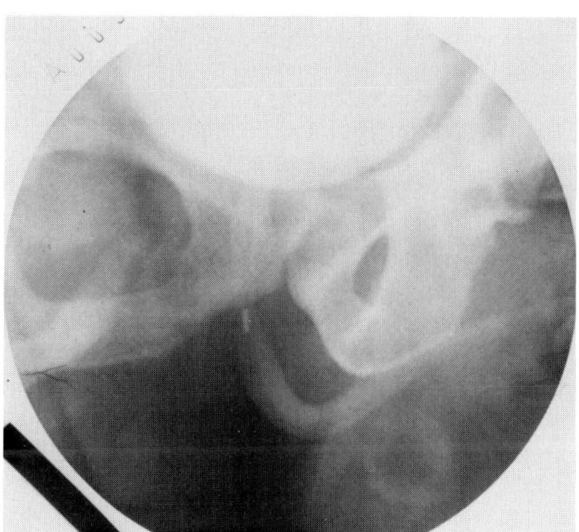

Figure 18-10. X-ray films of the same patient as in Figure 18-9. Note the rather narrow bladder neck, with a good voiding stream.

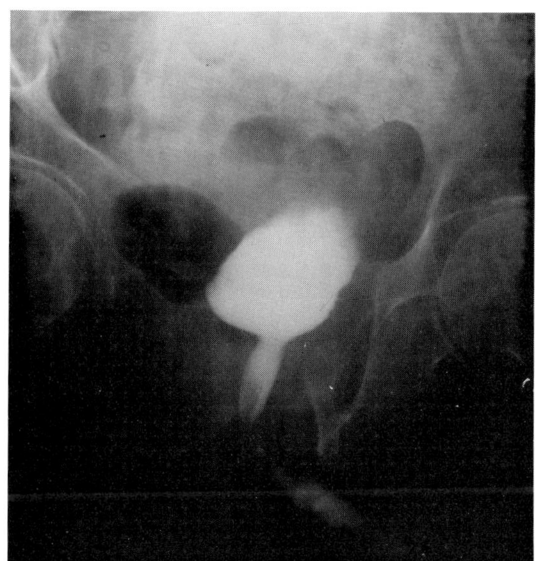

Figure 18-11. Voiding cystourethrogram of a 50-year-old complete L_2-L_3 male paraplegic. Bladder of small capacity is areflexic; note the wide open bladder neck due to concomitant sympathetic "denervation."

tion is associated with dyscoordination of smooth/striated muscle activity of the bladder outlet, appropriate sphincter dyssynergia of variable degree results (*26*).

Three grades of upper motor detrusor–sphincter dyssynergia were recognized in our urodynamic evaluations (*2,5,26*).

With *grade I dyssynergia* there is an unihibited but usually short-lived detrusor contraction; the striated sphincter response is a rapid rise followed by a sudden fall in urethral pressure and sphincter relaxation; bladder emptying is incomplete, however, owing to unsustained detrusor contraction. If trained to repeatedly stimulate the bladder to generate bouts of contraction by percussion, the Credé maneuver, coughing, rectal stimulation, or anal dilation, such patients may reasonably empty their bladders; good bladder emptying may be observed after bowel movements in the morning (Fig. 18–2).

With *grade II dyssynergia,* interrupted voiding is achieved by repeated short-lived detrusor contractions interrupted by sudden striated sphincter contraction(s); this unsustained contractile detrusor behavior results in frequent but incomplete voidings, high residual urine volumes, and interrupted voidings with low flow rates.

With *grade III dyssynergia* the detrusor pressure is high and becomes both phasic and oscillatory because the striated sphincter fails to relax; in fact, it relentlessly spasmodically contracts in a seesaw fashion that almost completely prevents satisfactory voiding. This voiding dysfunction may or may not be associated with opening of the bladder neck and, in either case, may cause marked autonomic dysreflexia in susceptible patients, an expression of severe dyssynergia (Figs. 18–6 and 18–7). EMG activity of the striated sphincter is only intermittent, and EMG silence occurs only if and when voiding takes place; "resting" EMG activity is recorded only while the detrusor is inactive.

In women, classic detrusor–striated urethral sphincter dyssynergia may not be seen since the striated sphincter is not fully developed (*28*). The voiding pattern observed in these patients often conforms with the above-described grade II dyssynergic pattern, which is due to frequent inhibition of detrusor activity by contractions of pelvic floor muscles; residual urine volumes are high under such settings. In all patterns of detrusor hyperreflexia associated with striated sphincter incoordination, the bladder later becomes heavily trabeculated, with the formation of cellules and diverticula. Vesicoureteral reflux is often seen with such types of dysfunction. If the bladder is severely spastic, residual urine may not be seen and the bladder wall becomes markedly thickened. All patterns of dysfunction can be influenced by infection, spasticity of the striated muscles, and any abnormal cutaneous stimuli secondary to infection or pressure sores. Sometimes severe constipation can result in abnormal and changing patterns of vesicourethral dysfunction.

Lower Motor Neuron Bladders

Lower motor neuron lesions result in flaccidity of the bladder and its outlet. The detrusor becomes inactive and areflexic; consequently, bladder wall compliance and vesical capacity become increased (*5,6*). Pressures in the outlet in both the internal sphincter (bladder neck) and the striated sphincter (membranous urethra) regions are markedly decreased. Periurethral striated muscles become nonresponsive to afferent pudendal reflex arc stimulation; stimulation of the glans penis or clitoris does not produce a urethral pressure increase or an EMG response of these muscles. If the sympathetic pathway is also involved because of extensive lesions at the thoracolumbar region, the bladder neck may become patulous and incompetent in association with a hypoactive detrusor and a hypoactive striated sphincter (*8*) (Fig. 18–11).

With partial lower motor neuron lesions, detrusor activity may be seen after filling the bladder to a large capacity, but its contractile response may be inadequate in magnitude and duration to expel urine completely. Detrusor contraction may be incomplete, unsustained, and of low pressure. It is our preference to call such a bladder a partial or incomplete lower motor bladder, rather than an upper motor one. We refrain from designating such a bladder "hyperreflexic" because in fact it is hyporeflexic; the pelvic floor is flaccid, and the bladder itself descends on voiding, which is achieved largely by the Valsalva maneuver. Consequently, periurethral striated muscles, though flaccid, may not relax completely.

Complete lower motor neuron lesions involving the bladder and its outlet produce features of total inactivity of both. Although the striated sphincter is completely paralyzed, it may still be obstructive during either the Valsalva or the Credé maneuvers to evacuate urine. With long-standing injuries and because of the patient's Valsalva type of voiding, the bladder base descends distally and thus may create malalignment or acute angulation of the prostatomembranous and bulbous urethral regions, with total obstruction in the striated sphincter region, Yet in a number of lower motor neuron bladders, the bladder neck remains closed and does not open with the Valsalva maneuver; the reason is unknown.

AUTONOMIC DYSREFLEXIA OR HYPERREFLEXIA

Uncontrolled sympathetic responses to stimuli below the level of a spinal cord lesion may cause autonomic dysreflexia. It is seen classically in patients with lesions above T_6, i.e., above the major splanchnic sympathetic outflow (*29–32*). The chances of developing autonomic dysreflexia are greater in patients with cervical lesions than in those with upper thoracic lesions; among a group of 213 patients with lesions of T_6 or above, autonomic dysreflexia was present in 48 percent (*33*). Autonomic dysreflexia manifests as a group of symptoms, mainly severe and pounding headache, piloerection, flushing of the face above the anatomic level of the lesion with sweating, and hypertension of a degree that may precipitate a seizure or cerebral hemorrhage; bradycardia also may be present. Autonomic dysreflexia usually starts to appear 6 to 8 weeks after the injury and may remain with the patient for the rest of his life (*33*).

Pathogenesis

Autonomic dysreflexia is not known to many medical practitioners, but the urologist should be aware of its possible presence in the patient with spinal cord injury at the T_6 level or higher because by far the most common cause of its sudden emergence in such a patient is vesical distension. The major causes of dysreflexia from the urologic standpoint are (a) detrusor–sphincter dyssynergia; (b) vesical distension by urine retention, from catheter obstruction, or during cystometry or cystoscopy; and (c) transurethral surgery or other manipulations of the lower urinary tract in all susceptible patients during surgery or the postoperative period. Other causes of dysreflexia include fecal impaction, fractures of long bones, visceral inflammations (e.g., appendicitis, cholecystitis, or pancreatitis), and occasionally pressure sores.

Norepinephrine release seems to be involved in the pathogenesis of autonomic dysreflexia (*31*). Serum levels of norepinephrine and dopamine-β-hydroxylase (the enzyme that converts dopamine to norepinephrine) are markedly elevated. Norepinephrine is known to have no effect on the heart rate, its major influence being through vasoconstriction of peripheral arterioles. Presumably, stimuli below the level of the cord lesion cause excitation of sympathetic pre- and postganglionic neurons that innervate peripheral blood vessels; subsequent release of norepinephrine at vascular receptor sites induces arteriolar vasoconstriction and high blood pressure, which remains unabated and continues to rise. Baroreceptors of the aortic arch and carotid sinuses, stimulated by the high blood pressure, reflexly cause bradycardia as well as vasodilation of the splanchnic bed. Dilation of arterioles of the splanchnic bed would normally absorb the shifted blood and regulate the blood pressure, but such vasodilation does not occur after spinal cord transection above T_6. Bradycardia, however, often occurs because it is mediated via the vagus nerve, which is not interrupted. Flushing of the face in autonomic dysreflexia is due to dilation of facial arterioles above the site of the lesion.

Management

It is always prudent to anticipate and prevent occurrence of autonomic dysreflexia in susceptible patients. Procedures expected to cause bladder distension, e.g., cystoscopy, cystolitholapaxy, or bladder outlet surgery, must be done under adequate anesthesia.

Spinal anesthesia is preferable because it blocks transmission of stimuli from the bladder and other pelvic organs (*34*). Insertion of an indwelling catheter or obstruction, e.g., by a blood clot, may induce autonomic dysreflexia. When a catheter is obstructed, it is removed immediately and adequate bladder drainage established. Pulmonary dysfunction and pulmonary edema have been reported as complications of autonomic dysreflexia (*35*) and should be watched for.

Patients known to have dysreflexia are prepared preoperatively by being given an alpha-adrenergic blocking agent a few days before bladder surgery is performed. Apart from a alpha-adrenergic blocking agents (*36*), chlorpromazine can be titrated more easily than nitroprusside and probably is a safer intravenous medication (*37*). Given in a dose of 1 to 2 mg intravenously every 3 to 4 hours, it has been effective and dependable. Other medications, e.g., phentolamine, hydralazine, diazoxide, and trimethaphan camsylate (Arfonad), have also been used intravenously (*29,37*). Recent observations of Lindan *et al.* (*37a*) suggest that Nifedipine, a calcium channel blocker can be administered both in prevention as well as in the management of an acute crisis.

UROLOGIC MANAGEMENT OF SPINAL CORD INJURY PATIENTS

Intermittent catheterization has been reestablished as the primary treatment of choice in spinal cord injury patients (*13,14,20*). It was abandoned near the end of World War I because of the occurrence of frequent sepsis (*38*). Despite the availability of antibiotics, rigid asepsis in catheterization is still preferred (*14*).

After the stage of spinal shock is over (8–10 weeks) and reflex voiding has been established the frequency of catheterization is reduced to fewer than three times per day, with a more liberal fluid intake instead of the originally restricted one. Physicians do differ, however, in the regimens favored for intermittent catheterization.

A few patients may prove unsuitable for intermittent catheterization because of skin sensitivity to antiseptic solutions, urethritis, or urethral stricture. Placement of a suprapubic cystocatheter may then be justified in the preliminary management (*13,39,40*).

Some time after spinal cord injury (4–6 months), 30 to 40 percent of patients still require a surgical procedure on the bladder outlet to achieve adequate vesical emptying (*13,41–45*); permanent suprapubic or indwelling catheters, however, are avoided at all costs. Bladder outlet surgery usually combines a striated urethral sphincterotomy and bladder neck incisions or resection. Life-long follow-up of such patients is required, as in more than 50 percent of them the need to repeat the surgery arises (*46*). Bladder outlet surgery, however, leads to and in fact aims at achieving urinary incontinence. Although this method may be acceptable to male patients who can use condom drainage, it certainly is not to women. Even in men other options for bladder rehabilitation, e.g., regulation of drinking habits or stimulation of "trigger points" at regular intervals, are evaluated and encouraged. After bladder surgery the voiding pressure is reduced, but bladder contractions remain unsustained. For this reason optional methods of bladder rehabilitation remain an essential part of patient management if vesical function is to be preserved and urinary infection avoided. Neuropharmacologic medications such as alpha-adrenergic blockers and anticholinergic and antispasmodic drugs may help keep a male or female patient "dry" (*27,47*).

Self-catheterization (or catheterization by a partner or health provider) has resurfaced as a viable alternative to bladder outlet surgery in the patient with spinal cord injury (*48*). This method of bladder drainage is certainly more attractive in many flaccid lower motor neuron bladders that cannot be emptied completely by the Valsalva maneuver. Self-catheterization has a distinct advantage in female patients (*27,47*). In general, sterile self-catheterization is indicated in the following groups of patients: (a) women (anticholinergic medications may be required); and (b) men who desire to maintain their fertility and protect it from bladder outlet surgery. Patients applying self-catheterization must have hand dexterity, self-discipline, and clean habits.

Bladder outlet surgery, however, remains as the favorable option in the following situations (*13,24,41–46,49*): tetraplegia, especially of a high cord level; autonomic dysreflexia; vesicoureteral reflux; recurrent infections with septicemia, fever, or epididymitis; and hydronephrosis with or without upper tract deterioration.

The urologic management of patients with spinal cord injury aims at prevention of urinary infection and protection of the upper urinary tracts. Each patient must be evaluated individually according to these guidelines (*50*). It must be remembered, however, that there remain a few patients who may best be treated by an indwelling catheter. These patients require a close follow-up with urine cytologies, cystoscopy, and bladder biopsies since it is known that prolonged indwelling catheters might lead to squamous metaplasia and squamous cell cancer (*51*).

REFERENCES

1. Roaf, R.: A study of the mechanics of spinal injuries. *J. Bone Joint Surg.* 42B:810, 1960.
2. Romanes, G. J.: The arterial blood supply of the human spinal cord. *Paraplegia* 2:199, 1965.
3. Hughes, J. T.: *Pathology of the Spinal Cord.* Saunders, London, 1978, pp. 91–101.
4. Barrett, H. J. M., and Jousse, A. T.: Post-traumatic syringomyelia (cystic myelopathy): injuries of the spine and spinal cord. In *Handbook of Clinical Neurology,* Vinken, P. J., and Bruyn, G. W. (eds.), Vol. 26. North Holland, Amsterdam, 1976, pp. 113–157.
5. Bors, E., and Comarr, A. E.: *Neurological Urology,* 1st ed. University Park Press, Baltimore, 1971, p. 129.
6. Thomas, D. G.: The urinary tract following spinal cord injury. In Williams, D. I., and Chisholm, G. D. (eds.), *Scientific Foundations of Urology,* 1st ed., Vol. 2. Year Book, Chicago, 1976, p. 59.
7. Blaivas, J. G., and Barbailias, G. A.: Characteristics of neural injury after abdominoperineal resection. *J. Urol.* 129:84, 1983.
8. Woodside, J. R., and McGuire, E. J.: Urethral hypotonicity after suprasacral spinal cord injury. *J. Urol.* 121:783, 1979.
9. Yalla, S. V., and Andriole, G. L.: Vesicourethral dysfunction following pelvic visceral ablative surgery. *J. Urol.* 132:503, 1984.
10. Hall, M.: *New Memoir on the Nervous System.* Bailliere, London, 1843.
11. Awad, S. A., Byniak, S. R., Downie, J. W., and Twiddy, A. A. S.: Urethral pressure profile during the spinal shock stage in man: a preliminary report. *J. Urol.* 117:91, 1977.
12. Rossier, A. B., Fam, B. A., DiBenedetto, M., and Sarkarati, M.: Urodynamics in spinal shock patients. *J. Urol.* 122:783, 1979.
13. Fam, B. A., Rossier, A. B., Blunt, K., Gabilondo, F. B., Sarkarati, M., Sethi, J., and Yalla, S. V.: Experience in the urologic management of 120 early spinal cord injury patients. *J. Urol.* 119:485, 1978.
14. Guttman, L., and Frankel, H.: The value of intermittent catheterization in the early management of traumatic paraplegia and tetraplegia. *Paraplegia* 4:63, 1966.
15. McCouch, G. P., Austin, G. M., Liu, C. N., and Liu, C. T.: Sprouting as a cause of spasticity. *J. Neurophysiol.* 21:205, 1958.
16. Bradley, W. E., Timm, G. W., and Scott, F. B.: Innervation of the detrusor muscle and urethra. *Urol. Clin. North Am.* 1:3, 1974.
17. Bradley, W. E., Rockswald, G. L., Timm, G. W., and Scott, F. B.: Neurology of micturition. *J. Urol.* 115:481, 1976.
18. Bors, E.: Neurogenic bladder. *Urol. Survey.* 7:177, 1957.
19. Rossier, A. B., Fan. B. A., DiBenedetto, M., and Sarkarati, M.: Urethrovesical function during spinal shock. *Urol. Res.* 8:53, 1980.
20. Pearman, J. W.: Urological followup of 99 spinal cord injured patients initially managed by intermittent catheterization. *Br. J. Urol.* 48:297, 1976.
21. Pearman, J. W., and Low, A. I.: The iced cystogram—a new technique for distinguishing obstruction at the level of the external sphincter from obstruction at the bladder neck. *Paraplegia* 12:153, 1974.
22. Rhodes, D. W., Scott, M. B., and Monow, J. W.: Use of the iced cystogram to differentiate bladder neck and external sphincter obstruction. *J. Urol.* 119:639, 1978.
23. Perkash, I.: Detrusor–sphincter dyssynergic responses. *J. Urol.* 120:469, 1978.
24. Perkash, I.: Problems of decatheterization in long-term spinal cord injury patient. *J. Urol.* 124:249, 1980.
25. Yalla, S. V., Rossier, A. B., and Fam, B. A.: Dyssynergic vesicourethral responses during bladder rehabilitation in spinal cord injury patients: effects of suprapubic percussion, Credé method and bethanechol chloride. *J. Urol.* 115:575, 1976.
26. Yalla, S. V., Blunt, K., Fam, B. A., Constantinople, N., and Gittes, R. F.: Detrusor urethral sphincter dyssynergia. *J. Urol.* 118:1026, 1977.
27. Yalla, S. V., and Dyro, F.: Periurethral striated muscle responses to afferent stimulation during voiding. In *Proceedings, International Continence Society, 2nd Joint Meeting,* Aachen, FRG, 1983 pp. 114–116.
28. Song, G. W., Fam. B. A., Lee, I. Y., Sarkarati, M., and Rossier, A. B.: Management of neurogenic bladder in female spinal cord injury patients. *J. Am. Paraplegia Soc.* 7:4, 1984.
29. Comarr, A. E.: Autonomic dysreflexia. *J. Am. Paraplegia Soc.* 7:4, 1984.
30. Kurnick, N. B.: Autonomic hyperreflexia and its control in patients with spinal cord lesions. *Ann. Intern. Med.* 44:678, 1956.
31. Mathias, C. J., Christensen, N. J., Corbett, J. L., Phil, D., Frankel, H. L., and Spalding, J. M. K.: Plasma catecholamines during paroxysmal neurogenic hypertension in quadriplegic man. *Circ. Res.* 39:204, 1976.
32. Scott, M. B., and Morrow, J. W.: Phenoxybenzamine in neurogenic bladder dysfunction after spinal cord injury. *J. Urol.* 119:483, 1978.
33. Lindan, R., Joiner, E., Freehafer, A. A., and Hazel, C.: Incidence and clinical features of autonomic

dysreflexia in patients with spinal cord injury. *Paraplegia* 18:285, 1980.
34. Broecker, B. H., Harnowsky, N., and Hackler, R. H.: Low spinal anesthesia for the prevention of autonomic dysreflexia in the spinal cord injury patient. *J. Urol.* 122:366, 1979.
35. Kiker, J. D., Woodside, J. R., and Jelinek, G. E.: Neurogenic pulmonary edema associated with autonomic dysreflexia. *J. Urol.* 128:1038, 1982.
36. McGuire, E. G., Wagner, F. M., and Weiss, R. M.: Treatment of autonomic dysreflexia with phenoxybenzamine. *J. Urol.* 115:53, 1976.
37. McGuire, E. J., and Rossier, A. B.: Treatment of acute autonomic dysreflexia. *J. Urol.* 129:1185, 1983.
37a. Lindan, R., Leffler, E. J., and Kedia, K. R.: A comparison of the efficacy of an alpha-1 adrenergic blocker and the slow calcium channel blocker in the control of autonomic dysreflexia. *Paraplegia* 23:34, 1985.
38. Walker, J. W. T.: The bladder in gunshot and other injuries of the spinal cord. *Lancet* 1:173, 1917.
39. Cook, J. B., and Smith, P. H.: Percutaneous suprapubic cystotomy after spinal cord injury. *Br. J. Urol.* 48:119, 1976.
40. Smith, P. H., Cook, J. B., and Burt, A. A.: Percutaneous cystotomy in paraplegia—a followup of 41 patients. *Paraplegia* 14:135, 1976.
41. Perkash, I.: Modified approach to sphincterotomy in spinal cord injury patients. *Paraplegia* 13:247, 1976.
42. Ross, J. C., Gibbon, N. O., and Donanski, M.: Division of the external sphincter in the treatment of the paraplegic bladder. *Br. J. Urol.* 30:204, 1958.
43. Ross, J. C., Gibbon, N. O. K., and Sunder, G. S.: Division of the external urethral sphincter in the neuropathic bladder: a 20 year review. *Br. J. Urol.* 48:649, 1976.
44. Whitmore, W. F., III, Yalla, S. V., Fam, B. A., and Gittes, R. F.: Experience with anteromedian (12 o'clock) external urethral sphincterotomy in 100 male subjects with neuropathic bladders. *Br. J. Urol.* 50:49, 1978.
45. Yalla, S. V., Fam, B. A., Gabilondo, F. B., Jacobs, S., DiBenedetto, M., Rossier, A. B., and Gittes, R. F.: Anteromedian external urethral sphincterotomy: technique, rationale and complications. *J. Urol.* 117:489, 1977.
46. Gershon, C., and O'Flynn, J. D.: Urological disability in quadriplegia: a study of treatment and followup in 92 patients. *Br. J. Urol.* 52:488, 1976.
47. Merritt, J. L., Lie, M. R., and Opitz, J. L.: Bladder retraining of paraplegic women. *Arch. Phys. Med. Rehabil.* 63:416, 1982.
48. Lapides, J., Diokno, A. C., Lowe, B. S., and Kalish, M. D.: Followup on unsterile intermittent self-catheterization. *J. Urol.* 111:184, 1974.
49. Emmett, J. L.: Transurethral in treatment of true and pseudo cord bladder. *J. Urol.* 53:545, 1945.
50. Wein, A. J., Raezer, D. M., and Benson, G. S.: Management of neurogenic bladder dysfunction in the adult. *Urology* 8:432, 1976.
51. Kaufman, J. F., Fam. B. A., Jacobs, S. C., Gabilondo, F. B., Yalla, S. V., Kane, J. P., and Rossier, A. B.: Bladder cancer and squamous metaplasia in spinal cord injury patients. *J. Urol.* 118:967, 1977.

19

Voiding Dysfunction in the Elderly

NEIL M. RESNICK, M.D.

The greatest obstacle to progress is the belief that no progress is possible.

SIR FRANCIS BACON

A striking transformation is occurring in the age composition of American society. Because of a decline in infant mortality and 25 percent decrease in the mortality rate for those over age 85 (*1*), individuals over age 65 have become part of the fastest growing segment of the population; each day their ranks swell by additional 1000 people. These demographic trends have led to a remarkable situation. Of all the people who have *ever* lived to age 65, more than two-thirds are currently walking the face of the earth (*2*).

Urinary incontinence is a major source of morbidity among America's elderly. Prevalence estimates vary widely, depending on which segment of the older population is examined. In the community setting, studies suggest that 5 to 15 percent of the elderly suffer from incontinence on at least a weekly basis; for one-third of these individuals, incontinence is severe enough to saturate clothing and disrupt social or domestic life (*3-7*). In the acute hospital setting, the prevalence of incontinence is higher, ranging between 20 and 35 percent (*8–10a*), and in the nursing home setting it is even higher, usually exceeding 50 percent (*11–14*).

The morbidity associated with incontinence in the elderly is substantial. Medically, it predisposes to cystitis, urosepsis, pressure sores, falls, fractures, and placement of an indwelling catheter. Psychosocially, it stigmatizes the sufferer and causes anxiety, embarrassment, isolation, depression, and regression (*15*). These effects make patients less likely to report new illness, less compliant with current therapy, and ultimately more likely to require institutionalization.

Economically, the costs are startling. Although exact costs are unknown, incontinence is estimated to account for one-third of Britain's nursing home budget (*16*) and for at least 10 to 15 percent of the nursing home budget in America (*17,18*). These figures translate into \$3 billion to \$8 billion annually, or between 1.5 and 4.0 times as much as we spend to dialyze every patient in the United States suffering from renal failure. The magnitude of the expense is further highlighted when one realizes that these estimates exclude the vast amount spent on appliances, pads, paraphernalia, physician visits, and pharmaceuticals by the 85 percent of incontinent elderly who are not institutionalized.

Despite its prevalence, morbidity, and expense, however, incontinence is a problem with which neither patients nor physicians feel comfortable. Numerous community surveys document that only a few elderly people with this malady seek medical care (*3-5,19*). When they do, it is a condition physicians add only infrequently to patient problem lists and even less frequently evaluate (*13*).

This neglect is particularly unfortunate as incontinence is no more a normal part of aging than is chest pain. Furthermore, it is largely remediable, even in the elderly (*3,8,10,20,21,21a,b*), if a carefully targeted approach is employed. However, this approach differs significantly from that used for younger patients because of the physiologic, pathologic, psychological, and pharmacologic changes that occur as individuals age. This chapter addresses many of these issues.

CHANGES WITH NORMAL AGING

To diagnose disease in the lower urinary tract of an older person, one must first be acquainted with the changes that occur as part of normal aging. Before considering the dearth of data available, it is worthwhile to focus on a few issues that have emerged from gerontologic research over the past few decades.

Theoretical issues

The first issue is the concept of normal aging (*22,23*). Although it is clear that one cannot compare sick elderly patients to healthy young medical students and conclude that the differences are due to aging alone, it is less clear what the proper definition of normal aging is. One approach accepts the mean value of a physiologic variable obtained from an unscreened population and adds a range of two standard deviations (SD). However, because 75 percent of individuals over age 65 have at least one serious chronic illness (*24*), average function does not necessarily imply normality. A second approach is to evaluate only patients who are neither acutely ill nor on medications known to affect the variable being examined. However, because they may have other illnesses or be on other medications, the relation between age and function may still be confounded. Finally, some investigators insist that only ideal aging should serve as a model, and that the only suitable subjects are those free from disease and taking no medications. This definition may engender a circular type of reasoning and result in only a few of the elderly being classified as normal. Nonetheless, each of the last two definitions is useful and appropriate under different circumstances if investigators carefully list the criteria used in their study. The important point is to separate an ineluctable age-related decline from superimposed pathologic changes that may be amenable to intervention.

A second issue concerns that concept of "old." Most physiologic variables seem to decline gradually and linearly with age and result in diminished physiologic reserve. However, these changes do not usually affect an individual's ability to adapt to stress until approximately age 75 to 80 (*25*). Additionally, because the variability of most physiologic parameters seems to increase with age (*22,23,25*), studies of aging physiology need to enlist more elderly subjects than young ones. They also need to use subjects over age 70, rather than those over age 55 or 60. Few studies examining the impact of age on the lower urinary tract have incorporated these guidelines.

A final lesson of research in gerontologic physiology is that cross-sectional studies, although easier to perform, have important limitations that must be considered (*22*). One such limitation is known as the "cohort effect." When investigators from the Framingham project examined the relation between age and weight, they found that weight appeared to decrease with age. However, the longitudinal data revealed a different phenomenon. Weight *increased* at all ages; it just increased at a slower rate in older people, accounting for the misleading conclusions from the cross-sectional data (*23*). This principle may apply to urologic research related to the aging process as well. Suppose that decreased bladder capacity is associated with frequent voiding and that social norms of previous decades encouraged housewives with ready access to toilets to void frequently. As social norms change, with women being encouraged to spend more time in the workplace (and less time voiding), bladder capacity may increase in working women, i.e., younger women. A cross-sectional study would imply that bladder capacity decreased with age, even though a longitudinal study would show no difference. Likewise, a cross-sectional study purporting to demonstrate an age-related decrease in urethral pressure may actually reflect a recent decrease in parity, improvement in obstetric practice, shortening of the duration of the second stage of labor, and a popularization of pelvic floor muscle exercises. Only data stratification or a longitudinal study would be able to tease these factors apart.

With these principles in mind, the data available on anatomic and physiologic changes with age may be easier to evaluate.

Anatomic Changes

Evidence for age-associated changes has been sought in bladder receptors, bladder collagen content, urothelium, urethral structure, and prostate size. Two studies evaluated bladder receptor changes with age, and no differences were found in either the number or affinity of cholinergic receptors in the rat bladder (*26, 26a*). On the other hand, autonomic innervation of the human bladder seems to decline with age (*26b*).

Two studies examined bladder collagen content in autopsy specimens (*27,28*). Too few specimens may have precluded meaningful conclusions in the first study. The second study may have confounded changes due to disease with those due to age, as few premortem functional data were available. A study in mice failed to show any age-related difference in bladder collagen or smooth muscle content (*29*).

Studies of the urothelium are equally sparse and difficult to interpret. An electron microscopic study of urothelium from patients aged 61 to 82 suggested that aged urothelium may fail to differentiate normally and thus may become more permeable (*30*). However, a study in mice failed to confirm this finding (*29*).

Mice have also served as a model to examine urethral changes with age. Investigators have found that urethral smooth muscle is replaced by increasing amounts of collagen (*31*). If true in humans, it would explain the changes in urethral function discussed below. Surprisingly, few human studies have been performed. Studies of vaginal exfoliative cytology have encountered a wide spectrum of atrophic changes in postmenopausal women. Some of these women have almost normal cellular maturation and estrogen effect. McLennan and McLennan found that 25 percent of women over age 75 had superficial well-estrogenized cells on cytologic analysis (*32*). Another study found frank vaginal atrophy in only 50 percent of individuals who had undergone menopause 10 years earlier (*33*). Research may provide a rationale for this finding, as it has been shown that 40 percent of postmenopausal women maintain moderate concentrations of circulating estrogen throughout life (*34*). The principal form and source of hormone, however, change with age. Estradiol, derived from ovarian secretion, is the primary form of estrogen in premenopausal women; estrone, derived primarily from peripheral conversion of precursors (*35*), is the main form of circulating estrogen in postmenopausal women (*36*). Thus vaginal and urethral atrophy are not universal concomitants of aging in women (*37,38*).

Prostate enlargement, however, is inevitable if a man lives long enough. Fifty percent of men aged 50 to 60 and 90 percent of those over age 80 harbor the condition (*39*). Although past evidence suggested that benign prostatic hypertrophy (BPH) was due to dihydrotestosterone accumulation in the prostate, more recent data have cast doubt on this hypothesis (*40*).

Microbiologic Changes

The prevalence of asymptomatic bacteriuria rises markedly and abruptly with age. The prevalence of bacteriuria in women aged 45 to 65 and in men aged 65 to 70 is roughly 3 percent (*41*). However, in a population of community-dwelling elderly people, Brocklehurst *et al.* found significant bacteriuria ($>10^5$/ml) in 20 percent of women over age 65 and in the same proportion of men over age 70 (*42*). Other investigators have found similar results (*43,44*), and not surprisingly the prevalence of significant bacteriuria in chronic care facilities is nearly doubled (*45,46*). The reasons for the high prevalence of bacteriuria in apparently healthy elderly persons have not yet been elucidated, but several studies have failed to find an association between asymptomatic bacteriuria and incontinence (*42,45,47, 47a*).

Symptoms of Dysfunction

Symptoms of lower urinary tract dysfunction are common in well-screened healthy elderly, as well as in randomly surveyed elderly subjects residing in the community. Precipitancy and urgency occur in 18 to 41 percent of the elderly, without a clear gender association (*6,42,48*). "Difficulty voiding" is acknowledged by 3 to 9 percent of women and by 13 to 18 percent of men in a community sample; slow stream, however, is present in 23 percent of healthy men who claimed to be asymptomatic when recruited to participate in a study (*7,42,48*). Urinary frequency is uncommon, affecting 9 to 29 percent of older people; the discrepancy between these two figures partly reflects the differing definitions of frequency that were employed (*7,42,48*). Nocturia, however, seems to be quite common: 61 percent of women and 71 percent of men living at home reported this symptom (*42*). Twenty-four to 29 percent voided at least twice per night, a proportion that in one study was tightly linked to advancing age (*7,42*). Another study of allegedly asymptomatic men reported that 53 percent of subjects voided at least once per night (*48*). Even allowing for the poor reproducibility of reporting documented in elderly populations, the prevalence of nocturia is high and may be due to several factors. It may reflect the fact that fluid excretion is handled differently by aged kidneys. One study found that older subjects excreted more than half of their daily ingested fluid load at night, whereas younger people excreted only 25 percent during the same period (*49*). The age-related and high prevalence of congestive heart failure may also be a contributing factor, but at least one study carefully excluded patients with this condition (*49*). Of course the extraordinarily high prevalence of BPH may also be implicated. Finally, both depression and the normal age-related alteration of sleep patterns may contribute to the high prevalence of nocturia. No study has shown a relation between any of these lower urinary tract symptoms and urinary tract infections.

Functional Changes

Several urodynamic studies have examined the impact of age on lower urinary tract function. Most are limited by considerations mentioned earlier, so a clear consensus is not yet possible and much more research is needed.

Uroflowmetry

The reproducibility of uroflowmetry in an elderly population is unknown but is certainly affected by patient cooperation, total bladder volume, the presence of a significant residual volume, the number of voidings studied, and if the patient strains to void. Although older patients are more likely to harbor residual urine (see below), are less able to cooperate, and perhaps are more likely to strain to void, no study has examined these parameters. Furthermore, most studies have not stated criteria for "normalcy," excluded pathology by urodynamic means, or examined many patients over age 70. Understandably, then, there is disagreement regarding the impact of age on uroflowmetry, especially in the case of women.

Some studies of uroflowmetry in women fail to demonstrate an age effect (*50–52*), whereas others do (*53,54*). Studies of men, on the other hand, all document a decrease in flow with age (*48,54–58*), although in one study it was minimal in men over age 45 (*58*). However, because no studies have evaluated patients with urodynamically normal outlets, the question remains unsettled. As a result, nomograms are still of limited and unproved value for elderly patients.

Urethral Profilometry

No studies of the changes with age in urethral profilometry have been reported for men. In continent women there is a consensus that maximal urethral pressure (MUP), maximal urethral closure pressure (MUCP), and functional urethral length decrease with age, but the data are not entirely clear (*59–62*). Edwards and Malvern, for instance, found a precipitous decrease in MUCP that begins in youth (*60*). Rud, on the other hand, found that MUCP increases until age 25 and then falls, but a closer look at the data discloses no clear decrease in pressures until beyond the age of 60 (*62*). These findings have been ascribed to reduced urethral vascularity, a decrease in alpha-adrenergic receptors, and soft tissue atrophy—all occurring secondary to low levels of circulating estrogens. The possible confounding influence of cohort effect was mentioned earlier.

Urethral Compliance

Using an innovative approach, Susset *et al.* examined changes in the compliance of the female urethra with age. None of these women was truly normal, as all presented with lower urinary tract symptoms. Nonetheless, the data are interesting and suggest that compliance decreases significantly with age (*63*). If confirmed in a normal population, it may prove to be the correlate of urethral structural changes summarized earlier.

Bladder Capacity

Only two studies have examined the change in bladder capacity with age. Brocklehurst *et al.*, using intermittent fill cystometry, evaluated 24 elderly women whose average age was 79 (*65*). Three-fourths of them were acutely hospitalized, and some had conditions known to affect bladder capacity; 10 percent had urinary tract infections (UTIs), 42 percent had uninhibited contractions, and some had diabetes, chronic renal failure, and depression. Whether patients with indwelling urethral catheters were excluded is not specified. In this group of subjects, half had bladder capacities under 250 ml. Andersen *et al.* evaluated 17 male volunteers aged 60 to 75 with a mean age of 66.5 (*48*). All initially denied lower urinary tract symptoms; use of medications was not specified. Bladder capacity averaged 360 ml in the eight subjects without uninhibited contractions, a significantly smaller amount than that documented in a younger group (*54*). However, the "normalcy" of this sample may be questioned, as a sizable proportion admitted to lower urinary symptoms when requestioned; 10 of 17 had a trabeculated bladder, and all had an elevated voiding pressure.

Resting Bladder Pressure

Two studies found no change with age in resting detrusor pressure (*61,62*).

Residual Urine

The two studies mentioned under Bladder Capacity also reported changes in residual volume. Brocklehurst *et al.* found that 88 percent of the women without prior incontinence or left cerebral hemispheric lesions had residual volumes of less than 100 ml; the median was 50 ml (*65*). Andersen *et al.* found an average residual volume of 28 ml with a range of 0 to 160 ml, but only one patient, who had a diverticulum, had a residual volume of more than 100 ml (*48*). Thus residual urine may increase with age but is still probably less than 50 ml.

Detrusor Contractility

In Andersen *et al.'s* small group of men with impaired uroflowmetry, voiding pressure was higher than normal (*48*). Whether this reflects an age effect or detrusor response to obstruction is uncertain. No studies have been reported for elderly women, and no studies in either gender have examined the impact of age on detrusor contractility.

Uninhibited Contractions

Andersen *et al.'s* series reported that 9 of 17 subjects had uninhibited contractions, again possibly due to obstruction (*48*). Studies of normal women revealed a much lower prevalence. In Brocklehurst *et al.'s* series, only 6 of 26 women had contractions over 10 cm H_2O, and 5 of the 26 had other neurologic reasons for them (*65*). Jones and Schoenberg found that 11 percent of 45 asymptomatic women aged 60 to 68, hospitalized for nonurologic reasons, had uninhibited contractions (*64*). Diokno *et al.* reported similar results; three women of 39 had uninhibited contractions (*7*).

Thus the literature on changes with age is scanty, and few firm conclusions can be drawn. Nonetheless, taken *in toto,* the results seem consistent with the hypothesis that the *reserve capacity* of the lower urinary tract, like that of all other senescent organ systems (*25*), *decreases with age* and thereby *predisposes* the elderly person to becoming incontinent. Thus even a relatively mild insult can decompensate the system. Because the elderly are more likely to face physiologic, pathologic, and pharmacologic insults, it is easy to understand why they are so likely to become incontinent.

CAUSES OF INCONTINENCE IN THE ELDERLY

Although urinary incontinence in the elderly is no more a normal condition than it is in younger patients, it differs in several ways. Unlike the situation in younger patients, it is unusual to find a single, isolated cause of incontinence in the elderly. Likewise, it is difficult to determine the most common causes of incontinence in the elderly as a group. These facts stem from two basic principles of geriatrics.

First, elderly individuals do not comprise a homogeneous group. As mentioned earlier, age-related declines in organ systems are gradual, progressive, and linear; and they generally occur independently of each other; i.e., cardiac, pulmonary, and renal function may be declining at different rates. Because each system declines at an independent rate and because variability in the rate of decline *increases* with age, older individuals differ more from each other physiologically than do younger individuals (*66*). Elderly individuals also suffer from more illnesses and use more medications than do younger people, which further exacerbate the physiologic differences. Finally, elderly patients in nursing homes, acute care hospitals, and the community differ substantially from each other. Even when matched for age, disease, and medications, the differences between individuals in each setting are substantial because their functional abilities and capacities are so disparate. Arthritis may mean mildly symptomatic swelling of the distal phalangeal joints to the person at home but crippling ankylosis and contracture to the patient in the nursing home; yet "arthritis" is the diagnosis for each. Hence it is unlikely that "the most common cause of incontinence in the elderly" will be a clinically relevant fact. The chief causes are likely to differ in different settings.

Second, multiple pathology is the rule in the elderly. The average community-dwelling elderly individual suffers from nearly four important disabilities (*67*), whereas the institutionalized patient suffers from nearly twice as many (*68*). If an older man with diabetes, prostatic enlargement, fecal impaction, and immobilization due to arthritis develops incontinence, which entity is to be impugned? If a patient who is continent despite compensated detrusor instability becomes incontinent after receiving a medication that clouds his sensorium or induces a diuresis, is the cause of the incontinence detrusor instability or the medication?

Finally, when interpreting the prevalence of causes of incontinence in the elderly, one must realize that referral and investigative biases, as well as difficulties in investigating the elderly, significantly influence the results reported. First, the elderly themselves are unlikely to tell caregivers of the problem; this situation is true of 80 percent of community-dwelling individuals (*4*) and may result from ageism, fear, depression, inadequate financial resources, and cognitive impairment (*69*). Second, research-quality urodynamic studies are more difficult to perform in elderly patients. Many patients have urinary tract infections that are difficult to eradicate. Others suffer from osteoporotic compression fractures and congestive heart failure, making it difficult for them to remain supine. Many women have atrophic urethritis, making catheter insertion uncomfortable, or vaginal stenosis, making urethral localization difficult. Many cannot stand because of osteoarthritis, fractures, amputations, or weakness. Many patients cannot cooperate because of depression or dementia, and many are unable to void on command. Most patients take medications for other conditions, medications that directly affect the lower urinary tract, and the high prevalence of detrusor overactivity makes it difficult to check for concomitant genuine stress incontinence. Because of these obstacles, no investigator has yet evaluated a representative sample of elderly incontinent patients, a fact that further confounds the interpretation of their results, especially as so few investigators explicitly characterized the patients they include or exclude.

Even with these caveats in mind, one still finds that studies of older patients document several differences in the etiology of incontinence in this population. These etiologies can be divided arbitrarily into causes of transient incontinence and established incontinence.

TRANSIENT INCONTINENCE

We have seen that the elderly are characterized by impaired homeostatic reserve, a greater propensity to face further pharmacologic or pathologic insults, and an increasing likelihood that these insults will cloud their sensorium or reduce their mobility. These traits make older patients more vulnerable than their younger counterparts and more likely to suffer from incontinence unrelated to dysfunction of the lower urinary tract. Three corollaries follow from this principle: Incontinence in older patients is more amenable to general medical ministration; urodynamic testing is necessary less often; and abnormalities detected during urodynamic evaluation may be neither the primary cause of the patient's incontinence nor require treatment in order to restore continence. Experience supports these contentions. Castleden *et al.* found that incontinence had resolved before it could be evaluated in 16 percent of elderly incontinent patients referred to their incontinence clinic (*70*). Resolution rates are even higher in acutely hospitalized patients. We prospectively evaluated patients over age 70 who were hospitalized for acute medical problems (*10*). We found that one-third of these patients were incontinent of urine, half of whom developed incontinence for the first time in association with their illness. Among the latter group, incontinence resolved in virtually all prior to discharge—with out urologic evaluation. Reasons for the resolution confirmed experience in other settings and can be remembered using the mnemonic DIAPPERS which represents delirium, infection, atrophic urethritis and vaginitis, pharmacologic causes, psychological causes, endocrine causes, restricted mobility, and stool impaction (*71*).

Delirium is defined as an acute confusional state. The patient may appear demented, but evaluation discloses a subacute or acute onset; and inattentiveness, stupor, or agitation is found on mental status examination. This confusion interferes with the patient's recognizing or caring about the need to get to a toilet. Delirium is common in the elderly and can result from any acute illness, medication, or toxin. If unrecognized and if the underlying illness is untreated, the mortality may exceed 25 percent (*72*). Because illnesses such as myocardial infarction, pneumonia, congestive heart failure, pulmonary edema, or cholecystitis may present as delirium, it is critical to search carefully for its precipitants rather than focusing on the urinary leakage (*71*). Resolution of the incontinence will accompany resolution of the confusion but may be delayed for more than a week.

Symptomatic urinary tract *infection* is another cause of incontinence, as an intense sense of urgency may overwhelm the ability of the older person to inhibit micturition (*21a,73*). Asymptomatic bacteriuria, alluded to earlier, does not seem to cause leakage (*42,45,47,47a*). However, because disease frequently presents atypically in the elderly, newly acquired incontinence may be the only atypical symptom of a symptomatic urinary tract infection. Thus if the initial evaluation of incontinence in the older individual discloses an infection, it should generally be treated (*71*).

Atrophic urethritis and vaginitis are quite common in elderly women (*21a,37,73–75*). They are widely alleged to produce both urge and stress incontinence, although some controversy exists on this point (*37,73,75,76*). Nonetheless, because this condition is easily diagnosed, occasionally associated with recurrent and refractory cystitis (*77*), and readily treated, therapy seems worthwhile.

Pharmacologic causes of incontinence are frequent because two-thirds of elderly patients ingest nonprescribed medications [often without their physician's knowledge (*78*)] and because offending agents are used ubiquitously in geriatric medicine. Five categories of medications are most commonly impugned: sedative hypnotics, potent diuretics, anticholinergic agents, adrenergically active agents, and calcium channel blockers.

Many sedative hypnotics undergo hepatic oxidation, a reaction that is significantly impaired with age, especially in men (*79*). As a result, diazepam, flurazepam, nitrazepam, and chlordiazepoxide may accumulate, cloud the sensorium, and thereby precipitate incontinence (*80*). Alcohol is another agent in this category and is frequently used by elderly individuals (*81*). It causes incontinence by clouding the sensorium and inducing a diuresis. The "loop diuretics" may overwhelm the patient's ability to get to the bathroom in time.

Medications with anticholinergic properties may lead to urinary retention, especially in patients predisposed to it by diabetes, spinal stenosis, or BPH. Medicines with anticholinergic side effects include neuroleptics (especially chlorpromazine and thioridazine), antidepressants (especially amitriptyline, doxepin, and imipramine), antiparkinsonian agents (benztropine mesylate and trihexyphenydyl), antispasmodic agents (Donnatal, propantheline, dicyclomine), antiarrhythmics [especially disopyramide (*82*)], opiates (including drugs such as diphenoxylate used in bowel preparations), antiemetics (e.g., prochlorperazine), and antihistamines (including agents available as hypnotics without prescription, e.g., diphenhydramine).

"Sympatholytics" such as prazosin, methyldopa, and reserpine are frequently used to treat hypertension, a condition found in 40 percent of the elderly (*83*). In elderly women, who are predisposed because of decreased urethral pressures and functional urethral lengths, these agents that further diminish urethral pressure may result in stress incontinence (*84,85*). On the other hand, sympathomimetic agents such as decongestants (Pseudoephedrine, phenylephrine) may induce urinary retention, especially when taken by elderly men with prostatic enlargement (*86,87*). These drugs, like the anticholinergic agents, must be carefully asked about, as they are contained in numerous "cold remedies" and are readily available without prescription. Finally, calcium channel entry blockers are commonly prescribed for the elderly; they suppress detrusor contractility (*88*) and can contribute to urinary retention.

Psychological causes of incontinence in elderly patients are poorly documented but not uncommonly seen. Incontinence can be used to seek attention or to manipulate others, or it may be a manifestation of depression so that the patient does not care about remaining dry. Treatment of the underlying psychological disorder may restore continence, but no trials have included older subjects.

Endocrine causes of polyuria may also cause incontinence, especially if they concomitantly cloud consciousness. Hypercalcemia and hyperglycemia are two such disorders.

Restricted mobility is a common cause of incontinence. It can be due to a flare in arthritis, an occult hip fracture, or enforced bed rest because of a vertebral compression fracture or a myocardial infarction. It may also be inflicted on the patient "poseyed" in bed for safety.

Stool impaction is the final reversible cause of incontinence, being found in 4 to 10 percent of patients referred to European incontinence clinics (*21a,70,74*) and in 7 percent of patients in our hospital series (and in 12 percent of those with new-onset incontinence) (*10*). It should be suspected particularly when the patient in an appropriate setting (immobile and on potentially offending medications) develops double incontinence with fecal oozing and a palpable bladder. Disimpaction restores continence.

Established Causes

Reports from a variety of investigators suggest that, with one possible exception (*89*), the established causes of incontinence in the elderly do not differ from those found in younger patients. The distribution of diagnoses in each series seems to depend heavily on referral bias, as well as on patient age and functional status. Most geriatricians evaluate patients whose average age is over 75 and who tend to be multiply-impaired, whereas gynecologists and urologists evaluate younger patients who are more likely to have correctable conditions. Also, especially in series reported by geriatricians, urodynamic investigation usually focuses more on bladder than on outlet function and rarely includes radiographic or electromyographic (EMG) evaluation. Thus in these series it is impossible to assess the contribution of outlet obstruction or incompetence to the high prevalence of detrusor overactivity. The distribution of detrusor hyperreflexia, as opposed to detrusor instability, is generally unspecified. This apparent "oversight" frequently occurs with good reason, however. Incontinent men with cervical spondylosis, Parkinson's disease, stroke, or dementia are also likely to suffer from some degree of outlet obstruction. Because the degree of obstruction correlates poorly with the presence of detrusor instability (*89a*), an investigator often finds it impossible to decide if detrusor overactivity in this instance should be termed hyperreflexia or instability (*90*). It is more than a mere exercise in nosology; it has definite therapeutic implications, as is discussed below.

Nonetheless, several conclusions can be drawn. Detrusor overactivity is quite common. Published series report rates of 39 to 100 percent (*20,21a,47,70,73,74,91–96a, b*), with most rates ranging between 50 and 70 percent. Stress incontinence is usually quite rare in geriatricians' series, occurring in less than 2 percent of patients (*21a,70,73,91,92,95,96*), but is found in 20 to 40 percent of patients studied in two surgical series (*20,74*). An American series (*97*) detected stress incontinence in 88 percent, but the age cutoff was 55, much lower than that employed by other investigators. Significantly, elderly women seem to be more likely than younger ones to have urethral sphincter incompetence (type III) as the cause of stress-induced leakage (*98,99*), a fact likely to have therapeutic implications. The higher prevalence of sphincteric incompetence is probably due to prior operative procedures, atrophic urethritis (with attendant decrease in urethral compliance), diabetes, and medications.

As in younger women, outlet obstruction in older women appears to be uncommon (*74,95,96*) but, except for one series (*96*), has not been sedulously searched for. Our preliminary data, based on the results of detailed urodynamic evaluation of 75 elderly and unselected nursing home residents (mean age 89 yrs.), document clearcut obstruction in 4 percent. Bladder neck obstruction was present in one woman, and distal urethral stenosis due to a fibrotic noncompliant urethra was present in two other women. The later finding coexisted with severe vaginal atrophy.

Because most series have included few men and because many of these men have undergone prior outlet surgery, the prevalence of obstruction in incontinent elderly men is unclear although certainly common. Interestingly, however, and despite the prevalence of disease metastatic to the vertebral column, no series has yet reported a case of detrusor–sphincter dyssynergia in older patients, although there is no reason to believe that it should not occur, and we have certainly seen it.

A noncontractile detrusor is reported in 6 to 14 percent of patients (*20,21a,70,95,96*), although the etiology is generally unspecified. Many series have also reported normal findings in 4 to 6 percent of patients (*70,74,95,96,98*).

Not surprisingly, mixed causes of incontinence, usually detrusor overactivity and stress incontinence, occur commonly in the elderly (*74,96,98*). Surprisingly, however, series of ambulatory patients (*70*), hospitalized patients (*94*), and institutionalized patients (*96*) have failed to find a close link between cognitive impairment and urodynamic diagnosis. In fact, in our series of elderly institutionalized incontinent patients, demented subjects were as likely as nondemented ones to suffer from outlet obstruction or stress incontinence. Furthermore, incontinence in demented subjects was no more likely than in nondemented ones to result from an overactive detrusor, which was detected in two-thirds of both groups. Additional support for this finding comes from examining the problem in another way: Fisher's group reported that 32 percent of their demented patients were continent without specific treatments (*100*). Thus the frequently heard comment that incontinence in elderly cognitively impaired patients is invariably due to detrusor hyperreflexia is incorrect. Berkson's bias (*101*) may explain why earlier series found different results. Because both cognitive impairment and incontinence independently predispose to institutionalization, studies conducted in long-term care facilities invariably find an exaggerated correlation between dementia and incontinence unless this bias is taken into account.

Finally, we have found that one-third of our frail elderly incontinent patients (mean age 89) and half of those with an overactive detrusor have bladders that are poorly contractile despite extensive trabeculation. We have termed this condition detrusor hyperactivity with impaired contractility (DHIC) (*89*). Compared to our patients with more typical "compensated" detrusor hyperreflexia, those with DHIC did not differ clinically. Eighty-four percent were women, and half of each group had severe impairments of mobility and cognition, whereas half were unimpaired. Although patients with DHIC had a longer duration of incontinence (44 versus 27 months) and were more likely to have experienced urinary retention (4 patients versus 0), neither difference reached statistical significance. Neither were patients with DHIC more likely to suffer from conditions that would impair detrusor function. Urodynamically, however, patients with DHIC differed markedly from those with compensated detrusor hyperreflexia. Significantly, there were no differences in the duration of the uninhibited contraction, the presence or degree of trabeculation and diverticulae, or the degree of diminished compliance. No differences in proprioception were detected (reduced in a few of both groups), and the bulbocavernosus reflex was present in all patients. There were no differences in EMG patterns: Most were normal; one from each group exhibited a few polyphasic potentials, but both patients had synergic sphincter function with intact reflexes.

It is of note that although residual volume was statistically higher in patients with DHIC, the overlap was great enough to limit its clinical utility. The reason appears to be that patients with DHIC were much more likely to use the Valsalva maneuver to augment voiding. Combined with the commonly found pelvic floor laxity and low urethral resistance present in the women, and the absence of a smooth muscle sphincter found in the men (because of prior transurethral resection of the prostate), the Valsalva maneuver enabled many of these patients to empty adequately. However, bladder contractility was markedly impaired, a condition unrelated to outlet obstruction, detrusor–sphincter dyssynergia, or slow sphincter relaxation, all of which were uniformly absent.

We found 10 additional patients with this condition in a series of 200 patients evaluated in our hospital-based urodynamic laboratory, a setting in which we see patients of all ages. Interestingly, all 10 of these patients with DHIC were over age 70. Thus it seems to be primarily a disorder of older patients and is quite common in an institutionalized setting. Furthermore, it may have significant therapeutic implications. First, because several of these patients developed urinary retention despite heightened detrusor reflex activity, DHIC must be added to the differential diagnosis of retention, especially as its therapy differs from that employed for outlet obstruction or underactive detrusor. Second, because contractility is impaired, the pharmacotherapeutic approach usually used for detrusor hyperreflexia may not be appropriate for DHIC. Third, because it represents a discrepancy between detrusor reflex and discrepancy between detrusor reflex and contractile function, it suggests that the terminology currently used for lower urinary tract pathology may need to be modified. There is no *a priori* reason to use one term, detrusor hyperreflexia, to encompass both reflex and contractile characteristics. Finally, the striking similarity between detrusor hyperreflexia and DHIC under resting conditions (diminished compliance; presence of trabeculation, diverticula, and uninhibited contractions; absence of obstruction and sphincter dyssynergia; similar cystometric capacities) coupled with the fact that the duration of incontinence in patients with DHIC was twice as long as in those with detrusor hyperreflexia suggests that DHIC may be the result of progressive deterioration of contractile function in patients with detrusor hyperreflexia. The final stage would then be a similar-appearing but acontractile bladder with diminished compliance. We have now seen six women with this condition. If this hypothesis is true, untreated detrusor hyperreflexia may not be as urologically benign as originally thought. Only a prospective study can test this hypothesis.

DIAGNOSTIC CONSIDERATIONS

Establishing the cause of incontinence in the elderly patient is often more difficult but frequently more rewarding than it is in younger patients. It is more difficult because of barriers to obtaining an accurate history and more rewarding because the diagnosis of a remediable cause outside the urinary tract is more likely and its reversal improves not only the patient's functional status but her incontinence as well.

Clinical Evaluation

Sufficient time must be allocated for the evaluation for several reasons. The relevant history is generally more complex because the patient may have multiple concurrent illnesses, may be taking numerous medications, and has frequently undergone several operations, each of which may be contributing to or causing the incontinence. In addition, even cognitively intact older patients often give an unreliable history (*12,98,102*). Milne *et al.* documented extensive variation in replies that healthy, community-dwelling elderly persons provided in response to a questionnaire dealing with physical symptoms. The questions were asked at baseline and repeated 2 months later by the same interviewer. The proportion of disagreement between replies related to bladder function ranged from 20 percent for nocturia to 71 percent for prostatic symptoms. There was a 60 percent discrepancy in subjects' responses to the question dealing with incontinence (*102*). Much of this variation is due to cognitive impairment, depression, patients' attitudes that these conditions are due to aging rather than to disease, and their fear of the diagnostic and therapeutic interventions that their responses might instigate (*69*). Hence the physician must be particularly sensitive to these issues and must rely more heavily on confirmatory reports from the family, as well as on medical records brought by the patient.

Even if the patient is severely cognitively impaired, a meaningful history may be obtainable from ancillary personnel. Nurses' aides may note that incontinence usually occurs when the patient is on the way to the bathroom, implying symptomatic urge incontinence. Alternatively, the staff may note that incontinence occurs only when the patient is lifted or strains. The staff can also specify the pattern, frequency, and severity of the patient's leakage. The patient's medical record provides the remainder of the relevant history.

Frequency/voiding charts completed by the patient, family, or nursing staff can be especially helpful for "teasing out" the cause of the incontinence. A patient who is wet only during the 4-hour period following breakfast may be incontinent because of the furosemide or the two cups of coffee she ingests. A patient whose 7 hours of sleep are disturbed by incontinence that only occurs an hour after retiring may be wet because of the alcohol she uses as a "nightcap." A wheelchair-bound male who sits napping for 4 hours in the afternoon without voiding or leaking, yet who wets every hour while supine at night, is more likely to suffer from congestive heart failure than prostatism (*71*). Finally, symptoms listed earlier of the reversible causes of incontinence must be carefully sought.

Because so many illnesses outside the lower urinary tract can cause incontinence, a complete physical examination must be performed. In addition, one must be able to recognize atrophic urethritis and vaginitis in the female patient. Vaginal signs of this entity include thinning of the mucosa, loss of the normal rugal pattern, punctate hemorrhages, easy friability, and friable adhesions of the posterior commissure. One must also realize that there are limitations to some aspects of the traditional neurourologic examination. For instance, anocutaneous and bulbocavernosus reflexes, as well as volitional control of the anal sphincters, are frequently weak or absent for other than neurologic reasons: The patient's inability to contract the anal sphincter may be due to the fact that no one has asked her to do so for 90 years!

The remainder of the clinical evaluation includes a metabolic survey to exclude hyperglycemia and hypercalcemia, urinalysis and culture, cystoscopy and urine cytologic examination if sterile hematuria is found, and determination of residual urine volume.

The accuracy of the clinical evaluation for determining the cause of incontinence in elderly patients is unknown. In a retrospective analysis, Hilton and Stanton thought that the etiology of incontinence could have been established without urodynamic studies in 60 percent of their elderly female subjects (*74*). In a prospective study, Eastwood *et al.* employed Hilton and Stanton's algorithm and were able to assign a correct diagnosis to 71 percent of elderly women (*95*).

Both groups of investigators pointed out that outlet obstruction and the etiology of stress-induced leakage were particularly difficult to diagnose, and Hilton and Stanton thus thought that 40 percent of their patients would have benefited from a urodynamic evaluation. These figures are similar to the diagnostic accuracy cited by most investigators who evaluate younger women. (No published data have addressed the accuracy of the clinical evaluation in elderly men.) Our data from institutionalized patients, however, revealed that the algorithm performed less well in this setting. We therefore devised and prospectively tested a simple algorithm for both institutionalized men and women. Surprisingly, in this setting, our algorithm led to the correct diagnosis of 82% of the cases and correctly guided treatment in 90% of cases. Significantly, none of the remaining patients would have been harmed by the incorrect treatment suggested by the algorithm (*95a*).

Urodynamic Evaluation

If the clinical evaluation does not establish the diagnosis, if reversal of the transient causes of incontinence does not restore continence, if empiric treatment has failed, if surgery is contemplated, of if empiric treatment carries with it a significant risk for the individual patient, urodynamic evaluation is performed if its outcome will affect therapy. Moreover, with the improved surgical techniques currently available, a urodynamic diagnosis of urethral hypermobility or outlet obstruction may have significant therapeutic implications, even in frail, demented patients. Additionally, accurate assessment spares the patient side effects of any medication targeted toward the wrong diagnosis.

The lack of normative data alluded to earlier may clearly complicate interpretation of urodynamic findings, but the clinical context is usually helpful. For instance, finding uninhibited contractions in an incontinent elderly woman has implications different from the same finding in an asymtomatic patient. In the former patient they should be treated.

Performing advanced urodynamic studies in elderly patients is feasible, safe, and probably reproducible (*96,98,103*). In fact, of the first 100 frail incontinent patients we investigated with uroflowmetry, provocative cystometry, and simultaneous videocystosphincterometry, the ages ranged from 77 to 100 years (mean 89), and half of them were severely demented, bedridden, and doubly incontinent. Nonetheless, all but two studies were completed at one sitting, with research-quality records obtained for each. Twenty-one studies were repeated, and all confirmed the original diagnoses with alterations in some physiologic parameters. None of the patients experienced urosepsis or other untoward events (*104*). Moreover, more than one-half of these patients were improved or cured by the treatment that was based on the urodynamic findings.

There is no consensus regarding the necessity for antibiotic prophylaxis when performing urodynamics in this population. Walter and Vejlsgaard, as well as Bergman and McCarthy, studied groups of young women undergoing urodynamic studies without prophylaxis. Using sterile technique, the investigators found a 2 to 4 percent rate of infection (*105,106*). Andersen and Vejlsgaard detected a 6 percent rate of infection in men aged 42 to 90 years who suffered from prostatism and underwent urodynamic studies without prophylaxis (*107*). On the other hand, Turck *et al.* investigated 39 sick elderly women and found that bacteriuria occurred after catheterization in 15 percent, one-third of whom subsequently developed pyelonephritis (*108*). In the absence of a controlled trial in this population, we have elected to use sterile technique and antibiotic prophylaxis for 48 hours following the study. None of the last 50 patients we have studied has developed bacteriuria on this regimen. We are conducting a prospective trial to see if this practice is necessary.

When urodynamically evaluating elderly patients, several points should be kept in mind. It is not sufficient to look for uninhibited contractions and then quit. Not only are uninhibited contractions common, they are usually not found in isolation, do not necessarily cause symptoms, and may not be the source of the patient's incontinence. Only a thorough evaluation can sort out which condition is most likely responsible for the problem and needs to be addressed. Examples abound. Detrusor instability may accompany genuine stress incontinence, yet it usually responds to an operative approach directed at the outlet (*109*). Detrusor instability may also accompany outlet obstruction; again the most appropriate therapy may be directed at the outlet. Stroke and prostatism frequently coexist, yet the therapeutic approach differs markedly. A study employing simultaneous videocystosphincterometry augmented by micturitional urethral profilometry (*110*) may be the best way to dissect out the relative contributions of each pathology.

Fluoroscopy is worthwhile for several reasons. Many elderly patients have an incompetent bladder neck. In men it may be due to prior prostatic surgery, and in elderly women it may be due to antihypertensive medications, diabetes, or prior surgical procedures. Simple urethral profilometry misses this finding; only fluoroscopically guided profilometry documents it (*111*). Fluoroscopy also aids in the assessment of ureteral reflux, stress leakage, and bladder trabeculation, diverticula, and masses. Although some of these data can be obtained from separately performed cystography, a simultaneous study with manometric monitoring resolves many diagnostic quandaries and permits omission of more painful EMG. Finally, it cannot be emphasized enough that interpretation of studies in this population is usually *more* difficult than in a younger population because so many abnormalities may be present concurrently. Omitting fluoroscopic monitoring only compounds the investigator's task.

Of course, performing urodynamic studies in this setting requires adaptation. Every attempt must be made to ensure the patient's comfort. Pads to cushion the patient's osteoporotic spine from the unforgiving firmness of the radiographic table, pillows to elevate the head of the patient who suffers from heart failure, foam rubber foot and heel pads to restrain excess leg motion, omission of stirrups for those with hip and knee osteoarthritis, warming of both the sterilizing solutions and the urodynamic suite, and a willingness to proceed slowly and to reiterate explanations to cognitively impaired patients are instrumental to a successful evaluation. Most helpful when evaluating the demented patient, however, is the addition of an extra person, usually an incontinence nurse specialist, whose sole role is to soothe, explain, coax, and divert the patient.

Urodynamic evaluations performed in this population are subject to several artifacts. Bacteriuria, as mentioned earlier, is extremely common. Although its effects on urodynamic findings are unknown, certainly symptomatic bacteriuria has been found by numerous investigators to have a significant impact (*106,112*). Additionally, the risk of inducing a bacteremia or urosepsis by instrumenting an infected bladder seems substantial. Finally, the elderly have a high prevalence of cardiac valve deformities, making them vulnerable to endocarditis. Thus it seems prudent to postpone urodynamic studies until bacteriuria has been eradicated; we wait until the urine has been sterile for 2 weeks.

Some components of the urodynamic evaluation itself can be deceptive in the elderly and need to be interpreted in the context of the entire study, Uroflowmetry, for instance, may be of limited value in many cases because elderly patients frequently cannot retain a quantity of fluid adequate to ensure the validity of the study. More often, however, a small voided volume is actually associated with a large, but clinically inapparent, residual volume. Thus, especially in the elderly, residual urine must always be known when interpreting flow rate. On the other hand, the propensity of many elderly to augment voiding by using a Valsalva maneuver may generate a relatively normal flow rate and a low residual volume despite poor detrusor mechanics. Unless the investigator carefully observes the patient or monitors abdominal pressure, a poorly contractile detrusor will be missed. Even the uroflow tracing may not provide a clue, as it can appear entirely normal. Thus urodynamic studies in elderly patients should always include intraabdominal pressure monitoring.

Another artifact is likely to occur when checking patients with DHIC for concomitant genuine stress incontinence, as stress maneuvers may trigger an uninhibited contraction. Not infrequently, this weak contraction dramatically alters the fluoroscopic configuration of the bladder without increasing bladder pressure. Because the contraction is associated with appropriate relaxation of the sphincter, one may mistakenly make a diagnosis of outlet incompetence. Use of fluoroscopic monitoring obviates the problem.

One other "artifact" must be mentioned. Impaired or absent proprioception in older patients does not necessarily imply the presence of peripheral nerve or spinal cord damage (*91*). Lesions in the thalamus and the frontal and parietal lobes are also associated with impaired proprioception.

Fortunately, at least one problem of urodynamics is minimized in elderly patients. Postural cystometry may not be necessary to detect uninhibited contractions, as more than 90 percent occur in the supine position (*74, 74a*).

Even after a urodynamic diagnosis has

been established, the therapeutic implication may not be straightforward. One problem arises in elderly women who are found to have both urethral hypermobility and detrusor overactivity. McGuire *et al.* have shown that treatment of the former usually alleviates the latter (*109*). However, it is not clear that neurologically mediated detrusor overactivity responds as well. Nor is it easy to establish the cause of detrusor overactivity in the elderly man with both a mild outlet obstruction and a neurologic abnormality (stroke, dementia, Parkinson's disease, cervical spondylosis, etc.). Because incontinence due to neurologically mediated detrusor hyperreflexia may worsen after prostatic resection (*100,113*), the distinction is important. Kimche *et al.* evaluated the utility of evoked response times in this situation and found promising results in their small series (*114*). In a somewhat related study, Reuther *et al.* employed intravesical installation of lidocaine in patients with outlet obstruction who did not have neurologic disease (*113*). Their intent was to differentiate idiopathic detrusor instability from that due to outlet obstruction, and their results in eight patients were promising. Because of the high prevalence of outlet obstruction in elderly men (*39,115*), combined with the cost and morbidity of prostatectomy in this age group, studies such as these are critical and need to be confirmed and extended.

THERAPEUTIC CONSIDERATIONS

In 1749 Allen stated that "[Incontinence] is a distemper very hard to be cured . . . , in old people it is altogether incurable, unless hot baths relieve them" (*116*). One hundred years later, Day noted that incontinence is "seldom susceptible of a cure" (*117*). Although modern investigators have offered more sanguine summaries, it is worthwhile noting that the modern pharmacopoeia of oxybutynin, bethanechol, and DDAVP differs little from the "astringent, nervine, and antiparalytick decoction" advocated by Allen in 1749. Fortunately, there is some evidence that treatments have improved over the centuries if only because we have abandoned remedies recommended by investigators in the interim: Sacral blisters (*118*), cerebrospinal fluid drainage (*118*), silver nitrate instillation (*37*), strychnia, carbonic acid, and chloroform (*118*).

Treatment of incontinence in the elderly is in many respects easier than it is in younger individuals. This rather surprising statement stems from the principle that has recurred throughout this chapter: Because of diminished homeostatic reserve, multiple pathology, and polypharmacy, the elderly are more likely to be incontinent because of dysfunction unrelated to the urinary tract. The limited efficacy of most available therapy is thus of less consequence to older patients. Rather, attention to the reversible conditions noted earlier is likely to prove beneficial. Nor is it necessary to completely reverse each condition (*90,119*). Slight improvement in several conditions can result in dramatic improvement in the patient's overall function as well as in amelioration of the incontinence (*71*). For instance, many patients have uninhibited contractions that are asymptomatic until other processes cloud their sensorium or interfere with their mobility (*94*). A typical example is an elderly woman with arthritis and mild heart failure who suffers a vertebral compression fracture, becomes bedridden, is treated with opiates, and becomes fecally impacted and incontinent. She does not need a urodynamic evaluation. Nor would the finding of uninhibited contractions be relevant. However, treatment of each of her conditions almost certainly would restore her continence. The conclusion is clear: *One does not need to abolish the urodynamic abnormality in order to restore continence* (*90*).

Before delving into specific modalities of treatment for established incontinence, it may be worthwhile to address a few methodologic issues that arise when assessing the therapeutic efficacy of various interventions for older patients.

The first issue is the question of efficacy itself. For most studies involving incontinent elderly patients, this question is difficult to answer because it depends on so many conditions. The cause of the incontinence must be correctly established, but we have seen how uncommonly elderly patients are thoroughly investigated. Outcome criteria must be reliable, but in this population we have seen how unreliable subjective reporting can be (*102*). This subjective unreliability is further compounded by depression and cognitive impairment, which interfere with patients keeping accurate diaries and contribute to their resisting repeated urodynamic evaluation. Moreover, because investigators frequently do not carefully scrutinize patients for nonurologic conditions, many studies have included patients with transient incontinence that would have resolved spontaneously. Each of these obstacles can be overcome and should not preclude performing further studies, but they do make interpretation of available studies difficult. On the other hand, it is hazardous to extrapolate from efficacy studies performed in healthy elderly, as these individuals are unlikely to be taking other medications or have other illnesses that would interfere with the therapy planned for a more realistic patient group. It is even more fallacious to extrapolate from results obtained on younger patients. Bladder function, outlet function, and the autonomic nervous system (*120*), as well as a host of other relevant variables, change substantially with age and may magnify or mitigate any response found in younger patients.

A second issue has to do with side effects. Only a dearth of studies have stratified side effects by age, despite the fact that they are likely to be strongly age-related (*121,122*). Drugs such as calcium channel blockers, imipramine, and prazosin potentiate orthostatic hypotension, a condition that afflicts 30 percent of patients above age 75 (*123*). This hypotension, combined with the increased prevalence of falls and osteoporosis found in the elderly (*124*), can result in a patient's becoming dry at the expense of a fractured hip, a condition associated with a 15 percent mortality rate (*125*). Diazepam may relax the striated sphincter; but because its hepatic metabolism is markedly impaired with age (*79*) the metabolites of a single tablet can be detected in the urine 3 weeks later. The likelihood that it will cause confusion is thus significant and well recognized (*80*). Anticholinergic medications can exacerbate xerostomia, glaucoma, constipation, dementia, and confusion, all of which are prevalent in the elderly. When one superimposes the increased probability that an adverse drug interaction will occur because of the multiple other drugs the patient may be taking, it is easy to understand how the therapeutic ratio of each drug in our armamentarium is likely to alter with age. The ratio is also likely to differ when a drug is given to healthy outpatients as opposed to frail institutionalized patients, yet patient's functional status and cognitive capacities are rarely specified in published trials.

A third issue is compliance. The drug may be effective and well tolerated; but when patients are prescribed more than three medications, compliance plummets. Yet 75 percent of people of age 65 take at least one prescribed drug regularly, and the average is 7.5 drugs per person (*126*). Cost is another contributing factor to poor rates of compliance. Medications represent the second largest out-of-pocket health expense borne by elderly patients (after physician visits) and are generally not covered by third-party payors.

A fourth issue relates to combination therapy. Oncologists design chemotherapeutic regimens to attack tumors in different ways. This approach maximizes efficacy while minimizing toxicity from each individual agent. This approach may be especially beneficial for older patients yet has been investigated infrequently.

Finally, many studies report reduced rates of incontinence. However, these studies must be interpreted with caution. A 50 percent reduction in the frequency of incontinence, from four episodes per day to two, may not make the patient appreciably happier (*15*), and it may be associated with significant expense and toxicity. Even complete restoration of continence in some elderly patients may be a disservice if it is accompanied by morbidity from an operation or toxicity from medications. As every good clinician knows, it is the patient, not the disease, that must be optimally treated.

Our approach to incontinence therefore is a stepped one. First, we search for and treat the reversible causes already alluded to. It is of note that we routinely determine the amount of residual urine in all of our patients, as symptoms of urinary retention can mimic those of detrusor overactivity or genuine stress incontinence. If the residual urine is elevated and a necessary neuroleptic medication is implicated, we first taper the drug to the lowest possible dose. If problems persist, we substitute another drug with less anticholinergic side effects. For psychosis, haloperidol has the least anticholinergic properties (*127*); for depression, desipramine is a reasonable choice. Other antidepressants, e.g., trazodone and alprazolam, are also appropriate substitutes and are devoid of anticholinergic side effects (*128*). Antihistamines used as soporifics; e.g., diphenhydramine, can be replaced by short-acting benzodiazepines such as oxazepam or triazolam. If presumed detrusor hyporeflexia persists despite substitution of medications with anticholinergic potency, adding bethanechol is occasionally effective (*129*).

Next, we deal with functional barriers to continence. Patients are advised about the diuretic effects of alcohol and theophylline. They are told that theophylline is contained in coffee and tea, and that they should schedule toileting appropriately or omit these beverages entirely. The amount of daily fluid intake optimal for the incontinent patient is unknown, but many elderly patients go to extremes. Some, encouraged by recommendations in many bladder training regimens, try to ingest 2 to 3 liters per day, which can clearly contribute to urinary leakage. Other patients severely restrict fluids. This practice is usually not beneficial and may even be harmful. The altered pattern of urinary excretion noted earlier mitigates the positive effects of fluid restriction; results from Hohlbrugger *et al.* raised the possibility that excessive urinary concentration may actually adversely modify detrusor excitability (*130*). The potentially harmful effects of fluid restriction are mediated by age-related decrease in thirst threshold (*131*), an age-related sluggishness in the renal response to fluid restriction (*132*), and in patients with dementia an increased tendency to develop hypernatremia (*133*). All of these effects predispose the patient to fluid and electrolyte abnormalities that induce confusion, exacerbate incontinence, and can be life-threatening.

Other barriers to continence are environmental. If patient's arthritis interferes with their manipulating buttons or zippers, Velcro fasteners or different styles of clothing can be tried. Physiotherapy may improve mobility. For patients with difficulty getting to a toilet, a bedside commode is used. For patients such as those with Parkinson's disease or stroke who have trouble getting on and off toilets, raised seats and handrails are valuable. Labeling bathrooms is useful for demented patients, and removing obstacles such as area rugs is worthwhile as well. For wheelchair-bound men a urinal is helpful. It should have a handle large enough that it can be used by patients with arthritic changes, and it should be light enough that it can be lifted without its contents spilling. For bedfast patients, small urinals or shallow plastic pans can be used (*134–136*). When dealing with cognitively impaired institutionalized patients, consulting with the nursing staff is essential to ensure that patients are being toileted at appropriate times and that they are left on the toilet long enough to be able to complete a void. Many a nursing aide has spent 20 minutes getting a patient to the commode only to allow her a few seconds to void.

If incontinence persists, the next step depends on the clinical evaluation. If the patient meets the criteria outlined earlier for urodynamic evaluation, such evaluation is the next step. However, if the clinical evaluation, augmented by a frequency/voiding record and residual volume determination, strongly suggests diagnosis of a condition that can be treated without surgery, we treat empirically. Only aspects of treatment germane to a geriatric population are discussed below.

Detrusor Overactivity

Few controlled trials of any therapy for detrusor overactivity have been performed in the elderly. Although some studies have included a few older patients, subject characteristics are usually unspecified, and results are rarely stratified by age. Experience, however, suggests a number of approaches, the multiplicity of which supports the fact that none is completely effective.

Pharmacologic approaches are similar to those used in younger populations with a few differences. For instance, although enthusiasm for flavoxate has waned (*137–139*), its minimal anticholinergic side effects and its lack of important interaction with other medications make it a desirable drug for an elderly patient—when it works.

Calcium channel blocking agents are another reasonable choice for the elderly incontinent patient, although evidence supporting their efficacy is also tenuous. The most favorable results yet reported in an elderly population were for flunarizine (*140*), but these results were attenuated significantly with time (*141*). If one chooses a calcium channel blocker, several considerations must be kept in mind. First, because the hepatic cytochrome P_{450} system is responsible for the metabolism of verapamil and diltiazem (*142*), and because its activity decreases with age (*79*), these drugs can be given on a less frequent, twice-daily basis (*142*). However, the decrement in P_{450} activity also increases the likelihood of an adverse drug reaction, as drugs such as cimetidine and propranolol inhibit it still further. Both agents can significantly impair the metabolism of verapamil and diltiazem. Another important drug interaction occurs with digoxin. Verapamil and diltiazem may increase serum digoxin levels by as much as 100 percent (*142*). Second, drug–disease interactions are also clinically relevant. Verapamil exacerbates constipation and has potent negative inotropic and chronotropic side effects; it must be used with caution in patients with congestive heart failure, sinus bradycardia, or conduction defects. Nifedipine has fewer negative inotropic properties because it is a potent vasodilator and induces a reflex tachycardia. However, it can induce or potentiate postural hypotension, which is common in the elderly, and must be used with caution in patients who are taking propranolol. Finally, calcium blockers may increase residual volume without suppressing detrusor overactivity (*88*).

Anticholinergic agents such as propantheline are best avoided in the elderly because of their myriad adverse effects, but agents that are primarily musculotropics, e.g., oxybutynin or imipramine (*143*), are better tolerated. Imipramine, however, is another agent that induces or exacerbates postural hypotension and must be used with caution. If one chooses to use a tricyclic agent, secondary amines such as desipramine are generally tolerated much better by the elderly than are tertiary amines such as imipramine or amitriptyline because they do not require phase I hepatic transformation (*128*). Doxepin, however, is both reasonably tolerated and perhaps the most effective of all the tricyclic agents for detrusor overactivity (*144*). Compared with imipramine, it is much less likely to cause postural hypotension (*144a*). Two final considerations apply to the elderly when using drugs with anticholinergic side effects. First, like the calcium blockers, these drugs may increase residual urine without diminishing detrusor overactivity or incontinence (*139,139a,b*). Second, they should be used as infrequently as possible in patients with confusion or dementia because of their propensity to exacerbate both. One option we have used successfully in this situation is combining a low dose of a tricyclic agent with a low dose of oxybutynin. Another option is to use either a calcium channel blocker or flavoxate. A final option is to change the route of administration; this has been tried recently with scopalamine patches (*144b*).

If the patient's incontinence is worse at night, the fact that the elderly excrete most of their daily ingested fluid load at night suggests that an antidiuretic such as DDAVP might be effective. This approach was tried in nursing home patients who showed improvement by using a bedpan (*139b*).

Nonpharmacologic interventions may be more promising alternatives for older patients. Bladder training has been proved effective in elderly subjects, even those with significant cognitive impairment. Sogbein and Awad, using a fixed voiding schedule, documented an 80 percent improvement in 85 percent of incontinent institutionalized geriatric patients (*47*). In another study involving confused elderly incontinent patients, Schnelle *et al.* tested the effect of prompted voiding plus social reinforcement. In a prospective controlled trial conducted in two community nursing homes, they found a 45 percent improvement in the treated group (*21*). In elderly patients without cognitive impairment, Abbey found an intensive habit retraining regimen successful in 22 of 23 subjects. Success was measured after 6 months of retraining and was maintained at 18 months (*145*). Reviews of various bladder training techniques explore these issues in greater depth (*146,146a*).

Biofeedback has received limited attention for elderly patients, although preliminary data are encouraging (*147*).

In an innovative approach, McGuire *et al.* used transcutaneous electrical stimulation of the peroneal or posterior tibial nerve to treat 22 young and middle-aged patients with detrusor overactivity. Electrical stimulation was administered using a portable unit similar to that used for pain control. Eighty-five percent of their patients improved or became dry using this device (*148*). Employing a different method, Fall reported a 73 percent success rate in premenopausal women treated with an inflatable intravaginal electrode over a prolonged period of time (*149*). Although neither technique was tried on elderly patients, and although both methods require adequate cognitive function, they may eventually prove beneficial in this population.

A more invasive but novel approach has been developed by Ewing *et al.* They reported that subtrigonal injection of phenol cured 23 of 30 patients with overactive detrusor function refractory to all other modalities (*150*). Blackford *et al.* confirmed these positive findings in 63 women with refractory detrusor instability. Significantly, in Blackford *et al.*'s series 69 percent of women over age 55 experienced a symptomatic response, whereas only 14 percent of those less than age 55 had a beneficial result. Other than a few urinary tract infections, morbidity was low, hospitalization was short, and efficacy was maintained for at least a year in 85 percent of those who initially responded. Of the 11 patients who relapsed, 9 were reinjected and 8 again responded (*151*). It should be emphasized, however, that other investigators had unfavorable results with this technique (*152a*) and, although it is relatively effective, simple, and safe, complications such as sciatic nerve palsy, trigonal ulcers, ureteral reflux, and chronic urinary retention have been reported and are more likely in inexperienced hands (*150–152*). The procedure has not been performed in men.

Stress Incontinence

The nonoperative options for genuine stress incontinence include weight reduction, pelvic floor muscle exercises, estrogen therapy, alpha-adrenergic agents, and occasionally a pessary.

Pelvic floor muscle exercises are difficult for many elderly women to learn, especially those with cognitive impairment. Nonetheless, a few studies have included carefully selected elderly women and have shown a beneficial response (*153–155, 155a,b*). Some of these series employed Kegel's perineometer to teach subjects the technique, but it is frequently not necessary. The mechanism mediating improvement in these patients has not been established, but many investigators believe it is related to strengthening of the striated muscle sphincter or to an alteration in its composition. In this context, Aniansson and Gustafsson have shown that, in response to physical training, the elderly experience an increase in muscle strength similar to that seen in younger subjects. Furthermore, muscle fiber composition can be altered by training: Type II fibers increase, largely due to an increase in Type IIA fibers (*156–158*).

Mohr *et al.* studied 46 postmenopausal women aged 42 to 92 years (average age 73) with a clinical diagnosis of stress incontinence. All could independently care for themselves, all lived at home, and all were wearing absorptive pads. The duration of their incontinence varied from 6 months to 5 years; most had a cystourethrocele, and half had undergone prior anterior vaginal repair. All were treated with estrogen and exercises. Of the 46 women, 44 reported marked alleviation of symptoms and no longer required pads; the improvement persisted for at least 6 to 36 months. Interestingly, incontinence recurred in 11 patients after stopping the exercise program but abated in all once exercise was reinstituted (*154*). Whether estrogen is needed, whether the exercises control severe leakage, and whether objective urodynamic improvement is necessary for cure remain unanswered questions, although Castleden *et al.* reported marked improvement in 14 of 19 women who exercised but did not use estrogen (*155*). Finally, Klarskow *et al.* investigating a younger group, found that 22 to 63 percent of women using these exercises could avoid surgery (*159*).

The facts that estrogen levels decrease with age, atrophic urethritis and vaginitis are found exclusively in postmenopausal women, estrogen receptors are present in the female urethra (*160,161*), and estrogen administration can reverse the findings of senile vaginal atrophy suggested that estrogen treatment might be beneficial for postmenopausal patients with stress incontinence. Most studies have substantiated this hypothesis (*37,162–169*), and studies showing no benefit generally used lower doses of estrogen (*76, 170*). Some studies have shown significant increases in urethral length, closure pressure, and maximal pressure (*165–169*), but most increases have been modest. The two studies of genuine stress incontinence that examined the issue more closely showed that improvement correlated best, albeit imperfectly, with a change in pressure/transmission ratios (*166,170*). Although Schreiter *et al.* suggested that estrogen sensitized the urethra to alpha-adrenergic stimuli in premenopausal women (*171*), other investigators have not confirmed this finding in postmenopausal patients (*169,170*). Thus if estrogen is given in adequate dosage for at least a month, most postmenopausal women seem to experience a beneficial effect. Estriol, administered either topically in a daily dose of 1 to 8 mg or intramuscularly in a monthly dose of 80 mg, seems to be the most effective treatment and avoids inducing endometrial proliferation (*172*). Because it is unavailable in the United States, however, topical conjugated estrogens (Premarin) can be used in a daily dose of 1 to 4 g. Alternatively, oral doses of Premarin 0.3 to 0.6 mg or ethinyl estradiol 10 to 20 μg (*21a*) can be given cyclically. Once an adequate response has occurred, the drug can usually be given as infrequently as once every 1 to 2 weeks. Note that these doses are inadequate treatment for osteoporosis (*173*).

Alpha-adrenergic agents have not been extensively studied in elderly patients with stress incontinence. It might be postulated that they would be less effective in older women because of the age-related reduction in urethral compliance, but it does not seem to be the case. However, although they may successfully augment the response to estrogen treatment in women with mild to moderate leakage (*168,169*), they are much less effective when administered alone (*168,169,174,175*) or when used for severe leakage (*176*). Most of these agents are difficult to use in elderly patients because they raise blood pressure and can induce anorexia, nausea, insomnia, restlessness, confusion, and hallucinations, as well as exacerbate coronary artery and peripheral vascular disease and hyperthyroidism (*174,176–179*). Some preparations, e.g., Ornade, include large doses of antihistamines, agents that exacerbate central nervous system side effects in this population and should therefore not be used. The only alpha-agonist that does not increase blood pressure is imipramine. However, as mentioned earlier, it can cause postural hypotension and thus lead to falls. If these agents are used, either phenylpropanolamine or imipramine is probably the drug of choice, depending on the patient, starting with slowly increasing doses while carefully monitoring side effects.

Although pessaries may exacerbate genuine stress incontinence in women with a large cystocele or uterine prolapse, in patients with less severe degrees of anatomic abnormality pessaries may actually ameliorate or alleviate the leakage. Bhatia *et al.* used pessaries to cure 12 such women, aged 33 to 72. Urodynamic evaluation revealed that the primary effect was to improve the pressure–transmission ratio by stabilizing the base of the bladder. Functional urethral length and closure pressures increased as well, even in the standing position, but these changes were less marked. Surprisingly, the pessary did not induce obstruction in any of the patients (*180*). Whether pessaries work as well in older women, who are more likely to have a less compliant urethra, vaginal stenosis, and anatomic abnormalities, is still unanswered.

The final nonsurgical approach to stress incontinence is electrical stimulation. Controlled reports (*181*) have not been optimistic, but the technique for optimally administering this method remains to be determined.

If the therapeutic interventions already mentioned, used singly or in combination, do not restore continence, surgical procedures should not be dismissed merely because of the patient's age. Numerous investigators have reported favorable results in elderly patients. For genuine stress incontinence many surgeons favor modified Pereyra suspension procedures and have published excellent results (*182–186,186a*). However, Stanton's group used a culposuspension procedure and obtained excellent results (*187,188*). They reported their long-term experience with 35 women aged 65 to 82: Half had undergone prior operative procedures, none had an overactive detrusor, none were cognitively impaired, all were medically suitable, and all had sufficient vaginal capacity and mobility. Eighty-nine percent were objectively cured at 3 to 5 years.

For patients with stress leakage due to sphincteric incompetence, in addition to the suspension procedures advocated by some investigators (*182,184*), others have advocated a pubovaginal sling procedure, teflon injection, or placement of an artifical sphincter. Patient selection characteristics, complications, and technique used for the pubovaginal sling have been reviewed by McGuire and Lytton (*99,189,189a*), but the success rate for older patients undergoing this procedure is unknown. Additionally, because of its obstructing nature and the associated risk of urinary retention, careful consideration must be given to the patient's or family's ability to cope with the possible need for subsequent intermittent catheterization(*189*).

Periurethral injection of teflon paste is a second option and has been used in patients over age 80 (*190–193*). It has been administered under local anesthesia (*191,193*) as well as under only sedation (*193*). Advantages include the fact that patients who fail to respond can undergo repeated injection, another type of operation, or even insertion of an artificial sphincter (*191*). Additionally, the hospital stay is short, and complications, including urinary retention, abscess, and urethritis are either transient or rare. One study found that success was not related to age, and that patients with an MUP of less than 30 cm H_2O were most likely to benefit (*192*). Nonetheless, it should be used only by experienced investigators in selected elderly patients with sphincteric insufficiency as the etiology of their stress incontinence. As with other procedures for stress incontinence, detrusor instability is only a relative contraindication (*99,109,189*).

More than 90 percent of the experience with the most advanced artificial sphincter, the AMS 800, has been restricted to men. Approximately 20 percent of these patients have been over age 70 (American Medical Systems, personal communication). Of these, 91 percent have been implanted at the bulbous urethral site. In this carefully selected sample, results have been similar to those found in younger patients. Clearly, adequate mental and manual capacity and motivation are mandatory (*194*), but in some elderly incontinent men an artificial sphincter may be a reasonable option. Although success is less likely and the operation more difficult (because the cuff must be implanted at the bladder neck), the sphincter can be utilized even in patients with an underactive detrusor if they are capable of self-catheterization (*195*). Experience with the sphincter in elderly women is still too limited to comment on (*196*).

The Kaufman prosthesis is an alternative to the dynamic AMS sphincter. Success has been reported in elderly men (*197*) and the good results confirmed (*198*).

Outlet Obstruction

Three differences are highlighted in the approach to outlet obstruction in frail elderly men. First, superimposed precipitants must be excluded, including fecal impaction, prescribed and nonprescribed medications (anticholinergic and alpha-adrenoceptor agonists), urinary infection (*106,112*), pernicious anemia, and bed rest with aggressive hydration and subsequent detrusor decompensation (*71*). In the unobstructed or mildly obstructed man, each of these factors can precipitate urinary retention. Removing the precipitant and temporarily decompressing the bladder may obviate the need for surgery. Second, the operative approach can be altered to permit surgery in these subjects. In this group of patients, even short-term benefits may result in significant improvement in their quality of life. Thus one need not necessarily extirpate the entire gland. An alternative approach is to resect just that portion of the gland that is causing the immediate obstruction. By altering the surgical goal in this manner, one can use a less stressful anesthetic approach and can even perform the procedure under local anesthesia (*199,199a*). Additional benefits include a shorter operative time and reduced likelihood of inducing hyponatremia and hyperammonemia —both potent causes of confusion in this population (*200*).

Finally, if an operative approach is still not feasible, alpha-adrenoceptor antagonists have been conclusively shown to improve pressure—flow patterns as well as symptoms (*201–204,204a–c*). The only discordant result was reported by Brook *et al.* in an unblinded study that did not measure pressure changes at an appropriate site (MUCP), did not correct flow for voided volume, and did not objectively measure subjective responses. Additionally, in this small study a patient who developed acute urinary retention while taking placebo was excluded from the analysis (*205*). Phenoxybenzamine should probably not be used because of its association with gastrointestinal malignancies in animal models. However, Hedlund *et al.* have provided convincing evidence that prazosin probably works as well as phenoxybenzamine with fewer side effects (*204*). The daily dose is 2 to 8 mg, and the patient must be monitored for postural hypotension. Note that although urologic trials of alpha-adrenoceptor antagonists have traditionally excluded patients with cardiovascular disease, it is not necessary in practice (*202*). In fact, these agents can be beneficial for patients with congestive heart failure or angina pectoris. They can even be used in the setting of an acute myocardial infarction, although medical consultation should always be enlisted. In many cases an alpha-antagonist administered for acute urinary retention (*202,206,207*) may be less stressful than urethral catheter for the patient with an acute myocardial infarction.

Underactive Detrusor

Similar to the situation for outlet obstruction, the initial approach to the patient with an underactive detrusor is to ensure that precipitants have been reversed. If detrusor hyporeflexia persists, the patient may be able to augment voiding by using the Credé or Valsalva maneuver. If detrusor areflexia is present and is accompanied by stress incontinence, these maneuvers may still help. Alpha-blockers and bethanechol are beneficial in some cases, although there are no data to suggest that the response to these agents differs from that found in younger patients (*208*). They are worth trying, particularly in situations where residual urine poses a threat and intermittent or indwelling catheterization is contraindicated, as in the patient with a prosthetic heart valve. Intermittent catheterization is feasible and acceptable for elderly patients (*209*), but it requires a dexterous and motivated patient or family. If necessary on more than a once- or twice-daily basis, it is usually not feasible for the institutionalized patient.

Palliative Measures

In addition to removing functional barriers to continence mentioned earlier, other palliative measures can be used. Condom catheters are associated with well-known complications such as balanitis, skin maceration, and irritation. They may also increase the risk of urinary infection (*210,211*). Equally important, they may reduce the patient's motivation to comply with bladder training or drug therapy. Still, in selected cases the condom catheter is helpful.

Selection of the optimal absorbent pad or diaper depends on the patient's situation. For those with adequate manual dexterity, a product employing a brief with an insertable pad may be superior to a diaper. If the patient's periodic urine losses are large, a thick pad with a large target area is best. For patients with smaller losses, the more compact but slower-absorbing gel-containing products may be a better choice, especially as the gel absorbs odor as well. For the hemiparetic patient, a side-opening product is easiest to use. If manual dexterity is a problem, a Velcro closure helps. For the bedfast patient, a launderable bed sheet is often the best choice (*212,213*). Details of numerous other products and appliances are available elsewhere (*8,135,214,215,215a*) and should become familiar to physicians dealing with incontinence.

Indwelling urethral catheters are rarely necessary if one applies the interventions listed above. Even in nursing home settings, the prevalence of catheters can be held to 2 percent or less (*13,98,216*). Temporary catheter placement is appropriate and helpful for managing fluid balance in the acutely ill patient, healing a refractory presacral pressure sore, and comforting the terminally ill patient. Long-term use is justified for nonoperative candidates with outlet obstruction and secondary renal insufficiency, some patients with detrusor–sphincter dyssynergia, and patients with refractory overflow incontinence due to an underactive detrusor. If indwelling urethral catheters are used, prophylactic antibiotics are contraindicated because they increase the likelihood that the inevitable bacteriuria will include more virulent organisms (*217*). Methenamine is useless in this setting because the acid hydrolysis necessary to form its active moiety, formaldehyde, requires contact with bladder urine for 45 to 90 minutes (*218*).

CONCLUSION

Despite its considerable prevalence, morbidity, and expense, urinary incontinence in the elderly has been neglected. This is an unfortunate situation because the disorder is usually remediable. The approach to it, however, differs significantly from that used for younger patients. Hopefully, the principles elaborated in this chapter will encourage a more vigorous and optimistic approach to the incontinent elderly patient and inspire investigators to pursue the problem further in the future.

ACKNOWLEDGMENTS

This work was supported in part by an Academic Award and a Teaching Nursing Home Award from the National Institute on Aging, NIH, as well as grants from the Commonwealth Fund and The Medical Foundation. I am also indebted to Ms. J. Longstreet for outstanding technical assistance.

REFERENCES

1. Rosenwaike, I., Yaffe, N., and Sagi, P. C.: The recent decline in mortality of the extreme aged. *Am. J. Public Health* 70:1074–1080, 1980.
2. Dans, P. E., and Kerr, M. R.: Gerontology and geriatrics in medical education. *N. Engl. J. Med.* 300:228–232, 1979.
3. Yarnell, J. W. G., and St. Leger, A. S.: The prevalence, severity, and factors associated with urinary incontinence in a random sample of the elderly. *Age Ageing* 8:81–85, 1979.
4. Thomas, T. M., Plymat, K. R., Blannin, J., and Meade, T. W.: Prevalence of urinary incontinence. *Br. Med. J.* 282:940–942, 1981.
5. Yarnell, J. W. G., Voyle, G. J., Richards, C. J., and Stephenson, T. P.: The prevalence and severity of urinary incontinence in women. *J. Epidemiol. Commun. Health* 35:71–74, 1981.
6. Resnick, N. M., Wetle, T. T., Scherr, P., Branch, L., and Taylor, J.: Urinary incontinence in community dwelling elderly: prevalence and correlates. *Abstracts, 16th Annual Meeting., International Continence Society,* Boston, 1986, pp. 76–78.
7. Diokno, A. C., Brock, B. M., Brown, M., and Herzog, A. R.: Prevalence of urinary incontinence and other urological symptoms in the non-institutionalized elderly. *J. Urol.* 136:1022–1025, 1986.
8. Willington, F. L. Problems in urinary incontinence in the aged. *Gerontol. Clin.* 11:330–365, 1969.
9. Sullivan, D. H., and Lindsay, R. W.: Urinary incontinence in the geriatric population of an acute care hospital. *J. Am. Geriatr. Soc.* 32:646–650, 1984.
10. Resnick, N. M., and Paillard, M.: Natural history of nosocomial incontinence. In *Proceedings of the 14th Annual Meeting, International Continence Society,* Innsbruck, 1984, pp. 471–472.
10a. Sier, H., Ouslander, J., and Orzeck, S.: Urinary incontinence among geriatric patients in an acute care hospital. *J.A.M.A.* 257:1767–1771, 1987.
11. Garibaldi, R. A., Brodine, S., and Matsumiya, S.: Infections among patients in nursing homes: policies, prevalence, and problesm. *N. Engl. J. Med.* 305:731–735, 1981.
12. Jewett, M. A. S., Fernie, G. R., Holliday, P. J., and Pim, M. E.: Urinary dysfunction in a geriatric long-term care population: prevalence and patterns. *J. Am. Geriatr. Soc.* 29:211–241, 1981.
13. Ouslander, J. G., Kane, R. L., and Abrass, I. B.: Urinary incontinence in elderly nursing home patients. *JAMA* 248:1194–1198, 1982.
14. Marron, K. R., Fillit, H., Peskowitz, M., and Silverstone, F. A.: The non-use of urethral catheterization in the management of urinary incontinence in the teaching nursing home. *J. Am. Geriatr. Soc.* 31:278–281, 1983.
15. Norton, C.: The effects of urinary incontinence in women. *Int. Rehabil. Med.* 4:9–12, 1982.
16. Brazda, J. F.: Washington report. *Nation's Health* 3:3, 1983.
17. Ouslander, J. G., and Kane, R. L.: The costs of urinary incontinence in nursing homes. *Med. Care* 22:69–79, 1984.
18. Hu, T-W.: Cost impact of incontinence in the long-term care facility. Paper presented at the symposium Incontinence—Rehabilitation and Management in the Long-Term Care Facility, Dallas, 1985.
19. Vetter, N. J., Jones, D. A., and Victor, C. R.: Urinary incontinence in the elderly at home. *Lancet* 2:1275–1277, 1981.
20. Fossberg, E., Sander, S., and Beisland, H. O.: Urinary incontinence in the elderly: a pilot study. *Scand. J. Urol. Nephrol.* [*Suppl.*] 60:51–53, 1981.
21. Schnelle, J. F., Traughber, B., Morgan, D. B., Embry, J. E., Binion, A. F., and Coleman, A.: Management of geriatric incontinence in nursing homes. *J. Appl. Behav. Anal.* 16:235–241, 1983.
21a. Overstall, P. W., Rounce, K., and Palmer, J. H.: Experience with an incontinence clinic. *J. Am. Geriatr. Soc.* 28:535–538, 1980.
21b. Castleden, C. M., Duffin, H. M., Asher, M. J., and Yeamanson, C. W.: Factors influencing outcome in elderly patients with urinary incontinence and detrusor instability. *Age Ageing.* 14:303–307, 1985.
22. Rowe, J. W.: Clinical research on aging: strategies and directions. *N. Engl. J. Med.* 297:1332–1336, 1977.
23. Rowe, J. W. Research in geriatrics and gerontology. In Somers, A. R., and Fabian, D. R. (eds.),

Geriatric Imperative. Appleton-Century-Crofts, New York 1981, pp. 91–104.
24. Kovar, M.: Health of the elderly and use of health services. *Public Health Rep.* 92:9–19, 1977.
25. Shock, N. W.: Age changes in physiological functions in the total animal: the role of tissue loss. In Strehler, B. L. (ed.), *The Biology of Aging, AIBS*, Washington, DC, 1960, pp. 258–264.
26. Hayes, E. E., McConnell, J. A., and Benson, G. S.: The effect of aging on cholinergic receptor binding in the rat urinary bladder. *Neurourol. Urodyn.* 2:311–315, 1983.
26a. Ordway, G. A., Esbenshade, T. A., Kolta, M.G., Gerald, M. C., and Wallace, L. J.: Effect of age on cholinergic muscarinic responsiveness and receptors in the rat urinary bladder. *J. Urol.* 136:492–496, 1986.
26b. Gilpin, S. A., Gilpin, C. J., Dixon, J. S., Gosling, J.A., and Kirby, R. S.: The effect of age on the autonomic innervation of the urinary bladder. *Br. J. Urol.* 58:378–381, 1986.
27. Swaiman, K. F., and Bradley, W. E.: Quantitation of collagen in the wall of the human urinary bladder. *J. Appl. Physiol.* 22:122, 1967.
28. Susset, J. G., Servot-Viguier, D., Lamy, F., Madernas, P. and Black, R.: Collagen in 155 human bladders. *Invest. Urol.* 16:204–206, 1978.
29. Phillips, J. I., and Davies, I.: The comparative morphology of the bladder and the urethra in young and old female C57BL/Icrfat mice. *Exp. Gerontol.* 15:551–562, 1980.
30. Jacob, J., Ludgate, C. M., Forde, J., and Tulloch, W. S.: Recent observations on the ultrastructure of human urothelium. *Cell Tissue Res.* 193:543–560, 1978.
31. Philips, J. I., and Davies, I.: A comparative morphometric analysis of the component tissues of the urethra in young and old female C57BL/Icrfat mice. *Invest. Urol.* 18:422–425, 1981.
32. McLennan, M. T., and McLennan, C. E.: Estrogenic status of mestruating and menopausal women assessed by cervicovaginal smears. *Obstet. Gynecol.* 37:325–331, 1971.
33. Meisels, A.: The menopause: a cytohormonal study. *Acta Cytol (Baltimore)* 10:49, 1966.
34. Jones, G. S., and Wentz, A. C.: Adolescence, menstruation, and the climacteric. In Danforth, D. N. (ed.), *Obstetrics and Gynecology*, 4th ed. Harper & Row, Philadelphia, 1982, pp. 157–181.
35. Siiteri, P. K., and MacDonald, P. C.: Role of extraglandular estrogen in human endocrinology. In Greep, R. O., and Astwood, E., (eds.) *Handbook of Physiology, Vol. 2: Endocrinology*, Section 1. American Physiological Society, Washington, DC, 1973, pp. 615–629.
36. Baird, D. T., and Guevara, A.: Concentration of unconcentrated estrone and estradiol in peripheral plasma in non-pregnant women thoughout the menstrual cycle, castrate and postmenopausal women and in men. *J. Clin. Endocrinol. Metab.* 29:149–156, 1969.
37. Salmon, U. J., Walter, R. I., and Geist, S. H.: The use of estrogens in the treatment of dysuria and incontinence in post-menopausal women. *Am. J. Obstet. Gynecol.* 42:845–851, 1941.
38. Smith, P.: Age changes in the female urethra. *Br. J. Urol.* 44:667–676, 1972.
39. Berry, S. J., Coffey, D. S., Walsh, P. C., and Ewing, L. L.: The development of human benign prostatic hyperplasia with age. *J. Urol.* 132:474–479, 1984.
40. Walsh, P. C., Hutchins, G. M., and Ewing, L. L.: Tissue content of dihydrotestosterone in human benign prostatic hyperplasia is not supranormal. *J. Clin. Invest.* 72:1772–1777, 1983.
41. Brocklehurst, J. C.: Aging of the human bladder. *Geriatrics* 27:154–170, 1972.
42. Brocklehurst, J. C., Dillane, J. B., Griffiths, L., and Fry, J.: The prevalence and symptomatology of urinary infection in an aged population. *Gerontol. Clin.* 10:242–253, 1968.
43. Sourander, L. B.: Urinary tract infection in the aged. *Ann. Med. Intern. Fenn.* 55(Suppl. 45):1–55, 1966.
44. Dontas, A. S., Kasviki-Charvati, P., Chem, L., Papanayiotou, P. C., and Marketos, S. G.: Bacteriuria and survival in old age. *N. Engl. J. Med.* 304:939–943, 1981.
45. Walkey, F. A., Judge, T. G., Thompson, J., and Sarkari, N. B. S.: Incidence of urinary infection in the elderly. *Scott. Med. J.* 12:411–414, 1967.
46. Brocklehurst, J. C., Bee, P., Jones, D., and Palmer, M. K.: Bacteriuria in geriatirc hospital patients: its correlates and management. *Age Ageing* 6:240–245, 1977.
47. Sogbein, S. K., and Awad, S. A.: Behavioral treatment of urinary incontinence in geriatric patients. *Can. Med. Assoc. J.* 127:863–864, 1982.
47a. Boscia, J. A., Kobasa, W. D., Abrutyn, E., Levison, M. E., Kaplan, A. M., and Kaye, D.: Lack of association between bacteriuria and symptoms in the elderly. *Am. J. Med.* 81:979–982, 1986.
48. Andersen, J. T., Jacobsen, O., Worm-Petersen, J., and Hald, T.: Bladder function in healthy elderly males. *Scand. J. Urol. Nephrol.* 12:123–127, 1978.
49. Kirkland, J. L., Lye, M., Levy, D. W., and Banerjee, A. K.: Patterns of urine flow and electrolyte excretion in healthy elderly people. *Br. Med. J.* 287:1665–1667, 1983.
50. Griffiths, D. J.: Urodynamic assessment of bladder function. *Br. J. Urol.* 49:29–36, 1977.
51. Drach, G. W., Ignatoff, J., and Layton, T.: Peak urinary flow rate: observations in female subjects and comparison to male subjects. *J. Urol.* 122:215–219, 1979.
52. Fantl, J. A., Smith, P. J., Schneider, V., Hurt, W. G., and Dunn, L. J.: Fluid weight uroflowmetry in women. *Am. J. Obstet. Gynecol.* 145:1017–1024. 1983.
53. Backman, K-A.: Urinary flow during micturition in normal women. *Acta Chir. Scand.* 130:357–370, 1965.
54. Frimodt-Moller, C.: A urodynamic study of micturition in healthy men and women. *Dan. Med. Bull.* 21:41–48, 1974.
55. Drach, G. W., and Binard, W. J.: Disposable peak urinary flow meter estimates lower urinary tract obstruction. *J. Urol.* 115:175–179, 1976.
56. Drach, G. W., Layton, T. N., and Binard, W. J.: Male peak urinary flow rate: relationships to volume voided and age. *J. Urol.* 122:210–214, 1979.
57. Drach, G. W., Layton, T., and Bottacini, M. R.: A

method of adjustment of male peak urinary flow rate for varying age and volume voided. *J. Urol.* 128:960–962, 1982.
58. Marshall, V. R., Ryall, R. L., Austin, M. L., and Sinclair, G. R: The use of urinary flow rates obtained from voided volumes less than 150 ml in the assessment of voiding ability. *Br. J. Urol.* 55:28–33, 1983.
59. Enhorning, G.: Simultaneous recording or intravesical and intra-urethral pressure. *Acta Chir. Scand.[Suppl.]* 276:1–64, 1961.
60. Edwards, L., and Malvern, J.: The urethral pressure profile: theoretical considerations and clinical application. *Br. J. Urol.* 46:325–336, 1974.
61. Henriksson, L., Andersson, K-E., and Ulmsten, U.: The urethral pressure profiles in continent and stress-incontinent women. *Scand. J. Urol. Nephrol.* 13:5–10, 1979.
62. Rud. T.: Urethral pressure profile in continent women from childhood to old age. *Acta Obstet. Gynecol. Scand.* 59:331–335, 1980.
63. Susset, J. G., Choniem, G. M., and Regnier, C. H.: Abnormal urethral compliance in females: diagnosis, results, and treatment. *J. Urol.* 129:1063–1065, 1983.
64. Jones, K. W., and Schoenberg, H. W.: Comparison of the incidence of bladder hyperreflexia in patients with benign prostatic hypertrophy and age-matched female controls. *J. Urol.* 133:425–426, 1985.
65. Brocklehurst, J. C., and Dillane, J. B.: Studies of the female bladder in old age. I. Cystometrograms in non-incontinent women. *Gerontol. Clin.* 8:285–305, 1966.
66. Bafitis, H., and Sargent, F.: Human physiological adaptability through the life sequence. *J. Gerontol.* 32:402–410, 1977.
67. Williamson, J., Stokoe, I. H., Gray, S., Fisher, M., Smith, A., McGhee, A., and Stephenson, E.: Old people at home: their unreported needs. *Lancet* 1:1117–1120, 1964.
68. Wilson, L. A., Lawson, I. R., and Brass, W.: Multiple disorders in the elderly: a clinical and statistical study. *Lancet* 2:841–843, 1962.
69. Besdine, R. W.: Geriatric medicine: an overview. In Eisdorfer, C. (ed.), *Annual Review of Gerontology and Geriatrics.* Springer, New York, 1980, pp. 135–153.
70. Castleden, C. M., Duffin, H. M., and Asher, M. J.: Clinical and urodynamic studies in 100 elderly incontinent patients. *Br. Med. J.*, 282:1103–1105, 1981.
71. Resnick, N. M.: Urinary incontinence in the elderly. *Med. Grand Rounds* 3:281–290, 1984.
72. Lipowski, Z. J.: Transient cognitive disorders in the elderly. *Am. J. Psychiatry* 140:1426–1436, 1983.
73. Wilson, T.S.: Incontinence of urine in the aged. *Lancet* 2:374–377, 1948.
74. Hilton, P., and Stanton, S.L.: Algorithmic method for assessing urinary incontinence in elderly women. *Br. Med. J.* 282:940–942, 1981.
74a. Eastwood, H. D. H.: Postural influences on urinary incontinence in the elderly. *Gerontology* 32:207–210, 1986.
75. Robinson, J. M.: Evaluation of methods for assessment of bladder and urethral function. In Brocklehurst, J. C. (ed.), *Urology in the Elderly.* Churchill Livingstone, New York, 1984, pp. 19–54.
76. Walter, S., Wolf, H., Barlebo, H., and Jensen, H. K.: Urinary incontinence in postmenopausal women treated with estrogens. *Urol. Int.* 33:135–143, 1978.
77. Parsons, C. L., and Schmidt, J. D.: Control of recurrent lower urinary tract infection in the postmenopausal woman. *J. Urol.* 128:1224–1226, 1982.
78. Lamy, P.: Over-the-counter medications: the drug interactions we overlook. *J. Am. Geriatri. Soc.* 30(Suppl.):S69–S75, 1982.
79. Greenblatt, D. J., Sellers, E. M., and Shader, R. I.: Drug disposition in old age. *N. Engl. J. Med.* 306:1081–1088, 1982.
80. Berg, S., Dehlin, O., Falkheden, T., Gatzinska, R., and Nordqvist, P.: Long-term study of hypnotic medication in geriatric patients: a study of dixyrazine, nitrazepam, and amylobarbitone. *Scand. J. Soc. Med.* 14(Suppl.):85–96, 1977.
81. Gerbino, P. P.: Complications of alcohol use combined with drug therapy in the elderly. *J. Am. Geriatr, Soc.* 30(Suppl.):S88–S93, 1982.
82. Danziger, L. H., and Horn, J. R.: Disopyramide-induced urinary retention: report of nine cases and review of the literature. *Arch. Intern. Med.* 143:1683–1686, 1983.
83. Gordon, T.: *Blood Pressure of Adults by Age and Sex.* National Center for Health Statistics, Washington, DC, 1964, 11(4).
84. Kiruluta, G., Mercer, A. R., and Winsor, G. M.: Prazosin as cause of urinary incontinence. *Urology* 18:618–619, 1981.
85. Raz, S.: Adrenergic influence on the internal urinary sphincter. *Isr. J. Med. Sci.* 10:608, 1974.
86. Valentine, J. J., and Fitzgerald, J. S.: Retention of urine due to ephedrine. *J. Urol.* 34:314, 1935.
87. Balyeat, R. M., and Rinkel, H. J.: Urinary retention due to the use of ephedrine. *JAMA* 98:1545, 1932.
88. Forman, A., Andersson, K-E., Henriksson, L., Rud, T., and Ulmsten, U.: Effects of nifedipine on the smooth muscle of the human urinary tract in vitro and in vivo. *Acta Pharmacol. Toxicol. (Copenh.)* 43:111–118, 1978.
89. Resnick, N. M., and Yalla, S. V.: Detrusor hyperactivity with impaired contractile function. An unrecognized but common cause of incontinence in elderly patients. *JAMA*, 257:3076–3081, 1987.
89a. Coolsaet, B., and Blok, C.: Detrusor properties related to prostatism. *Neurourol. and Urodyn.* 5:435–447, 1986.
90. Resnick, N. M., and Yalla, S. V.: Management of urinary incontinence in the elderly. *N. Engl. J. Med.* 313:800–805, 1985.
91. Brocklehurst, J. C., and Dillane, J. B.: Studies of the female bladder in old age. II. Cystometrograms in 100 incontinent women. *Gerontol. Clin.* 8:306–319, 1966.
92. Langworthy, O. R., Jarvis, J. A., and Lewis, L. G.: Incontinent patients in chronic hospital. *South. Med. J.* 40:969–973, 1937.
93. James, M. H.: Disorders of micturition in the elderly. *Age Ageing* 8:285–288, 1979.

94. Eastwood, H. D. H.: Urodynamic studies in the management of urinary incontinence in the elderly. *Age Ageing* 8:41–48, 1979.
95. Eastwood, H. D. H., and Warrell, R.: Urinary incontinence in the elderly female: prediction in diagnosis and outcome of management. *Age Ageing* 13:230–234, 1984.
95a. Resnick, N. M., Yalla, S. V., Laurino, E., and Prout, V.: Evaluation of a clinical algorithm to identify the causes of incontinence in the elderly. *J. Urol.* 135:168A, 1986.
96. Resnick, N. M., Yalla, S. V., and Reilly, C. H.: Causes and correlates of urinary incontinence in extremely aged patients: new insights. *J. Urol.* 133:329A, 1985.
96a. Thompson, J.: Cystometry in the investigation of urinary incontinence. In: W. F. Anderson, and B. Isaacs (eds.), *Current Achievements in Geriatrics*. London: Cassell, 1964, pp. 105–114.
96b. Ouslander, J. G., Hepps, K., Raz, S., and Su, H. L.: Genitourinary dysfunction in a geriatric outpatient population. *J. Amer. Geriatr. Soc.* 34:507–514, 1986.
97. Bennett, C. J., Diokno, A. C., Wells, T., and Brink, C.: Urinary incontinence in elderly female patients. In *Proceedings of the 14th Annual Meeting, International Continence Society,* Innsbruck, 1984, pp. 76–77.
98. Fossberg, E., Beisland, H. O., and Sander, S.: Urinary incontinence in old age. *Ann. Chir. Gynaecol.* 71:228–231, 1982.
99. McGuire, E. J.: Retropubic operative procedures for stress urinary incontinence. In Raz, S., (ed.), *Female Urology*. Philadelphia, Saunders, 1983, pp. 241–251.
100. Barkin, M., Dolfin, D., Herschorn, S., Comisarow, R., and Fisher, R.: Voiding dysfunction in institutionalized elderly men: the influence of previous prostatectomy. *J. Urol.* 130:258–259, 1983.
101. Berkson, J.: Limitations to the application of fourfold table analysis to hospital data. *Biometrics Bull.* 2:47–53, 1966.
102. Milne, J. S., Hope, K., and Williamson, J.: Variability in replies to a questionaire on symptoms of physical illness. *J. Chronic. Dis.* 22:805–810, 1970.
103. Abrams, P., Feneley, R., and Torrens, M.: Geriatric problems. In Abrams, P., Feneley, R., and Torrens, M. (eds.), *Urodynamics*. Springer-Verlag, New York, 1983, pp. 156–164.
104. Resnick, N. M., Yalla, S. V., and Laurino, E.: Feasibility, safety and reproducibility of urodynamics in the elderly. *J. Urol.* 137:189A., 1987.
105. Walter, S., and Vejlsgaard, R.: Diagnostic catheterization and bacteriuria in women with urinary incontinence. *Br. J. Urol.* 50:106–108, 1978.
106. Bergman, A., and McCarthy, T. A.: Antibiotic prophylaxis after intrumentation for urodynamic testing. *Br. J. Urol.* 55:568–569, 1983.
107. Andersen, J. T., and Vejlsgaard, R.: The risk of inducing bacteriuria in urodynamic and uroradiological studies of men with prostatism. *Scand. J. Urol. Nephrol.* 14:229–232, 1980.
108. Turck, M., Goffe, B., and Petersdorf, R. G.: The urethral catheter and urinary tract infection. *J. Urol.* 88:834–837, 1962.
109. McGuire, E. J., Lytton, B., Kohorn, E. I., and Pepe, V.: The value of urodynamic testing in stress urinary incontinence. *J. Urol.* 124:256–258, 1980.
110. Yalla, S. V., and Resnick, N. M.: Vesicourethral static pressure profile during voiding: methodology and clinical utility. *World J. Urol.* 2:196–202, 1984.
111. McGuire, E. J.: Combined radiographic and manometric assessment of urethral sphincter function. *J. Urol.* 118:632–635, 1977.
112. Stanton, S.: Lower urinary tract infection and its effects on vesical and urethral function. In Ostergard, D. R. (ed.), *Gynecologic Urology and Urodynamics*. Williams & Wilkins, Baltimore, 1980.
113. Reuther, K., Aagard, J., and Jensen, K. S.: Lignocaine test and detrusor instability. *Br. J. Urol.* 55:493–494, 1983.
114. Kimche, D., Saar, M., and Lask, D. Evoked response studies in detrusor hyperreflexia due to infravesical obstruction in neurological patients. *J. Urol.* 133:641–643, 1985.
115. Lytton, B., Emery, J. M., and Harvard, B. M.: The incidence of benign prostatic obstruction. *J. Urol.* 99:639–645, 1968.
116. Allen, J.: *Synopsis Medicinae*. Vol. 1. London, Printed for W. Innys, W. Meadows, R. Manby; and H. S. Cox and the executor of H. Pemberton 1949.
117. Day, G. E.: *A Practical Treatise on the Domestic Management and Most Important Diseases of Advanced Life*. T. and W. Boone, London, 1849, p. 252.
118. Kirshen, A. J., and Cape, R. D. T.: A history of urinary incontinence: or, 400 years of incontinence—are we any drier? *J. Am. Geriatr. Soc.* 32:686–688, 1984.
119. Williams, M. E., and Hadler, N. M.: The illness as the focus of geriatric medicine. *N. Engl. J. Med.* 308:1357–1360, 1983.
120. Rowe, J. W., and Troen, B. R.: Sympathetic nervous system and aging in man. *Endocr. Rev.* 1:167–179, 1980.
121. Hurwitz, M.: Predisposing factors in adverse reactions to drugs. *Br. Med. J.* 1:536–539, 1969.
122. Caranasos, G. J., Stewart, R. B., and Cluff, L.E.: Drug-induced illness leading to hospitalization. *JAMA* 288:713–717, 1974.
123. Caird, F. I., Andrews, G. R., and Kennedy, R. D.: Effect of posture on blood pressure in the elderly. *Br. Heart J.* 527–530, 1973.
124. Knowleden, J., Buhr, A. J., and Dunbar, O.: Incidence of fractures in persons over 35 years of age. *Br. J. Prev. Soc. Med.* 18:130–141, 1964.
125. Gallagher, J. C., Melton, L. M., Riggs, B. L., and Bergstrath, E.: Epidemiology of fractures of the proximal femur in Rochester, Minnesota. *Clin. Orthop.* 150:163–171, 1980.
126. Goldsmith, M. F.: Research on aging burgeons as more Americans grow older. *JAMA* 253:1369–1405, 1985.
127. Spira, N., Dysken, M. W., Lazarus, L. W., Davis, J. M., and Salzman, C.: Treatment of agitation and psychosis. In Salzman, C. (ed.), *Clinical Geriatric Psychopharmacology*. McGraw-Hill, New York, 1984, pp. 49–76.

128. Salzman, C., and van der Kolk, C.: Treatment of depression. In Salzman, C. (ed.), *Clinical Geriatric Psychopharmacology*. McGraw-Hill, New York, 1984, pp. 77–115.
129. Everett, H. C.: The use of bethanechol chloride with tricyclic antidepressants. *Am. J. Psychiatry* 132:1202–1204, 1975.
130. Hohlbrugger, G., Lentsch, P., and Madersbacher, H.: Intravesical ions and osmolarity influence the volume pressure response in the normal rat bladder der and is more pronounced in experimental cystitis. In *Proceedings of the 14th Annual Meeting, International Continence Society,* Innsbruck. 1984, pp. 224–225.
131. Phillips, P. A., Rolls, B. J., Ledingham, J. G. G., *et al.:* Reduced thirst after water deprivation in healthy elderly men. *N. Engl. J. Med.* 311:753–759, 1984.
132. Epstein, M., and Hollenberg, N. K.: Age as a determinant of renal sodium conservation in normal men. *J. Lab. Clin. Med.* 87:411, 1976.
133. Aycinena, P., and Robertson, G. L.: Deficiencies of thirst and vasopressin secretion in the hyperosmolar syndrome. *Clin. Res.* 30:538A, 1982.
134. Wells, T.: Promoting urinary incontinence in the elderly in hospital. *Nursing Times* 71:1908–1909, 1975.
135. Castleden, C. M., and Duffin, H. M.: Guidelines for controlling urinary incontinence without drugs or catheters. *Age Ageing* 10:186–190, 1981.
136. Mandelstam, D.: Disability and incontinence. *Int. Rehabil. Med.* 4:3–7, 1982.
137. Finkbeiner, A. E., and Bissada, N. K.: Drug therapy for lower urinary tract dysfunction. *Urol. Clin. North Am.* 7:3–16, 1980.
138. Briggs, R. S., Castleden, C. M., and Asher, M. J.: The effect of flavoxate on uninhibited detrusor contractions and urinary incontinence in the elderly. *J. Urol.* 123:665–666, 1980.
139. Robinson, J. M., and Brocklehurst, J. C.: Emepronium bromide and flavoxate hydrochloride in the treatment of urinary incontinence associated with detrusor instability in elderly women. *Br. J. Urol.* 55:371–376, 1983.
139a. Zorzilto, M. L., Jewett, M. A. S., Fernie, G. R., Holliday, P. J., and Bartlett, S.: Effectiveness of propantheline bromide in the treatment of geriatric patients with detrusor instability. *Neurourol. and Urodyn.* 5:133–140, 1986.
139b. Dequecker, J.: Drug treatment of urinary incontinence in the elderly. *Gerontol Clin.* 7:311–317, 1965.
140. Palmer, J. H., Worth, P. H. L., and Exton-Smith, A. N.: Flunarizine: a once-daily therapy for urinary incontinence. *Lancet* 2:279–281, 1981.
141. Palmer, J. H., Worth, P. H. L., and Exton-Smith, A. N.: Flunarizine—short term fact—long term fantasy? Abstract presented at British Foundation for Age Research, November, 1982.
142. McAllister, R. G., Jr., Hamann, S. R., and Blouin, R. A.: Pharmacokinetics of calcium-entry blockers. *Am. J. Cardiol.* 55:30B–40B, 1985.
143. Castleden, C. M., George, C. F., Renwick, A. G., and Asher, M. J.: Imipramine—a possible alternative to current therapy for urinary incontinence in the eldery. *J. Urol.* 125:318–320, 1981.
144. Levin, R. M., and Wein, A. J.: Comparative effects of five tricyclic compounds on the rabbit urinary bladder. *Neurourol. Urodyn.* 3:127–131, 1984.
144a. Neshkes, R. E., Gerner, R., and Jarvik, L. F.: Orthostatic effect of imipramine and doxepin in depressed geriatric outpatients. *J. Clin. Psychopharmacol.* 5:102–106, 1985.
144b. Wiener, L. B., Baun, N. H., and Suarez, G. M.: New method for management of detrusor instability: Transdermal scopalamine. *Urology* 28:208–210, 1986.
145. Abbey, J. C.: Treatment of aged urinary incontinence: an exploratory study. *J. Am. Geriatr. Soc.* (in press.)
146. Hadley, E.: Bladder training and related therapies for urinary incontinence in older people. *JAMA.,* 256:372–379, 1986.
146a. Burgio, K. L., and Burgio, L. D.: Behavior therapies for urinary incontinence in the elderly. *Clinics in Geriat. Med.* 2:809–827. 1986.
147. Ehrman, J. S.: Use of biofeedback to treat incontinence. *J. Am. Geriatr. Soc.* 31:182–184, 1983.
148. McGuire, E. J., Shi-Chun, Z., Horwinski, E. R., and Lytton B.: Treatment of motor and sensory detrusor instability by electrical stimulation. *J. Urol.* 129:78–79, 1983.
149. Fall, M.: Does electrostimulation cure urinary incontinence. *J. Urol.* 131:664–667, 1984.
150. Ewing, R., Bultitude, M. I., and Shuttleworth, K. E. D.: Subtrigonal phenol injection for urge incontinence secondary to detrusor instability in females. *Br. J. Urol.* 54:689–692, 1982.
151. Blackford, H. N., Murray, K., Stephenson, T. P., and Mundy, A. R.: Results of transvesical infiltration of the pelvic plexuses with phenol in 116 patients. *Br. J. Urol.* 56:647–649, 1984.
152. Ewing, R., Bultitude, M. I., and Shuttleworth, K. E. D.: Subtrigonal phenol injection therapy for incontinence in female patients with multiple sclerosis. *Lancet* 1:1304–1305, 1983.
152a. Nordling, J., Steven, K., Meyhoff, H. H., and Hald, T.: Subtrigonal phenol injection: Lack of effect in the treatment of detrusor hyperactivity, *Neurourol. and Urodyn.* 5:449–451, 1986.
153. Kegel, A. H.: Physiologic therapy for urinary stress incontinence. *JAMA* 146:915–917, 1951.
154. Mohr, J. A., Rogers, J. Jr., Brown, T. N., and Starkweather, G.: Stress urinary incontinence: a simple and practical approach to diagnosis and treatment. *J. Am. Geriatr. Soc.* 31:476–478, 1983.
155. Castleden, C. M., Duffin, H. M., and Mitchell, E. P.: The effect of physiotherapy on stress incontinence. *Age Ageing* 13:235–237, 1984.
155a. Burgio, K. L., Whitehead, W. E., and Engel, B. T.: Urinary incontinence in the elderly. Bladder sphincter biofeedback and toileting skills training. *Ann. Int. Med.* 103:507–515,1985.
155b. Burton, J. R., Pearce, K. L., Burgio, K. L., Engel, B. T., and Whitehead, W. E.: Comparison of biofeedback to a program of education self-management as treatment for urinary incontinence in elderly ambulatory patients. *Abstract. 16th Annual Meeting of International Continence Society,* Boston, 1986, pp. 84–86.
156. Aniansson, A., Grimby, G., Hedberg, M., and Krotkiewski, M.: Muscle morphology, enzyme ac-

tivity, and muscle strength in elderly men and women. *Clin. Physiol.* 1:73–86, 1981.
157. Aniansson, A., and Gustafsson, E.: Physical training in elderly men with special reference to quadriceps muscle strength and morphology. *Clin. Physiol.* 1:87–98, 1981.
158. Aniansson, A., Ljungberg, P., Rundgren, A., and Wetterqvist, H.: Effect of a training programme for pensioners on condition and muscular strength. *Arch. Gerontol. Geriatr.* 3:229–241, 1984.
159. Klarshkow, P., Belving, D., Bischoff, N., *et al.*: Pelvic floor exercise versus surgery for female urinary stress incontinence: preliminary results. In *Proceedings of the 14th Annual Meeting, International Continence Society*, Innsbruck. 1984, pp. 159–161.
160. Iosif, C. S., Batra, S., Ek, A., and Astedt, B.: Estrogen receptors in the human female lower urinary tract. *Am. J. Obstet. Gynecol.* 141:817–820, 1981.
161. Wilson, P. D., Barker, G., Barnard, R. J., and Siddle, N. C.: Steroid hormone receptors in the female lower urinary tract. *Urol. Int.* 39:5–8, 1984.
162. Siegel, I., Zelinger, B. B., and Kanter, A. E.: Estrogen therapy for urogenital conditions in the aged. *Am. J. Obstet. Gynecol.* 84:505–507, 1962.
163. Judge, T. G.: The use of quinestradol in elderly incontinent women, a preliminary report. *Gerontol. Clin.* 11:159–164, 1969.
164. Raz, S., Zeigler, M., and Caine, M.: The role of female hormones in stress incontinence. In *XVI Congres de la Societe Internationale Urologie*. Vol. 2. Paris, 1973.
165. Faber, P., and Heidenreich, J.: Treatment of stress incontinence with estrogen in postmenopausal women. *Urol. Int.* 32:221–223, 1977.
166. Rud, T.: The effects of estrogens and gestagens on the urethral pressure profile in urinary continent and stress incontinent women. *Acta Obstet. Gynecol. Scand.* 59:265–270, 1980.
167. Beisland, H. O., Fossberg, E., and Sander, S.: Combined treatment with estriol and alpha-adrenergic stimulation in elderly female patients with urinary incontinence: a pilot study. *J. Oslo City Hosp.* 31:39–42, 1981.
168. Kiesswetter, H., Hennrich, F., and Englisch, M.: Clinical and urodynamic assessment of pharmacologic therapy of stress incontinence. *Urol. Int.* 38:58–63, 1983.
169. Beisland, H.O., Fossberg, E., Moer, A., and Sander, S.: Urethral sphincteric insufficiency in postmenopausal females: treatment with phenylpropanolamine and estriol separately and in combination: urodynamic and clinical evaluation. *Urol. Int.* 39:211–216, 1984.
170. Ek, A., Andersson, K-E., Gullberg, B., and Ulmsten, U.: Effects of oestradiol and combined norephedrin and oestradiol treatment on female stress incontinence. *Zentralbl. Gynakol.* 102:839–844, 1980.
171. Schreiter, F., Fuchs, P., and Stockamp, K.: Estrogenic sensitivity of alpha-receptors in the urethra musculature. *Urol. Int.* 31:13–18, 1976.
172. Tzingounis, V. A., Aksu, M. F., and Greenblatt, R. B.: Estriol in the management of the menopause. *JAMA* 239:1638–1641, 1978.
173. Genant, H. K., Cann, C., Ettinger, B., *et al.*: Quantitative computed tomography of vertebral spongiosa: a sensitive method for detecting early bone loss after oophorectomy. *Ann. Intern. Med.* 97:699–705, 1982.
174. Fossberg, E., Beisland, H. O., and Lundgren, R. A.: Stress incontinence in females: treatment with phenylpropanolamine: a urodynamic and pharmacological evaluation. *Urol. Int.* 38:293–299, 1983.
175. Stewart, B. H., Banowsky, L. H. W., and Montague, D. K.: Stress incontinence: conservative therapy with sympathomimetic drugs. *J. Urol.* 115:558–559, 1976.
176. Obrink, A., and Bunne, G.: The effect of alpha-adrenergic stimulation in stress incontinence. *Scand. J. Urol. Nephrol.* 12:205–208, 1978.
177. Lose, G., and Lindholm, P.: Clinical and urodynamic effects of norfenefrine in women with stress incontinence. *Urol. Int.* 39:298–302, 1984.
178. Woodhouse, C. R. J., and Tiptaft, R. C.: Mazindol in the control of micturition. *Br. J. Urol.* 55:636–638, 1983.
179. Tiptaft, R. C., Woodhouse, C. R. J., and Badenoch, D. F.: Mazindol for nocturnal enuresis. *Br. J. Urol.* 56:641–643, 1984.
180. Bhatia, N. N., Bergman, A., and Gunning, J. E.: Urodynamic effects of a vaginal pessary in women with stress urinary incontinence. *Am. J. Obstet. Gynecol.* 147:876–884, 1983.
181. Shepherd, A. M., Tribe, E., and Bainton, D.: Maximum perineal stimulation: a controlled study. *Br. J. Urol.* 56:644–646, 1984.
182. Stamey, T. A.: Endoscopic suspension of the vesical neck for urinary incontinence in females: report on 203 consecutive patients. *Ann. Surg.* 192:465–471, 1980.
183. Mundy, A. R.: A trial comparing the Stamey bladder neck suspension procedure with colposuspension for the treatment of stress incontinence. *Br. J. Urol.* 55:687–690, 1983.
184. Leach, G. E., and Raz, S.: Modified Pereyra bladder neck suspension after previously-failed anti-incontinence surgery: surgical technique and results with long-term follow-up. *Urology* 23:359–362, 1984.
185. Ashken, M. H., Abrams, P. H., and Lawrence, W. T.: Stamey endoscopic bladder neck suspension for stress incontinence. *Br. J. Urol.* 56:629–634, 1984.
186. Gaum, L., Ricciotti, N. A., and Fair, W. R.: Endoscopic bladder neck suspension for stress urinary incontinence. *J. Urol.* 132:1119–1121, 1984.
86a. Barendam, T. G., and Leach, G.: Surgical management of female incontinence. *Sem. Urol.* 5:94–107, 1987.
187. Stanton, S., and Cardozo, L.: Surgical treatment of incontinence in elderly women. *Surg. Gynecol. Obstet.* 150:555–557, 1980.
188. Gillon, G., and Stanton, S.: Long-term follow-up of surgery for urinary incontinence in elderly women. *Br. J. Urol.* 56:478–481, 1984.
189. McGuire, E. J., and Lytton, B.: Pubovaginal sling procedure for stress incontinence. *J. Urol.* 119:82–84, 1978.
189a. McGuire, E. J., Bennett, C. J., Konnak, J. A., Sonda, L. P., and Savastano, J.: Experience with

pubovaginal slings for urinary incontinence at the University of Michigan. *J. Urol.* 138:525–526, 1987.

190. Politano, V. A., Small, M. P., Harper, J. M., and Lynne, C. M.: Periurethral Teflon injection for urinary incontinence. *J. Urol.* 111:180–183, 1974.
191. Politano, V.: Periurethral polytetrafluoroethylene injection for urinary incontinence. *J. Urol.* 127:439–442, 1982.
192. Lim, K. B., Ball, A. J., and Feneley, R. C. L.: periurethral Teflon injections: a simple treatment for urinary incontinence. *Br. J. Urol.* 55:208–210, 1983.
193. Schulman, C. C., Simon, J., Wespes, E., and Germeau, F.: Endoscopic injections of Teflon to treat urinary incontinence in women. *Br. Med. J.* 288:192, 1984.
194. Furlow, W. L., and Barrett, D. M.: Management of complicated sphincteric incontinence: artificial urinary sphincter. In Barrett, D. M., and Wein, A. J. (eds.), *Controversies in Neuro-urology.* Churchill Livingstone, New York, 1984, pp. 407–422.
195. Barrett, D. M., and Furlow, W. L.: Incontinence, intermittent self-catheterization and artificial genitourinary sphincter. *J. Urol.* 132:268–269, 1984.
196. Furlow, W. L., and Barrett, D. M.: The artificial urinary sphincter: experience with the AS 800 pump-control assembly for single-stage primary deactivation and activation—a preliminary report. *Mayo Clin. Proc.* 60:255–258, 1985.
197. Kaufman, J. J.: Treatment of post-prostatectomy urinary incontinence using a silicone gel prosthesis. *Br. J. Urol.* 45:646–653, 1973.
198. Fowler, J. W., and Auld, C. D.: The control of male stress incontinence by implantable prosthesis. *Br. J. Urol.* 57:175–180, 1985.
199. Orandi, A.: Urological endoscopic surgery under local anesthesia: a cost-reducing idea. *J. Urol.* 132:1146–1147, 1984.

199a. Orandi, A.: Transurethral incision of prostate (TULP): 646 cases in 15 years—a chronological appraisal. *Br. J. Urol.* 57:703–707, 1985.

200. Hoekstra, P. T., Kahnoski, R., McCamish, M. A. Bergen, W., and Heetderks, D. R.: Transurethral prostatic resection syndrome—a new perspective: encephalopathy with associated hyperammonemia. *J. Urol.* 130:704–707, 1983.
201. Caine, M., Perlberg, S., and Meretyk, S.: A placebo-controlled double-blind study of the effect of phenoxybenzamine in benign prostatic obstruction. *Br. J. Urol.* 50:551–554, 1978.
202. Caine, M., Perlberg, S., and Shapiro, A.: Phenoxybenzamine for benign prostatic obstruction: review of 200 cases. *Urology* 17:542–546, 1981.
203. Gerstenberg, T., Blaabjerg, J., Nielsen, M. L., and Clausen, S.: Phenoxybenzamine reduces bladder outlet obstruction in benign prostatic hyperplasia: urodynamic investigation. *Invest. Urol.* 18:29–31, 1980.
204. Hedlund, H., Andersson, K-E., and Ek, A.: Effects of prazosin in patients with benign prostatic obstruction. *J. Urol.* 130:275–278, 1983.

204a. Griffiths, D. J., and Schroder, F. H.: Phenoxybenzamine in prostatic obstruction. *Urol. Int.* 39:241–242, 1984.

204b. Ramsay, J. W. A., Scott, G. I., and Whitefield, H. N.: A double blind controlled trial of a new alpha-1 blocking drug in the treatment of bladder outflow obstruction. *Br. J. Urol.* 57:657–659, 1985.

204c. Abrams, P. H., Shah, P. J. R., Stone, R., and Choa, R. G.: Bladder outflow obstruction treated with phenoxy-benzamine. *Br. J. Urol.* 54:527–530, 1982.

205. Brooks, M. E., Sidi, A. A., Hanani, Y., and Braf, Z. F.: Ineffectiveness of phenoxybenzamine in treatment of benign prostatic hypertrophy: a controlled study. *Urology* 21:474–478, 1983.
206. Leventhal, A., and Pfau, A.: Pharmacologic management of postoperative overdistention of the bladder. *Surg. Gynecol. Obstet.* 146:347–348, 1978.
207. Reuther, K., and Aagard, J.: Acute retention of urine due to benign prostatic obstruction treated with alpha-adrenergic blockers. *Urol. Int.* 39:114–115, 1984.
208. Downie, J. W.: Bethanechol chloride in urology—a discussion of the issues. *Neurourol. Urodyn.* 3:211–222, 1984.
209. Bennett, C. J., and Diokno, A. C.: Clean intermittent self-catheterization in the elderly. *Urology* 24:43–45, 1984.
210. Hirsch, D. D., Fainstein, V., and Musher, D. M.: Do condom catheter collecting systems cause urinary tract infection. *JAMA* 242:340–341, 1979.
211. Johnson, E. T.: The condom catheter: urinary tract infection and other complications. *South. Med. J.* 76:579–582, 1983.
212. Thomas, S., and Hubbard, J. K.: A laboratory evaluation of incontinence underpads. *Nursing Times* 75:1136–1139, 1979.
213. Williams, T. F., Foerster, J. E., Proctor, J. K., Hahn, A., Izzo, A. J., and Elliott, G. A.: A new double-layered launderable bed sheet for patients with urinary incontinence. *J. Am. Geriatr. Soc.* 29:520–524, 1981.
214. Mandelstam, D.: *Incontinence and Its Management.* Croom Helm, London, 1980.
215. Association of Continence Advisors: *Directory of Aids.* London, 1983.

215a. Brink, C. A., and Wells, T. J.: Environmental support for incontinence. *Clin. Geriat. Med.* 2(4):829–840, 1986.

216. Marron, K. R., Fillit, H., Peskowitz, M., and Silverstone, F. A.: The nonuse of urethral catheterization in the management of urinary incontinence in the teaching nursing home. *J. Am. Geriatr. Soc.* 31:278–281, 1983.
217. Kass, E. H.: Asymptomatic infections of the urinary tract. *Trans. Assoc. Am. Physicians* 69:56–63, 1956.
218. Warren, J. W., Muncie, H. L., Bergquist, E. J., and Hoopes, J. M.: Sequelae and management of urinary infection in the patient requiring chronic catheterization. *J. Urol.* 125:1–8, 1981.

20

Abnormalities of Vesicourethral Function Following Radical Pelvic Extirpative Surgery

EDWARD J. McGUIRE, M.D., SUBBARAO V. YALLA, M.D., AND AHMAD ELBADAWI, M.D.

Most patients after abdominoperineal rectal resection or radical hysterectomy, and a few after low anterior resection of the colon, experience difficulty with reflex vesical function. Although in most patients this difficulty resolves, it persists in 16 to 20 percent of patients, manifested by urinary retention, usually associated with incontinence as well as difficulty in initiating and sustaining the urinary stream (*1*). The standard method of treatment of this symptomatology in men is transurethral resection of the prostate or suprapubic prostatectomy. Some authors have recommended that prostatectomy be performed as an integral part of an abdominoperineal resection simply because urinary complications during the postoperative period are so common. It should be kept in mind that the first patient who underwent a Marshall-Marchetti-Krantz procedure was a man who suffered from virtually total urinary incontinence after an abdominoperineal resection. We are therefore in somewhat of a dilemma when faced with a patient with incontinence or residual urine, a slow stream and difficulty of voiding after a radical pelvic extirpative procedure. The basis of the dilemma is that it is difficult to determine whether the symptoms and findings are due to obstruction or are the result of vesicourethral denervation.

The usual hallmarks of obstructive uropathy, including vesical trabeculation, urinary tract infection, difficulty of voiding, slow urinary stream, poor flow rate, residual urine and incontinence, are also common to parasympathetic "denervation." Men who require abdominoperineal resection generally fall into the age group that has some degree of prostatic hypertrophy. It must be emphasized that endoscopic demonstration of prostatic hypertrophy is not tantamount to a diagnosis of obstructive uropathy. Although this concept may be perfectly valid, in practice most urologists use endoscopic criteria to diagnose obstructive uropathy. Although a skilled urologist certainly is able to use this method in routine cases of men suffering from obstructive prostatism, endoscopy as the sole method of diagnosis is unreliable in those who have neurogenic vesical dysfunction. Women are so rarely the victims of obstructive uropathy that endoscopy is not used in them to make that diagnosis. Since the usual treatment of obstructive uropathy in women is urethral dilatation (which often does not work), little harm is done unless the patient is selected for a more invasive procedure such as YV-plasty.

BACKGROUND NEUROLOGY

During pelvic extirpative surgery injury to parasympathetic pathways may occur at the rectal level, where the inferior hypogastric plexuses (incorporating both parasympathetics and sympathetic postganglionic nerves) are situated parasagitally on either side of the rectum. Damage may also occur to sympathetic nerve fibers that are carried through the superior hypogastric nerve plexus in the region of the pelvic brim, medial to the ureters and lateral to the rectum. In some patients perirectal neural plexuses may be involved even before surgery by an infiltrative rectal tumor, in which case the vesicourethral dysfunction may be present preoperatively (*2*). Moreover, mobilization of the anus in the perineum can lead to injury of somatic branches of the pudendal nerves.

Depending on the extent of dissection, therefore, varying degrees of damage to sympathetic, parasympathetic, and somatic nerves may occur during abdominoperineal resections. Such damage may be a complete or incomplete neural injury or simply a neural traction injury (neurapraxia). Extensive neural injuries are not seen with less extensive procedures such as proctocolectomy and low anterior rectal resection. Vesicourethral dysfunction after radical hysterectomy is predominantly related to parasympathetic loss. It has been suggested that the frequency of sympathetic denervation in women depends on the extent of dissection in the vicinity of cardinal ligaments and the amount of their resection (*3*). The spectrum of vesicourethral abnormalities seen in patients after extensive pelvic surgery is thus broad and variable; despite all the statistics accumulated in the literature, the true incidence of such abnormalities remains undetermined.

Neural Factors Influencing Urethral Closing Pressure

The combination of altered vesical compliance and a fixed or relatively fixed urethral resistance constitutes the constellation of lower urinary tract findings encountered following radical pelvic extirpative surgery. Part of the urethral closing pressure is clearly related to sacral pudendal (somatic) neural influence. The principal effects of pudendal nerve activity is pressure in the "high pressure zone," which is demonstrable by urethral closure pressure profilometry. Radiographically, volitional pudendal nerve-mediated contraction of the striated urethral sphincter is manifested by an increase in visible coaptation over an area about 1 cm distal to the verumontanum, extending to the bulbous urethra. Complete sacral rhizotomy eliminates the volitional ability to contract the striated sphincter and reduces peak urethral closing pressure values recorded from the mid-urethral high-pressure zone, with loss of action potentials and induction of denervation potentials from pelvic floor musculature and extrinsic (not the intrinsic) striated urethral sphincter (*4*). Whether sacral rhizotomy annuls intrinsic striated urethral sphincter function is not conclusively known at present.

Although complete sacral rhizotomy has a demonstrable effect on the mid-urethral high-pressure zone, it does not influence closing pressure or radiographic closure of the urethra from the bladder neck to the area of the volitional sphincter. Following sacral rhizotomy, however, alpha-adrenergic blocking agents can diminish residual closing pressures, as can sympathectomy in experimental animals (*4*). Following sacral rhizotomy, continence is maintained at the bladder neck and the proximal urethral sphincter mechanism (prostatic) urethra in men and proximal segment of the urethra in women), remains perfectly competent and functional radiographically and manometrically.

The parasympathetic pathway via the pelvic nerves can elicit an increase in sphincteric pressure, with filling of the bladder, as well as sphincter relaxation with loss of pressure during detrusor contraction. Virtually all reflex bladder and urethral responses to filling can be eliminated by excision of the $S_{2\text{-}4}$ dorsal root ganglia. Pelvic nerve-conveyed parasympathetic motor fibers mediate detrusor contraction and appear to be involved in consequent opening of the bladder outlet by relaxation. How preganglionic–postganglionic discharge across pelvic ganglia of the pelvic plexus, which induces bladder contractility, also leads to urethral smooth muscle relaxation to open the bladder outlet with loss of intrinsic urethral closing pressure is not clear at this time. Mechanisms of intraganglionic or peripheral preterminal functional interaction of postganglionic sympathetic and parasympathetic axons through axoaxonal synapses in the vesicourethral muscularis demonstrated morphologically and pharmacologically, may be responsible (*5–11*).

The result of pelvic nerve injury at the time of radical extirpative surgery is more than a simple loss of reflex bladder contractility; it includes loss of reflex urethral responses to bladder filling as well as any urethral responses that generally accompany reflex bladder contractility. In addition to annulling reflex bladder contractility, pelvic nerve transection apparently frees postganglionic parasympathetic axons and their neuroeffector junctions with detrusor muscle cells from the inhibitory control of higher spinal and supraspinal neural centers. With time, the detrusor becomes less compliant, or hypertonic in response to filling. It appears that this hypertonic response is in part due to the mural fibrosis and in part is neuromuscular in origin, as it can be influenced by bethanechol as well as anticholinergic agents.

Sacral rhizotomy is done deliberately as a treatment of some spinal cord injury patients to prevent contractile reflex detrusor responses. The procedure, however, does not influence smooth urethral sphincter function, which can be diminished only by concurrent administration of alpha-adrenergic blocking agents; the lack of smooth sphincter function with a widely open bladder neck and prostatic urethra in men or the first 1.5 cm of the urethra in women appears to be due to injury to sympathetic nerve fibers that mingle with those of the pelvic nerve in the pelvic plexus. Primary sympathetic pathways to the lower urinary tract are along the hypogastric nerves (*8,9,12*). Albert et al. demonstrated that urethral smooth sphincter hypofunction can be recorded following hypogastric nerve section, although loss of internal sphincter pressure is not complete (*13*). Their findings are inconsistent with clinical data demonstrating complete loss of urethral smooth muscle sphincter function that occurs after peripheral pelvic nerve injury combined with sympathetic nerve injury; there are also reports of isolated thoracolumbar sympathetic cell mass destruction leading to total loss of internal (smooth muscle) sphincter function (*14*).

Urodynamic Abnormalities

The type of postoperative vesicourethral dysfunction depends on the extent of neural damage that may occur during the surgical procedure and the time at which the urodynamic evaluation is performed. In other words, the resultant dysfunctions vary with the postoperative time and can be classified as early and transient, delayed, or persistent (*15,16*).

Within a week or two after an extensive extirpative pelvic procedure, e.g., abdominoperineal rectal resection, the bladder capacity may be markedly reduced (Figs. 20–1 and 20–2). Other features during the

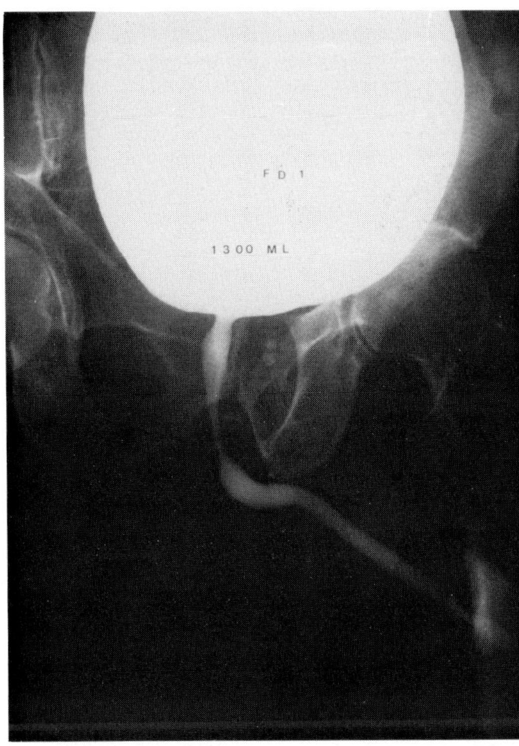

Figure 20–1. Preoperative bladder capacity of 1300 ml is suspected to result from a partial parasympathetic lesion caused by disk disease or infiltrative rectal cancer. (From Yalla, S. V., and Andriole, G.: *J. Urol.* 132:503, 1984. Copyright © 1984, The Williams & Wilkins Co., Baltimore.)

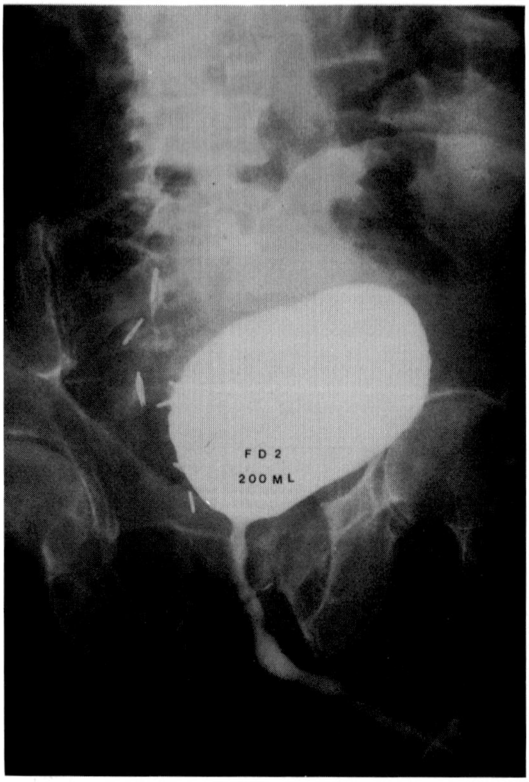

Figure 20–2. Two weeks after abdominoperineal rectal resection, there is markedly diminished bladder capacity and an incompetent posterior urethra; contrast medium passively seeps out. (From Yalla, S. V., and Andriole, G.: *J. Urol.* 132:503, 1984. Copyright © 1984, The William & Wilkins Co., Baltimore.)

immediate postoperative period may be detrusor hypertonia, indicating reduced vesical compliance, diminished proprioception, and detrusor hypoactivity or inactivity (Fig. 20–3). With neurogenic detrusor dysfunction, these features have been ascribed to damage to the parasympathetic innervation, probably with damage of sympathetic innervation, particularly its beta-adrenergic component. Others workers suggested that reduced vesical capacity and detrusor hypertonia may be caused by the surgical trauma to vesical smooth muscle and the resultant edema in vesical and perivesical tissues (*3*). We have seen functional changes of the posterior urethra characterized by incompetence of the bladder neck, prostatic urethra, and membranous urethral region, in addition to vesical hypertonia and diminished bladder capacity (Figs. 20–3 and 20–4). Urethral closure pressure profiles (UCPPs) are stunted compared to pressure profiles observed preoperatively (Figs. 20–4 and 20–5). The patient may be totally incontinent during the immediate postoperative period. Similar abnormalities, related to parasympathetic and sympathetic "denervation," may be seen after radical hysterectomy, depending on the extent of surgery.

Delayed and Persistent Voiding Abnormalities After Extirpative Pelvic Surgery

Vesicourethral dysfunctions following pelvic visceral surgery may become stabilized, and some that occur during the immediate postoperative period may regress (*17*). Changes secondary to neurapraxia could be transient and may disappear a few months after surgery (*17*); it is especially true with somatic neural traction injury during abdominoperineal resections, where gradual restoration of membranous urethral pressures have been seen. Despite such restorations, persistent findings of increased bladder capacity and detrusor hypo- or inactivity suggest persistent parasympathetic "denervation." Incompetence of the bladder neck may or may not be seen in such patients.

In several studies bladder biopsies from patients following abdominoperineal rectal resections have been examined. Patients with a "denervated" long-term decentralized bladder had greater density of cholinergic detrusor innervation than those studied immediately after surgery (*17*). These studies also revealed that there was no change in the density of adrenergic detrusor innervation in the patients immediately after surgery or after prolonged postoperative periods.

"DENERVATION" SUPERSENSITIVITY TESTS

"Denervation" supersensitivity tests have been used by a few workers to identify parasympathetic and sympathetic lesions following abdominoperineal rectal resection and radical hysterectomy (*19,20*). Gerstenberg et al. have utilized denervation supersensitivity tests and identified a loss of

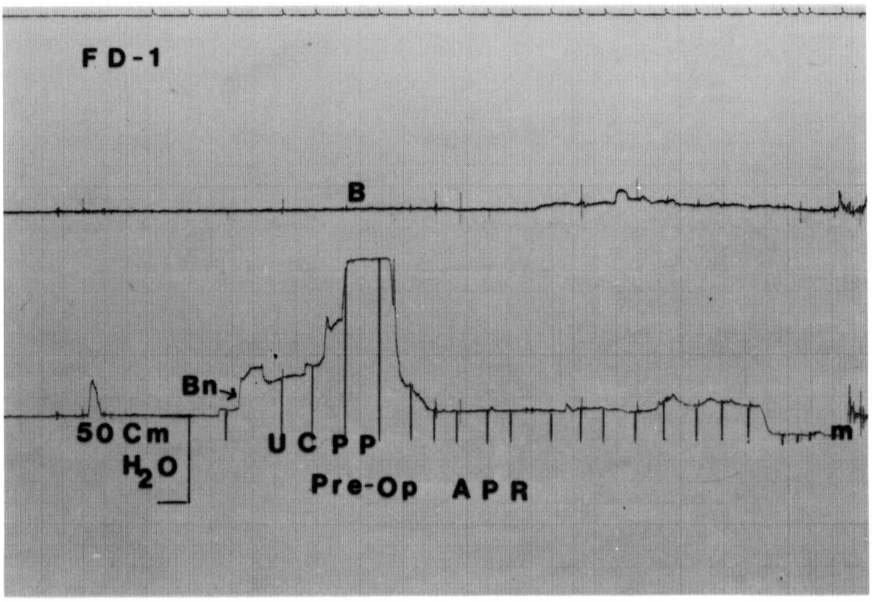

Figure 20–3. Preoperative urethral closure pressure profile (UCPP) shows normal pressure configuration. *B* = bladder. *Bn* = bladder neck. *m* = meatus. (From Yalla, S. V., and Andriole, G.: *J. Urol.* 132:503, 1984. Copyright © 1984, The Williams & Wilkins Co., Baltimore.)

parasympathetic influence after abdominoperineal rectal resection (*21*). In these studies, which were conducted both pre- and postoperatively, it was believed that only 2 of 10 male patients developed neurogenic vesical paresis. The question that now arises is how many of these patients had false-negative tests, which are known to occur following a parasympathetic decentralization? To understand the correlation between denervation supersensitivity and actual loss of effector parasympathetic innervation, bladder biopsies and cholinergic receptor assays should be investigated. At-

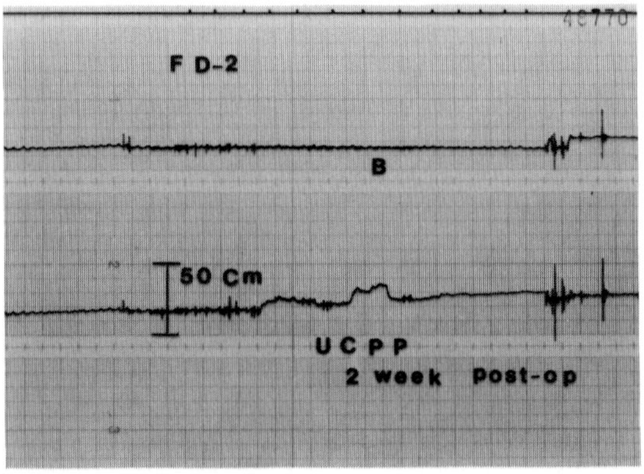

Figure 20–4. UCPP of the same patient as in Figure 20–3 shown around 2 weeks after AP rectal resection. Compared to the preoperative UCPP shown in Figure 20–3, there is no closure pressure in the urethra. (From Yalla, S. V., and Andriole, G.: *J. Urol.* 132:503, 1984. Copyright © 1984, The Williams & Wilkins Co., Baltimore.)

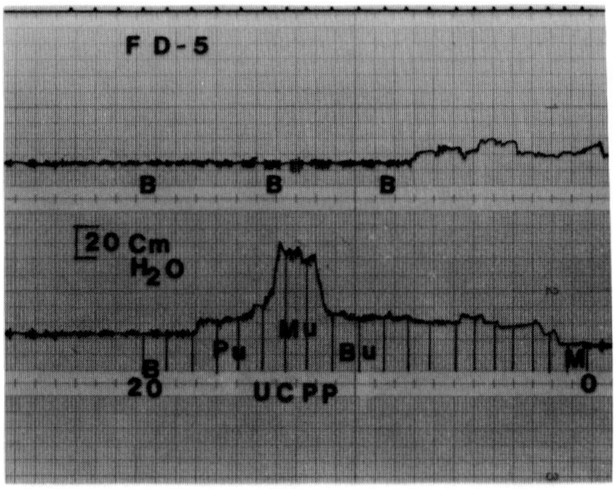

Figure 20–5. Same patient as in Figures 20–3 and 20–4, studied 8 weeks after AP rectal resection shows recovery of the urethral closure pressure, especially in the membranous urethral region (*Mu*). Patient also regained continence. *B* = bladder. *Pu* = Prostate urethra. *Bu* = bulb, *M* = meatus. (From Yalla, S. V., and Andriole, G.: *J. Urol.* 132:503, 1984. Copyright © 1984, The Williams & Wilkins Co., Baltimore.)

tempts have also been made to recognize urethral denervation supersensitivity to norepinephrine following radical hysterectomy (*19*); a positive test is implied if a rise in maximum urethral pressure exceeding 20 cm H_2O occurs during intravenous norepinephrine infusion.

In patients who sustained permanent injury to the pelvic nerves during extirpative pelvic surgery, Blaivas and Barbalias (*22*) and McGuire et al. (*23*) reported that incompetence of the proximal urethral sphincter is relatively common. The findings in such patients are predictable and usually typical: (a) The areflexic detrusor becomes gradually hypertonic, but striated sphincter function is reasonably well preserved, as the pudendal nerve is rarely injured by intrapelvic operations (Fig. 20–6). (b) The bladder continues to fill until intrinsic intravesical pressure is approximately equal to the striated sphincter resistance, at which time urinary leakage occurs. (c) The sensation of bladder distension and fullness is often preserved.

The relation between ureteral efflux and vesical pressure appears to be relatively straightforward insofar as the latter is determined by the degree of urethral resistance offered by its striated sphincter. Experimental and human data in two studies demonstrated that intraureteral resistance to perfusion is linearly related to intravesical pressure

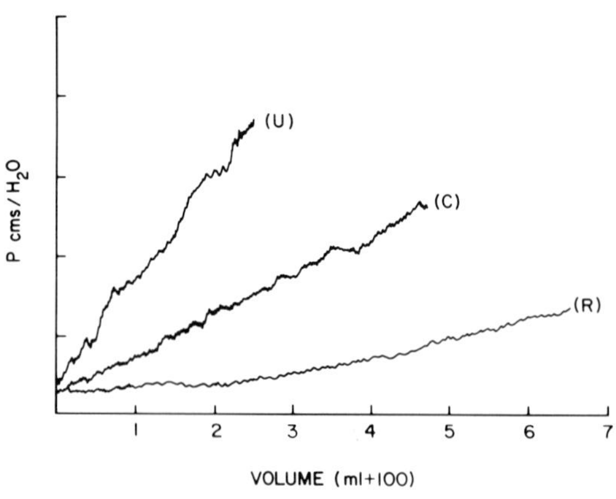

Figure 20–6. CO_2 cystometrogram 6 months after AP rectal resection in a 68-year-old man. Note the steep pressure volume curve used as the control (*C*), the steeper curve after bethanechol administration (*U*), and flattening of the curve after glycopyrrolate (*R*) administration.

(*23,24*). Even in the absence of vesicoureteral reflux, ureteral perfusion pressures increase markedly with an increase in bladder pressure. There are basically two ways to approach the problem of dilated ureters and impending renal compromise: (a) to decrease urethral resistance offered by the striated sphincter; or (b) to rely on anticholinergic agents to diminish vesicotonic responses to filling in an effort to gain vesical reservoir capacity and utilize intermittent self-catheterization frequently enough to void sustained intravesical pressures of more than 40 cm H_2O. The precise pressure at which the average adult ureter becomes dilated and unable to coapt is not known, but presumably that pressure is higher than what it is in children, in whom it has been established that 40 cm H_2O pressure is required for that to occur (*25*). Unless all involved pressures are clearly known, it probably is better to avoid reaching bladder volumes that induce pressures of more than 40 cm H_2O.

EVALUATION

An areflexic bladder can be diagnosed by cystometrography, particularly if supplemented with administration of bethanechol chloride or glycopyrrolate, which, respectively, increase and decrease the bladder tonic response to filling. The sensation of bladder fullness, but not urgency, is usually recognized by the patient. A cystometrogram with an electromyogram (EMG) demonstrates poor EMG responses to filling despite a gradual increase in intravesical pressure.

MANAGEMENT

The goals of treatment are basically preservation of continence and protection of upper urinary tract function. In patients without internal sphincter function, it may be necessary to augment urethral resistance in the proximal urethra to provide a stress-competent urethra. This goal can be accomplished with a Scott artificial sphincter in men and a pubovaginal sling procedure in women. Before undertaking these procedures it is necessary to ensure that adequate bladder reservoir capacity is present. A cystometrogram should demonstrate a flat bladder pressure filling curve to approximately 400 ml before sphincter-augmenting procedures are planned. With contracted bladders, after prolonged catheter or suprapubic tube drainage it may be necessary to gain reservoir capacity by performing an augmentation cystoplasty.

REFERENCES

1. McGuire, E. J.: Neurovesical dysfunction after abdominoperineal resection. *Surg. Clin. North Am.* 60:1207, 1980.
2. Fowler, J. W., Bremner, D. N., and Moffat, L. E. F: The incidence and consequences of damage to the parasympathetic nerve supply to the bladder after abdominoperineal resection of the rectum for carcinoma. *Br. J. Urol.* 50:95, 1978.
3. Forney, J. P.: The effect of radical hysterectomy on bladder physiology. *Am. J. Obstet. Gynecol.* 138:374, 1980.
4. McGuire, E. J., and Morrissey, S.: The development of neurogenic vesical dysfunction after experimental spinal cord injury or sacral rhizotomy in non-human primates. *J. Urol.* 128:1390, 1982.
5. Elbadawi, A., and Schenk, E. A.: A new theory of the innervation of bladder musculature: the innervation apparatus of the ureterovesical junction. *J. Urol.* 105:368, 1971.
6. Elbadawi, A., and Schenk, E. A.: A new theory of the innervation of urinary bladder musculature. III. Postganglionic synapses in ureterovesicourethral autonomic pathways. *J. Urol.* 105:372, 1971.
7. Elbadawi, A.: Ultrastructure of vesicourethral innervation. III. Axoaxonal synapses between postganglionic cholinergic axons and probably SIF-cell derived processes in feline lissosphincter. *J. Urol.* 133:524, 1985.
8. DeGroat, W. C., and Saum, W. R.: Synaptic transmission in parasympathetic ganglia in the urinary bladder of the cat. *J. Physiol. (Lond.)* 256:137, 1976.
9. Elbadawi, A.: Ultrastructure of vesicourethral innervation. I. Neuroeffector and cell junctions in the male internal sphincter. *J. Urol.* 128:180, 1982.
10. Mattiasson, A., Andersson, K. E., and Sjögren, C.: Adrenoceptors and cholinoceptors controlling noradrenaline release from adrenergic nerves in the urethra of rabbit and man. *J. Urol.* 131:1190, 1984.
11. Elbadawi, A.: Ultrastructure of vesicourethral innervation. II. Postganglionic axoaxonal synapses in intrinsic innervation of the vesicourethral lissosphincter: a new structural and functional concept in micturition. *J. Urol.* 131:781, 1984.
12. Elbadawi, A.: Neuromuscular mechanisms of micturition. In Yalla, S. V., McGuire, E., Elbadawi, A., and Blaivas, J. (eds.), *Principles and Practice of Urodynamics and Neurourology*. Macmillan, New York, 1987.
13. Albert, N. E., Sparks, F. C., and McGuire, E. J.: Effect of pelvic and retroperitoneal surgery on the urethral pressure profile and perineal floor electromyogram in dogs. *Invest. Urol.* 15:140, 1977.
14. Woodside, J. R., and McGuire, E. J.: Urethral hypotonicity following suprasacral spinal cord injury. *J. Urol.* 121:783, 1979.
15. Woodside, J. R., and McGuire, E. J.: Detrusor hypotonicity as a late complication of a Wertheim hysterectomy. *J. Urol.* 127:1143, 1982.
16. Yalla, S. V., and Andriole, G.: Vesicourethral dysfunction following pelvic visceral ablative surgery. *J. Urol.* 132:503, 1984.
17. Neal, D. E., Bogue, R., and Williams, R. E.: Histological appearances of the nerves of the bladder in patients with denervation of the bladder after excision of the rectum. *Br. J. Urol.* 54:658, 1982.
18. Mundy, A. R.: An anatomical explanation for bladder dysfunction following rectal and uterine surgery. *Br. J. Urol.* 54:504, 1982.
19. Koyanagi, T.: Denervation supersensitivity of the urethra to alpha-adrenergics in the chronic neurogenic bladder. *Urol. Res.* 6:89, 1978.
20. Blaivas, J. G., Labib, K. B., Michalik, S. J., and Zayed, A. A. H.: Failure of bethanechol denervation supersensitivity as a diagnostic aid. *J. Urol.* 123:199, 1980.
21. Gerstenberg, T. C., Nielsen, M. L., Clausen, S, Blaabjerg, J., and Lindenberg, J.: Bladder function after abdominoperineal resection of the rectum for anorectal cancer: urodynamic investigation before and after operation in a consecutive series. *Ann. Surg.* 191:81, 1980.
22. Blaivas, J. G., and Barbalias, G. A.: Characteristics of neural injury after abdominoperineal resection. *J. Urol.* 129:84, 1983.
23. McGuire, E. J., Savastano, J., and Morrissey, S.: Bladder and ureteral pressure relationships in non-human primates. *J. Urol.* 130:374, 1983.
24. Coolsaet, B. R. L. A., VanVenrooij, G. E. P. M., and Blok, C.: Detrusor pressure versus wall stress in relation to ureterovesical resistance. *Neurourol. Urodyn.* 1:105, 1982.
25. McGuire, E. J., Woodside, J. R., Borden, T. A., and Weiss, R. M.: Prognostic value of urodynamic testing in myelodysplastic patients. *J. Urol.* 126:205, 1981.

21

Urodynamics of Radical Prostatectomy and Enteric Substitution Cystoplasty

SUBBARAO V. YALLA, M.D., AND KEVIN LOUGHLIN, M.D.

RADICAL PROSTATECTOMY AND RECONSTRUCTION

Retropubic and perineal approaches are commonly used for removing the prostate and the seminal vesicles in patients with surgically curable carcinoma of the prostate. During this procedure vesicourethral continuity is established by anastomosing the wider bladder neck with the narrower membranous urethra. In order to avoid tension on the anastomosis, some degree of mobilization of the bladder neck and the base of the bladder is inevitable. After radical prostatovesiculectomy, varying degrees of neurologic and mechanical changes may occur in relation to the reconstructed lower urinary tract. These changes can be related to the surgical dissection in the vicinity of the base of the bladder and the injury that may occur to some of the branches of the sympathetics and parasympathetic nerves. During perineal radical prostatectomy the terminal branches of the pudendal nerve innervating the periurethral striated musculature may also be injured. In addition, mechanical trauma to the periurethral striated musculature may occur while dissecting the apical region of the prostate. Postoperatively, therefore, the continence and the conduit behavior of the reconstructed lower urinary tract depend on the functional integrity of the muscular and neural structures that escape surgical injury.

After vesicourethral reconstruction, the continence mechanisms depend entirely on the extrinsic and the intrinsic forces that operate in the vicinity of the newly constructed vesicourethral junction. The integrity of the residual intrinsic factors that operate in the vicinity of the membranous urethra further depend on the extent of distal resection carried out at the membranous urethra while performing radical prostatectomy. It has been known from the cadaveric studies that the volume of prostatic tissue present distal to the verumontanum varies (*1*). Therefore during performance of a radical prostatectomy, if the prostatic tissue is abundant in the vicinity of the apex of the prostate and encroaches on the membranous urethra, there could be great damage to the intrinsic mechanisms in the vicinity of the membranous urethra while carrying out distal transection. Under these circumstances, anastomosis of the bladder neck to the remaining compromised membranous urethra may lead to passive urinary incontinence.

Passive incontinence also depends on the functional integrity of periurethral striated musculature, which reinforces the intrinsic mechanisms at the membranous urethral region by creating passive external compression. If the patient had peripheral neuropathy leading to weak periurethral and pelvic floor musculature, this external periurethral reinforcement, which is needed for passive continence mechanisms, would not be available. When a patient with peripheral neuropathy that involves the function of the periurethral musculature (as suggested by the weak bulbocavernosus reflex and poor voluntary contractions of the periurethral musculature) is subject to prostatic transection encroaching on the membranous urethra, the chances of this patient becoming incontinent are high. Also, when these factors are combined with the perineal approach, the chances of attaining adequate postoperative passive continence are slim.

Rudy *et al.*, in a prospective clinical and urodynamic study, found that the incidence of incontinence following radical prostatectomy was 87 percent using strict urodynamic criteria (*2*). They recognized, however, that only 13 percent of their patients had significant clinical incontinence that ultimately required treatment. In another study, the postoperative urethral closure pressure profiles (UCPP) revealed that the closure pressure in the urethra proximal to the anastomosis were practically negligible; and some degree of closure pressures were observed only in the vicinity of the membranous urethral region (*3*). The studies also suggested that continence in the postoperative patients depended on the length of the functional urethral segment that showed adequate closure pressure. Patients with shorter segments and lower pressures were found to be incontinent. O'Donnell *et al.* reported that the incidence of incontinence was significantly less (6%) in 34 patients with nerve-sparing radical prostatectomy (*3a*). They studied a total of 68 patients, 34 of whom had conventional radical prostatectomy (without nerve sparing). This latter group had 30% incontinence. They observed that the functional urethral length and maximum urethral closure pressures were significantly less in the conventional radical prostatectomy group.

Despite the above-mentioned observations, we do not understand why some patients after radical prostatectomy are continent and the remaining are incontinent. We have looked at this problem more closely by performing pre- and postoperative evaluations at our center (*4*). The studies included a voiding cystourethrogram, uroflowmetry, cystometry, UCPP, tests of the voluntary control of the periurethral striated musculature and the bulbocavernosus reflex, electromyography (EMG), sacral evoked potentials testing, and a micturitional voiding pressure profile. All patients who developed incontinence were longitudinally studied at periodic intervals.

Our observations revealed that patients who retained their continence mechanisms postoperatively belong essentially to the retropubic surgery group. These continent patients, although deprived of proximal sphincter mechanisms in the vicinity of the bladder neck and the prostatic urethra, have recovered normal urethral closure pressures in the membranous urethral region. The closure pressures in this segment of the urethra were more than 50 to 60 cm H_2O. Voluntary control on the periurethral musculature (both magnitude and duration) was intact, and the patients all had normal bulbocavernosus reflexes. All these continent patients had normal proprioception, and the cystometry was unchanged postoperatively. When detrusor contraction was initiated, simultaneous reflex relaxation of the periurethral musculature was seen. It was shown by diminution of closure pressures in the membranous urethral region and attenuation EMG activity of the periurethral striated musculature when detrusor contraction appeared. In this continent group voiding was continuous, and patients were able to voluntarily interrupt voiding.

Incontinence was seen in those who had shown preoperative functional abnormalities of the periurethral musculature. In the group with radical perineal prostatectomy, six of eight patients became incontinent. Each of these six postoperative patients showed diminution of the UCPP, and the functional urethral length in each was markedly diminished. The patients also had poor voluntary control of the periurethral musculature. They could not maintain striated sphincter contractions for more than 5 seconds. In patients with severe incontinence the bladder capacity became smaller. These patients, in addition, showed evidence of detrusor hypertonia and overflow incontinence with smaller volumes of bladder filling. There was no evidence of reflex relaxation of the periurethral musculature when pressures in the bladder increased during the onset of detrusor contraction. The degree of incontinence was more severe in patients who had preexisting weakness of the periurethral musculature preoperatively.

In a prospective study in 33 men with prostate cancer by Leach and associates (*4a*), diminished bladder wall compliance was noted 1 year following radical prostatectomy in 50% of the incontinent men (4 out of 8). They urodynamically documented a very high incidence of urinary incontinence (93%) at 3 months postoperatively.

A study by Krauss and Associates (*5*) on 17 patients who had had radical perineal prostatectomy showed that all patients had a shortened functional urethral length and decreased maximal urethral closure pressures. In the standing position further shortening of functional length was observed in patients with incontinence. Cystometry showed lower detrusor contraction pressures. Moreover, 20 percent of their 30 patients developed some degree of incontinence. It appears that continence mechanisms are compromised to a severe degree and more so if there were preexisting functional abnormalities.

Turner-Warwick (*6*) believed that the continence mechanisms following radical prostatectomy tend to be precarious because of the ablation of the proximal sphincter mechanism, as well as most of the distal intrinsic mechanisms. He suggested that closing tonus of the extrinsic periurethral muscles alone are insufficient for intact continence. Donker (*7*) believed that the smooth muscles of the distal urethra, together with the "longitudinal sphincter externus" are the important factors for the preservation of continence after prostatectomy. Following intravenous administration of sympatheticolytic agents after radical prostatectomy, patients who were continent became incontinent.

ENTERIC SUBSTITUTION CYSTOPLASTY

The essential urodynamic features in patients who undergo enteric augmentation cystoplasty depend on the disease for which augmentation cystoplasty was performed and on the mechanics of the recently constructed enterovesical augmentation. Patients with preoperative neurogenic vesicourethral abnormalities may demonstrate complex postoperative problems. On the other hand, in patients with nonobstructive bladder outlet, the problems secondary to enteric augmentation appear to be predictable. Abnormal voiding patterns are observed in all these patients. Nevertheless, the patients are symptomatically better, and with proper postoperative rehabilitation these procedures are well tolerated by most of the patients.

Augmentation cystoplasty is usually carried out with ileal, cecal, ileocecal, or colonic bowel segments. Currently, ileal or ileocecal segment augmentations are being carried out with great enthusiasm. The UCPP in this group of patients are unchanged unless the bladder neck is encroached on by additional procedures such as bladder neck incisions of YV-plasties. These patients continue to have some degree of proprioception when the trigone is left intact and undisturbed in these procedures. Cystometry may show undulating pressure activity representative of bowel contractions; they are of varying amplitude and duration and cannot be inhibited. Similar observations have been made by Turner-Warwick and Handley-Ashken (*8*). Voiding is usually accomplished by abdominal straining. As most of the detrusor of the bladder was removed in these procedures, reflex relaxation of the bladder outlet that occurs during efficient normal voiding may not be seen. However, the patient in the course of time will learn to relax to a certain extent and effectively expel the urine with abdominal straining. Gittes believed that preservation of trigone may facilitate outlet relaxation (R. F. Gittes, personal communication).

Although severe neuropathic vesicourethral dysfunctions have been regarded as contraindications for augmentation cystoplasty, some workers believe these procedures can be performed with successful results (*9*). They have advised intermittent catheterization and artificial sphincter for managing urethral sphincter dyssynergia and sphincter incompetence, respectively. Light and Englemann conducted detailed studies in 14 patients whose lower urinary tract was reconstructed with bowel (*9*). Eleven of the patients had artificial urinary sphincter. These authors observed the onset of peristaltic contractions in ileocecal and cecal segments when they were filled to 150 to 600 ml. The mean pressure was 60 cm H_2O when the volume was increased to 250 to 1400 ml. All patients voided with the Valsalva maneuver, the flow rates ranging between 20 to 48 ml/s. With sigmoid bowels, the threshold volume at which contractions appeared was low (the mean was 25 ml). The patients with ileal cup patch reconstructions showed low-amplitude or no bowel contractions. Their capacity markedly increased (200–450 ml). They also had good continence, unlike the patients who had high-pressure bowel contractions of long duration. Thuroff et al. (*10*). described favorable results in 22 patients who had "Mainz pouch" reconstruction involving utilization of cecum, ascending colon, and two terminal ileal loops. They are split open on their antimesenteric border and anastomosed side to side to create a pouch. It is believed that longitudinal transection of circular muscle fibers in the bowel would produce a low-pressure reservoir of good capacity.

Turner-Warwick and Handley-Ashken (*8*) stressed the importance of urodynamic follow-up of these patients to check their voiding efficiency. These authors believed that large residual urine, urine infections, mucous retention, stone formation, and pyelonephritis may occur in this group of patients. They carefully studied several patients with enterocystoplasty and noted that pressure studies tended to be uniform and predictable in these segments. They found that the voiding flow pattern tended to be slow and intermittent even with the efficiently performed voiding cystoplasty. A normally opening bladder neck may fail to open after subtotal cystoplasty with bowel replacement. They called it iatrogenic, dyssynergic bladder neck obstruction. They believed, particularly in men, that bladder neck incisions or sometimes selective sphincterotomy confined to the intrinsic urethral mechanisms may be useful for improving the voiding efficiency. They also suggested that follow-up of these patients can be performed using voiding videocystographic methods without pressure measurements.

More detailed studies were performed by Gleason and associates (*11*) on patients with ileocecal cystoplasty. Based on their urodynamic data, they believed that the relaxation, or the opening of bladder neck during voiding, depends on the intactness of the bladder and its contained volume. They suggested that the fluid in the normal bladder acts as a scaffold against the wall of the detrusor and fixes itself, which in turn generates tension for pulling open the bladder neck. They therefore suggested that in patients with ileocecocystoplasty the cecal pouch acts as a vent to the bladder, thereby allowing the fluid mobility: It removes the fixation necessary to develop adequate intramural tension. This abnormality after cecocystoplasty would result in micturition with high energy loss probably secondary to the failure of bladder neck opening. In the few patients we studied, we observed that both the bladder neck and the periurethral musculature at the membranous urethral region in men failed to relax adequately. The patients had to void against a nonrelaxing bladder neck as well as the nonrelaxed membranous urethral region. The studies by Gleason and associates showed, in both male and female patients, high energy losses (more than 90 percent) with low residual (exit) energy. On the other hand, their studies in normal patients with intact detrusors revealed that the losses of energy were about 50 percent in women and about 70 percent in men. Their studies also indicated that the amount of bladder resection did not have any impact on the amount of energy loss after ileocecocystoplasty. In contradiction to the stable energy loss that persisted throughout micturition in normal subjects, the patients with ileocecocystoplasty demonstrated an increasing loss as micturition proceeded. In these patients there was an inverse relation between instantaneous bladder volume and energy loss. As the bladder volume decreased during voiding, the energy losses tended to increase to a point when the voiding stopped.

Several innovative enteric vesical substitutions incorporating long ileal or ileocecal segments are being increasingly used to create large urinary reservoirs with low pressures. These procedures are reinforced with continent and/or antireflux ileal intussusceptions or continent ileal plications (*12–14*). The precise mechanisms underlying the interaction of these enteric reservoirs with the continent and/or antireflux segments are not clear.

REFERENCES

1. Shah, P. J. R., Abrams, P. H., Feneley, R. C. L., and Green, N. A.: The influence of prostatic anatomy and the differing results of prostatectomy according to the surgical approach. *Br. J. Urol.* 51:549, 1979.
2. Rudy, D. C., Woodside, J. R., and Crawford, E. D.: Urodynamic evaluations of incontinence in patients undergoing modified Campbell radical prostatectomy: a prospective study. *J. Urol.* 132:708, 1984.
3. Hauri, D.: Urinary continence after radical prostatectomy. *Urol. Int.* 32:149, 1977.

3a. O'Donnell, P. D., and Finan, B.: Urinary continence following nerve sparing radical prostatectomy. *Abstract 487., J. Urol.* 127:225a, 1987.

4. Yalla, S. V., and Andriole, G.: Alterations of urinary continence mechanisms following radical prostatectomy. In *Proceedings of AUA Meeting,* Las Vegas, 1983.

4a. Leach, G. E., Yip, C. M., Donovan, B. J., and Kaswick, J.: A prospective study of bladder and urethral function before and after radical retropubic prostatectomy. *Abstract 64., Neurourol. Urodyn.* 6:64, 1987.

5. Krauss, D., Paletsky, S. H., and Lilien, O. M.: Urodynamics of post-radical perineal prostatectomy incontinence. *J. Urol.* 124:263, 1980.
6. Turner-Warwick, R.: Discussion of the function of the bladder neck. In Lutzeyer, W., and Melchior, L. (eds.), *Urodynamics—Upper and Lower Urinary Tract.* Springer-Verlag, New York, 1978, pp. 268–269.
7. Donker, P.: Discussion on the function of the bladder neck. In Lutzeyer, W., and Melchior, H. (eds.), *Urodynamics—Upper and Lower Urinary Tract.* Springer-Verlag, New York, 1973, pp. 268–269.
8. Turner-Warwick, R. T., and Handley-Ashken, M.: The functional results of practical subtotal and total cystoplasty with special reference to ureterocecocystoplasty, selective sphincterotomy and cystocystoplasty. *Br. J. Urol.* 39:3, 1967.
9. Light, J.K., and Engelmann, U. H.: Reconstruction of the lower urinary tract: observations on bowel dynamics and the artificial urinary sphincter. *J. Urol.* 133:594, 1985.
10. Thuroff, J. W., Alken, P., Riedmiller, H., Engelmann, U. H., and Hohenfellner, R.: The Mainz-pouch for bladder augmentation and continent urinary diversion. In *Proceedings of International Continence Society,* London, 1985, pp. 278–279.
11. Gleason, D. M., Bottaccini, M. R., Byrne, R. C., and Gittes, R. F.: Energy balance of voiding post ileocecocystoplasty. In Lutzeyer, W., and Melchior, H. (eds.), *Urodynamics—Upper and Lower Urinary Tract.* Springer-Verlag, New York, 1978, pp. 327–336.
12. Goldwasser, B., and Webster, G. D.: Continent urinary diversion. *J. Urol.* 134:227, 1985.
13. Kock, N. G., Nilson, A. E., Nilsson, L. O., Norlen, L. J., and Philipson, B. M.: Urinary diversion via a continent ileal reservoir: Clinical results in 12 patients. *J. Urol.* 128, 469, 1982.
14. Rowland, R. G., Mitchell, M. E., Bihrle, R., Kahnoski, R. J., and Piser, J. A.: Indiana continent urinary reservoir. *J. Urol.,* 137:1136, 1987.

22

Neurologic Dysfunctions

JERRY G. BLAIVAS, M.D.

Urinary bladder symptoms in patients afflicted with neurologic diseases are usually attributed to the underlying condition, yet this is often not the case. These patients develop common urologic conditions such as urinary tract infection, bladder and prostate cancer, and benign prostatic hypertrophy at approximately the same rate as patients without neurologic disorders. Thus in a patient with a known neurologic disorder, it is important to exlude these common urologic conditions as the cause of the patient's symptoms prior to instituting treatment. The diagnosis and treatment require a clear understanding of the neurophysiology of micturition and knowledge of how various neurologic lesions affect normal physiology. Moreover, one must be able to evaluate the intricacies and nuances of diagnostic urodynamic techniques and apply those principles to diagnosis and treatment.

Although most of these topics have been well covered in the preceding chapters, certain points bear reemphasis. The *micturition reflex* is a coordinated voiding contraction characterized by relaxation of the external urethral sphincter, contraction of the detrusor, and opening of the bladder outlet (*1*). The reflex is organized in the rostral brainstem and requires participation of the parasympathetic and somatic components of the sacral spinal cord as well as the thoracolumbar sympathetics (*1–3*). Interruption of the neural pathways connecting the "brainstem micturition center" to the "sacral micturition center" usually results in detrusor external sphincter dyssynergia or other manifestations of poor coordination of the micturition reflex, such as weak, poorly sustained detrusor contractions (*1, 4–6*). Common diseases that result in neurologic lesions of this type include multiple sclerosis, myelodysplasia and tumors, disc, or arteriovenous malformations of the cervical and thoracic segments of the spinal cord. Patients with untreated detrusor external sphincter dyssynergia are at considerable risk for developing serious urologic complications such as vesicoureteral reflux, hydronephrosis, urolithiasis, and sepsis (*7*).

Neurologic lesions above the pons usually leave the micturition reflex intact, and when they affect voiding at all they generally result in loss of voluntary control of the micturition reflex. Thus in these patients micturition is physiologically normal: There is a coordinated relaxation of the sphincter during detrusor contraction, but the patient has simply lost the ability to either initiate or prevent voiding (*1,8*). Such lesions include cerebrovascular accident, tumor, Parkinson's disease, normal-pressure hydrocephalus and a variety of miscellaneous conditions. In general, these patients suffer the consequences of urinary incontinence; but unless they are treated with an indwelling vesical catheter, they are at little risk for developing urologic complications.

Neurologic lesions that interfere with sacral reflex arcs may be caused by herniated discs, diabetic neuropathy, multiple sclerosis, and spinal cord tumors. They are also commonly encountered after extensive pelvic surgery such as abdominoperineal resection of the rectum and radical hysterectomy, but in these cases there is usually an associated sympathetic lesion as well (*9–13*). With complete parasympathetic lesions the bladder usually becomes "areflexic," although there may be weak, poorly sustained detrusor contractions known as autonomous waves (*14*). Despite these contractions, voiding is usually incomplete and obstructive because the vesical neck remains competent and does not open (*15*). In many cases the detrusor also develops poor compliance (there is a steep rise in detrusor pressure during bladder filling). At present, the pathophysiology of this poor compliance has not been well delineated. Some authors have suggested an active muscular hypertonicity (*16,17*), whereas others believe the etiology to be alterations in the passive viscoelastic properties of the detrusor wall (*18–20*). Regardless of the cause, McGuire *et al.* clearly demonstrated the deleterious effects that this pressure rise exerts on the upper urinary tract (*21*). When in addition to a parasympathetic lesion there is a sympathetic one, the proximal urethra loses its sphincteric function. Proximal urethral pressure becomes isobaric with detrusor pressure, and when viewed radiographically the vesical neck is open. Clinically, this situation results in incomplete bladder emptying (due to the acontractile detrusor) and sphincteric incontinence (due to the nonfunctioning proximal urethra) (*9,11–13,22,23*).

TREATMENT OVERVIEW

Although the ultimate goal of therapy is restoration of normal voiding, it is usually not possible unless the neurologic condition is cured or remits, or if the symptoms are caused by coincidental urologic condition such as benign prostatic hypertrophy. The social and emotional consequences of urinary bladder symptoms, particularly incontinence, must always be weighed against the risks to the patient's general health imposed by the proposed therapy. For example, women with mild but uncontrollable incontinence due to refractory detrusor instability may be better managed with menstrual pads (a treatment that poses no threat to their health) than with an indwelling vesical catheter (which predisposes to urinary infection, obstruction, and urolithiasis). On the other hand, patients with mild symptoms, e.g., men with detrusor external sphincter dyssynergia, may require more monitoring and even ablative surgery because of the high risk of urologic complications (*1*).

On the basis of clinical and urodynamic findings, urinary bladder symptoms may be classified as filling/storage abnormalities, emptying abnormalities, or combinations of the two (*24,25*). Treatment is directed at the underlying urodynamic abnormality responsible for the symptom (*26*). Thus if a patient complains of urinary incontinence and the symptoms are reproduced during the urodynamic study and found to be due to involuntary detrusor contractions (a pure storage problem), therapy is directed at abolishing the detrusor hyperreflexia. On the other hand, if incontinence is found to be due to involuntary detrusor contractions associated with bladder outlet obstruction, abolition of the detrusor contractions is likely to result in urinary retention. Relief of the obstruction may result in disappearance of the detrusor hyperreflexia and thus may obviate the need for further treatment.

MULTIPLE SCLEROSIS

Multiple sclerosis is primarily a disease of young and middle-aged adults with a predilection for women. The underlying pathophysiology is characterized by impairment of nerve conduction due to the presence of focal demyelination (*27*). The slowing of nerve conduction, which is exacerbated by increased temperature, results in varying and bizarre neurologic abnormalities that tend to exacerbate and remit over time. The demyelinating plaques have a predilection for the white matter of the cervical spinal cord, particularly in the posterior and lateral columns (*28,29*). Because these pathways subserve vesical and urethral function, it is not surprising that neurologic involvement of the bladder and its sphincter is common (*30–32*). Autopsy studies of patients with multiple sclerosis have revealed an almost constant presence of demyelination in the cervical spinal cord, but the lumbar cord was involved in only approximately 40 percent and the sacral cord in 18 percent (*28,29*). From these data one would predict that most patients would have detrusor hyperreflexia and detrusor external sphincter dyssynergia, which is indeed the case.

Urinary bladder complaints are prominent

in approximately 50 to 80 percent of patients with multiple sclerosis (*25,33–37*). Bladder involvement is part of the presenting symptom complex in approximately 10 percent of cases and, on rare occasion is the sole initial complaint (*36*). In general, bladder symptoms correlate reasonably well with the severity of the neurologic findings but not with the age of the patient or the duration of multiple sclerosis. The relation between bladder symptoms and neurologic findings has not been extensively studied. Philp *et al.* (*38*) found no correlation between neurologic findings and bladder symptoms, but Awad *et al.* (*34*) found a statistical correlation between (a) detrusor hyperreflexia and areflexia and pyramidal lesions, and (b) detrusor areflexia and cerebellar lesions. No such correlation was found between sphincteric dysfunction and specific neurologic lesions. Several series have documented a poor correlation between specific urinary bladder symptoms and the underlying urodynamic abnormality (*35,39*), although in Awad *et al.'s* series (*34*) there was a correlation between urge incontinence and detrusor hyperreflexia and between hesitancy and detrusor areflexia. The specific reasons for this discrepancy are not well documented; but even in patients without neurologic disorders the bladder often bears false witness to the underlying pathophysiology (*26*). Accordingly, in addition to the usual urologic history and physical examination, urodynamic studies are considered an essential part of the diagnostic evaluation. Of particular importance is the identification of specific urodynamic parameters that, unless properly treated, forebode an ominous outcome. Studies suggest that with multiple sclerosis there are three major factors predisposing to urologic complications (hydronephrosis, vesicoureteral reflux, urolithiasis, and urosepsis): (a) the presence of an indwelling catheter, (b) the presence of detrusor–external sphincter dyssynergia in men, and (c) the presence of poor vesical compliance with its attendant high detrusor pressures 40 cm H_2O (*7,21*).

Blaivas and Barbalias in a prospective study found that virtually all of the multiple sclerosis patients who developed urologic complications were either women who were managed with indwelling vesical catheters because of incapacitating incontinence or men with detrusor external sphincter dyssynergia (*7*). McGuire *et al.* convincingly demonstrated the deleterious effects of high intravesical filling pressures on the upper urinary tract (*21*). In a series of 42 children with myelodysplasia followed for a mean of 7 years, there was significant upper urinary tract damage (hydronephrosis or vesicoureteral reflux) in 80 percent of the patients whose intravesical filling pressure exceeded 40 cm H_2O but in only 9 percent of those with lower filling pressures. Despite the rather clear-cut association between urologic complications, indwelling vesical catheters, and detrusor external sphincter dyssynergia, the overall incidence of urologic complications and their morbidity and mortality in multiple sclerosis patients remains the subject of controversy, as discussed below.

MORBIDITY AND MORTALITY

Postkanzer *et al.*, in a study of all documented cases of multiple sclerosis in two counties in the United Kingdom, found that the disease shortens the life expectancy of men by approximately 10 years and of women by 14 years, but they did not mention the role of urologic complications (*40*). Leibowitz *et al.* determined that the cause of death was urologic in only 5 percent of deaths due to multiple sclerosis (*41*). In a Veterans Administration study, Samellas and Rubin stated that "death in 12 of 20 cases (55%) of multiple sclerosis in which autopsies were performed was ascribed to hydronephrosis, pyelonephritis, and/or septicemia arising from in the urinary tract" (*42*). Upper tract obstruction, pyelonephritis, or stones was evident in 19 percent of those patients who underwent excretory urography. Other series have documented upper urinary tract abnormalities in 15 to 25 percent of patients who had bladder symptoms (*25,43,44*).

All of the morbidity data are based on studies of patients with persistent bladder symptoms, most of whom had undergone many years of urologic treatment. In most series no entry criteria were defined and prior modes of therapy not outlined. Thus it is impossible to assess the relative contribution of the disease process itself, compared to iatrogenic complications from therapy, in the genesis of urologic complications. In a preliminary study of the natural history of bladder symptoms in multiple sclerosis patients, we found that virtually all urologic complications arose in men with detrusor external sphincter dyssynergia or in patients of either sex who were treated with an indwelling vesical catheter. Women with detrusor external sphincter dyssynergia did not seem at increased risk. (*7*).

Urodynamic Findings

There are no reported data on urodynamic findings in unselected patients with multiple sclerosis. Accordingly, the data presented here represent the results of urodynamic evaluations of multiple sclerosis patients who were tested because of persistent lower urinary tract symptoms. In most series the commonest urodynamic abnormality was the presence of detrusor hyperreflexia, which varied from approximately 50 to 99 percent (*25,33,35,37–39,45–49*). Of the patients with detrusor hyperreflexia, detrusor external sphincter dyssynergia was seen in 30 to 66 percent. An acontractile detrusor during cystometry was seen in 1 to 40 percent and in most there was increased external sphincter activity during bladder filling. When attempting to void, these patients generally strain, increasing their intraabdominal and intravesical pressures equally, but they are unable to relax the external sphincter or open the vesical neck. Occasionally patients have incontinence associated with sudden, complete, and involuntary relaxation of the external urethral sphincter without a measurable rise in detrusor pressure. Although this condition has been called urethral instability (*50*), it is my opinion that this phenomenon represents an involuntary micturition reflex in which urethral resistance is so low that the detrusor contraction does not record a rise in pressure. The distinction between urethral and detrusor instability is important because therapy must be directed at abolishing the detrusor hyperreflexia rather than "strengthening the sphincter."

Bladder symptoms and urodynamic findings in these patients may change as the disease itself waxes and wanes. Wheller *et al.* described 18 multiple sclerosis patients who had repeat urodynamic studies because of changing bladder symptoms (*51*). Fifty-five percent of the patients had different urodynamic findings on the repeat examination. In most instances the repeat examination documented the development of detrusor–external sphincter dyssynergia, and no patient with preexisting dyssynergia demonstrated any improvement. It has been our experience that once detrusor sphincter dyssynergia develops it rarely remits, but occasionally detrusor–external sphincter dyssynergia is present intermittently during a single urodynamic study (*35,52,53*).

Treatment

Treatment of bladder disturbances in multiple sclerosis patients requires a clear-cut understanding of the underlying pathophysiology. Several authors have demonstrated a rather poor correlation between symptoms and urodynamic findings, (*25,35,51*). Accordingly, empiric therapy, without knowledge of the etiology, is often unsuccessful and may even be harmful. There are several reasons why therapy for persistent bladder symptoms should not be instituted until urodynamic studies have documented their cause. First, and most important, the urodynamic study may demonstrate an abnormality such as detrusor–external sphincter dyssynergia, which unless treated and monitored aggressively, may lead to serious urologic complications (*7*). Unfortunately, empiric therapy may actually cause symptomatic improvement while accentuating the risk factors. For example, a patient with detrusor–sphincter dyssynergia who is treated with anticholinergics may notice improvement in the incontinence while at the same time residual urine increases as does the potential for serious infection. Second, urodynamic demonstration of the etiology of a symptom provides the clinician with a degree of confidence about therapy that cannot be obtained when the patient is treated empirically. If a patient complains of urinary frequency and urgency, for example, and is treated empirically with anticholinergics, how does one evaluate the clinical response? If the patient claims he is no better in 1 week, should the dosage be increased or should another drug be used? Are the symptoms really due to detrusor hyperreflexia or is there bladder outlet obstruction with secondary detrusor instability? If it is known beforehand that the problem is one of uncomplicated detrusor instability, the drugs can be increased with relative impunity; if this information is not at hand, it is difficult to make a clinical judgment.

Therapeutic decisions are further complicated in multiple sclerosis by the fact that the disease itself is subject to exacerbations and remissions, and that when they occur the underlying urologic pathology may change. For example, several authors have documented patients with detrusor hyperreflexia reverting to normal or changing to detrusor areflexia and even more than one urodynamic pattern being present within a single urodynamic investigation (*31,51*). These considerations dictate that no patient with multiple sclerosis undergo ablative or irreversible surgery until it is clear that the neurologic condition is either stable or progressive over time and that there is no reasonable hope for recovery. Unfortunately, there are no firm guidelines to allow one to predict if there is a reasonable chance for neurologic recovery. Most patients with exacerbating and remitting forms of multiple sclerosis continue in that pattern for long periods of time; these patients are best managed conservatively for as long as possible. Patients with stable or gradually progressive disease rarely have significant neurologic recovery. If these patients have a persistent neurourologic problem for at least 2 years, ablative or irreversible surgery may be considered if conservative therapy has failed.

DIABETES MELLITUS

Peripheral and autonomic neuropathies are well-known complications of diabetes mellitus. The primary pathologic process that causes the neuropathy is a metabolic derangement of the Schwann cell, which results in segmental demyelinization and impairment of nerve conduction (*54–56*). Involvement of the lower urinary tract by diabetic neuropathy has been termed "diabetic cystopathy" by Frimødt-Moller (*57,58*). The most prominent clinical feature of diabetic cystopathy is its insidious onset and progression with only minimal symptomatology. The first symptom is usually impairment of bladder sensation, which results in a gradual increase in the time interval between voiding. This condition may progress to the point where the patient voids only once or twice a day, by the clock, without any awareness of the need to void at all. With further progression the patient may require abdominal straining to initiate and maintain micturition, and the strength and force of the stream may become impaired. Unselected diabetics generally do not complain of bladder symptoms (*59,60*); but if specifically questioned, 25 to 50 percent recount the usual symptoms of diabetic cystopathy (*57,58,61–64*). When unselected diabetic patients have undergone routine urodynamic studies the incidence of diabetic cystopathy has ranged from 27 to 85 percent (*61–63,65–67*). In Frimødt-Moller's study, diabetic cystopathy correlated with the duration of diabetes (generally occurring approximately 10 years after onset) but not with the severity of the diabetes as judged by the amount or type pharmacologic treatment (*57,58*). Diabetic cystopathy almost always coexists with signs of peripheral neuropathy (*61,63,64,66–69*).

Urodynamic Findings

The principal urodynamic findings with diabetic cystopathy include impaired bladder sensation, increased cystometric bladder capacity, decreased detrusor contractility, and impaired uroflow. Historically, abnormalities of vesical sensation have been difficult to evaluate. During cystometry a qualitative assessment of sensation has been made by measuring the bladder volume at the first awareness of bladder filling, first urge to void, the feeling that micturition is imminent, and bladder capacity (*58,61–64,70,71*). Normal values of the first sensation of bladder filling varied in these series from 200 to 600 ml. In this regard, it is difficult to assess the real significance of these qualitative methods. Carlsson and Sundin suggested that the first sensation of bladder filling normally occurs at approximately 50 percent of bladder capacity (*71*). Using these criteria, abnormalities of bladder sensation are seen in most unselected diabetic patients.

Frimødt-Moller and Hald, in an attempt to assess bladder sensation in a more quantitative way, developed a technique to measure the electrical perception threshold (EPT) (*72*). The bladder mucosa was electrically stimulated via a specially designed catheter electrode, and the current at which the patient first experienced the tingling sensation was defined as the EPT. Normal patients experienced the EPT at currents below 10 mA. Values above 15 mA were considered pathologic. Furthermore, these authors found that the EPT increased with age. It is a nonspecific test of bladder sensation and cannot distinguish diabetic neuropathy from other causes of impaired sensation.

Increased bladder capacity has been documented in many studies, but, like assessment of bladder sensation, quantitative data are difficult to extrapolate from one series to another (*57,58,61,64,73*). Frimødt-Moller compared bladder capacity and micturition volume in normal volunteers and unselected diabetics (*57,58,73*). He found that there was a significant difference in both bladder capacity (913 ml for diabetics, 625 ml for normal controls) and micturition volume (655 ml for diabetics, 513 ml for normal controls). However, large-capacity bladders are not necessarily pathologic. Weir and Jaques found that of 3500 patients referred for urodynamic evaluation, 109 had cystometric bladder capacities in excess of 800 ml, which was more than 2 SD from the mean value (500 ml) of the larger group (*74*). Bladder sensation was not assessed in this series, but of the whole group one-third were found to be urodynamically normal despite the large capacity. All of these patients had cystometric bladder capacities between 800 and 1500 ml. Of the patients with large-capacity bladders only 4.8 percent had diabetes mellitus, and of those, one was urodynamically normal, one had an acontractile bladder, one had impaired detrusor contractility, and two had instability.

Impaired detrusor contractility is widely accepted as one of the manifestations of diabetic cystopathy, but there has been little documentation of it in the literature. In Frimødt-Moller's series there was no statistical difference in voiding pressure between normal age- and sex- matched controls (45 cm H_2O) and unselected diabetic patients (*57,58,73*). Norlen *et al.*, on the other hand, reported that 6 of 12 diabetics awaiting renal transplantation because of diabetic nephropathy had impaired detrusor contractility (*69*).

Detrusor instability has not been reported in any of the series on diabetic cystopathy; however, unpublished data from our laboratory suggest that as many as 25 percent of symptomatic diabetics may have detrusor instability. Other unpublished reports have found a similar incidence of instability (*75*). Moreover, two of the five diabetic patients with large-capacity bladders in the study by Weir and Jaques (*74*) also had detrusor instability, as did 1 of the 12 patients in Norlen *et al.*'s series (*69*).

Differential Diagnosis

The most important condition that can mimic the findings of diabetic cystopathy is bladder outlet obstruction, which may coexist with diabetic cystopathy. In the series of Frimødt-Moller diabetic cystopathy was found in 38 percent and bladder outlet obstruction (mostly benign prostatic hypertrophy) in 26 percent of 124 patients (*58,73*). Other series have reported a similar incidence of bladder outlet obstruction, but sophisticated urodynamic studies were not performed to document this clinical impression (*63,68*).

Because both diabetic cystopathy and bladder outlet obstruction usually result in impaired uroflow, screening uroflowmetry is of little help in making this distinction. However, simultaneous measurement of detrusor pressure and uroflow is usually definitive. Bladder outlet obstruction is documented by measuring a high or normal detrusor pressure in the presence of an impaired urinary flow rate. With diabetic cystopathy the detrusor pressure during voiding is low. Occasionally, patients with poor detrusor contractility due to diabetic cystopathy also have bladder outlet obstruction. The only means for diagnosing obstruction in these instances is to perform the micturitional static urethral pressure profile, as described by Yalla *et al.* (*76,77*).

Treatment

Treatment of bladder disturbances in diabetics requires a precise knowledge of the underlying pathophysiology. Of particular importance is the distinction between diabetic cystopathy and bladder outlet obstruction because empiric bladder outlet reducing procedures, e.g., prostatectomy, which usually alleviates the symptoms of patients with prostatic obstruction, is of no value in patients who have only impaired detrusor contractility and may prove harmful.

To date, there have been no controlled clinical trials reported for diabetic cystopathy. Accordingly, most of the remaining recommendations are based on personal observations. Autopsy studies have demonstrated that chronic pyelonephritis occurs at a rate four to five times higher than that in the nondiabetic population (*78,79*). Moreover, the incidence of bacteriuria and urinary tract infections is much higher in diabetics (*58,73,80*). Whether the increased rate of urinary tract infection is due to diabetic cystopathy or other manifestations of diabetes is not known. Nevertheless, the association of a large postvoid residual urine volume, bacteriuria, and urinary tract infection is well known, and if these risk factors are present they demand treatment.

Treatment Guidelines. *Asymptomatic Patients with Diabetic Cystopathy.* Because there are few data on the natural history of untreated asymptomatic diabetic cystopathy, and because there seem to be few short-term complications from this condition, either no treatment at all or conservative, reversible, noninvasive therapy is instituted. Scheduled, timed voiding is a simple and effective means for dealing with the sensory abnormality that leads to infrequent voiding. Double or triple voiding may permit emptying of a bladder that otherwise leaves a large residual. Straining to void may be helpful in some patients, but harmful in others. To test the efficacy of straining, a simple uroflow may be obtained and the patient instructed to strain in the midst of voiding. If the flow improves, straining should be recommended; if it causes a fall in uroflow, the patient should be specifically instructed not to strain. Patients with excessively large bladder capacities or residual urine should have urodynamic studies performed to determine whether there are other risk factors that need treatment. Of particular importance is the presence of bladder outlet obstruction, detrusor hypertonicity, or poor bladder compliance because of the danger of upper tract damage (*21*). In addition, if asymptomatic bacteriuria is present it should be treated with culture-specific antibiotics.

Symptomatic Patients with Diabetic Cystopathy. The mainstay of treatment for symptomatic diabetic cystopathy is clean intermittent self-catheterization (CISC) (*81*). If infection is present it should be treated with culture-specific antibiotics in conjunction with CISC. A number of other treatment regimens have been recommended over the years and many have gained both popularity and credibility. Parasympathetic agonists such as bethanechol chloride have been recommended to promote bladder emptying (*82–84*). However, most clinical studies have shown that bethanechol does not significantly improve voiding (*85–89*). The investigators whose studies show a beneficial effect from bethanechol seem to agree that there must be at least partial integrity of the lower motor neuron to permit "reflex bladder function" in order for the drug to be effective. Thus patients with complete lower motor neuron lesions or detrusor areflexia are not candidates for treatment with cholinergic medications.

Effective treatment regimens with bethanechol have required much higher dosages, usually administered subcutaneously, than recommended by the Federal Drug Administration. Sonda *et al.* recommended subcutaneous doses of 2.5 to 10.0 mg bethanechol every 4 hours to initiate treatment in patients with severely decompensated bladders (*84*). It is best accomplished in conjunction with intermittent catheterization in an inpatient environment because of the likelihood of severe parasympathetic side effects from the medication. If the patient is unable to void satisfactorily after 3 days, bethanechol is discontinued and the patient continued on intermittent catheterization. Oral maintenance doses averaged 50 mg four times per day, but higher dosages were often necessary.

Alpha-adrenolytic agents, alone and in combination with cholinergic agonists, have been employed to decrease outlet resistance and thus promote bladder emptying; a sound body of experimental evidence exists to support their use (*90,91*). However, most studies of alpha-adrenolytic agents have been performed on patients with bladder outlet obstruction due to benign prostatic hypertrophy or detrusor external sphincter dyssynergia (*23,92–94*). In one study of patients with "autonomous bladders", Norlen found that alpha-adrenolytic therapy in the form of phenoxybenzamine increased bladder capacity and at the same time reduced residual urine (*14*). Phenoxybenzamine has been shown to be mutagenic in mice and is no longer recommended for prolonged usage. Another agent, prazosin, is a postsynaptic alpha-adrenergic blocking agent that has fewer side effects than phenoxybenzamine and is not known to be mutagenic. Two milligrams prazosin seem to be equivalent to 10 mg of oral phenoxybenzamine (*91*).

Transurethral bladder neck or prostatic resection has been recommended even in young diabetics to reduce residual urine, and favorable results have been reported (*64,95–97*). However, no urodynamic data other than cystometry were reported in these series; the successes were generally judged by a fall in residual urine volume. Moreover, no data were presented to ensure that these patients did not have concomitant bladder outlet obstruction. It has been our unpublished experience that patients who have poor urinary flow and impaired bladder emptying due to impairment of detrusor contractility do poorly after transurethral vesical neck incision or prostatic resection.

Reduction cystoplasty and vesicoplication are two other surgical procedures recommended for the treatment of large-capacity, low-pressure bladders with high residual urine (*98*). However, in our experience, the large capacity and retention recur within a year. Moreover, there were no data in any of these studies to suggest that the patients being treated did in fact have diabetic cystopathy.

Another time-honored treatment for impaired bladder emptying is the use of the Credé maneuver (*64*). However, in a prospective urodynamic evaluation of the Credé manuever, we found that even on theoretical grounds it would be effective in only about 1 percent of patients (*99*). In order for the Credé maneuver to be therapeutically useful, the increase in intravesical pressure must not be completely transmitted to the flow-controlling zone in the urethra; the vesical neck must open, and the external sphincter must relax. Because these phenomena rarely accompany the Credé maneuver, it is only rarely useful; and in patients in whom the high intravesical pressures meet outlet resistance, it may prove to be harmful.

SUPRASPINAL NEUROLOGIC LESIONS

The effect of specific supraspinal neurologic lesions on vesicourethral function has not been well evaluated. Most suprapontine lesions, when they affect micturition, result in detrusor hyperreflexia with variable control of the external urethral sphincter, but urinary retention with an acontractile detrusor is occasionally seen as well.

In a clinical urodynamic study of 550 patients with detailed neurologic examination, 25 percent of patients with suprapontine neurologic lesions were found to have an acontractile bladder, and the remainder had either detrusor hyperreflexia with synergistic relaxation of the external urethral sphincter or normal micturition. No patient with a suprapontine lesion had detrusor–external sphincter dyssynergia; conversely, all patients with detrusor–external sphincter dyssynergia were found to have suprasacral lesions of the spinal cord (*1*). Of the patients with detrusor hyperreflexia, 50 percent retained voluntary control of the external sphincter despite the fact they were unable to prevent the onset of the involuntary detrusor contraction. These patients were able to interrupt the urinary stream by voluntarily contracting the sphincter. In half of those patients the involuntary detrusor contraction subsided once the sphincter contracted; but in the other half the detrusor contraction continued unabated, and once they could no longer maintain the sphincter contraction incontinence ensued.

In another study (*8*) of incontinent patients with suprapontine lesions, all were found to have detrusor hyperreflexia, but only 2 of the 18 patients had voluntary control of the external urethral sphincter: One had an isolated unilateral lesion of the frontal lobe and one a lesion of the parietal lobe.

Treatment Overview

Urinary bladder symptoms in patients with supraspinal neurologic lesions are usually due to either detrusor hyperreflexia with relaxation of the external urethral sphincter or a nonneurologic cause such as benign prostatic hypertrophy or stress urinary incontinence. When the etiology is of nonneurogenic origin, treatment is dictated by the same guidelines one uses in patients without neurologic disorders. A difficult therapeutic problem arises when a patient with a known suprasacral neurologic disorder and detrusor hyperreflexia also has an obstructing prostate. Detrusor instability is seen in at least 60 percent of men with obstructing prostatism without neurologic disorders, and it subsides in approximately half of them after successful surgery to relieve the obstruction (*45,100,101*). However, age-matched controls without benign prostatic hypertrophy had an identical incidence of instability (*101*). On the basis of these data it seems impossible, with current technology, to differentiate between neurogenic and nonneurogenic involuntary detrusor contractions. Nevertheless, certain guidelines may be useful when recommending prostatic surgery for these patients. If the patient has involuntary detrusor contractions of which he is totally unaware that result in urinary incontinence and he is unable to voluntarily contract the external sphincter when attempting to inhibit micturition, he will almost assuredly have incontinence after prostatectomy. On the other hand, if the patient senses the involuntary detrusor contraction as an urge to void and is able to voluntarily contract the external sphincter and interrupt the stream when attempting to inhibit micturition, that patient, in our unpublished experience, has at least a 50 percent chance of retaining continence after transurethral prostatectomy.

When it is determined that incontinence is due only to the neurologic lesion, it is managed as previously described, beginning with anticholinergics. It bears reemphasis that without treatment these patients are not at increased risk for developing urologic complications. They generally void normally from a physiologic standpoint; they simply lack control. Thus the only condition that needs to be treated is the incontinence, and if the degree of incontinence is socially acceptable no treatment is mandated. However, it is impossible to treat patients for incontinence whose mental status is such that they are either unaware or unconcerned.

Frontal Lobe Lesions

Isolated lesions of the frontal lobe are usually due to tumors, strokes, or aneurysms of the anterior communicating artery. Andrew and associates (*102,103*) found that lesions of the superomedial portion of the frontal lobe, the anterior portion of the cingulate gyrus, the genu of the corpus callosum, and the intervening white matter resulted in a characteristic syndrome. The patients had urinary incontinence due to detrusor hyperreflexia, and they lost the usual sensations of the urge to void, the feeling that micturition is imminent, and even the awareness the micturition is in progress. There are few data concerning sphincter abnormalities in these patients; however, Khan *et al.* (*8*) and Blaivas (*9*) found that voluntary sphincter control is independently preserved in at least some of them. The effect of unilateral versus bilateral and dominant versus nondominant lesions has not been studied.

Parkinson's Disease

Parkinson's disease is a degenerative disorder that chiefly affects the pigmented neurons of the substantia nigra. It results in a relative dopamine deficiency and a predominance of cholinergic activity on the corpus striatum. The classic symptoms consist in the clinical triad of bradykinesia, tremor, and skeletal rigidity. Yahr estimated the annual prevalence at 100 to 150 cases per 100,000 population (*104*).

The incidence of urinary bladder symptoms in Parkinson's disease is usually reported to be approximately 25 percent. Most symptomatic patients are found to have detrusor hyperreflexia at cystometry (*46,105–108*). Voluntary control of the external urethral sphincter was reportedly preserved in half the patients with detrusor hyperreflexia in one series (*46*). Pavalakis *et al.* reported that 75 percent of patients with detrusor hyperreflexia have "appropriate sphincter relaxation," but it was not clear if these patients retained voluntary sphincter control (*106*). They also described two patients with "sphincter bradykinesia" characterized by delayed relaxation of the external sphincter during the detrusor contraction.

Moreover, almost 60 percent of the men had diminished urinary flow rates consistent with a diagnosis of concomitant bladder outlet obstruction.

Because arteriosclerotic cerebrovascular disease is common in patients with Parkinson's disease, it is difficult to determine the etiology of the urodynamic abnormalities. In the study by Andersen *et al.* (*46*), because of the lack of age-matched controls, the authors were unable to determine whether the detrusor hyperreflexia was due to Parkinson's disease, other supraspinal neurologic lesions, or benign prostatic hypertrophy. On the basis of comparing cystometrograms before and after thalamic stimulation and ablation studies in animals (*109,110*) and thalamotomy in humans (*105,107*), it has been suggested that the net effect of the basal ganglia on micturition is one of inhibition. Accordingly, neurologic lesions that involve the basal ganglia are thought to release the micturition reflex from cortical inhibition, thereby resulting in detrusor hyperreflexia.

Shy-Drager Syndrome

Shy-Drager syndrome is an uncommon degenerative disorder that results in atrophy of the cerebellum, brainstem, peripheral autonomic ganglia, and the thoracolumbar preganglionic sympathetic neurons (*111*). The condition presents with progressive clinical features of Parkinsonism coupled with orthostatic hypotension and erectile impotence. Urinary symptoms are almost universal but nonspecific. Only a few reports of urodynamic studies have been published, most of which have shown detrusor hyperreflexia. Our experience has been quite different (*111a*). All of the patients we have seen have had the same urodynamic findings: (a) detrusor areflexia (sometimes with "autonomous waves") and (b) open vesical neck and isobaric proximal urethral segment and EMG evidence of lower motor neuron disease of the external urethral and external anal sphincter. These patients have had incontinence due to sphincter malfunction and incomplete bladder emptying due to an acontractile detrusor. Vesical neck obstruction has been reported by others, but vesical neck resection or transurethral prostatectomy has resulted in urinary incontinence or continued retention in most patients (*112–115*). Anticholinergics and intermittent catheterization was successful in one patient (*115*), but most patients are unable to catheterize themselves because of their cerebellar disease. Unfortunately, most patients have been relegated to indwelling vesical catheters.

Lumbar Disc Disease

Urinary bladder symptoms are present in approximately 10 percent of patients with lumbar disc disease (*116–118*). The symptoms are generally mild in nature and include urinary frequency, hesitancy, and a feeling of incomplete emptying. The sensation of the urge to void may be lost and replaced by a sensation of suprapubic fullness. Occasionally, acute urinary retention occurs. When lumbar disc disease is accompanied by signs of cauda equina compression, the pathophysiology is straightforward (*116*). However, even in the absence of these signs, bladder dysfunction is not uncommon (*118*). Cystometric abnormalities have been demonstrated in more than 80 percent of unselected patients with lumbar disc disease requiring treatment, yet less than 15 percent of these patients admitted having any any bladder symptoms at all (*118*). In that series 96 percent of the cystometrograms reverted to normal within 2 years, and most of the symptomatic patients were rendered asymptomatic. Aho *et al* retrospectively evaluated 18 patients who underwent emergency lumbar disc surgery because of acute cauda equina syndrome (*116*). The duration of symptoms ranged from 1 to 7 days. All of the patients reported "inability to void normally," and 15 of them had partial or complete urinary retention. Preoperative cystometry was performed in eight. All had impairment of bladder sensations and detrusor areflexia. Sixteen patients had postoperative cystometry that was performed 6 months to 3 years after surgery (mean, 16 months). Eleven of the 16 had persistent sensory impairment and detrusor areflexia. However, three of the patients with detrusor areflexia developed normal cystometry at follow-up. Overall, 11 of the 18 patients reported no bladder symptoms at follow-up despite the abnormal cystometric findings.

Two of the patients complained of "slight dripping of urine," but the problem was not evaluated further.

McGuire also reported on the rare occurrence of sphincteric incontinence (presumably due to neurologic impairment of the vesical neck and proximal urethral smooth muscle) in patients with herniated discs (*12*). Clinically, these patients had signs of somatic, sympathetic, and parasympathetic nerve injury, a triad that is difficult to explain on the basis of lumbosacral disc disease.

On rare occasions, urinary bladder symptoms are the sole complaint of patients with lumbar disc disease or other occult neurologic disorders (*52,53,119,120*). Emmett and Love reported on 35 patients who they believed to have vesical dysfunction caused by occult herniated lumbar discs (*120*). There were 30 women and 5 men with a variety of obstructive and irritative symptoms ranging from complete urinary retention to frequency and urgency. The hallmark of the diagnosis was the presence of the "classic cystoscopic findings," which included: (a) diminished vesical sensation; (b) loss of the normal "desire to void," which was replaced by a vague sense of abdominal fullness; (c) absence of pain or discomfort when the cystoscope is "prodded" against the trigone; (d) absence of vesical trabeculation; and (e) increased bladder capacity. Surprisingly, the neurologic examination was generally unremarkable, and other signs of nerve root compression, e.g., positive straight leg raising, were often absent. Nevertheless, all of these patients underwent myelography because of the cystoscopic findings. Forty percent were found to have centrally protruding discs, 46 percent had equivocal findings, and 6 percent had a negative myelogram. All patients underwent surgical exploration and were found to have centrally protruding discs. The site of the disc was L_4 in 29 patients (83%), L_3 in two, L_4 in two, L_4 and L_5 in one, and no herniation was found in one. The patients were followed for approximately 1 year, and the overall clinical results were as follows: 49 percent returned to normal, 20 percent were improved from a urologic standpoint but developed back pain that was not present preoperatively, and 31 percent were unimproved by the surgery.

Check *et al.* (*119*) reported a series of eight patients whose clinical histories were similar to those reported by Emmett and Love (*120*). In addition to the clinical and cystoscopic examinations, these patients underwent urodynamic evaluation. All voided by abdominal straining and had acontractile detrusors at cystometry. Urinary flow rate was markedly diminished, and during micturition they were unable to relax the striated muscles of the pelvic floor. They all had large postvoid residual urine volumes. Five of the eight patients had negative myelograms, and all underwent exploratory surgery. A midline protruded disc was found in six patients, five at L_4 and one at L_5. Postoperatively all patients had transitory improvement of bladder symptoms, and the improvement persisted in five. Of the five with persistent improvement, three underwent urodynamic studies, which were unchanged in two and normal in one.

As the results of these studies attest, relatively little is known about the true incidence, natural history, or treatment of vesicourethral dysfunction caused by lumbar disc disease. It seems evident that certain patients with disc disease do develop "neurogenic bladder," and that when a cauda equina syndrome is present the diagnosis is clear-cut. However, only a few patients present with so clear a clinical picture, and those patients usually require surgery. A more difficult diagnostic problem arises when patients have the "classic findings" described by Emmett and Love (*120*) but no objective signs of neurogenic impairment. It is my opinion that, in the absence of objective signs of neuropathy, further invasive neurologic work-up and surgical exploration are unwarranted. However, when subtle neurologic findings are present, complete neurologic investigation is mandatory. These subtle but objective findings include: absence of the bulbocavernosus reflex, diminished perianal sensation, diminished anal sphincter tone and control, EMG findings consistent with neurologic disorders, and an unexplained "open" vesical neck during cystography (*12,35,52,53*).

The most rational treatment for patients with urinary bladder symptoms due to lumbar disc disease is to treat the underlying disorder. Unfortunately, there is a paucity of data with respect to the efficacy of such treatment. In most patients without significant bladder symptoms the abnormal cystometric findings revert to normal, but in patients with significant bladder symptoms preoperatively the results are less encouraging. At the present time it seems reasonable to perform surgery for cauda equina syndrome due to ruptured disc; our experience suggests, however, a high incidence of persistent symptoms after back surgery. At the present time, it seems reasonable to recommend surgery when bladder symptoms are severe, but when they are mild a more conservative approach should be undertaken.

Guillain-Barré Syndrome

The Guillain-Barré syndrome is characterized by a symmetrically progressive paralysis that usually reaches maximum by 4 weeks followed by a gradual but complete recovery over the course of approximately 6 months. The pathology is a polyradiculopathy, which primarily involves demyelination of the junction of the anterior and posterior spinal nerve roots (*121*). The brunt of the demyelination involves the anterior root, accounting for the clinical observation that the predominant finding is one of motor neuropathy with little if any sensory involvement. Although the incidence of vesicourethral involvement has ranged from 0 to 40 percent, it is rarely a significant clinical problem (*121–126*). Virtually all of the reported patients with urologic symptoms had some degree of urinary retention as the major symptom and, of the eight who underwent urodynamic studies, four were found to have evidence of lower motor neuron disease involving both the detrusor (detrusor areflexia, impaired sensation, and a positive bethanechol test) and the striated external sphincter (increased number of polyphasic potentials and poor recruitment). The remaining patients were inexplicably found to have detrusor hyperreflexia accompanied by relaxation of the external urethral sphincter. Two of these patients also had a positive Babinski reflex, which is indicative of pyramidal tract involvement and is not part of the usual findings in the Guillain-Barré syndrome (*51,127,128*). Treatment is initiated with intermittent catheterization until the neurologic process resolves.

REFERENCES

1. Blaivas, J. G.: The Neurophysiology of micturition: a clinical study of 550 patients, *J. Urol.* 127:958, 1982.
2. Bradley, W. E., and Conway, C. J.: Bladder representation in the pontine mesencephalic reticular formation. *Exp. Neurol.* 16:237, 1966.
3. DeGroat, W. C., Booth, A. M., Krier, J., Milner, R. J., Morgan, C., and Nadelhaft, I.: Neural control of the urinary bladder and large intestine. In McBrooks, C., Koizumi, K., and Sato, A., (eds), *Integrative Functions of the Autonomic Nervous System.* Elsvier, Amsterdam, 1979, Chap. 4.
4. Blaivas, J. G., Sinha, H. P., Zayed, A. A. H., and Labib, K. B.: Detrusor–external sphincter dyssynergia. *J. Urol.* 125:542, 1981.
5. Blaivas, J. G., and Fisher, D. M.: Combined radiographic and urodynamic monitoring: advances in technique. *J. Urol.* 125:693, 1981.
6. McGuire, E. J., and Brady, S.: Detrusor–sphincter dyssynergia, *J. Urol.* 121:774, 1979.
7. Blaivas, J. G., and Barbalias, G. A.: Detrusor–external sphincter dyssynergia in men with multiple sclerosis: an ominous urological condition. *J. Urol.* 131:91, 1984.
8. Khan, Z., Hertanu, J., Yang, W. C., Melman, A. M., and Leiter, E.: Predictive correlation of urodynamic dysfunction in brain injury after cerebrovascular accident. *J. Urol.* 126:86, 1981.
9. Blaivas, J. G., and Katz, G. P.: The role of urodynamic testing in evaluating subtle neurologic lesions. In *Proceeding of the International Continence Society, Twelfth Annual Meeting,* Leiden, 1982, pp. 43–45.
9a. Blaivas, J. G., and Barbalias, G. A.: Characteristics of neural injury after abdominal perineal resection of the rectum. *J. Urol.* 129:84, 1983.
10. Chang, P. L., and Fan, H. A.: Urodynamic studies before and/or after abdominoperineal resection of the rectum for carcinoma. *J. Urol.* 130:948, 1983.
11. Gerstenberg, T. C., Nielsen, M. L., Clausen, S., Blaabjerg, J., and Lindenberhg, J.: Bladder function after abdominoperineal resection of the rectum for anorectal cancer: urodynamic investigation before and after operation in a consecutive series. *Ann. Surg.* 191:81, 1980.
12. McGuire, E. J.: Urodynamic evaluation after abdominal perineal resection and lumbar intervertebral disc herniation. *Urology* 6:663, 1975.
13. Yalla, S. V., and Andriole, G.: Vesicourethral dysfunction following pelvic visceral ablative surgery. *J. Urol.* 132:503, 1984.
14. Norlen, L.: The autonomous bladder: a clinical and experimental study. *Scand. J. Urol. Nephrol.* [*Suppl.*]36:1, 1976.
15. McGuire, E. J., and Wagner, F. C., Jr.: The effects of sacral denervation on bladder and urethral function. *Surg. Gynecol. Obstet.* 144:343, 1977.
16. McGuire, E. J., and Savastano, J. A.: Effect of alpha adrenergic blockade, and anticholinergic agents on the decentralized primate. *Neurourol. Urodyn.* 4:2, 1985.
17. Maggi, C., Santicioli, P., and Meli, A.: Sympa-

thetic inhibition of reflex activation of bladder motility during filling at a physiological like rate in urethane anaesthetized rats. *Neurourol. Urodyn.* 4:2, 1985.
18. Ghoniem, G. M., Regnier, C. H., Biancani, P., Johnson, L., and Susset, J.: Effect of bilateral sacral decentralization on detrusor contractility and passive properties in dog. *Neurourol. Urodyn.* 3:23, 1984.
19. Klevmark, B.: Motility of the urinary bladder in cats during filling at physiologic rates. I. Intravesical pressure patterns studies by a new method of cystometry. *Acta Physiol. Scand.* 90:565, 1974.
20. Klevmark, B. J.: Motility of the urinary bladder in cats during filling at physiologic rates. II. Effects of extrinsic bladder denervation on intramural tension and on intravesical pressure patterns. *Acta Physiol. Scand.* 101:176, 1977.
21. McGuire, E. J., Woodside, J. R., Borden, T. A., and Weiss, R. M.: Prognostic value of urodynamic testing in myelodyplastic patients. *J. Urol.* 124:205, 1981.
22. Blaivas, J. G., and Barbalias, G. A.: Characteristics of neural injury after abdominal perineal resection of the rectum. *J. Urol.* 129:84, 1983.
23. Gerstenberg, T., Blaaberg, J. M., Nielsen, M. L., and Clausen, S.: Phenoxybenzamine reduces bladder outlet obstruction in benign prostatic obstruction: a urodynamic investigation. *Invest. Urol.* 18:29, 1980.
24. Wein, A. J.: Classification of neurogenic voiding dysfunction. *J. Urol.* 125:605–609, 1981.
25. Blaivas, J. G.: Management of bladder dysfunction in multiple sclerosis. *Neurology* 30:12–18, 1980.
26. Katz, G. P., and Blaivas, J. G.: A diagnostic dilemma: when urodynamic findings differ from the clinical impression. *J. Urol.* 129:1170, 1983.
27. MacDonald, W. I.: Pathophysiology in multiple sclerosis. *Brain* 97:179–196, 1974.
28. Fog, T.: Topographic distribution of plaques in the spinal cord in multiple sclerosis. *Arch. Neurol. Psychiatry* 63:382–414, 1950.
29. Oppenheimer, D. R.: The cervical cord in multiple sclerosis, *Neuropathol. Appl. Neurobiol.* 4: 151–162, 1978.
30. Barrington, F. J. F.: The localization of the paths serving micturition in the spinal cord of the cat. *Brain* 56:126, 1933.
31. Nathan, P. W., and Smith, N. C.: The centripetal pathway from the bladder and urethra within the spinal cord. *J. Neurol. Neurosurg. Psychiatry* 14:262, 1951.
32. Nathan, P. W., and Smith, N. C.: The centrifugal pathway for micturition with the spinal cord. *J. Neurol. Neurosurg. Psychiatry* 21:177, 1958.
33. Andersen, J. T., and Bradley, W. E.: Abnormalities of detrusor and sphincter dysfunction in multiple sclerosis. *Br. J. Urol.* 48:193–198, 1976.
34. Awad, S. A., Downie, J. W., Sogbein, S. K., Murray, J. T., and Field, C. A.: Relationship between neurologic and urologic status in patients with multiple sclerosis. *J. Urol.* 132:499, 1984.
35. Blaivas, J. G., Bhimani, G., and Labib, K. L.: Vesicourethral dysfunction in multiple sclerosis. *J. Urol.* 122:342–347, 1979.
36. Miller, H., Simpson, C. A., and Yeates, W. K.: Bladder dysfunction in multiple sclerosis. *Br. Med. J.* 1:1265, 1965.
37. Piazza, D. H., and Diokno, A. C.: Review of neurogenic bladder in multiple sclerosis, *Urology* 14:33, 1979.
38. Philp, T., Read, D. J., and Higson, R. H.: The urodynamic characteristics of multiple sclerosis. *Br. J. Urol.* 53:672–675, 1981.
39. Goldstein, I., Siroky, M. B., Sax, D. S., and Krane, R. J.: Neurourologic abnormalities in multiple sclerosis. *J. Urol.* 128:541, 1982.
40. Postkanzer, D. C., Schapira, K., and Miller, H.: Epidemiology of multiple sclerosis in the countries of Northumberland and Durham. *J. Neurol. Neurosurg. Psychiatry* 26:368, 1963.
41. Leibowitz, U., Kahana, E., Jacobson, S. G., and Alter, M.: The cause of death in multiple sclerosis. In Leibowitz, U. (ed.), *Progress in Multiple Sclerosis: Research and Treatment.* Academic Press, New York, 1972, pp. 196–209.
42. Samellas, W., and Rubin, B.: Management of upper urinary tract complications in multiple sclerosis by means of urinary diversion to an ileal conduit. *J. Urol.* 93:548, 1965.
43. Damansky, M., and Sutcliffe-Kerr, A.: Paraplegia of nontraumatic origin and disseminated multiple sclerosis: urinary complications, their nature and treatment. *Acta Neuro. Psychiatr. Belg.* 64:495, 1964.
44. Jameson, R. M.: Management of the bladder in nontraumatic paraplegia. *Paraplegia* 12:92, 1974.
45. Anderson, J. T.: Detrusor hyperreflexia in benign infravesical obstruction. *J. Urol.* 115:532, 1976.
46. Anderson, J. T., Helbjorn, S., Frimødt-Moller, C., Walter, S., and Worm-Petersen, J.: Disturbances of micturition in Parkinson's disease. *Acta Neurol. Scand.* 53:161–170, 1976.
47. Bradley, W. E., Logothetis, J. L., and Timm, G. W.: Cystometric and sphincter abnormalities in multiple sclerosis: *Neurology* 23:1131–1139, 1973.
48. Ketalaer, P., Leruitte, A., and Vereecken, R. L.: Striated sphincter urethral and anal sphincter electromyography during cystometry in multiple sclerosis. *Electromyogr. Clin. Neurophysiol.* 17:427, 1977.
49. Summers, J. L.: Neurogenic bladder in the woman with multiple sclerosis, *J. Urol.* 120:555, 1978.
50. McGuire, E. M.: The neuropathic urethra. In Mundy, A. R., Stephenson, T. P., and Wein, A. J., (eds.), *Urodynamics: Principles, Practice and Application.* Chruchill Livingstone, Edingburgh, 1984.
51. Wheller, S., Siroky, M. B., Pavlakis, A. J., Goldstein, I., and Krane, R. J.: The changing neurourologic pattern of multiple sclerosis. *J. Urol.* 130:1123, 1983.
52. Blaivas, J. G., Labib, K. B., and Scott, R. M.: Urodynamic evaluation as a test of sacral cord function. *Urology* 9:682, 1979.
53. Blaivas, J. G.: A critical appraisal of specific diagnostic techniques. In *Clinical Neurourology.* Little, Brown, Boston, 1979.
54. Thomas, P. K., and Lascelles, R. G.: The pathology of diabetic neuropathy. *J. Med.* 35:489, 1978.
55. Faerman, I., Glacer, C. M., Celemer, D. M., Jadzinsky, M., Fox, D., Maler, M., and Alverex, E.:

Autonomic nervous system and diabetes: histological and histochemical study of the autonomic nerve fibers of the urinary bladder in diabetic patients. Diabetes 22:255, 1973.
56. Ellenberg, M.: Neurologic changes in early diabetes. *Adv. Metab. Disord.* 2:459, 1973.
57. Frimødt-Moller, C., and Hald, T.: A new method for quantitative evaluation of bladder sensibility. *Scand. J. Urol. Nephrol.* 15:135–142, 1972.
58. Frimødt-Moller, C.: Diabetic cystopathy. I. A clinical study on the frequency of bladder dysfunction in diabetes. *Dan. Med. Bull.* 23:279, 1976.
59. Spring, M., and Hymes, J.: Neurogenic bladder dysfunction as a complication of diabetes. *Diabetes* 2:199, 1953.
60. Martin, M. M.: Diabetic neuropathy: a clinical study of 150 cases. *Brain* 76:594, 1953.
61. Ellenberg, M., and Weber, H.: The incipient asymptomatic diabetic bladder. *Diabetes* 16:331, 1967.
62. Faerman, I., Maler, M., Jadzinski, M., Fox, D., Alvarex, E., Zilbervarg, J., Cibeira, J. B., and Colinas, R.: Asymptomatic neurogenic bladder in juvenile diabetes. *Diabetologia* 7:169, 1971.
63. Fagerberg, S. E., Koch, N. G., Petersen, I., and Stener, I.: Urinary bladder disturbances in diabetics. *Scand. J. Urol. Nephrol.* 1:19, 1967.
64. Kahan, M., Goldberg, P. D., and Mandel, E. E.: Neurogenic vesical dysfunction in diabetes mellitus. *New York J. Med.* 2:2448, 1970.
65. Bossi, L., and Caffaralli, E.: Tube vesicali in diabetici con neuropatia studio clinico e radiologico. *Minerva Radiol.* 13:40, 1968.
66. Larcan, A., Huriet, C., Vaillandet, M., and Fauchier, J. P., Les manifestations vesicales au cours due diabetes: interet de la cystomanometrie. *Presse Med.* 73:273, 1965.
67. Reed, P. I., Buck, A. C., McRea, C. U., Siddig, Y. K., Chisholm, G. D., and Fraser, T. R.: Vesicourethral dysfunction and neuropathy in diabetes. In *Proceedings VIII Congress of the International Diabetes Federation,* Brussels, 1973.
68. Bartley, O., Brolin, I., Fagerberg, S. E., and Wilhemsen, L.: Neurogenic disorders of the bladder in diabetes mellitus. *Acta Med. Scand.* 108:187, 1966.
69. Norlen, L., Blaivas, J. G., and Gabel, H.: Cystopathy in patients with severe diabetic nephropathy. *Diabetes Nephrol.* 1983.
70. Bradley, W. E., Timm, G. W., and Scott, F. B.: Cystometry. V. Bladder sensation. *Urology.* 6:654, 1975.
71. Carlsson, C. A., and Sundin, T.: *Neurogenic Bladder Disease.* Elanders, Götteberg, 1974.
72. Frimødt-Moller, C., and Hald, T.: Clinical urodynamics, methods and results. *Scand. J. Urol. Nephrol.* 6:143, 1972.
73. Frimødt-Moller, C.: Diabetic cystopathy. II. Relationship to some late diabetic manifestations. *Dan. Med. Bull.* 23:279, 1976.
74. Weir, J., and Jaques, P. F.: Large capacity bladder, a urodynamic survey. *Urology* 4:544–548, 1974.
75. Rocca Rosetti, S., Boccafoschi, C., Maurel, A., and Marega, D.: Physiopathology of the diabetic bladder. Presented at the Annual Meeting of the Italian Urodynamics Society, Sorrento, 1982.
76. Yalla, S. V., Sharma, G. V. R. K., and Barsamian, E. M.: Micturitional urethral pressure profile during voiding and the implications. *J. Urol.* 124:649, 1980.
77. Yalla, S. V., Waters, W. B., Snyder, H., Varady, S., and Blute, R.: Urodynamic localization of isolated bladder neck obstruction in men: studies with micturitional vesourethral static pressure profile. *J. Urol.* 125:677, 1981.
78. Robbins, S. L., and Tucker, A. W., Jr. The cause of death in diabetes: a report of 307 autopsied cases. *N. Engl. J. Med.* 231:865, 1944.
79. Edmonson, H. A., Martin, H. E., and Evans, N.: Necrosis of renal papillae and acute pyelonephritis in diabetes mellitus. *Arch. Intern. Med.* 79:148, 1947.
80. Vejlsgaard, R.: Bakteruiri, Thesis, Copenhagen, Fadl, 1973.
81. Lapides, J., Diokno, A. C., Gould, F. R., and Lowe, B. S.: Further observations of self catheterization. *J. Urol.* 116:169, 1976.
82. Downie, J. W., Moochhala, S. M., and Bialik, J. G.: The role of reflexes in modifying the response to bethanechol chloride: a basis for selectivity of action on the bladder. *Neurourol. Urodyn.* 2:301, 1983.
83. Downie, J. W.: Bethanechol chloride in urology—a discussion of issues. *Neurourol. Urodyn.* 3:211, 1984.
84. Sonda, L. P., Gershon, C., Diokno, A. C., and Lapides, J.: Further observations on the cystometric and uroflowmetric effects of bethanechol chloride on the human bladder. *J. Urol.* 122:775–777, 1979.
85. Barrett, D. M.: The effect of oral bethanechol chloride on voiding in female patients with excessive residual urine: a randomized double blind study. *J. Urol.* 126:640, 1981.
86. Light, K. J., and Scott, F. B.: Bethanechol chloride and the traumatic cord bladder. *J. Urol.* 128:85, 1982.
87. Wein, A. J., Hanno, P. M., Dixon, D. O., Raezer, D. M., and Benson, G. S.: The effect of oral bethanechol chloride on the cystometrogram of the normal male adult. *J. Urol.* 120:330, 1978.
88. Wein, A. J., Malloy, T. P., Shofer, F., and Raezer, D. M.: The effects of bethanechol chloride on urodynamic parameters in normal women and women with significant residual urine volumes. *J. Urol.* 124:397, 1980.
89. Yalla, S. V., Rossier, A. B., and Fam, B.: Dyssynergia vesicourethral responses during bladder rehabilitation in spinal cord injury patients: effect of suprapubic percussion, Credé method and bethanechol chloride. *J. Urol.* 115:575, 1976.
90. Norlen, L., and Sundin, T.: Alpha-adrenolytic treatment in patients with autonomous bladders. *Acta Pharmacol. Toxicol. (Copenh.)* 43:31, 1978.
91. Norlen, L.: Influence of the sympathetic nervous system on the lower urinary tract and clinical implications. *Neurol. Urodyn.* 1:125, 1982.
92. Caine, M., Pfau, A., and Perlberg, S.: The use of alpha adrenergic blockers in benign prostatic obstruction. *Br. J. Urol.* 48:255, 1976.
93. Caine, M., Perlberg, S., and Meretyk, S.: A placebo controlled double-blind study of the effect

of phenoxybenzamine in benign prostatic obstruction. *Br. J. Urol.* 50:551, 1978.
94. Caine, M., Perlberg, A., and Shapira, A.: Phenoxybenzamine for benign prostatic obstruction. *Urology* 17:542, 1981.
95. Emmett, J. L., Daut, R. V., and Sprague, R. G.: Transurethral resection for neurogenic vesical dysfunction in cases of diabetic neuropathy. *J. Urol.* 61:244, 1949.
96. Weinberg, S. R.: Transurethral resection of the vesical neck for relief of diabetic neurogenic dysfunction of the bladder. *N.Y. State J. Med.* 56:882, 1956.
97. Zincke, H., Cambell, J. T., and Furlow, W. L.: Neurogenic vesical dysfunction in diabetes mellitus. *Br. J. Urol.* 11:448, 1974.
98. Stewart, H. H.: The surgical treatment of severe chronic retention without large diverticula. *Br. J. Urol.* 38:685, 1966.
99. Barbalias, G. A., Klauber, G. T., and Blaivas, J. G.: Critical evaluation of the Credé manuever: urodynamic study of 207 patients. *J. Urol.* 130:720, 1983.
100. Abrams, P. H., Farrar, D. J., Turner-Warwick, R. T., Whiteside, C. G., and Feneley, R. C., L.: The results of prostatectomy: a symptomatic and urodynamic analysis of 152 patients. *J. Urol.* 121:640, 1979.
101. Anderson, J. T.: Prostatism: clinical, radiologic, and urodynamic aspects. *Neurourol. Urodyn.* 1:241–293, 1982.
102. Andrew, J., and Nathan, P. W.: Lesions of the anterior frontal lobes and disturbances of micturition and defecation. *Brain* 87:233, 1964.
103. Andrew, J., Nathan, P. W., and Spanos, N. C.: Disturbances of micturition and defecation due to aneurysms of anterior communicating or anterior cerebral arteries. *J. Neurosurg.* 24:1, 1966.
104. Yahr, M. D.: Parkinson's disease—overview of its current status. *Mt. Sinai J. Med.* 44:183, 1977.
105. Murnaghan, G. F.: Neurogenic disorders of the bladder in parkinsonism, *Br. J. Urol.* 33:403, 1961.
106. Pavalakis, A. J., Siroky, M. B., and Siroky, R. J.: Neurourologic findings in Parkinson's disease. *J. Urol.* 129:80–83, 1983.
107. Porter, R. W., and Bors, E. M.: Neurogenic bladder in parkinsonism: effect of thalamotomy. *J. Neurosurg.* 34:27, 1971.
108. Schneider, E., Patras, L., and Fischer, P. A.: Neurogene Blasenstorungen bei Morbus Parkinson. *Fortschr. Neurol. Psychiatr.* 46:260–268, 1978.
109. Lewin, R. J., and Porter, R. W.: Inhibition of spontaneous bladder activity by stimulation of the globus pallidus. *Neurology* 15:1049, 1965.
110. Lewin, R. J., Dillard, G. V., and Porter, R. W.: Extrapyramidal inhibition of the urinary bladder. *Brain Res.* 4:301, 1967.
111. Bannister, R., and Oppenheimer, D. R.: Degenerative diseases of the nervous system associated with autonomic failure. *Brain* 95:457, 1972.
111a. Salinas, J. M., Berger, Y., de la Rocha, R. E., and Blaivas, J. G.: Urologic evaluation in the Shy-Drager syndrome. *J. Urol.* 135:741, 1986.
112. Lockhart, J. L., Webster, G. D., Sheremata, W., Camuzzi, F. A., and Carrion, H. C.: Neurogenic bladder dysfunction in the Shy Drager syndrome. *J. Urol.* 126:119, 1981.
113. Sakuta, M., Nakanishi, T., and Tokokura, Y. M.: Anal muscle electromyograms differ in amyotrophic lateral sclerosis and Shy Drager syndrome. *Neurology* 28:1289, 1978.
114. Singh, N., and Fahn, S.: Electrophysiologic studies in the Shy Drager syndrome. *Neurology* 30:394, 1980.
115. Wulfsoh, A., and Rubenstein, A. M.: The management of Shy-Drager syndrome with propantheline and Intermittent catheterization. *J. Urol.* 126:122, 1981.
116. Aho, A. J., Auranen, A. M., and Pesonen, K.: Analysis of cauda equina symptoms in patients with lumbar disc prolapse. *Acta Chir Scand.* 135:413, 1969.
117. Konturi, M., Harviaiment, M., and Larmi, T. R.: Atonic bladder in lumbar disc herniation. *Acta Chir. Scand.* [*Suppl.*] 35:232, 1966.
118. Rosomoff, H. L., Johnson, J. D. H., Gallo, A. E., Ludmer, M., Givens, F. T., Carnery, F. T., and Kuehn, C. A.: Cystometry as an adjunct in the evaluation of lumbar disc syndromes. *J. Neurosurg.* 33:68, 1970.
119. Cheek, W. R., Anchondo, H., Raso, E., and Scott, R.: Neurogenic bladder and the lumbar spine. *Urology* 2:July, 1973.
120. Emmett, J. L., and Love, J. G.,: Vesical dysfunction caused by protruded lumbar disk. *J. Urol.* 105:86, 1971.
121. Haymaker, W., and Kernohan, J. W.: The Landry-Guillain-Barré syndrome: a clinicopathologic report of 50 fatal cases and a critique of the literature. *Medicine (Baltimore)*, 28:519, 1949.
122. Soffer; D., Feldman, A., and Alter, M.: Clinical features of Guillain-Barré syndrome. *J. Neurol. Sci.* 37:135, 1978.
123. Osler, L. D., and Sodell, A. D.: The Guillain-Barré syndrome: the need for exact diagnostic criteria. *N. Engl. J. Med.* 262:964, 1960.
124. Lichtenfeld, P.: Autonomic dysfunction in the Guillain-Barré syndrome. *Am. J. Med.* 50:772, 1971.
125. Swash, M.: Clinical aspects of Guillain-Barré syndrome: a review. *J. R. Soc. Med.* 72:670, 1979.
126. Samantray, S. K., Johnson, S. C., Mathai, K. V., and Pulimood, B. M.: Landry Guillain Barré Strohl syndrome, a study of 302 cases. *Med. J. Aust.* 2:184, 1977.
127. Kogan, B. A., Solomon, M. H., and Diokno, A. C.: Urinary retention secondary to Guillain-Barré syndrome. *J. Urol.* 131:917, 1984.
128. Wheeler, J. S., Siroky, M. B., Pavlakis, A. M., and Krane, R. J.: The urodynamic aspects of the Guillain-Barré syndrome. *J. Urol.* 131:917, 1984.

23

Psychogenic Voiding Dysfunction

MIKE B. SIROKY, M.D., AND ROBERT J. KRANE, M.D.

Patients complaining of voiding dysfunction of obscure etiology constitute a significant portion of urologic outpatient practice. Because standard clinical investigation has by and large failed to elucidate the etiology in this group of patients, urodynamic techniques have been increasingly utilized. There is no question that urodynamics has been helpful in understanding the mechanisms of symptom production and therefore in managing these symptoms. However, understanding the source of these symptoms requires a broader viewpoint than urodynamics alone can provide. The aims of this chapter are to provide an overview of the problem in the adult in terms of incidence and diagnosis and to highlight the contribution of urodynamics to its management.

Definition and Prevalence

Psychogenic voiding dysfunction is a diagnosis of exclusion. Thus it is defined more in terms of what it is *not* than in terms of what it is. This method is necessarily so because the recognition of psychologic disturbance is imprecise; and, even if obviously present, its relation to genitourinary symptomatology is difficult to demonstrate. Psychogenic voiding dysfunction is a clinical syndrome characterized by urologic symptoms in the absence of organic genitourinary or neurologic pathology. A correlation between the onset of the syndrome and psychologic disturbance can be demonstrated. Furthermore, the syndrome is characterized by a significant response to behavioral, psychologic or psychopharmacologic therapies. This definition of the problem is in fact a somewhat narrow one as it excludes those patients found to have some deviation from normal (mucosal erythema, vesical neck polyps, trigonitis) that has nothing to do with their symptoms.

The possible relations between organic disease, psychologic disturbance, and symptomatology are indicated in Figure 23–1. An organic lesion (e.g., bladder tumor) leading directly to a symptom (e.g., hematuria) is the sequence of events that physicians are trained to recognize. However, consider the situation in which the same patient, on being told of the presence of a tumor, develops a short-lived episode of urinary urgency and frequency. Are the symptoms due to the organic lesion, the psychologic disturbance, or both? Now consider the situation in which no organic pathology exists but a psychologic disturbance per se is the cause of urgency and frequency. This situation is probably the most common form of psychogenic voiding dysfunction seen for urodynamic referral because it tends to be the most chronic. Finally, we need to consider the situation wherein a psychologic disturbance is possibly the cause of organic changes in the urinary tract (? interstitial cystitis, ? chronic retention of urine with damage to the detrusor). In the latter circumstance, separation of cause and effect becomes extremely difficult if not impossible.

The prevalence of psychosomatic complaints in urologic practice has been estimated at 50 percent (*1*). This high prevalence should not be surprising when one considers the psychosexual implications of the acts of micturition and reproduction. A

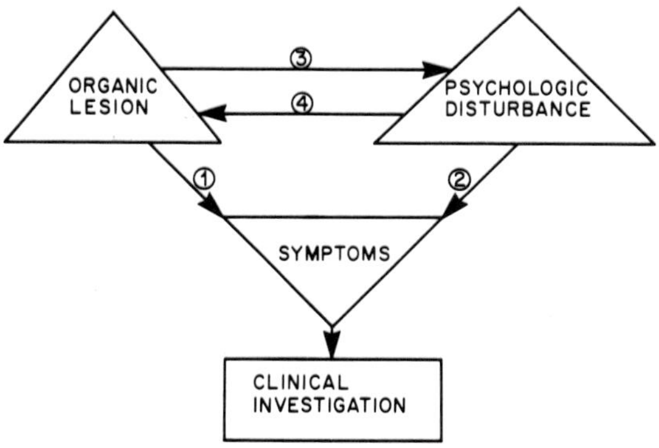

Figure 23–1. Possible relations between organic disease, psychologic disturbance, and symptoms. See text for further discussion.

review of our experience indicates that, for both men and women, psychogenic voiding dysfunction constitutes approximately 20 percent of urodynamic referrals. Because the cases referred for urodynamic study tend to be the most chronic and refractory to standard therapy, the prevalence in general urologic practice is undoubtedly higher.

PSYCHOGENIC URINARY RETENTION

Incidence

Acute urinary retention in women (due to any cause) is generally thought to be rare. However, in a review of 3 years' experience in Bristol, U.K., Doran and Roberts (*2*) were able to identify 103 cases. Of these, 33 occurred postpartum and 25 postoperatively. Of the remaining 45 cases, 17 (38%) were due to gynecologic causes (pelvic mass), 15 (33%) were due to urologic causes (obstruction and infection), 7 (16%) were neurogenic, and only 3 (7%) were thought to be definitely psychiatric. However, as Frewen (*3*) has pointed out, if postpartum/postoperative retention is included as psychosomatic manifestation, the proportion with psychogenic etiology rises to 59% of women with "idiopathic" urinary retention. This experience emphasizes that psychogenic urinary retention is a diagnosis to be made only after thorough investigation has ruled out organic causes (Table 23–1).

Table 23–1. Organic Causes of Urinary Retention in Women

Postpartum
Postoperative
Pelvic mass
Procidentia
Bladder neck obstruction
Urethral obstruction
Multiple sclerosis
Herpes zoster
Herniated disc
Fecal impaction

Etiology:

This condition afflicts women almost exclusively (*4*), although a similar syndrome has been described in adult men (*5*) as well as young boys (*6*). Smith mentioned that it may occur in male homosexuals following acute psychosexual stress (*7*). The psychiatric literature is replete with case studies of urinary retention secondary to various psychologic causes (Table 23–2). The psychosexual nature of many of these psychologic insults is apparent.

Objective evidence of a psychologic disorder in patients presenting with idiopathic urinary retention was first provided by Larson *et al.* in 1963 (*4*). Of 37 patients evaluated by the Minnesota Multiphasic Personality Inventory (MMPI), 12 patients had evidence of hysterical neurosis and 8 were found to be psychotic. In our experience, a psychosocial insult leading to urinary retention could be identified in approximately 50 percent of cases using clinical examination only (*8*).

Table 23–2. Psychologic Causes of Urinary Retention in Women Reported in the Literature

Hysteria
Psychosis
Rape
Incest
Abortion
Pelvic surgery
Sterility
Marriage
Death of close relative
Hostility toward parents

Clinical Presentation

The patient typically presents to an emergency room claiming that she has not passed urine for a long time. She may be anxious or overwrought, but more often she displays a remarkable lack of concern regarding her situation (*la belle indifference*). For this reason, taking a history from these patients requires direct and pointed questioning, as they rarely offer information spontaneously. The bladder is easily palpable and may be tender. Evidence of hydronephrosis or uremia is generally absent. On catheterization, a large volume of clear urine is drawn from the bladder.

Differential Diagnosis

It cannot be overemphasized that a careful exclusion of organic disease is mandatory in these patients (Table 23–1). Even if a patient is obviously a hysteric, she may still have organic pathology as the cause of her symptoms. Therefore thorough neurologic, gynecologic, urologic, and rectal examinations are performed in all cases.

As noted above, not all cases of psychogenic, urinary retention are due to hysteria; some are secondary to well-defined traumatic events in an individual's life (e.g., abortion). Hysteria is a specific psychiatric diagnosis with characteristic findings. The implication of a diagnosis of hysteria is that of a *life-long* disorder of which urinary retention is only one of many manifestations. Thus hysterical urinary retention is a particular subgroup within the broader diagnostic category of psychogenic urinary retention.

Hysteria is a chronic, lifelong, psychologic disorder that is seen almost exclusively in women and is characterized by repetitive, dramatic somaticization. It has its onset usually prior to age 30 and extends over many years. The patient has complaints involving multiple organs for which no physical cause can be found. The reporting of symptoms tends to be markedly exaggerated ("It's like someone put a knife in my urethra"). There is typically a long history of multiple diagnostic procedures, hospitalizations, or surgical operations with negative or unconvincing findings. Paul Briquet in 1859 offered the following terse description, "They may spend a year or more in bed, completely incapacitated. They are always sick, abort easily, or if they go to term, give birth to more hysterics" (*9*).

Perley and Guze (*10*) devised criteria as an aid to the specific diagnosis of hysteria (Table 23–3). Patients who fulfill these criteria have been found on long-term follow-up to have stability of their hysterical nature; i.e., they do not spontaneously improve. The ability to make a specific diagnosis of hysteria is enormously helpful for managing these patients from a urologic viewpoint. The realization that the patient has a chronic psychologic disorder should temper the physician's enthusiasm for risky diagnostic or therapeutic procedures.

Urodynamic Findings

There is scant information in the literature regarding the urodynamic findings in psychogenic urinary retention (Table 23–4). Blaivas and Labib (*11*) reported on 16 women with acute urinary retention of whom 9 were thought to have psychogenic causes. Barrett (*12*) studied six patients with psychogenic urinary retention (one man, five women) of whom four were schizophrenic. Our experience with 15 female patients included 9 patients who manifested evidence of hysteria (*8*). Most of these patients are in the early portion of their reproductive years.

Bladder sensation is generally normal, although Barrett (*12*) described it as "delayed." The bladder is areflexic with variable amounts of abdominal straining. Perineal electromyography (EMG) demonstrates no evidence of denervation with increased activity during attempts to void. It is important to note that this pattern, far from being specific for psychogenic retention, is commonly seen in female patients during urodynamic testing. Therefore the examiner must attempt to determine if this pattern is representative of the patient's retentive history.

Bethanechol supersensitivity is always absent in our and Barrett's (*12*) experience. However, false-positive bethanechol supersensitivity has been reported in some of these patients (*11*). Electromyography is similarly normal, with no evidence of neuro-

Table 23–3. Criteria for Diagnosis of Hysteria

Age at onset <30 years
Dramatic, complex medical history
A minimum of 25 symptoms in at least nine of the following groups

- Group 1
  - Headaches
  - Sickly most of life
- Group 2
  - Blindness
  - Paralysis
  - Anesthesia
  - Aphonia
  - Fits or convulsions
  - Unconsciousness
  - Amnesia
  - Deafness
  - Hallucinations (in absence of psychosis)
  - Urinary retention
  - Trouble walking
  - Other conversion symptoms
- Group 3
  - Fatigue
  - Lump in throat
  - Fainting spells
  - Visual blurring
  - Weakness
  - Dysuria
- Group 4
  - Breathing difficulty
  - Palpitations
  - Anxiety attacks
  - Chest pain
  - Dizziness
- Group 5
  - Anorexia
  - Weight loss
  - Marked fluctuations in weight
  - Nausea
  - Abdominal bloating
  - Food intolerances
  - Diarrhea
  - Constipation
- Group 6
  - Abdominal pain
  - Vomiting
- Group 7
  - Dysmenorrhea
  - Menstrual irregularity
  - Amenorrhea
  - Excessive bleeding
- Group 8
  - Sexual indifference
  - Frigidity
  - Dyspareunia
  - Other sexual difficulties
  - Vomiting during 9-month pregnancy or hospitalized for hyperemesis gravidarum
- Group 9
  - Back pain
  - Joint pain
  - Extremity pain
  - Burning pains of the sexual organs, mouth, or rectum
  - Other bodily pains
- Group 10
  - Nervousness
  - Fears
  - Depressed feelings
  - Need to quit working or inability to carry on regular duties because of feeling sick
  - Cries easily
  - Feeling of hopelessness
  - Thinking a good deal about dying
  - Wanting to die
  - Thinking of suicide
  - Suicide attempts

Hospitalizations and operations (additionally confirmatory but not obligatory)

Table 23–4. Literature Review of Female Urinary Retention Studied Urodynamically

AUTHOR	NO. OF PTS.	MEAN AGE (RANGE)	CYSTOMETROGRAM (ML) *Sensation*	*Capacity*	EMG ACTIVITY	PSYCHIATRIC HISTORY
Blaivas & Labib (*11*)	9	32 (22–66)	435	679	Increased	2 Hysteria 5 Depressive neurosis
Barrett (*12*)	6	33 (22–66)	Delayed	1183	Increased	4 Schizophrenia
Krane & Siroky (*13*)	15	20 (15–42)	200	—	Increased	9 Hysteria

pathic changes. The normal response to vesical filling (increased perineal activity) is present or even exaggerated. When attempting to void, these patients typically fail to relax their perineal muscles, and some even increase their EMG activity during straining maneuvers.

In an attempt to develop a diagnostic aid for the assessment of psychogenic urinary retention, we described the use of intravenous diazepam in conjunction with cystometry (*13*). The test is based on the ability of diazepam to relax skeletal muscle as well as its better known anxiolytic effect. If psychologic mechanisms are producing inhibition of the detrusor reflex and perineal muscle spasm, diazepam should counteract these effects and enable some of these individuals to void normally. Diazepam (0.1 mg/kg) is given by slow intravenous injection after the initial cystometrogram (CMG). Within 2 to 3 minutes of injection, most subjects report some somnolence or lightheadedness. The cystometric examination is repeated at this point. All 13 patients in whom we performed this test demonstrated a marked reduction in perineal EMG activity. In 8 patients (62%), a sustained detrusor contraction was observed. In those patients demonstrating a normal detrusor contraction under these circumstances, neurogenic areflexia was thus ruled out.

We have developed a list of diagnostic clinical criteria for this disorder (Table 23–5). The purpose of these criteria is primarily to differentiate functional (psychogenic) urinary retention from retention secondary to occult neurologic lesions such as herniated intervertebral disc, spinal cord meningioma, multiple sclerosis, diabetic neuropathy, and herpes zoster. The most important urodynamic criteria are a negative bethanechol test, normal sphincter EMG, and a positive diazepam test. As discussed above, the diazepam test is helpful when positive but does not rule out psychogenic retention when negative.

Table 23–5. Suggested Clinical Criteria for Diagnosis of Psychogenic (Including Hysterical) Urinary Retention in Women

1. Normal neurologic examination
   a. Bulbocavernosus reflex
   b. Perineal sensation
   c. Voluntary sphincter contraction
2. Urodynamic findings
   a. Underactive detrusor/increased EMG activity
   b. Normal bladder sensation
   c. Negative bethanechol test
   d. No sphincter denervation
   e. Positive diazepam test
3. Normal pelvic, vaginal, and rectal examinations
4. Normal cystoscopic examination
5. Positive psychiatric history (preexisting psychiatric condition or identification of specific psychosocial precipitant)

Treatment

The treatment of psychogenic retention is essentially nonoperative and conservative. A variety of procedures have been described, including transurethral resection of the vesical neck, urethral dilatation, internal urethrotomy, pudendal nerve block, and even pudendal neurectomy (*14*). These therapies are based on the presumed presence of urethral obstruction. There is little if any evidence for organic obstruction of the urethra. However, as discussed above, functional obstruction by the striated perineal muscles is a component of this syndrome. For this reason, procedures such as urethral dilatation or internal urethrotomy are occasionally effective. However, because we believe that the most important mechanism in this disorder is supraspinal inhibition of the detrusor reflex, intermittent catheterization has been our primary modality of treatment. Wherever possible and appropriate, intermittent self-catheterization is combined with psychologic treatment, consultation, or biofeedback. Drug therapy using bethanechol, phenoxybenzamine, or diazepam has in our experience yielded disappointing results.

The institution of intermittent self-catheterization is generally straight forward. The major problem is in achieving acceptance by the patient of a psychological basis for her disorder. Such acceptance is somewhat facilitated by a thorough search for all possible organic causes including neurologic consultation. The question of psychiatric intervention must be raised carefully once the treatment program of self-catheterization has been established. Inquiries into emotional factors that may have contributed to the onset of retention may be made and psychiatric consultation suggested. Certainly the unexpected arrival of the psychiatrist in the patient's room may be resented by the patient and result in outright rejection of psychotherapy. Furthermore, it may result in a difficult subsequent relationship between patient and urologist. In this regard, it is important that the patient be assured that she is not being abandoned by the urologist and that her urinary retention will continue to receive appropriate attention.

The combination of intermittent self-catheterization, psychologic support from the urologist, and psychotherapy usually results in restoration of normal voiding, although it may require a long time. Using a similar approach, Barrett has reported that 50 percent of patients resume normal voiding, 30 percent are improved, and 20 percent continue to need intermittent catheterization (*12*).

PSYCHOGENIC FREQUENCY AND URGENCY

Definition

The syndrome of psychogenic frequency and urgency consists primarily of urinary frequency, urgency, and occasional urge incontinence in the absence of intrinsic lower urinary tract or neurologic disease. Additional symptoms may include dysuria, post-void urgency, suprapubic pain or pressure, and perineal ache. The symptoms are usually long-standing, tend to wax and wane, and are present primarily in the daytime. The syndrome occurs in both men and women. In men it is usually labeled "prostatitis," and in women it may be referred to as urethral syndrome, psychosomatic cystitis, spastic bladder reaction, or unstable bladder. The average age of male patients with this syndrome is 36.7 years (*5*); female patients are slightly younger (35.7 years) (*15*). Both men and women, in our experience, have onset of symptoms about 6 years prior to urodynamic referral, and a significant number (about 15%) report the presence of symptoms throughout adult life.

Symptoms

Symptoms may be divided into three groups: pain or discomfort, frequency/urgency, and hesitancy/weak stream. Pain or discomfort is an important component of the syndrome in men (Table 23–6), constituting 51 percent of all complaints and noted in 69 percent of patients (*5*). The most frequent site is the urethra or penis; the pain is typically described as burning, and is not necessarily associated with voiding. In women (Table 23–7) voiding dysfunction predominates with frequency and urgency of micturition comprising 50 percent of all symptoms and manifesting in most patients (86%). Incontinence of some degree was noted in 75 female patients (54%). The most reasonable explanation for the different distribution of symptoms in men and women appears to be the greater ability of men to counteract unstable bladder contractions by perineal muscle spasm. This situation would explain the frequent presence of various pain syndromes in men (suprapubic, perineal) with rare incontinence, in contrast to the much greater incidence of urge incontinence in women with unstable bladders. George and Slade (*16*) also noted the relatively greater incidence of pain syndromes in men with psychosomatic voiding disorders.

Etiology

Causes considered in the etiology of this syndrome include, in women, infection, urethral trauma during intercourse, meatal stenosis, bladder neck or urethral obstruction, pelvic congestion, and allergic mechanisms; in men they include urethritis, prostatitis (infectious and inflammatory), and bladder neck obstruction. The evidence sup-

Table 23–6. Summary of Symptoms Noted in 42 Males with Psychosomatic Genitourinary Complaints

SYMPTOM	NO.
Pain or discomfort	29
Penis/urethra	15
Scrotum	10
low back	9
suprapubic/groin	8
sex-related	6
perineal	2
Frequency/urgency	28
Hesitancy/weak stream	20
Total No. of Symptoms	98

Table 23–7. Summary of Symptoms Noted in 140 Women with Psychogenic Voiding Complaints, Excluding Patients in Complete Retention

SYMPTOM	NO.
Frequency/urgency	120
Incontinence	75
Hesitancy/weak stream	44
Total No. of symptoms	239

porting or negating the role of some of these factors deserves careful consideration.

Urinary tract infection is often supposed to be the cause of episodic frequency and urgency in women. However, careful studies of the incidence of bacteriuria in this syndrome have failed to show convincingly that infection is the cause (*17–19*). Between 55 and 75 percent of these patients are free of infection. Moreover, even in patients with bacteriuria, symptoms often persist or quickly recur despite its eradication with antibiotics. Nonbacterial infections, especially those due to chlamydial organisms, have been reported in "urethral syndrome" (*20*), but such infection has not been shown to be present in most patients. It has been suggested that bacteriuria is not necessarily always present; infection may be limited to the urethra or vaginal introitus (*21*). However, the incidence of introital colonization is similar in normal women (23%) and in patients with recurrent infections (28%) (*21*). The mere presence or persistence of perineal organisms is not associated with an increased probability of infection (*22*). In conclusion, mechanisms other than infection must be considered in symptomatic abacteriuric women.

The close temporal relation between sexual intercourse and the onset of irritative urinary symptoms is well known. It has led to the supposition that urethral trauma leads to displacement of urethral bacteria into the bladder. Indeed, it has been shown that this phenomenon occurs with surprising frequency (55%) in normal women (*23*). However, the bacteriuria is transient and clears spontaneously within 48 hours without causing symptoms. Hence this phenomenon cannot explain why some women develop irritative symptoms following intercourse whereas most do not.

The idea that outflow obstruction is a factor in producing frequency and urgency has long existed in urology (*24*). Studies have found, however, that outlet obstruction is rare in women with recurrent frequency/urgency (<10%) (*19*). In fact, obstructive symptoms are more common in abacteriuric patients than in those with infection (*17*). Outflow obstruction in thus seen to be quite rare in women, and even when present it does not explain the presence of bacteriuria.

In men, symptoms of recurrent perigenital pain or voiding symptoms are most frequently ascribed to "prostatitis," i.e., prostatic infection or inflammation. Careful bacteriologic studies in these patients have demonstrated an infectious etiology in only 15 percent of cases (*25,26*). In a survey of 105 men presenting with "chronic prostatitis," Smart *et al.* (*27*) found gram-negative infection in 23 percent, outflow obstruction in 16 percent, urethral stricture in 5 percent, and carcinoma *in situ* of the bladder in 2 percent. Nevertheless, a group constituting 25 percent of the series remained in whom neuroticism was the only obvious cause. This group was significantly younger (38 years of age) than patients with bacterial prostatitis (56 years of age) and had a higher incidence of sexual complaints. It is this group with which we are concerned in this chapter.

Psychodynamics

In one series of women with persistent frequency/urgency, 50 patients underwent psychiatric interviews and standardized psychometric testing (*18*). It was found that 60 percent manifested significant anxiety or depression compared to 6 percent of controls. Psychometric variables such as free-floating anxiety and somatization were noted to be higher in the patients than in controls. Hysteria and obsessionality scores in the patient population approach those of psychiatrically ill patients. In our own experience (*15*), anxiety neurosis and depression were noted in 38 percent of women with persistent frequency/urgency. In addition, there is a higher than expected incidence of functional gastrointestinal complaints, migraine, low back pain, and dyspareunia.

Men without detectable physical abnormality have been found to be significantly more neurotic than those with such abnormality (*27*). It has been noted that most of these patients are obsessively concerned with their work or personal health (*16*). In our experience (*5*), psychiatric or social disturbance is present in more than 50 percent, including chronic anxiety neurosis, depression, cancerphobia, marital discord, and high-pressure occupations. Upper gastrointestinal complaints are noted in 25 percent, and 15 percent have psychogenic impotence.

Urodynamics

In women the most significant urodynamic abnormality is detrusor instability. This finding, reported in 15 to 30 percent of patients complaining of frequency/urgency, is important because a good response to anticholinergic treatment can be expected. Bladder instability appears to be correlated with the presence of trabeculation but not with outflow obstruction. In our experience (*15*), detrusor hyperactivity is present in about 51 percent of women with persistent frequency/urgency. This incidence is higher than generally reported in the literature and may be due to the highly selected nature of our patient population. A smaller proportion (37%) demonstrated acontractile detrusor, and the remainder had normal studies (12%).

The urodynamic diagnosis of bladder instability rests on filling and provocative cystometry. According to most reports, about half of unstable bladders become manifest upon simple filling. The rest become apparent only upon provocative maneuvers such as coughing, a change in position, or catheter removal. Several forms of bladder instability have been noted: (a) phasic contractions, (b) poor compliance, and (c) unstable urethra. The first of these forms involves one or more well developed contractions that occur during filling cystometry and is the most common type. The second manifests as a steeply rising curve with or without superimposed contractions. Why some of these patients have poor bladder wall compliance is unclear at present, but it may represent structural changes secondary to detrusor hypertrophy (? fibrosis, ? ischemia). Finally, in some patients provocative maneuvers may induce reflex urethral relaxation without detrusor contraction. The patients usually report marked urgency at such times, termed urethral instability (*28*).

As mentioned above, underactive detrusor was fairly commonly observed (37%) in women with functional voiding disorders. It is often difficult to assess the significance of hypoactive detrusor in women as it is seen in 44 percent of normal women, presumably due to anxiety induced by the examination itself (*29*). It is therefore important to determine if the finding of detrusor inactivity is representative of the patient's voiding symptomatology. The correlation of cystometric findings with symptoms in our series of women with functional voiding problems is shown in Table 23–8. This analysis indicates a statistically significant correlation ($p < 0.01$ by chi-square analysis) between, on one hand, acontractile detrusor and obstructive symptoms and, on the other hand, hyperactivity and irritative symptoms. Thus it seems reasonable to conclude that the finding of underactive detrusor, when corroborated by purely obstructive symptoms, is a clinically significant observation. Of 52 women with underactive detrusor, 18 (35%) had purely obstructive symptoms and 11 (21%) had both obstructive and irritative symptoms. The remainder (44%) demonstrated underactive detrusor during urodynamic testing but had purely irritative symptoms.

Perineal electromyography (EMG) failed to reveal evidence of neuropathy in any patient. The patients with bladder instability

Table 23–8. Correlation of Cystometrogram Findings with Symptoms in 140 Women

SYMPTOM	DETRUSOR INSTABILITY	ACONTRACTILE DETRUSOR	NORMAL	TOTAL
Frequency/urgency	62	23	11	96
Hesitancy/weak stream	1	18	1	20
Combined	8	11	5	24
Total	71 (51%)	52 (37%)	17 (12%)	140

demonstrated complete relaxation of their perineal musculature during detrusor contraction. Those with underactive detrusor demonstrated persistent guarding by EMG during attempts to void, which was characteristically accentuated during abdominal straining.

The urodynamic pattern is somewhat different in men and may be described as the reverse of that observed in women (*5*). Bladder underactivity was observed in 50 percent of the men (compared to 37 percent of women), and bladder hyperactivity occurred in 38 percent of the men (compared to 51 percent of the women). Approximately 12 percent of the men had normal studies. The incidence of underactive bladder in this group of men is tenfold higher than that noted in normal controls (5%) (*29*) and appears to characterize well the pathophysiology in this syndrome. Pain was noted as frequently in those with underactivity as in those with hyperactivity. Uroflowmetry correlated well with cystometric findings, as 86 percent of patients with acontractility has an abnormal flow pattern compared to 20 percent of patients with hyperactivity. This finding indicates that weak or absent detrusor contraction is characteristic in this group of patients.

Treatment

The major contribution of urodynamic examination in psychogenic voiding disorders has been to provide guidance for initial therapy as well as objective documentation of treatment efficacy. A variety of therapeutic strategies are available and may be grouped by the urodynamic abnormality they are intended to correct (Table 23–9). The therapies include pharmacologic, psychologic, electrical, and surgical modalities as well as self-catheterization.

Pharmacologic therapy of detrusor instability utilizes agents with a variety of actions, although the anticholinergic/musculotropic drugs remain the mainstay of treatment. This regimen is based on the supposition that detrusor contraction is predominantly under cholinergic control. In an *in vitro* study of these agents, Benson *et al.* found propantheline to be a potent pure anticholinergic, flavoxate hydrochloride to be a weak anticholinergic/antispasmodic, and imipramine to be a potent anticholinergic as well as antispasmodic (*30*). Clinically, there are few controlled studies comparing the efficacy of the various preparations with each other. However, subjective improvement is reported in 50 to 80 percent of patients with detrusor instability treated with anticholinergic or antispasmodic drugs. It should be noted, however, that urodynamic improvement occurs in a far lower proportion (40%) (*31*). In addition, the placebo response rate ranges from 40 to 50 percent (*32,33*). Therefore, it seems likely that about half of the symptomatic response to anticholinergic/antispasmodic treatment is due to placebo effect.

Our practice is to use propantheline bromide in doses ranging from 45 to 120 mg per 24 hours, although occasionally higher doses are required. Dosage is gradually increased until adequate therapeutic effect is achieved

Table 23–9. Treatment Options for Functional Voiding Disorders Based on Urodynamic Findings

DETRUSOR INSTABILITY	ACONTRACTILE DETRUSOR
Pharmacologic therapy	Pharmacologic therapy
Psychologic therapy	Psychologic therapy
Bladder drill	Behavior modification
Biofeedback	Biofeedback
Psychotherapy	Psychotherapy
Functional electrical stimulation	Intermittent self-catheterization
Surgical therapy	Surgical therapy
Bladder distension	Bladder stimulation
Denervation procedures	Bladder reduction
Bladder augmentation	Urinary diversion
Urinary diversion	

or side effects become intolerable. The most common side effect is dryness of the mouth, noted in more than 80 percent of our patients. This side effect is sometimes severe, even producing dysphagia. Other side effects include visual blurring, drowsiness, dizziness, and constipation. In refractory patients we have added imipramine (100 mg per 24 hours). Imipramine may also be combined with propantheline to permit a lower dose of propantheline to be used when severe side effects are a problem. Anticholinergics are contraindicated for angle-closure glaucoma and gastrointestinal obstruction. They should be used with caution in patients with tachycardia.

The use of sympathomimetic agents has been suggested for bladder instability based on their ability to improve urethral tone (alpha effect) as well as suppress detrusor contraction (beta effect) (*34*). Insufficient experience has accumulated with this approach to assess its usefulness. Other approaches have included prostaglandin inhibitors (*35*), baclofen (*33*), and bromocriptine (*32*). In most of these trials the efficacy of the drug in question was not significantly greater than that of placebo.

One promising avenue currently under investigation is the use of calcium channel blockers. Because it is well know that calcium plays an important role in muscle contraction, calcium antagonists can be expected to be useful for treating smooth and striated muscle spasm. Ekman *et al.* have reported excellent initial experience using terodilene in women with unstable bladder (*36*). Further experience is needed, but this group of drugs appears promising.

Pharmacologic treatment of psychogenic detrusor areflexia is in general disappointing. The strategy has generally been to increase detrusor contractility, decrease outlet resistance, or both. Bethanechol chloride continues to be widely used to facilitate bladder emptying. There is no question that 5 mg of bethanechol given subcutaneously increases intravesical pressure and decreases cystometric capacity (*37*). Oral doses of 50 mg or less produce little change in cystometric parameters. It is our experience that oral bethanechol is of little use in psychogenic detrusor areflexia and sometimes produces increased bladder pain. Another possible approach was reported by Bultitude *et al.* (*38*), who found that intravesical instillation of prostaglandin E_2 (0.5 mg) in women with urinary retention resulted in improvement in about two-thirds. This finding was substantiated in another report by these authors in 1980 (*39*). The prostaglandins appear to act by increasing detrusor tone and require an intact sacral reflex arc to be effective.

Pharmacologic attempts to decrease outlet resistance are aimed either at the smooth muscle or the striated muscle sphincter. Alpha-adrenergic blocking agents such as phenoxybenzamine, prazosin, and α-methyldopa have been used to reduce outflow resistance at the level of the smooth muscle sphincter, primarily in neurogenic bladder dysfunction. There is little experience with these drugs in psychogenic detrusor areflexia. Therapy aimed at the striated sphincter seems to be more promising in functional disorders charcterized by failure to empty. However, no pharmacologic agent is available that can selectively relax the external urethral sphincter. This group of drugs, which includes diazepam, methocarbamol, dantrolene, and baclofen, may produce drowsiness, dizziness, and muscle weakness despite their differing modes of action.

We have had considerable experience with the use of diazepam in both male and female patients with psychogenic voiding disorders. For example, oral diazepam (6–18 mg/day) was used in 18 male patients with underactive detrusor and perineal floor spasm; significant improvement was observed in 15 patients (*5*). It is unclear whether this effect was due to the skeletal muscle relaxant, the antianxiety component, or the placebo effects of the drug. Nevertheless, the therapeutic effect appeared to be genuine, as most patients after ceasing therapy were soon symptomatic again. Similar results have been obtained in carefully selected female patients.

Psychologic techniques have been applied for both detrusor instability and acontractile detrusor. Perhaps the best known of these techniques is the "bladder drill" described by Frewen for detrusor instability (*40*). This technique involves instruction to the patient that she keep a record of diurnal voidings and reward herself for increasing the interval between them by consious suppression of the detrusor. Frewen has reported a success rate in excess of 80 percent using this simple technique. Biofeedback has also been used for detrusor instability (*41*). With this technique a visual or auditory signal is transmitted to the patient that is proportional to the intravesical pressure. The patient can then use this feedback to practice conscious suppression of the bladder. This technique also has a high success rate of about 80 percent subjective improvement and 50 percent cystometric improvement. Bladder drill may be considered a simple form of biofeedback in which paper and pencil take the place of complex electronic equipment. The advantage of any form of biofeedback is simplicity, safety, and success. The disadvantage is that it is not applicable to all patients, requiring a well motivated, insightful individual to be successful. For example, Cardozo *et al.* found that the extremely hostile patient could be predicted to fail biofeedback therapy (*41*).

Self-catheterization, discussed previously in the context of urinary retention, may also be applied to the patient with underactive detrusor who is not in retention. Patients with functional voiding disorders characterized by abdominal straining and perineal spasm not infrequently are able to completely empty their bladder. Nevertheless, they may complain of suprapubic ache, burning on urination, constant urge to void, and so forth. One striking finding is that their symptoms are completely alleviated by placing a Foley catheter in preparation for urodynamic study. This measure is successful despite the fact that there is little or no residual urine found. We have found an intermittent self-catheterization program, sometimes in combination with anticholinergic/antispasmodic medications, to be quite useful in such patients. Self-catheterization is obviously merely a temporizing maneuver in this situation, but it permits the patient to participate in biofeedback therapy relatively free of disabling symptoms.

In patients who fail pharmacologic or other conservative treatment of detrusor hyperactivity, *functional electrical stimulation* may be considered. Using nonimplantable anal or vaginal electrodes, electrical stimulation causes direct contraction of the perineal floor as well as indirect inhibition of detrusor contractions. It is therefore a theoretically attractive method of treating difficult cases of detrusor instability. Nevertheless, the method has seen relatively limited application in idiopathic detrusor instability, being used primarily for the treatment of neurogenic incontinence. Godec *et al.* reported a success rate of 92 percent in carefully selected patients (*42*), most of whom had neurogenic detrusor hyperreflexia. It seems that electrical stimulation should receive further trial in functional voiding disorders characterized by detrusor instability.

Surgical therapy is occasionally indicated in refractory cases of detrusor instability. We include under this heading bladder distension, denervation procedures, bladder augmentation, and urinary (supravesical) diversion. Cystodistension is performed by raising the intravesical pressure to a level equivalent to the systolic blood pressure (*43*). It is done under continuous epidural anesthesia for four successive periods of 30 minutes each. The procedure has been applied in idiopathic detrusor instability, interstitial cystitis, and neuropathic detrusor hyperreflexia with varying results. Only 20 percent of patients with bladder instability are symptomatically improved at 1 year (*44*). Bladder rupture occurs as a complication in 5 percent of cases. Bladder distension therapy may be considered a form of denervation procedure, as degeneration of unmyelinated nerve fibers has been demonstrated to occur in the bladder wall following distension (*45*).

Surgical denervation may be accomplished by sacral neurectomy (*46*), transvaginal neurectomy (*47*), and cystolysis or cystocystoplasty (*48*). Sacral neurectomy has been applied to relatively few patients with idiopathic instability, and it is difficult to assess its usefulness. The most common approach is selective ablation of the anterior S_3 nerve root bilaterally, which produces increased bladder capacity with sphincter impairment in most cases. However, the long-term results (2 years) with idiopathic instability are poor, especially with respect to nocturnal enuresis (*46*).

In contrast, denervation performed close to the bladder itself appears to be more successful, which may be due to the fact that sensory as well as motor fibers are cut. Ingleman-Sundberg divided the perivesical plexus through an incision in the vaginal wall (*47*). The procedure is said to improve symptoms of detrusor instability in about 70 percent of patients on long-term follow-up. Similarly, bladder transection has been reported to improve more than 50 percent of patients with severe detrusor instability, even though the instability is not abolished on cystometrogram follow-up (*49*).

Finally, augmentation cystoplasty has been performed in a few patients with idiopathic detrusor instability. A critical review by the UCLA group indicates that these cases tend to respond much less satisfactorily (20%) than cases of neurogenic, interstitial, or tuberculous etiology (*50*). Rarely, supravesical diversion is the only option for severely refractory cases of incontinence due to detrusor instability.

REFERENCES

1. Karafin, L., and Kendall, A. R.: Psychosomatic problems in urology. In Karafin, L., and Kendall, A. R. (eds.), *Urology*. Vol. 2. Harper & Row, Hagerstown, 1974.
2. Doran, J., and Roberts, M: Acute urinary retention in the female. *Br. J. Urol.* 47:793–796, 1976.
3. Frewen, W.: Evaluation of psychogenic urinary retention in the female. *GU* February: 30–34, 1979.
4. Larson, J. W., Swenson, W. M., Utz, D. C., and Steinhilber, R. M.: Psychogenic urinary retention in women. *JAMA* 184:111, 1963.
5. Siroky, M. B., Goldstein, I., and Krane, R. J.: Functional voiding disorders in men. *J. Urol.* 126:200–204, 1981.
6. Kahn, A. U.: Psychogenic urinary retention in a boy. *J. Urol.* 106:432–434, 1971.
7. Smith, D. R.: Psychosomatic urinary frequency and retention. In Smith, D. R. (ed.), *General Urology*, 8th ed. Lange, Los Altos, CA, 1975, p. 473.
8. Krane, R. J., and Siroky, M. B.: Psychogenic voiding dysfunction in the adult female. In Raz, S. (ed.), *Female Urology*. Saunders, Philadelphia, 1983.
9. Mai, F. M., and Merskey, H.: Briquet's treatise on hysteria: a synopsis and commentary. *Arch. Gen. Psychiatry* 37:1401–1405, 1980.
10. Perley, M. J., and Guze, S. B.: Hysteria—the stability and usefulness of clinical criteria: a quantitative study based on a follow-up period of six to eight years in 39 patients. *N. Engl. J. Med.* 266:421–426, 1962.
11. Blaivas, J. G., and Labib, K. B.: Acute urinary retention in women: complete urodynamics evaluation. *Urology* 10:383–389, 1977.
12. Barrett, D. M.: Evaluation of psychogenic urinary retention. *J. Urol.* 120:191–192, 1978.
13. Krane, R. J., and Siroky, M. B.: Hysterical urinary retention in the female. *Proc. I. C. S.* 9:21–25, 1979.
14. Allan, T. O.: Psychogenic urinary retention. *South. Med. J.* 65:302–302, 1972.
15. Pavlakis, A. P., Wheeler, J. S., Jr., Siroky, M. B., and Krane, R. J.: Functional voiding disorders in females. *Neurourol. Urodyn.* 5:145–151, 1986.
16. George, N. J. R., and Slade, N.: Hesitancy and poor stream in younger men without outflow obstruction—the anxious bladder. *Br. J. Urol.* 51:506–509, 1979.
17. Rees, D. L. P., Whitfield, H. N., Islam, A. K. M., Doyle, P. T., Mayo, M. E., and Wickham, J. E. A.: Urodynamic findings in adult females with frequency and dysuria. *Br. J. Urol.* 47:853–859, 1976.
18. Rees, D. L. P., and Farhoumand, N.: Psychiatric aspects of recurrent cystitis in women. *Br. J. Urol.* 49:651–658, 1971.
19. Rees, D. L. P., Wickham. J. E. A., and Whitfield, H. N.: Bladder instability in women with recurrent cystitis. *Br. J. Urol.* 50:524–528, 1978.
20. Trait, A. I., and Rees, E.: Urethral syndrome associated with chlamydial infection of urethra and cervix. *Br. J. Urol.* 50:425–426, 1971.
21. O'Grady, F. W., Richards, B., McSherry, M. A., O'Farrell, S. M., and Catell, W. R.: Introital enterobacteria, urinary infection and the urethral syndrome. *Lancet* 2:1208–1210, 1970.
22. Neto, N. R., Rangel, P. E., DeSilva, R. P., and Lemos, G. C.: Relation between the vaginal, introital and perianal flora in recurrent cystitis in women. *Urol. Int.* 33:260–266, 1978.
23. Buckley, R. M., Jr., McGurkin, M., and MacGregor, R. R.: Urine bacterial counts after sexual intercourse. *N. Engl. J. Med.* 298:321–323, 1978.
24. Bugbee, H. G.: Frequency of urination in women. *JAMA* 68:693–694, 1917.
25. Fritjofsson, A., Kihl, B., and Danielson, D.: Chronic prostato-vesiculitis: incidence and significance of bacterial findings. *Scand. J. Urol. Nephrol.* 8:173–178, 1974.
26. Mardh, P. A., and Colleen, S.: Search for uro-genital tract infections in patients with symptoms of prostatitis. *Scand. J. Urol. Nephrol.* 9:8–16, 1975.
27. Smart, C. J., Jenkins, J. D., and Lloyd, R. S.: The painful prostate. *Br. J. Urol.* 47:861–869, 1976.
28. McGuire, E. J.: Reflex urethral instability. *Br. J. Urol.* 50:200–204, 1978.
29. Merrill, D. C., Bradley, W. E., and Markland, C.: Air cystometry. II. A clinical evaluation of normal adults. *J. Urol.* 108:85–88, 1974.
30. Benson, G. S., Sarshik, S. A., Raezer, D.M., and Wein, A. J.: Bladder muscle contractility: comparative effects and mechanisms of action of atropine, propantheline, flavoxate and imipramine. *Urology* 9:31–35, 1977.
31. Noisey, C. U., Stephenson, T. P., and Brendler, C. B.: The urodynamic and subjective results of treatment of detrusor instability with oxybutinin chloride. *Br. J. Urol.* 52:472–475, 1980.
32. Abrams, P. H., and Dunn, M.: A double-blind trial of bromocriptine in idiopathic detrusor instability. *Br. J. Urol.* 51:24–27, 1979.
33. Taylor, M. C., and Bates, C. P.: A double-blind trial cross-over trial of baclofen a new treatment for the unstable bladder syndrome. *Br. J. Urol.* 51:504–505, 1979.
34. Cardozo, L. D., and Stanton, S. L.: A comparison between bromocriptine and indomethacin in the treatment of detrusor instability. *J. Urol.* 123:399–401, 1980.

35. Norlen, L., Sundin, T., and Waagstein, F.: Beta adrenoceptor stimulation of the human urinary bladder in vivo. *Acta Pharmacol. Toxicol. (Copenh.)* 43:26–30, 1978.
36. Ekman, G., Andersson, K. E., Rud, T., and Ulmsten, U.: A double blind crossover study of the effects of terodilene in women with unstable bladder. *Acta Pharmacol. Toxicol. (Copenh.)* 46:39–45, 1980.
37. Wein, A. J., Malloy, T. R., Shafer, F., and Raezer, D. M.: The effects of bethanechol chloride on urodynamic parameters in normal women and in women with significant residual urine volumes. *J. Urol.* 124:397–399, 1980.
38. Bultitude, M. I., Hills, N. H., and Shuttleworth, K. E. D.: Clinical and experimental studies on the action of prostaglandins and their synthesis inhibitors on detrusor muscle in vitro and in vivo. *Br. J. Urol.* 48:631–637, 1976.
39. Desmond, A. D., Bultitude, M. I., Hills, N. H., and Shuttleworth, K. E. D.: Clinical experience with intravesical prostaglandin E_2: a prospective study of 36 patients. *Br. J. Urol.* 52:357–366, 1980.
40. Frewen, W. K.: The management of urgency and frequency of micturition. *Br. J. Urol.* 52:367–369, 1980.
41. Cardozo, L. D., Abrams, P., Stanton, S. L., and Fenely, R. C. L.: Idiopathic bladder unstability treated by biofeedback. *Br. J. Urol.* 50:321–523, 1978.
42. Godec, C., Cass, A. S., and Ayala, G. F.: Electrical stimulation for incontinence: technique, selection and results. *Urology* 7:388–397, 1976.
43. Ramsden, P. D., Smith, J. C., Dunn, M., and Ardran, G. M.: Distention therapy for unstable bladder. *Br. J. Urol.* 48:623–629, 1976.
44. Smith, J. C.: The place of prolonged bladder distention in the treatment of bladder instability and other disorders. *Br. J. Urol.* 53:283–283, 1976.
45. Sehn, J. T.: Anatomic effect of distention therapy in unstable bladder: a new approach. *Urology* 11:581–587, 1978.
46. Torrens, M., and Hald, T: Bladder denervation procedures. *Urol. Clin. North Am.* 6:283–297, 1979.
47. Ingleman-Sundberg, A.: Partial bladder denervation for detrusor dyssynergia. *Clin. Obstet. Gynecol.* 21:797–805, 1978.
48. Essenhigh, D. W., and Yeates, W. K.: Transection of the bladder with particular reference to enuresis. *Br. J. Urol.* 45:299–305, 1973.
49. Hindmarsh, J. R., Essenhigh, D. W., and Yeates, W. K.: Bladder transection for adult enuresis. *Br. J. Urol.* 49:515–521, 1977.
50. Smith, R. B., Van Cangh, P., Skinner, D. G., Kaufman, J. J., and Goodwin, W. E.: Augmentation enterocystoplasty: a critical review. *J. Urol.* 118:35–39, 1977.

24

Upper Urinary Tract Dysfunction

BO COOLSAET, M.D., Ph.D.

Pathologic changes all along the lower and upper urinary tract may cause dysfunction of the upper urinary tract. Organic and functional dynamic disturbances affect proximal parts of the urinary unit. The degree of inadequacy to transport urine in the proximal part depends on: (a) the amount of urine that must be transported; (b) the remaining dynamic properties of the unit; and (c) if present, the degree of functional or organic obstruction (*1*)

ACUTE COMPLETE OUTFLOW OBSTRUCTION

Acute complete outflow obstruction is the best reproducible model to be investigated. Standardization, however, is still influenced by the diuretic load that exists prior to the obstruction. Acute obstruction causes a back-up of urine. The proximal part of the unit reacts by increasing intraluminal baseline pressure, which can increase to the level of the filtration and secretory pressure of the nephrons. This pressure is between 65 and 90 cm H_2O. Backing up of urine increases the urine volume and dilates the system. The wall is stretched and wall stress increases, which induces increased frequency of the action potentials. The evoked contractions become more forceful.

Contractions become weaker after approximately 5 minutes, and the frequency of action potentials decreases. Baseline pressure initially increases but subsequently decreases to the level of the renal secretory pressure. After such acute trauma, the system develops a number of defense mechanisms.

1. Urine production is lowered by a reduction in glomerular filtration and tubular secretion.
2. Back-flow pathways are developed via pyelovenous and pyelolymphatic channels. Distension impedes coaptation of the caliceal walls during contraction, which allows pyelocaliceal and calicotubular backflow via the collecting tubules.
3. The pressure decrease is further enhanced by progressive dilatation, stress relaxation of the wall, and weakening of the contractions.

Long-standing complete obstruction results in nearly complete loss of parenchyma due to a reduction in blood supply and destruction of the tubular and glomerular system. The muscular coat is nearly completely replaced by connective tissue.

Temporary acute obstruction is frequently caused by ureteral stones.

Rapid relief of obstruction allows nearly complete restoration of normal dynamics at short notice. However, the longer the occlusion exists, the more the proximal part of the system is threatened and the more nephron function is lost.

PARTIAL CHRONICALLY IMPAIRED OUTFLOW

Partial chronically impaired outflow induces more balanced morphologic and dynamic changes, depending on the amount of increase of outflow resistance, the flow rate, and the time the obstruction exists. The system develops a series of protecting mechanisms. A delicate balance exists between urine production, wall activity, and geometry of the system. Baseline pressure in chronic dilated upper tract systems is low. Hence parenchymal atrophy is not caused by high baseline pressure but, rather, by other mechanisms that are not completely understood.

Dilatation is probably one of these mechanisms. It allows pyelotubular back-flow which causes reduced concentrating ability in the distal tubules and vascular changes. However, distal tubular damage does not occur in some systems despite the dilatation.

Possibly, transient recurrent episodes of increased urinary production or transient increased outflow resistance result in recurrent high pressure episodes. Uncomplicated wide upper tract systems generally develop higher pressure during forced diuresis than controls.

Renal damage might also be caused by hemodynamic changes due to mechanisms other than pressure. However, reduced glomerular filtration rate and renal plasma flow occur later in the course of chronically impaired outflow (*2*).

The greatest threat to the renal parenchyma is the combination of obstruction with infection, although under these circumstances the system maximally tries to protect the renal parenchyma. Indeed, dilated systems that had been complicated by infection are unable to build up high pressures even at maximal diuretic load.

The dynamics of the dilated and elongated upper tract system changes dramatically. A wide variety of situations can be observed, however, depending on the amount and the duration of increased outflow resistance.

Indeed, in some wide systems dynamics are nearly normal. The wall shows muscle hypertrophy, which contributes to the generation of slightly higher pressures. Coaptation of the urethral wall at the contraction ring still occurs.

In the case of a more pronounced increase of outflow resistance or in longer-standing disease, however, the hypertrophic muscle coat is gradually changed. Smooth muscle bundles become widely separated by connective tissue (*3*). Clusters of collagen separate adjacent muscle bundles, and close contact areas are separated. Because of the increased dilatation and collagen infiltration in the wall, coaptation at the rear end of the bolus is no longer possible. Transport function then becomes seriously disturbed. Intraureteric regurgitation of urine through the peristaltic contraction wave further dilates the system (Fig. 24–1). Generation of pressure by the contraction ring progressively decreases according to the Laplace equation. The more the system dilates, the less is the intraluminal pressure generation, and the less effective is the propulsive property of the contraction ring.

These events gradually enhance collagen formation in the muscle coat, resulting in an increasing loss of contractile capabilities. The partial chronically impaired outflow can be caused by organic or functional outflow disturbances localized along the urinary tract. Urethral diverticula, urethral valves, detrusor–sphincter dyssynergia, detrusor–bladder neck dyssynergia, bladder neck obstruction, neurogenic detrusor dysfunction, detrusor instability, low compliance bladders, high compliance bladders, dysfunction of the distal ureteral segment, vesicoureteral reflux, retroperitoneal fibrosis, tumors, vascular obstruction, and many other situations can result in similar upper tract dysfunction. Although in the normal person pacemaker function is probably controlled by atypical cells that generate the highest frequency of action potentials at the fornix, with chronically dilated systems this frequency gradient is mostly lost. Hence latent pacemaker cells can take over pacemaker function and initiate dystopic orthograde peristaltic contractions. They can also generate retrograde contractions. Whether these functional changes are secondary to the dilatation or vice versa is not certain. With many "hydronephrotic" systems or so-called primary obstructed megaureters, no organic obstruction is found. Investigation on the nondilated distal "adynamic" part showed spontaneous phasic activity with a frequency of seven or eight contractions per minute.

This part also shows hypertonic responses to norepinephrine, histamine, and serotonin. These observations point to the probability

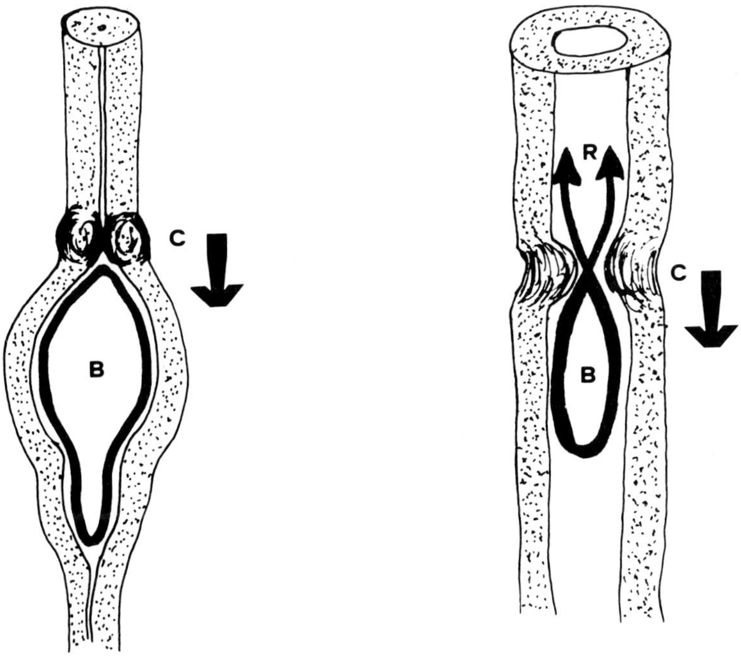

Figure 24–1. In the normal ureter (left) the contraction ring (*c*) propulses the bolus (*B*) toward the bladder, and the ureteral wall coapts and prevents regurgitation. In some wide ureters (right) coaptation of the wall is no longer possible causing regurgitation of urine through the peristaltic contraction wave.

of hyperdynamic, rather than adynamic, dysfunction of the distal part.

It becomes more and more obvious that dysfunction of the peristaltic activity is involved early in the process, which furthermore enhances secondary changes of the wall in the cranial part. Dysfunction in this part causes hypertrophy with collagen infiltration. Wide upper tract systems, however, also occur in the absence of increased outflow resistance. They appear to be congenital variations or secondary to intrauterine temporary impairment. Their dynamic function is grossly similar to that in normal individuals; parenchymal function remains normal and stable in most of the uncomplicated wide systems (*4*). Urinary tract infections might seriously disturb this delicate balance.

The impact of an uncomplicated, wide system on parenchymal function seems not to be harmful over the course of a few years. However, long-term follow-up (> 5 years) is not yet available.

DYSFUNCTION AND INFECTION

Upper urinary tract infection dramatically interferes with peristaltic activity (*5*). The action of bacterial products causes the upper tract to finally become a dilated aperistaltic tube. The effect of bacterial infection varies according to the bacterial type, its concentration, and the resistance factors of the host's excretory system.

Endotoxin and other products produced by *Eschirichia Coli, Citrobacter, Pseudomonas, Aerobacter,* and *Proteus* act directly on upper tract peristaltic mechanisms. In addition, they enhance inflammatory edema, which increases outflow resistance. These effects seriously interfere with the effect of treatment of the bacterial infection. Abolished or incomplete peristalsis, dyskynesias, and retrograde peristalsis, outflow obstruction by inflammatory edema, cause stasis of residual urine in the upper tract. Stasis, regurgitation, and impaired washout seriously impede the effect of antibacterial treatment. After the infection has been adequately treated, peristaltic activity returns to normal after 2 to 7 days. Long-standing upper tract infections, however, cause replacement of muscle bundles in the muscle coat by acontractile cicatricial connective tissue.

Intravesical release of toxic products might offend the active intramural antireflux mechanism. Hence reflux of urine in the ureter may be caused by, among other factors, endovesical toxic infection.

CONCLUSION

Upper urinary tract dysfunction may be due to intrinsic or extrinsic factors; transport function has essentially changed in these characteristic properties. Unidirectional flow is disturbed by intraureteric reflux and retrograde or reversed peristalsis. Stasis occurs mostly in a dilated system: contraction waves are no longer coordinated, resulting in less effective forces. The exact mechanism of impaired nephron function remains to be investigated. Changes of upper tract dynamics must be within certain limits to protect renal parenchyma and prevent calculus formation, infection, and pain. Further investigation of upper urinary tract dynamics is essential for the rational prevention of renal insufficiency.

REFERENCES

1. Rose, J., and Gillenwater, J.: Effects of obstruction on ureteral function. *Urology* 12:139, 1978.
2. Vaughan, E. D., Sorenson, E. J., and Gillenwater, J.: The renal hemodynamic response to chronic unilateral complete ureteral occlusion. *Invest. Urol.* 8:78, 1970.
3. Hanna, M. K., Jeffs, R. D., Sturgess, J. M., and Barkin, M.: Ureteral structure and ultrastructure. IV. The dilated ureter, clinicopathologic correlation. *J. Urol.* 117:28, 1977.
4. Bratt, C. G., Aurell, M., and Nilsson, S.: Renal function in patients with hydronephrosis. *Br. J. Urol.* 49:249, 1977.
5. Boyarsky, S., Labay, P., and Teague, N.: Aperistaltic ureter in upper urinary tract infection: cause or effect? *Urology* 12:134, 1978.

Section Four

Pharmacology, Rehabilitation, and Other Methods of Management

25

Clinical Neuropharmacology of the Lower Urinary Tract

ALAN J. WEIN, M.D.

Application of knowledge regarding the neuropharmacology and neurophysiology of the urinary bladder and bladder outlet has resulted in rational pharmacologic therapy that is useful in the management of many types of voiding dysfunction. It is the intention of this chapter to briefly summarize both the relevant pharmacologic principles on which this therapy is based and the current data as to the actual efficacy of various drugs within a functional scheme of therapy for disorders of micturition.

NEUROPHARMACOLOGY OF THE LOWER URINARY TRACT

The lower urinary tract performs two basic functions: storage and emptying of urine. The physiology of this micturition cycle has been described by many qualified authors, and each has described his own particular concept of the neuroanatomy and neurophysiology of the smooth and striated muscular structures involved, the peripheral autonomic and somatic neural factors involved, and the spinal and supraspinal influences that are necessary for and participate in the organization of normal bladder filling/storage and emptying (see Chapter 1). There are significant disagreements regarding the finer details, and the interrelations and correlations, of the relevant neuromorphology, neurophysiology, and neuropharmacology. However, it is important to understand that exact agreement regarding the neuromorphologic and neurophysiologic details is *not* necessary for understanding the pharmacologic principles involved in drug-induced alteration of voiding function.

Neurotransmitters and most drugs produce their effects by first combining with specialized functional cell components called receptors, generally located on the cell membrane. The drug–receptor interaction alters the function of the cell component and initiates the series of biochemical and physiologic changes that characterize the effects produced by the agent. The term "cholinergic" refers to those receptor sites where acetylcholine is the neurotransmitter. Peripheral cholinergic fibers are generally thought to include somatic motor fibers, preganglionic autonomic fibers, and postganglionic parasympathetic fibers (*1,2*). Cholinergic receptor sites are further classified as "muscarinic" and "nicotinic." The effects of cholinergic stimulation at autonomic effector cells, e.g., bladder smooth muscle cells, are referred to as muscarinic actions, as the alkaloid muscarine was characterized originally as having a relatively selective action at these sites, producing qualitatively the same effects as acetylcholine. Atropine characteristically exhibits a complete blocking action at muscarinic receptor sites (*3*). Nicotinic effects refer to the initial low-dose stimulation and subsequent high-dose blockade of autonomic ganglia and of the motor end-plates of skeletal muscle by cholinergic stimulation, actions comparable to those of nicotine.

The smooth muscle of the bladder and urethra in a variety of experimental animals and in man has been shown to contain typical atropine-sensitive muscarinic receptor sites (*4–8*). Quantitation of these receptor sites using a specific radioligand assay shows quite clearly that muscarinic receptor sites are more common in the bladder body than in the bladder base (*9*). A sustained bladder contraction is generally produced by stimulation of the parasympathetic pelvic nerves (*10,11*). The potent muscarinic blocking agent atropine only partially antagonizes the bladder response to this stimulus or to direct electrical stimulation of bladder smooth muscle strips, although it completely antagonizes the response of bladder smooth muscle strips to exogenously administered acetylcholine. The most attractive explanation for this relative "atropine resistance" phenomenon is that a portion of the neurotransmitter released by pelvic nerve stimulation is noncholinergic in nature (*10*). Burnstock (*12*) has proposed that this "missing" contractile neurotransmitter is purinergic, i.e., that the noncholinergic-induced portion of the bladder contraction is secondary to the neural liberation of adenosine triphosphate (ATP). There are a number of other substances that have been theorized to be released upon pelvic nerve stimulation and that have been proposed as alternate excitatory neurotransmitters or neuromodulators, notably histamine, various prostaglandins, and serotonin. Most of the agents discussed under the heading Inhibiting Bladder Contractility, below, are agents that inhibit muscarinic cholinergic receptor sites. These agents, though helpful, leave much to be desired in terms of efficacy in certain situations, and there certainly exists a potential pharmacologic basis for attempting to further inhibit bladder contractility by inhibiting the various other types of receptor sites thought to be responsible for the noncholinergic portion of the contractile response elicited through pelvic nerve efferent impulses. Unfortunately, clinically useful agents of this type are either unavailable (as in the case of ATP) or have not been shown to produce consistently useful clinical effects, at least at this time.

Receptor sites where norepinephrine (NE) is the neurotransmitter are termed "adrenergic" and include most postganglionic sympathetic fibers as well as the fibers of certain central nervous system (CNS) tracts (*2*). Adrenergic receptor sites are further classified as "alpha" or "beta" on the basis of the differential effects elicited by a series of catecholamines (*2,13,14*). Classically, alpha-adrenergic effects consist in vasoconstriction and contraction of smooth musculature; these actions are stimulated most potently by NE and epinephrine (EPI) and cannot be elicited by isoproterenol (ISO). Alpha-adrenergic effects are inhibited by phentolamine and phenoxybenzamine. Beta-adrenergic effects are classically considered to include cardiac stimulation, vasodilation, and smooth muscle relaxation; they are stimulated most potently by ISO and EPI, and least by NE. There has been a great deal of attention paid to the identification and subclassification of adrenergic receptors (*13–16*). At the present time, the generally accepted convention is that alpha-1-receptors include typical postsynaptic alpha-receptors, which mediate smooth muscle contraction. Alpha-2-receptors include a group of presynaptic (located on the postganglionic fiber), autoregulatory receptors whose function is that of a negative feedback mechanism for the release of NE in response to postganglionic neural stimulation. Alpha-2-receptors also include some less typical adrenergic receptors such as those that exist on human platelets. Beta-receptors can also be subdivided into beta-1- and beta-2-receptors on the basis of the relative selectivity of effects of certain agonists and antagonists. Beta-1-receptors are located chiefly at cardiac sites, produce inotropy when stimulated, are stimulated more potently by ISO than EPI and NE (equipotent), and are preferentially inhibited by metoprolol. Beta-2-receptors are present primarily in smooth muscle and gland cells, cause inhibition of smooth muscle contractility when stimulated, are stimulated most potently by ISO and more so by EPI than by NE, and are somewhat selectively inhibited by butoxamine. In general, the effect of activation of alpha-1-receptors in smooth muscle is excitatory, whereas that of beta-2-receptors inhibitory. Activation of alpha-2-receptors inhibits the neural release of NE (and therefore may decrease an alpha-1 effect caused by neural stimulation).

Whether one believes that there is or is not significant innervation of the bladder and proximal urethral smooth musculature by postganglionic fibers of the sympathetic nervous system, one must acknowledge the existence of alpha- and beta-adrenergic receptor sites in these areas (*5,6,17–19*). They have been quantitated with radioligand assays, and the conclusions have been generally similar to those drawn from isolated muscle strip experiments (*20*). The human bladder body contains both alpha- and beta-adrenergic receptors, with the beta variety being the more common. Stimulation of the beta-receptor sites in this area results in relaxation. The bladder base and proximal urethra contain predominantly alpha-receptors, though beta-receptors are present. Thus whatever the physiologic role of the sympathetic nervous system in bladder filling, urine storage, and bladder emptying, alpha-adrenergic agonists have at least the potential to facilitate urine storage at a peripheral level by stimulating contractile receptors in the bladder base and proximal outlet, thereby facilitating functional closure of this area. Significant activation of the beta-receptors in the bladder body would directly inhibit bladder muscle contractility and increase urine storage. In cats at least, a further adrenergic mechanism exists whereby bladder contractility can be inhibited. DeGroat and Saum described depression of neural transmission in bladder parasympathetic ganglia by postganglionic sympathetic neuronal stimuli (*21,22*). This effect, though inhibitory, is mediated by alpha-receptors and is blocked by alpha-antagonists. Although there has been speculation regarding such a mechanism in man, no studies have yet been carried out that would confirm or refute its existence. If it does in fact exist, it represents another potential pharmacologic mechanism for altering bladder contractility.

Most of the agents that alter the urodynamics of the lower urinary tract affect synthesis, transport, storage, or release of neurotransmitter, affect combination of the neurotransmitter with postjunctional receptors, or affect the inactivation, degradation, or reuptake of neurotransmitter. It is obvious that the complex metabolic changes that occur after receptor activation are also potential sites of pharmacologic stimulation, inhibition, or modulation. Calcium plays an important role in excitation–contraction coupling in striated, cardiac, and smooth muscle cells (*23*). The dependence of contractile activity on the inflow of calcium from extracellular sources or on its release from intracellular stores varies from tissue to tissue, but interference with these processes, interference with intracellular calcium utilizing mechanisms, or acceleration of calcium extrusion from the cells are potential mechanisms for mediation of at least vascular smooth muscle relaxation (*24*). Therapy affecting such mechanisms that are "metabolically distal" to the membrane receptor sites, whether concerned with calcium metabolism or other as yet unexplored factors influencing contractility, are also obvious potential sites of pharmacologic stimulation, inhibition, or modulation.

Finally, the knowledge "explosion" in the field of neuropeptide physiology has also provided potential insights into lower urinary tract function and its pharmacologic alteration. Endogenous encephalins are thought to exert a tonic inhibitory effect on the micturition reflex (*25,26*), and agents such as narcotic antagonists offer a possibility for stimulating reflex bladder activity (*27–29*). Vasoactive intestinal polypeptide (VIP) is inhibitory *in vitro* to bladder smooth muscle activity, and a decreased concentration of VIP in bladder tissue may be associated with the unstable bladder syndrome (*30*), raising another possibility for future therapeutic alterations to influence bladder contractility.

THERAPY TO FACILITATE BLADDER EMPTYING

Increasing Intravesical Pressure

Parasympathetic Agents. Agents that imitate the actions of acetylcholine might be expected to be useful in the management of patients who exhibit failure to empty due to inadequate bladder contractility. Acetylcholine itself cannot be used for therapeutic purposes because of actions at the central and ganglionic levels, as well as at the peripheral neuromuscular junction, and because of its rapid hydrolysis by acetylcholinesterase and nonspecific cholinesterase (*31*). Bethanechol chloride is cholinesterase-resistant and causes *in vitro* contraction of smooth muscle from the bladder body and base (*5*). Current recommendations for its use for postoperative urinary retention are for subcutaneous doses of 5 to 10 mg in an awake, alert patient with no outlet obstruction. For more than 30 years it has been used in the treatment of the atonic or hypotonic bladder (*32*) and has been reported to be effective in achieving "rehabilitation" of the chronically atonic or hypotonic detrusor (*33–36*). For this purpose it is recommended that the drug be initially administered subcutaneously in a dose of 5 to 10 mg (usually 7.5 mg) every 4 to 6 hours. It is done preferably with the patient on some intermittent bladder decompression regimen. The patient is asked to try to void 20 to 30 minutes after each subcutaneous dose; and when the residual urine has decreased to an acceptable level, the dose is decreased by 2.5 mg and ultimately changed to an oral dose of 50 mg four times daily. In cases of partial bladder emptying, a therapeutic trial of oral dose of 25 to 100 mg four times daily is utilized in conjunction with attempted voiding every 4 hours with abdominal straining and the Credé maneuver. Bethanechol has been used also to stimulate or facilitate the development of reflex bladder contractions in patients with suprasacral spinal cord injury (*35–37*).

Twiddy *et al.* (*38*) in fact concluded that, in cats at least, intact pelvic reflex pathways are required for bethanechol to produce what they described as a brisk and sustained increase in intravesical pressure during bladder filling.

Urodynamically, attempts to facilitate bladder emptying in patients where bethanechol was the only variable have been generally disappointing. A pharmacologically active subcutaneous dose (5 mg) did not demonstrate significant changes in flow parameters or residual urine in women with a residual urine volume equal to or more than 20 percent of bladder capacity but no evidence of neurologic disease or outlet obstruction, or in a group of 27 "normal" women of approximately the same mean age (*13*). A similar dose failed likewise to produce urodynamic evidence of improved emptying in patients with a positive bethanechol supersensitivity test (*3*). This dosage did increase the intravesical pressure at all points along the filling limb of the cystometrogram and decreased the bladder capacity threshold, findings previously described by others (*36,39*). Although bethanechol chloride in adequate doses is capable of eliciting an increase in tension in bladder smooth muscle such as one would expect from *in vitro* studies, its ability to stimulate or facilitate a true physiologic-like bladder contraction in most patients with neurogenic or nonneurogenic disease has been unimpressive in our experience. Similar sentiments, at least with respect to its use in neurogenic bladder dysfunction, have been expressed by Gibbon (*40*), Merrill and Rotta (*41*), Yalla *et al.* (*42*), and Light and Scott (*43*). It is difficult to find reproducible urodynamic data that support recommendations for the usage of bethanechol chloride in any specific category of patients who exhibit failure to empty. Invariably, long-term studies in such patients are neither prospective nor double-blind, and they do not exclude the effects of other simultaneous regimens, such as treatment of urinary infection, bladder decompression by continuous or intermittent catheterization, timed voiding with the Credé maneuver, and other types of treatment affecting the bladder or outlet. Short-term studies in which the drugs was the *only* variable have generally failed to demonstrate significant efficacy in terms of flow and residual urine volume data. Whether repeated doses of bethanechol or any other cholinergic agonist can achieve a clinical effect that a single dose cannot is speculative. If it is not the case, the long-term response to therapy could be predicted by a urodynamic assessment before and after a single subcutaneous dose or a short oral trial. It is generally agreed, even by proponents of the use of bethanechol, that oral doses of 50 mg or less have little if any effect on even cystometric parameters (*44–46*). It is also generally agreed that, at least in a denervated bladder, a 200-mg oral dose is required to produce the same effect as a 5-mg subcutaneous dose (*44,47*)

Philp and associates (*47*) reported that a 4-mg oral dose of carbachol, a cholinergic agonist that also possesses some ganglionic stimulating properties, had a much greater effect on urodynamic parameters than a 50-mg oral dose of bethanechol without an apparent increase in side effects. This agent is available only as an optic solution in the United States. Anticholinesterase agents, which inhibit the enzymatic degradation of acetylcholine, also have the net effect of producing or enhancing cholinergic stimulation. Cameron reported that distigmine bromide, a long-acting anticholinesterase, was effective in preventing postoperative urinary retention (*48*). Philp and Thomas have reported that parenteral, but not oral, distigmine improved voiding efficiency in patients with neurogenic bladder dysfunction with reflex detrusor activity (*49*). They recommended a 0.5-mg intramuscular dose of this agent per day. It is also available as a 5-mg oral preparation.

No agreement exists as to whether cholinergic stimulation produces an increase in urethral resistance (*50,51*). It appears that pharmacologically active doses do in fact increase urethral closure pressure, at least in patients with neurogenic bladder dysfunction with detrusor hyperreflexia (*52*). If such a phenomenon does occur, a logical question is whether cholinergic agonists could be combined with agents to decrease outlet resistance to facilitate emptying. Khanna (*7*) reported that a combination of a total daily oral dose of bethanechol of 50 to 100 mg with 20 to 30 mg of oral phenoxybenzamine (see below) produced satisfactory results in a group of patients with an atonic bladder and functional outlet obstruction. Our own experience in this situation with such combined pharmacologic therapy, utilizing even 200 mg of oral bethanechol daily, has been extremely disappointing. Certainly most would agree that a daily dose of 50 to 100 mg rarely affects any urodynamic parameter at all (*39,44,45,47*).

The potential side effects of the cholinergic agonists and the anticholinesterase agents are similar and include flushing, nausea, vomiting, diarrhea, gastrointestinal cramps, bronchospasm, headache, salivation, sweating, and difficulty with visual accommodation (*31*). Intramuscular or intravenous use of bethanechol is contraindicated, as such use can precipitate acute and severe side effects resulting in acute circulatory failure and cardiac arrest. Contraindications to the use of these general categories of drug include bronchial asthma, peptic ulcer, bowel obstruction, enteritis, history of recent gastrointestinal surgery, cardiac arrhythmia, hyperthyroidism, and any type of bladder outlet obstruction.

Prostaglandins. Bultitude *et al.* hypothesized that both prostaglandins and acetylcholine were necessary for the maintenance of bladder tone and spontaneous bladder activity (*53*). They summarized their supporting evidence as follows: (a) prostaglandins (PGs) are produced by the bladder, (b) PGE_2 and $PGF_{2\alpha}$ cause a dose-related contraction in *in vitro* bladder strips, and (c) inhibitors of prostaglandin synthesis cause a decrease in bladder tone and spontaneous activity. Other experiments have suggested that prostaglandins may contribute to purinergic excitation of rabbbit and guinea pig bladder (*54,55*). Instillation of 0.5 mg PGE_2 into the bladders of women with varying degrees of urinary retention was reported to result in acute emptying and to improve long-term emptying in two-thirds of the patients studied (*53*). Desmond *et al.* reported results with this agent in patients whose bladder exhibited no contractile activity or in whom bladder contractility was relatively impaired (*56*). PGE_2, 1.5 mg in diluent, was infused intravesically and left for 1 hour. Of 36 patients, 20 showed a strongly positive and 6 a weakly positive immediate response. Fourteen patients showed prolonged beneficial effects, all but one of whom had shown a strongly positive immediate response. Stratification of the data revealed that an intact sacral reflex arc was a prerequisite for any type of positive response. The authors noted additionally that the effects of PGE_2 appeared to be additive or synergistic with cholinergic stimulation in some patients. Vaidyanathan *et al.* reported that intravesical instillation of 7.5 mg of 15 (*S*)-15-methyl-$PGF_{2\alpha}$ produced reflex voiding in some patients with incomplete suprasacral spinal cord lesions (*27*). The favorable response to a single dose of drug, when present, lasted for 1 day to 2.5 months. Other reliable investigators, including Stanton (*57*) and Delaere *et al.* (*58*), have reported no success with this type of treatment. Prostaglandins have a relatively short half-life, and it is difficult to understand how any effects after a single application can last up to even several months. If such does occur, it must be the result of a "triggering effect" on some as yet unknown physiologic or metabolic mechanism. Potential side effects of prostaglandin usage include bronchospasm, chills, hypotension, tachycardia, cardiac arrhythmia, convulsions, hypocalcemia, and diarrhea (*59*).

Blockers of Inhibition. DeGroat and co-workers (*11,21,22*) have demonstrated a sympathetic reflex that, at least in the cat, promotes urine storage by exerting an inhibitory effect on pelvic parasympathetic ganglionic transmission. This effect, although inhibitory, is alpha-adrenergic in nature. Some have suggested on this basis that alpha-adrenergic blockade, in addition to decreasing outlet resistance (see appropriate section), may in fact facilitate transmission through these ganglia and thereby enhance bladder contractility. Guanethidine (*60*) and methyldopa (*61*) have been used with this rationale with at least some good initial results, but here have been no subsequent reports of such efficacy in adequately controlled trials.

Likewise, on this basis, Raz and Smith have advocated a trial of an alpha-adrenergic blocking agent for the treatment of nonobstructive urinary retention (*62*). Although we and others have had occasional anecdotal success using this or another exotic approach, we caution against the assumption that improvement during administration of a drug occurs solely *because* of it.

Decreasing Outlet Resistance

At the Level of the Smooth Sphincter. The observation that sympatholytic drugs are capable of facilitating emptying in certain patients was first made by Kleeman in 1970 (*63*). Krane and Olsson described the concept of a physiologic internal sphincter, controlled partially by tonic stimulation of contractile alpha-receptors in the smooth musculature of the bladder neck and proximal urethra via the sympathetic nervous system (*64,65*). They further hypothesized that some obstructions that occur at this level during detrusor contraction are a result of inadequate opening of the bladder neck or of an inadequate decrease in resistance in the area of the proximal urethra. They also theorized and presented evidence that alpha-adrenergic blockade could be useful for promoting emptying in such a patient with an adequate bladder contraction but without anatomic obstruction or detrusor–striated sphincter dyssynergia. Abel *et al.* (*66*) called attention to the fact that such a functional obstruction, which they too presumed to be mediated by the sympathetic nervous system, could be maximal in the urethra, rather than at the bladder neck, and coined the term "neuropathic urethra." The implication that alpha-adrenergic blockade could be useful in certain patients with a failure to empty despite an adequate increase in intravesical pressure was subsequently supported by others (*67–70*). Successful results—usually defined as an increase in flow rate, a decrease in residual urine, and improved upper tract appearance (where pathologic)—could often be correlated with an objective decrease in urethral closure pressure profile. Although one would expect success with such therapy to be most evident in patients without detrusor–striated sphincter dyssynergia, as reported by Hachen (*71*), Mobley (*72*) reported a startling 86 percent success rate in 21 patients with a reflex neurogenic bladder, with corresponding success rates of 66 percent for what was termed "flaccid" and 57 percent for what was termed "autonomous" neurogenic bladder dysfunction. Success was defined as a postvoid residual urine volume of consistently less than 100 ml. Scott and Morrow (*73*), on the other hand, noted excellent results with phenoxybenzamine therapy in 9 of 10 patients with a flaccid bladder and a flaccid external sphincter, a single patient with an upper motor neuron bladder with intact sympathetic innervation, only 8 of 21 patients with hyperreflexia and autonomic dysreflexia, and none of six patients with an upper motor neuron bladder and sympathetic denervation (lesion between T10 and L2). Harrison *et al.* (*74*) reported significant improvement in residual urine volume in 10 of 14 patients with neuropathic bladder dysfunction and increased outlet resistance of unspecified type treated with an alpha-blocker.

There is a rationale for the addition of alpha-adrenolytic therapy in the patient with inadequate emptying secondary to neurogenic voiding dysfunction after conventional pharmacologic treatment has failed. It has been reported that parasympathetic decentralization leads to a marked increase in adrenergic innervation of the bladder, with a resultant conversion of the usual beta response of the bladder body in response to sympathetic stimulation to an alpha effect (*75–77*). Although the alterations in innervation have been disputed (*78*), the alteration in receptor function has not. Koyanagi showed supersensitivity of the urethra to alpha-adrenergic stimulation in a group of patients with autonomous neurogenic bladders (*79,80*). This finding implies a similar change in adrenergic receptor function in the urethra with parasympathetic decentralization. Parsons and Turton provided a different pharmacologic explanation for a similar type of neuropathic urethra (*81*). They ascribed the cause to adrenergic supersensitivity of the urethral smooth muscle caused by sympathetic decentralization, resulting in an inappropriately high sensitivity to alterations in circulating catecholamine levels brought about as a part of normal cardiovascular homeostasis. Nordling *et al.* described a similar phenomenon in women after radical hysterectomy and ascribed this change to damage to the sympathetic innervation of the lower urinary tract (*82*).

In addition to the effect on smooth muscle, it has been suggested that alpha-adrenergic blocking agents may decrease perineal striated muscle activity, and that this action may contribute to their effect in decreasing outlet resistance (*83*). If this suggestion is so, it seems that such a mechanism must be a central one or must be mediated by noninnervated receptors, as adrenergic innervation of the striated urethral sphincter seems lacking (*84, 85*).

There has been another group of patients in whom alpha-adrenergic antagonists have been reported to be of value. These patients are predominantly male, *without* neurologic disease *or* anatomic obstruction of any type, and they exhibit a failure to empty despite adequate bladder contraction and a lack of striated sphincter dyssynergia. These individuals, adult and pediatric, can often be improved with alpha-adrenergic blocking agents, and their voiding dysfunction has variously been termed bladder neck dysfunction and bladder neck dyssynergy (*86–88*).

The phentolamine stimulation test can usually predict the effectiveness of alpha-adrenolytic therapy in a given situation (*89*). Flow rates are measured before and after an intravenous dose of 5 mg, and the values are plotted on a nomogram that relates flow rate to volume voided. An increase of 0.8 units on the nomogram predicts improved voiding with oral alpha-blocker therapy.

Phenoxybenzamine is the alpha-adrenolytic agent that was most commonly used in the treatment of voiding dysfunction (*50*). The initial adult dosage of this agent is 10 mg daily. An electrocardiogram and supine and standing blood pressure measurements are recommended prior to initiating therapy. The dose may be increased by 10 mg every 4 to 5 days to a recommended maximum of 60 mg daily. Daily doses larger than 10 mg are generally divided and given every 8 to 12 hours. The maximum effect of a particular dose usually becomes apparent only after a week following the initiation of or a change in therapy. After discontinuation, the effects of daily administration persist for about the same period of time. In our experience, patients who responded favorably to this agent generally did so at doses of less than 30 mg and did not respond to dose increases with incremental improvement. Some patients who responded to 10 mg daily could be maintained on an even lower dose. Potential side effects include orthostatic hypotension, reflex tachycardia, nasal congestion, diarrhea, miosis, sedation, and nausea and vomiting (secondary to local irritation) (*14*). Ejaculatory failure, due to lack of seminal emission and not to retrograde ejaculation, frequently occurs (*89*) but with no adverse effect on erection.

Those who still use phenoxybenzamine for long-term therapy should be aware of the adverse *in vitro* and *in vivo* mutagenicity studies with this agent (*90*). These reports indicated that phenoxybenzamine produced increases in gene mutation in *in vitro* systems employing *Salmonella* and mouse lymphoma cells, but that it did not increase the frequency of micronuclei in mouse bone marrow cells *in vivo*. Furthermore, a letter from the manufacturer has indicated a dose-related incidence of gastrointestinal tumors in rats (*91*). Although this agent has been in use for some 30 years in humans without adverse epidemiologic associations, it is obvious that one must now carefully consider the potential medicolegal ramifications of long-term phenoxybenzamine therapy, especially in young individuals.

Prazosin hydrochloride is one of a new class of antihypertensive agents with an affinity for postsynaptic alpha-1-receptors, at least in vascular smooth muscle (*14,92,93*). This agent has little affinity for alpha-2-receptors, in contrast to the classic alpha-adrenergic blocking agents such as phentolamine and phenoxybenzamine, both of which have blocking properties at both alpha-1- and alpha-2-receptor sites. Prazosin has been shown to cause alpha-1 blockade in the smooth muscle of the canine and human urethra (*94,95*); moreover, it has been used successfully and safely to lower outlet resistance in some patients (*95*). In this respect, it is theoretically preferable to phenoxybenzamine because of its relatively selective action at postsynaptic receptor sites. It also produces less tachycardia because of a lesser increase in plasma norepinephrine. Therapy with prazosin is generally begun in daily divided doses of 2 to 3 mg. The dose may be gradually increased to a maximum of 20 mg daily, although we seldom use more than 12 to 15 mg daily in three divided doses. The exact daily dose that is equivalent to the "standard" 10-mg dose of phenoxybenzamine for voiding dysfunction is as yet unknown, but it seems to be 9 to 12 mg in most patients. The potential side effects of prazosin are consequent to its alpha-1 blockade. Additionally, there occasionally occurs the "first-dose phenomenon," a symptom complex of faintness, dizziness, palpitation, and infrequently syncopy, thought to be due to acute postural hypotension. The incidence of this phenomenon can be minimized by restricting the initial dose of the drug to 1 mg and by administering this dose at bedtime. Other side effects associated with chronic prazosin therapy are generally mild and rarely necessitate withdrawal of the drug (*93*). Thus far, reports of adverse effects on seminal emission have been sparse.

Other agents with some alpha-adrenergic blocking properties at various levels of neural organization have urologic side effects that may be therapeutically useful in certain circumstances. Methyldopa is an antihypertensive agent that is converted to α-methyl norepinephrine, which functions as a false neurotransmitter at a central and perhaps peripheral level, with the end result being a decreased peripheral sympathetic effect (*16,96*). Raz *et al.* have reported improved emptying in patients with neurogenic bladder dysfunction with this agent (*97*). Clonidine is another antihypertensive agent whose net effect is a decreased peripheral sympathetic effect, reflected in the urinary tract by a decrease in the urethral closure pressure profile (UCPP) (*78*). Other commonly used pharmacologic agents with significant alpha-adrenergic blocking properties include chlorpromazine and haloperidol (*14*).

Beta-adrenergic stimulation has been shown experimentally to decrease the urethral pressure profile and, by inference, urethral resistance (*18*). The beta-receptors of urethral smooth muscle are of the beta-2 type, producing a decrease in smooth muscle tension upon stimulation. This reaction accounts for the decrease in urethral closure pressure after administration of terbutaline, a relatively specific beta-2-agonist (*98*). Whether this drug or other pharmacologically similar agents will prove useful for facilitating bladder emptying by decreasing outlet resistance remains to be investigated.

At the Level of the Striated Sphincter. There is no class of pharmacologic agents that selectively relaxes the striated musculature of the pelvic floor. Chlordiazepoxide, methocarbamol, orphenadrine, and diazepam belong to a group of agents classified as centrally acting muscle relaxants (*99*). Effective total daily doses of diazepam, the most widely used agent of this group, range from 6 to 60 mg. The primary side effect of all members of this group is sedation, which many believe is primarily responsible for their muscle relaxing effect when administered orally. Only a few studies have actually shown any advantage of these agents, insofar as their purely striated muscle relaxing activity is concerned, over a placebo or aspirin (*100*). In general, we have not found the recommended oral doses to be effective in controlling the classic type of striated sphincter dyssynergia secondary to true neurologic disease. If the etiology of incomplete emptying in a neurologically normal patient is obscure, and the patient has what appears to be inadequate relaxation of the pelvic floor striated musculature, trial with an agent such as diazepam may be worthwhile. The theoretical rationale in such circumstances is either that there is relaxation of the pelvic floor striated musculature (a) during bladder contraction or (b) after removing a stimulus that is inhibitory to bladder activity. Improvement under such circumstances may simply be due, however, to the drug's antianxiety effect or to the intensive explanation, encouragement, and modified biofeedback therapy that usually accompanies this type of treatment in such patients.

Dantrolene sodium is a skeletal muscle relaxant that has been shown to dissociate excitation–contraction coupling at a site distal to the neuromuscular end-plate in the sarcoplasmic reticulum (*99*). It has been shown to have therapeutic benefits in chronic spasticity associated with CNS disorders. The drug has been used in patients with classic detrusor striated sphincter dyssynergia and was initially reported as being successful in improving voiding function in these patients (*101*). It is recommended that adult therapy be begun at a dose of 25 mg twice daily, increasing the dose weekly by 50- to 100-mg increments up to a daily maximum of 400 mg given in divided doses. Hackler *et al.* achieved improvement in voiding function in approximately half of their patients treated with dantrolene but found that such improvement required doses of 600 mg per day (*102*). Although the drug has no autonomic side effects, it may induce a generalized weakness severe enough to compromise its therapeutic benefits, especially at high doses. Other potential side effects include euphoria, dizziness, diarrhea, and hepatotoxicity. The liver toxicity is seemingly related to long-term usage of high doses and has unfortunately apparently resulted in some fatalities.

Baclofen is an agent thought to hyperpolarize primary afferent fiber terminals in the spinal cord (*99*) and to inhibit mono- and polysynaptic spinal reflex activity (*103,104*). It has been found useful in the treatment of skeletal spasticity due to a variety of causes (*105,106*). Treatment is started at an initial dose of 5 mg three times daily, and the dose is doubled every 3 days until a daily total dose of 60 mg is reached. The manufacturer recommends that the total daily dose not exceed 20 mg four times daily. Florante *et al.* (*107*) reported that 73 percent of their patients with voiding dysfunction secondary to acute and chronic spinal cord injury showed decreased striated sphincter responses and decreased residual urine volume following treatment, but with an average daily oral dose of 120 mg. Hachen and Krucker (*108*) found a 75-mg daily oral dose to be ineffective in patients with striated sphincter dyssynergia and traumatic paraplegia, whereas a daily intravenous dose of 20 mg was highly effective. Potential side effects of baclofen include drowsiness, insomnia, rash, pruritus, dizziness, and weakness. Hallucinations sometimes occur after abrupt withdrawal.

THERAPY TO FACILITATE URINE STORAGE

Inhibiting Bladder Contractility

Anticholinergic Agents. Because at least a major portion of the neurohumoral stimulus for physiologic bladder contraction is acetylcholine-induced stimulation of postganglionic parasympathetic cholinergic receptor sites on bladder smooth muscle, atropine and its cogeners depress true detrusor hyperreflexia of any etiology (*109–112*). In patients with detrusor hyperreflexia, the volume to the first involuntary contraction is generally increased, the amplitude of the contractions decreased, and the total bladder capacity increased, with a proportionate reduction in symptomatology. Interestingly, bladder compliance in normal individuals and those with detrusor hyperreflexia, in whom the initial slope of the filling curve on cystometry is normal prior to the involuntary contraction, does not seem to be significantly altered (*112*). The effect of these agents on intravesical pressure during filling in those patients who exhibit only decreased compliance has not been well studied. In patients with detrusor hyperreflexia, although significant clinical improvement is often achieved, only partial inhibition generally results because of the phenomenon of atropine resistance (see Neuropharmacology of the Lower Urinary Tract, above). Outlet resistance, reflected by intraurethral pressure measurements, does not seem to be affected by anticholinergic therapy (*113*). The potentially troublesome side effects of all antimuscarinic agents include inhibition of salivary secretion (dry mouth), blockade of the iris sphincter muscle (pupillary dilation) and the len's ciliary muscle to cholinergic stimulation (blurred vision for near objects), tachycardia, drowsiness, and inhibition of gut motility (*3*). Those agents that possess some ganglionic blocking activity may also cause orthostatic hypotension at high doses. Antimuscarinic agents are generally contraindicated in patients with narrow-angle glaucoma and must be used with caution in patients with significant bladder outlet obstruction, as complete urinary retention may be precipitated.

Although atropine sulfate is available as a 0.5-mg tablet, and it and all related anticholinergics are well absorbed from the gastrointestinal tract, propantheline bromide is the oral agent that is most commonly used to produce an antimuscarinic effect in the lower urinary tract. The usual adult oral dosage is 15 to 30 mg every 4 to 6 hours. Oral administration in the fasting state rather than with or after meals is preferable from the standpoint of bioavailability (*114*). The clinical efficacy can generally be predicted by observation of the effect of a parenteral dose on the cystometrogram (*111*). The parenteral preparation is no longer available, at least in many hospitals in the United States, and atropine or glycopyrrolate may be used instead. For such studies, we generally use 0.2 mg of glycopyrrolate (available as a 1-ml single-dose vial) (*115,116*). There seems to be little difference between the antimuscarinic effects on bladder smooth muscle of propantheline and those of other antimuscarinic agents. Although there are obviously many other considerations that account for the activity of a given dose of drug at its site of action, there is no oral drug available whose direct antimuscarinic binding potential, at least *in vitro*, approximates that of atropine better than the long-available and relatively inexpensive propantheline bromide (*117*.).

It seems that an agent with a significant ganglionic blocking effect as well as such an action at the peripheral receptor level might be more effective in suppressing bladder contractility. Methantheline has a higher ratio of ganglionic blocking to antimuscarinic activity than does propantheline, but the latter drug, clinical dose per dose, seems to be at least as potent in each respect (*3*). Methantheline does have similar effects on the lower urinary tract, however, and some clinicians still prefer it, in doses of 50 to 100 mg four times a day, over other anticholinergic agents (*118,119*). Emepronium bromide is an anticholinergic agent that has been reported to have activity at both peripheral and ganglionic levels (*120,121*). It has been reported to increase bladder capacity in patients with detrusor hyperreflexia while decreasing intravesical pressure and urinary flow (*122*). Recommended oral dosages range from 100 mg three times daily to 200 mg four times daily (*123*). However, Ritch *et al.* (*124*) failed to show any significant effect with oral therapy (200 mg three times daily), although they did demonstrate a good end-organ response with parenteral administration (50 mg intramuscularly). Cardozo and Stanton (*125*) likewise found a clinically significant effect with a parenteral dose of 50 mg. Bladder responses to an intramuscular dose of 0.3 mg/kg, however, were found to be insignificant by Perera *et al.* (*126*). In elderly patients with urinary incontinence and involuntary bladder contractions, Hansen *et al.* (*127*) found no difference between the effects of oral emepronium 200 mg three times daily and placebo, although there was a significant overall subjective cure or improvement (both groups) rate of 79 percent. Potential side effects of this agent are predominantly antimuscarinic, but they also include mucosal alteration, sometimes leading to oral ulcers and esophagitis. This agent is not available for use in the United States.

Musculotropic Relaxants (Antispasmodics). The agents that comprise the relatively exotic sounding category of musculotropic relaxants come under the general heading of direct-acting smooth muscle depressants. Their "antispasmodic" activity is reportedly directly on the smooth muscle at a site that is metabolically distal to the cholinergic receptor mechanism (*50,128*). Although in the laboratory all three of the agents to be discussed do relax smooth muscle by a papavarine-like activity, all have been found to possess variable antimuscarinic and local anesthetic properties as well. There is still some question as to how much of their clinical efficacy is due simply to their atropine-like effect. If in fact any of these agents do exert a clinically significant inhibitory effect that is independent of an antimuscarinic action, there exists a therapeutic rationale for combining their use with that of a relatively pure antimuscarinic agent.

Oxybutynin chloride has been described as a moderately potent anticholinergic agent with strong independent musculotropic relaxant activity as well as local anesthetic activity (*129–132*). This agent has been used successfully to relieve urinary discomfort and "bladder spasm" following endoscopic resection (*133,134*) and to successfully depress detrusor hyperreflexia in patients with neurogenic bladder dysfunction (*135*). A randomized double-blind control study in 30 patients with detrusor instability comparing oxybutynin 5 mg three times daily and placebo was carried out by Moisey *et al.* (*136*). Of 23 patients who completed the study with oxybutynin, 17 had symptomatic improvement and 9 had evidence of urodynamic improvement, mainly an increase in bladder volume at first contraction and an increase in total bladder capacity. The recommended adult dose of oxybutynin is 5 mg three or four times daily. The potential side effects are the same as those of propantheline.

Dicyclomine hydrochloride is another agent reported to possess a direct relaxant effect on smooth muscle in addition to an antimuscarinic action (*137–139*). An oral dose of 20 mg three times daily in adults has been reported to increase bladder capacity in patients with detrusor hyperreflexia (*140*). Our own experience suggests that the individual dose must often be raised to at least 30 mg to achieve a good clinical effect. The potential side effects are antimuscarinic ones.

Flavoxate hydrochloride is another compound that has been reported to have a direct inhibitory action on smooth muscle in addition to anticholinergic and local analgesic properties (*141,412*). Favorable clinical effects have been noted in patients with frequency, urgency, and incontinence, and in those with urodynamically documented detrusor hyperreflexia (*120,143,144*). However, Briggs *et al.* (*145*) reported essentially no effect of this agent on detrusor hyperreflexia in an elderly population, an experience that would coincide with our own subjective impression of limited clinical efficacy in situations where other less expensive agents have failed (*146*). However, as with all agents in this group, a short clinical trial may be worthwhile. The recommended adult dose is 100 to 200 mg three or four times daily. Reported side effects are rare and primarily antimuscarinic in nature.

Beta-Adrenergic Agonists. The presence of beta-2-adrenergic receptors in human bladder muscle has prompted attempts to increase bladder capacity with beta-adrenergic stimulation. Such stimulation can cause significant increases in the capacity of animal bladders that contain a moderate density of beta-receptors (*147*). *In vitro* studies show a strong dose-related relaxant effect of beta-2-agonists on the bladder body of rabbits but little effect on the bladder base or proximal urethra (*148*). Terbutaline in oral doses of 5 mg three times daily has been reported to have a "good clinical effect" in some patients with urgency incontinence but no significant effect on the bladders of neurologically normal humans without voiding difficulty (*149*). Although these results are compatible with those in other organ systems (beta-adrenergic stimulation causes no acute change in total lung capacity in normal humans, but it does favorably affect patients with bronchial asthma), few if any adequate studies are available on the effects of beta-adrenergic stimulation in patients with detrusor hyperactivity.

Alpha-Adrenergic Antagonists. Jensen has reported an increased alpha-adrenergic effect in patients' bladders he characterized as uninhibited (*150*). He reported short- and long-term administration of prazosin to increase bladder capacity and decrease the amplitude of contractions in this category of patients (*150,151*). Rohner *et al.* reported a change in the normal beta response of canine bladder body to an alpha response in response to bladder outlet obstruction (*152*). Perlberg and Caine (*153*) studied the *in vitro* response of bladder dome muscle from patients with obstructive prostatic hypertrophy and found an alpha-adrenergic response to norepinephrine (instead of the usual beta response) in 23 percent of 47 patients. They speculated as to a potential relation between irritative symptoms in these patients and this altered adrenergic response. They further theorized that at least some of the symptomatic improvement in irritative symptoms seen in patients with benign prostatic hypertrophy treated with alpha-adrenergic blocking agents may be due to a direct effect of these agents on bladder muscle, rather than to their effect on outflow resistance.

Prostaglandin Inhibitors. As mentioned previously, prostaglandins are one class of compound with a potentially important role in excitatory neurotransmission in the lower urinary tract. Thus there are multiple mechanisms whereby inhibitors of prostaglandin synthesis might decrease bladder contractility. Cardozo *et al.* reported such effects in a double-blind placebo study of 30 women with detrusor instability utilizing the prostaglandin synthetase inhibitor flurbiprofen in an oral dose of 50 mg three times daily (*154*). Abnormal bladder activity, however, was not abolished in significantly more drug-treated than placebo-treated patients, and actual bladder capacity likewise showed no change. It was concluded that the drug did not abolish detrusor hyperreflexia but delayed the intravesical pressure rise to a greater level of distension. Forty-three percent of the patients experienced side effects from the drug, primarily nausea, vomiting, headache, indigestion, gastric distress, constipation, and rash. Cardozo and Stanton reported symptomatic improvement in patients with detrusor instability given indomethacin, another prostaglandin synthetase inhibitor, in oral doses of 50 to 200 mg daily (*155*). It was a short-term study with no cystometric data, and the drug was compared only to bromocriptine. The incidence of side effects was high, although no patient had to stop treatment because of them. Numerous prostaglandin inhibitors exist, most of which fall under the heading of nonsteroidal antiinflammatory drugs. The most common such agent, aspirin, is only a relatively weak inhibitor of prostaglandin synthesis.

Calcium Antagonists. The rationale underlying the potential use of calcium antagonists for the inhibition of bladder contractility has been described previously. The calcium antagonist nifedipine has been shown to effectively inhibit contraction induced by several mechanisms in human and guinea pig bladder muscle (*156,157*). This agent has been shown to be capable also of completely blocking the noncholinergic portion of the contraction produced by electrical field stimulation in rabbit bladder (*158*).

Terodiline, an agent with both calcium blocking and anticholinergic properties, caused complete inhibition of the response of rabbit bladder to electrical field stimulation (*158*). This agent in low concentrations seemed to have mainly an antimuscarinic action, whereas at higher concentrations a calcium antagonist effect became evident. *In vitro* experiments appeared to show that these two effects are at least additive with regard to bladder contractility. If the calcium antagonist properties of terodiline contribute to its *in vivo* clinical effectiveness and if the drug is actually more effective in decreasing bladder contractility than standard antimuscarinic agents alone remain to be established. Rud *et al.* (*159*) reported that terodiline in oral doses of 12.5 mg two or three times daily produced a marked decrease in the number of hyperreflexic contractions in a group of seven women with urgency incontinence and two with nocturnal enuresis. Bladder capacity was approximately doubled, and the amplitude of the contractions was decreased. In a double-blind crossover study in 12 women with motor urge incontinence, Ekman *et al.* (*160*) reported an increase in bladder capacity and in the volume at which the sensation of urgency was experienced in all but one of the patients treated with terodiline, whereas placebo treatment had no effect on either objective or subjective parameters.

Palmer *et al.* (*161*) reported a double-blind placebo trial with a single 20-mg daily dose of flunarizine in 14 women with urinary frequency, incontinence, and urodynamically proved detrusor instability. A statistically significant decrease in urgency was produced in the flunarizine-treated group, but there was no change in the frequency of micturition. Although there was a trend toward improvement of cystometric parameters, it was not statistically significant at the 0.05 level.

The side effects produced in patients who have been treated with calcium antagonists for voiding dysfunction have been small in number, but the potential side effects of these agents can be of considerable magnitude. They are hypotension, facial flushing, headache, dizziness, abdominal discomfort, constipation, nausea, skin rash, weakness, palpitations, and heart block. Although work in this area is obviously in its infancy, this class of agents may yet prove to be a promising alternative or addition to existing treatment for the inhibition of bladder contractility.

Increasing Outlet Resistance

Alpha-Adrenergic Agonists. Various orally administered pharmacologic agents are available to produce alpha-adrenergic stimulation with relatively mild side effects. Potential side effects of all of the agents that produce a peripheral alpha-adrenergic sympathetic effect include (a) blood pressure elevation and (b) anxiety and insomnia due to CNS stimulation. They may also cause headache, tremor, weakness, dizziness, respiratory difficulties, palpitations, and cardiac arrhythmias. All of these agents must be used with caution in patients with hypertension, cardiovascular disease, and hyperthyroidism (*13*).

Ephedrine is a noncatecholamine sympathomimetic agent that owes part of its peripheral action to the release of norepinephrine but which also directly stimulates both alpha- and beta-adrenergic receptors (*13*). The oral adult dosage is 25 to 50 mg four times daily. Some tachyphylaxis develops to its peripheral actions, probably as a result of depletion of norepinephrine stores.

Pseudoephedrine (Sudafed) is a stereoisomer of ephedrine used for similar indications with similar precautions (*50*). The adult dose is 30 to 60 mg four times daily, and the 30-mg dose form is available in the United States without a prescription.

Norephedrine chloride in a dose of 75 to 100 mg was shown to acutely increase maximum urethral pressure (MUP) and maximum urethral closure pressure (MUCP) in women with urinary stress incontinence (*162*). At a 300-ml bladder volume, the MUP rose from 82 to 100 cm H_2O and the MUCP rose from 63 to 93 cm H_2O. The functional profile length did not change significantly. A 14-day double-blind crossover study comparing the effects of norephedrine to placebo showed that reduction of urinary leakage with the drug compared with placebo occurred in 12 of 22 patients. The MUP and MUCP were increased over those seen with placebo by only 10 and 14 percent, respectively, however.

Obrink and Bunne noted that 100 mg of norephedrine chloride twice daily did not improve severe stress incontinence sufficiently to offer an alternative to surgical treatment (*163*). They further noted in their group of 10 such patients that the MUCP was not influenced at rest or with stress at low or moderate bladder volumes.

Diokno and Taub reported a good to excellent response in 27 of 38 patients with sphincteric incontinence treated with ephedrine sulfate (*164*). They noted that beneficial effects were most often achieved in those with minimal to moderate wetting, and that little benefit was achieved in patients with severe stress incontinence.

Phenylpropanolamine hydrochloride shares the pharmacologic properties of ephedrine and is approximately equal in peripheral potency while causing less central stimulation (*13*). Utilizing doses of 50 mg three times daily, Awad *et al.* found that after 4 weeks of therapy 11 of 13 women and 6 of 7 men with stress incontinence (severity not noted) were significantly improved (*165*). The MUCP was increased from a mean of 47 cm H_2O to 72 cm H_2O in the empty bladder and from 43 cm H_2O to 58 cm H_2O with a full bladder. Phenylpropanolamine 50 mg was combined with 8 mg of chlorpheniramine (an antihistamine) and 2.5 mg of isopropamide (an antimuscarinic) as a sustained-release capsule called Ornade, used primarily for the relief of symptoms of allergic rhinitis. Using one capsule twice daily, Stewart *et al.* found that of 77 women with urinary stress incontinence 18 were completely cured, 28 were much better, 6 were slightly better, and 25 were no better (*166*). In 11 men with postprostatectomy stress incontinence, the numbers in the corresponding categories were 1, 2, 1, and 7. Subsequently, Montague and Stewart carried out urethral profilometry in 12 women with moderate to marked stress incontinence and 6 women with no history of incontinence (*167*). The MUP increased more than 20 percent in 11 of the incontinent women and in only 1 in the continent group. Rees and Ransley reported on the use of Ornade in 83 children with daytime wetting from a variety of causes (*168*). Of 24 children with bladder neck incompetence, 41 percent were cured, 29 percent had minimal symptoms, and 12 percent were improved. Interestingly, of 31 patients with bladder instability, the corresponding improved percentages were 24, 24, and 20. The latter beneficial effect may have been due to the anticholinergic in the preparation. Treatment had to be discontinued in 8 children because of side effects; 23 other children had mild, transient side effects. Major surgery was avoided by drug treatment in 4 children. The formulation of Ornade has now been changed such that each capsule contains 75 mg of phenylpropanolamine and 12 mg of chlorpheniramine. It is also available as a liquid.

Midodrine is a long-acting alpha-adrenergic stimulator reported to be useful in the treatment of seminal emission and ejaculation disorders following retroperitoneal lymphadenectomy (*169*). Treatment with 5 mg b.i.d. for 4 weeks in 20 women with stress incontinence produced a cure in one and improvement in 14 (*170*). The mean MUCP rose by 8.3 percent, and the planimetric index of the continence area on profilometry increased 9 percent. This agent is not yet available for general use in the United States.

Although some clinicians report spectacular cure and improvement rates with alpha-adrenergic agonists in women with stress urinary incontinence, our own experience coincides with that of those who report that treatment with such agents often produces improvement but rarely total dryness in cases of severe or even moderate stress incontinence. A clinical trial is certainly worthwhile, however, and at the least assures the patient that the possibility of one type of nonsurgical therapy has been explored.

Beta-Adrenergic Antagonists. Theoretically, beta-adrenergic blocking agents might be expected to "unmask" or potentiate an alpha-adrenergic effect, thereby increasing outlet resistance. Gleason *et al.* (*171*) reported success in treating certain patients with stress urinary incontinence with propranolol, a beta-adrenergic blocking agent, with oral doses of 10 mg four times daily. The beneficial effect, however, manifested only after 4 to 10 weeks of treatment, a fact that is difficult to explain on a pharmacologic basis, as the cardiac effects occur rather promptly after administration. However, the hypotensive effects of propranolol do not usually appear as rapidly (*13*). Such treatment has been suggested as an alternative method (to alpha-adrenergic stimulation) of pharmacologic therapy in patients with hypertension and stress incontinence. Few if any subsequent reports have appeared to support this approach, however, and it should be noted that others have been unable to show significant increases in urethral profilometry pressures in normal women after administration of a beta-adrenergic blocking agent (*172*). Although 10 mg four times daily is a relatively small dose of propranolol, it should be remembered that the major potential side effects are related to the drug's therapeutic beta-adrenergic blocking effects. Heart failure may develop as well as an increase in airway resistance; asthma is contraindication to the use of this drug. Abrupt discontinuation may precipitate an exacerbation of anginal attacks and rebound hypertension (*13*).

Effect of Imipramine on the Lower Urinary Tract

Some authors have found tricyclic antidepressants, particularly imipramine hydrochloride, to be particularly useful agents for facilitating urinary storage (*173–176*). All of these agents possess varying degrees of at least three major pharmacologic actions (*177–180*): (a) central and peripheral anticholinergic actions at some but not all sites; (b) blockade of the active transport system in the presynaptic nerve ending that is responsible for reuptake of the released amine neurotransmitter serotonin and norepinephrine; and (c) a sedative effect, an action that occurs presumably on a central basis but is perhaps related to their antihistaminic properties. There is also evidence that they sensitize alpha-2-receptors on central noradrenergic neurons (*181,182*). Paradoxically, they have also been shown to have alpha-1-adrenergic and serotonin receptor blocking properties.

Imipramine has prominent systemic anticholinergic effects (*179*). However, it appears to have only a weak antimuscarinic effect on bladder smooth muscle (*110,183,184*), similar to its effect on salivary gland function (*185*). A strong direct inhibitory effect on bladder smooth muscle does exist, however, that is neither anticholinergic nor adrenergic (*132,146, 183–185*). It may be due to a local anesthetic-like action at the nerve terminals in the adjacent effector membrane, an effect that seems to occur also in cardiac muscle (*186*), or to inhibition of the participation of calcium in the excitation–contraction coupling process (*184*). Clinically, the drug seems effective in decreasing bladder contractility and increasing outlet resistance (*175,176,185,187,188*). Trying to correlate the mechanism of action with the clinical effect, one might postulate that the increase in outlet resistance is due to a peripheral blockade of norepinephrine reuptake, which would tend to produce or enhance an alpha-adrenergic effect in the smooth muscle of the bladder base and proximal urethra. Theoretically, at least, this latter action, if indeed it occurs in the lower urinary tract as it does centrally, might tend to also stimulate predominantly beta-adrenergic receptors in bladder body smooth musculature, an action that would further facilitate urine storage by decreasing the excitability of smooth muscle in that area.

Castleden *et al.* (*176*) began therapy in elderly patients with detrusor instability with a single 25-mg nighttime dose that was increased every third day by 25 mg until the patient was continent, had side effects, or reached a dosage of 150 mg. Six of ten patients became continent; and in those who underwent repeat cystometry, bladder capacity increased by a mean of 105 ml and bladder pressure at capacity decreased by a mean of 30 cm H_2O. Our usual adult dose of imipramine for voiding dysfunction is 25 mg four times daily; half that dose is given to elderly patients. In our experience, the effects of imipramine on the lower urinary tract are often additive to those of the atropine-like agents. Consequently, a combination of imipramine and propantheline is sometimes especially useful to decrease bladder contractility (*175*). If imipramine is to be used in conjunction with an atropine-like agent, it should be noted that the anticholinergic side effects of the drugs may be additive.

It has been known for many years that imipramine is relatively effective in the treatment of childhood nocturnal enuresis (*189–191*). Doses have ranged from 10 to 50 mg daily. Whether the mechanism of action is the same as that of imipramine in decreasing bladder contractility or increasing outlet resistance, or it is centrally mediated, is unknown. Korczyn and Kish (*192*) have presented evidence that the antienuretic effect is neither on a peripheral anticholinergic basis nor on the same basis as whatever effects are responsible for the drug's antidepressant action. The antienuretic effect occurs soon after initial administration of the drug, whereas the antidepressant effects generally take 2 to 4 weeks to develop.

When used in the generally larger doses employed for antidepressant activity, the most frequent side effects of this group of agents are those attributable to their systemic anticholinergic activity. Allergic phenomena, including rash, elevated liver function studies, obstructive jaundice, and agranulocytosis may also occur, but rarely. CNS side effects may include weakness, fatigue, a parkinsonian effect, a fine tremor most noted in the upper extremities, and a manic or schizophrenic picture. Sedation may also result from an antihistaminic effect. Postural hypotension may be seen, presumably on the basis of alpha-1-receptor blockade. Antidepressants can be shown electrophysiologically and hemodynamically to have a depressant effect on the myocardium shortly after their institution (*193,194*). Whether cardiotoxicity will prove to be a legitimate concern in patients receiving somewhat smaller doses for lower urinary tract dysfunction remains to be seen.

If imipramine or any of the tricyclic antidepressants is to be prescribed for the treatment of voiding dysfunction, the patient should be thoroughly informed of the usual indications, the potential side effects, and, in the United States, of the fact that this drug is not approved by the federal regulatory agency for this purpose. The onset of significant side effects (severe abdominal distress, nausea, vomiting, headache, lethargy, and irritability) following abrupt cessation of high-dose imipramine in children suggests that the drug should be discontinued gradually, especially in patients receiving high doses (*195*). Tricyclic antidepressants can also cause excess sweating of obscure etiology and a delay of orgasm and orgasmic impotence, whose cause is likewise unclear (*179*). The use of imipramine is contraindicated in patients receiving monoamine oxidase inhibitors, as severe CNS toxicity (hyperpyrexia, seizures, and coma) can be precipitated.

Estrogen Therapy

Caine and Raz (*196*) reported that a daily dose of 2.5 mg of Premarin improved stress incontinence and increased urethral pressures in postmenopausal patients, effects they attributed to (a) mucosal proliferation with a consequently improved "mucosal seal effect" and (b) enhancement of the alpha-adrenergic contractile response of urethral smooth musculature to endogenous catecholamines. Schreiter *et al.* (*197*) reported similar benefits after 10 days of treatment with daily divided doses of 6 mg of estriol. They showed also that the effects of estrogen and exogenous alpha-adrenergic stimulation were additive. Hodgson *et al.* (*198*) reported that the sensitivity of the rabbit urethra to alpha-adrenergic stimulation was estrogen-dependent, as castration caused decreased sensitivity, and treatment with low levels of estrogen reversed the defect.

Rud (*199*) studied the effects of 4- and 8-mg daily doses of estriol on 30 women with an average age of 61 years, 24 of whom had stress urinary incontinence. Profilometry parameters were recorded at a bladder volume of 200 ml with microtransducer technique. Small but statistically significant changes occurred in the maximum urethral pressure (from 59 to 63 cm H_2O), functional urethral length (from 25 to 28 mm), and in actual urethral length (fromm 33 to 37 mm). No statistically significant change occurred in urethral closure pressure (from 37 to 39 cm H_2O). Eight of the 24 incontinent patients experienced subjective and objective improvement, 9 experienced subjective improvement only, and 7 experienced neither subjective nor objective improvement. There was no correlation between subjective or objective improvement and the previously mentioned urodynamic parameters. However, in 18 patients pressure transmission to the urethra was recorded during cough, and in 7 of these patients it improved. All of these patients had subjective improvement, and 5 were shown to be objectively dry. Rud pointed out that it is difficult to believe that the small changes in urodynamic parameters, even though statistically significant, are directly related to resumption of continence. He pointed out also that the increased pressure/transmission ratio might be due to factors outside the urethra—either in the pelvic floor striated musculature or in the periurethral vasculature or supporting tissues. Interestingly, he found no changes in urodynamic parameters in five continent and three stress incontinent women with cystic glandular hyperplasia treated with a single injection of 1000 mg of intramuscular progesterone, except that the pressure/transmission ratio was lower in the three patients in whom this parameter was measured. Rud also recorded profilometric parameters during the menstrual cycle in six women (*200*). There was no change in any profilometric parameter during the menstrual cycle and no correlation between estrogen levels and maximum urethral pressure. It may be, as he suggested, that at physiologic levels estrogens have little influence on urodynamic parameters related to continence and that only pharmacologic doses cause urodynamically significant change. Furthermore, pharmacologic doses may alter responses to other exogenous autonomic stimulation, particularly alpha-adrenergic agents, as the previously described laboratory experiments by Hodgson *et al.* suggested (*198*).

Parenteral estrogen administration can change the alpha-adrenergic receptor content and the autonomic innervation of the lower urinary tract of immature female rabbits (*9,201*). Whether these experiments have any clinical significance is unknown. Certainly, estrogen therapy seems capable of (a) facilitating urinary storage in some women by increasing outlet resistance and (b) having an augmentative or perhaps additive effect to alpha-adrenergic therapy in this regard. Whether the levels achieved by commonly utilized oral or parenteral estrogen preparations or by estrogen vaginal creams (which simply provide a convenient vehicle for systemic absorption) actually increase the alpha-adrenergic receptor content of the smooth muscle of the bladder outlet or the "mucosal seal effect" is still a matter for speculation. The potential long-term effects of such treatment must be carefully considered, however, in the light of the current controversy over whether estrogen therapy predisposes to the development of endometrial carcinoma in menopausal and postmenopausal women.

REFERENCES

1. Koelle, G.: Parasympathomimetic agents. In Goodman, L. S., and Gilman, A. (eds.), *The Pharmacologic Basis of Therapeutics*. Macmillan, New York, 1975, pp. 467–476.
2. Mayer, S.: Neurohumoral transmission and the autonomic nervous system. In Gilman, A. G., Goodman, L. A. and Gilman, A. (eds.), *The Pharmacological Basis of Therapeutics*. Macmillan, New York, 1980, pp. 56–90.

3. Weiner, N.: Atropine, scopolamine and related antimuscarinic drugs. In Gilman, A. G., Goodman, L. S., and Gilman, A. (eds.), *The Pharmacological Basis of Therapeutics*. Macmillan, New York, 1980, pp. 120–137.
4. Todd, J., and Mach, A.: A study of human bladder detrusor muscle. *Br. J. Urol.* 41(Suppl.):448, 1969.
5. Raezer, D., Wein, A., Jacobowitz, D., and Corriere, J., Jr.: Autonomic innervation of canine urinary bladder: cholinergic and adrenergic contributions and interaction of sympathetic and parasympathetic systems in bladder function. *Urology* 2:211, 1973.
6. Nergardh, A.: Autonomic receptor functions in lower urinary tract: a survey of recent experimental results. *J. Urol.* 113:180, 1975.
7. Khanna, O.: Disorders of micturition: neuropharmacologic basis and results of drug therapy. *Urology* 8:316, 1976.
8. Benson, G., Wein, A., Raezer, D., and Corriere, J., Jr.: Adrenergic and cholinergic stimulation and blockade of the human bladder base. *J. Urol.* 116:174, 1976.
9. Levin, R., Shofer, F., and Wein, A.: Cholinergic, adrenergic and purinergic response of sequential strips of rabbit urinary bladder. *J. Pharmacol. Exp. Ther.* 212:536, 1980.
10. Wein, A., and Raezer, D.: Physiology of micturition. In Krane, R., and Siroky, M. (eds.), *Clinical Neurourology*. Little, Brown, Boston, 1979, pp. 1–33.
11. DeGroat, W., and Booth, A.: Physiology of the bladder and urethra. *Ann. Intern. Med.* 92:312, 1980.
12. Burnstock, G.: Past and current evidence of the purinergic nerve hypothesis. In Baer, H. P., and Drummon, G. I. (eds.), *Physiological and Regulatory Functions of Adenosine and Adenine Nucleotides*. Raven Press, New York, 1979, pp. 3–32.
13. Weiner, N.: Norepinephrine, epinephrine and the sympathomimetic amines. In Gilman, A. G., Goodman, L. S., and Gilman, A. (eds.), *The Pharmacological Basis of Therapeutics*. Macmillan, New York, 1980, pp. 138–175.
14. Weiner, N.: Drugs that inhibit adrenergic nerves and block adrenergic receptors. In Gilman, A. G., Goodman, L. S., and Gilman, A. (eds.), *The Pharmacological Basis of Therapeutics*. Macmillan, New York, 1980, pp. 176–210.
15. Hoffman, B., and Lefkowitz, R.: Alpha adrenergic receptor subtypes. *N. Engl. J. Med.* 302:1390, 1980.
16. Weinshiebaum, R.: Antihypertensive drugs that alter adrenergic function. *Mayo Clin. Proc.* 55:390, 1980.
17. Edvardsen, P.: Nervous control of the urinary bladder in cats. *Acta Physiol. Scand.* 72:157, 1968.
18. Raz, S., and Caine, M.: Adrenergic receptors in the female canine urethra. *Invest. Urol.* 9:319, 1971.
19. Awad, S., Bruce, A., Carro-Ciampi, G., Downie, J., and Lin, M.: Distribution of alpha and beta adrenoreceptors in human urinary bladder. *Br. J. Pharmacol.* 50:545, 1974.
20. Wein, A., and Levin, R.: Adrenergic receptor density in the human urinary bladder as compared to that of the dog and rabbit. *Surg. Forum* 30:576, 1979.
21. DeGroat, W., and Saum, W.: Sympathetic inhibition of the urinary bladder and of pelvic ganglionic transmission in the cat. *J. Physiol. (Lond.)* 220:297, 1972.
22. DeGroat, W., and Saum, W.: Synaptic transmission in parasympathetic ganglia in the urinary bladder of the cat. *J. Physiol. (Lond.)* 256:137, 1976.
23. Andersson, K.: Effects of calcium and calcium antagonists on the excitation contraction coupling in striated and smooth muscle. *Acta Pharmacol. Toxicol. (Copenh.)* 43:5, 1978.
24. Movsesian, M.: Calcium physiology in smooth muscle. *Prog. Cardiovasc. Dis.* 25:211, 1982.
25. Roppolo, J., Booth, A., and DeGroat, W.: The effects of naloxone on the neural control of the urinary bladder of the cat. *Brain Res.* 264:355, 1983.
26. DeGroat, W., and Booth, A.: Autonomic systems to the urinary bladder and sexual organs. In Dyck, P., Thomas, P., Lambert, E., and Bunge, E. (eds.), *Peripheral Neuropathy*. Saunders, Philadelphia, 1984, pp. 285–299.
27. Vaidyanathan, S., Rao, M., Chary, K., Sharma, P., and Das, N.: Enhancement of detrusor reflex activity by naloxone in patients with chronic neurogenic bladder dysfunction: preliminary report. *J. Urol.* 126:500, 1981.
28. Vaidyanathan, S., Rao, M., Mapa, M., Bapna, B., Chary, K., and Swamy, R.: Study of instillation of 15(S)-15 methyl prostaglandin F-2 alpha in patients with neurogenic bladder dysfunction. *J. Urol.* 126:81–85, 1981.
29. Thor, K., Rappolo, J., and DeGroat, W.: Naloxone induced micturition in unanesthetized paraplegic cats. *J. Urol.* 129:202, 1981.
30. Mundy, A.: Neuropeptides in lower urinary tract function. *World J. Urol.* 2:211, 1984.
31. Taylor, P.: Cholinergic agonists. In Gilman, A. G., Goodman, L. S., and Gilman, A. (eds.), *The Pharmacological Basis of Therapeutics*. Macmillan, New York, 1980, pp. 91–99.
32. Lee, L.: The clinical use of urecholine in dysfunctions of the bladder. *J. Urol.* 62:300, 1949.
33. Lapides, J.: Urecholine regimen for rehabilitating the atonic bladder. *J. Urol.* 91:648, 1964.
34. Lapides, J.: Neurogenic bladder: principles of treatment. *Urol. Clin. North Am.* 1:81, 1974.
35. Diokno, A., and Koppenhoeffer, R.: Bethanechol choloride in neurogenic bladder dysfunction. *Urology* 8:455, 1976.
36. Sonda, L., Gershon, C., Diokno, A., and Lapides, J.: Further observations on the cystometric and uroflowmetric effects of bethanechol chloride on the human bladder. *J. Urol.* 122:775, 1979.
37. Perkash, I.: Intermittent catheterization and bladder rehabilitation in spinal cord injury patients. *J. Urol.* 114:230, 1975.
38. Twiddy, D., Downie, J., and Awad, S.: Response of the bladder to bethanechol after acute spinal cord transection in cats. *J. Pharmacol. Expe. Ther.* 215:500, 1980.

39. Lapides, J., Friend, C., Ajemian, E., and Sonda, L.: Comparison of action of oral and parenteral bethanechol chloride upon the urinary bladder. *Invest. Urol.* 1:94, 1963.
40. Gibbon, N.: Urinary incontinence in disorders of the nervous system. *Br. J. Urol.* 37:624, 1975.
41. Merrill, D., and Rotta, J.: A clinical evaluation of detrusor denervation supersensitivity using air cystometry. *J. Urol.* 111:27, 1974.
42. Yalla, S., Blunt, K., Fam, B., Gabilondo, F., DiBenedetto, M., and Gittes, R.: Detrusor–sphincter dyssynergia. *J. Urol.* 118:1026, 1977.
43. Light, J., and Scott, F.: Bethanechol chloride and the traumatic cord bladder. *J. Urol.* 128:85, 1982.
44. Diokno, A., and Lapides, J.: Action of oral and parenteral bethanechol on decompensated bladder. *Urology* 10:23, 1977.
45. Wein, A., Hanno, P., Dixon, D., Raezer, D., and Benson, G.: The effect of oral bethanechol chloride on the cystometrogram of the normal adult male. *J. Urol.* 120:330, 1978.
46. Barrett, D.: The effect of oral bethanechol chloride on voiding in female patients with excessive residual urine: a randomized double-blind study. *J. Urol.* 126:640, 1981.
47. Philp, N., Thomas, D., and Clarke, S.: Drug effects on the voiding cystometrogram: a comparison of oral bethanechol and carbachol. *Br. J. Urol.* 52:484, 1980.
48. Cameron, M.: Distigmine bromide (Ubretid) in the prevention of postoperative retention of urine. *J. Obstet. Gynaecol. Br. Commonw.* 73:847, 1966.
49. Philp, N. H., and Thomas, D.: The effect of distigmine bromide on voiding in male paraplegic patients with reflex micturition. *Br. J. Urol.* 52:492, 1980.
50. Wein, A.: Pharmacology of the bladder and urethra. In Stanton S. L., and Tanagho, E. A. (eds.), *Surgery of Female Incontinence.* Springer-Verlag, New York, 1980, pp. 185–199.
51. Wein, A., Malloy, T., Shofer, F., and Raezer, D.: The effects of bethanechol chloride on urodynamic parameters in normal women and in women with significant residual urine volumes. *J. Urol.* 124:397, 1980.
52. Sporer, A., Leyson, J., and Martin, B.: Effects of bethanechol chloride on the external urethral sphincter in spinal cord injury patients. *J. Urol.* 120:62, 1978.
53. Bultitude, M., Hills, N., and Shuttleworth, K.: Clinical and experimental studies on the action of prostaglandins and their synthesis inhibitors on detrusor muscle in-vitro and in-vivo. *Br. J. Urol.* 48:631, 1976.
54. Andersson, K., Husted, S., and Sjogren, C.: Contribution of prostaglandins to the adenosine triphosphate induced contraction of rabbit urinary bladder. *Br. J. Pharmacol.* 70:443, 1980.
55. Anderson, G.: Evidence for a prostaglandin link in the purinergic activation of rabbit bladder smooth muscle. *J. Pharmacol. Exp. Ther.* 220:347, 1982.
56. Desmond, A., Bultitude, M., Hills, N., and Shuttleworth, K.: Clinical experience with intravesical prostaglandin E_2: a prospective study of 36 patients. *Br. J. Urol.* 53:357, 1980.
57. Stanton, S.: Diseases of the urinary system: drugs acting on the bladder and urethra. *Br. Med. J.* 1:1607, 1978.
58. Delaere, K., Thomas, C., Moonen, T., and Debruyne, F.: The value of prostaglandin E_2 and $F_{2\alpha}$ in women with abnormalities of bladder emptying. *Br. J. Urol.* 53:306, 1981.
59. Moncada, S., Flower, R., and Vane, J.: Prostaglandins, prostacyclin and thromboxane A_2. In Gilman, A. G., Goodman, L. S., and Gilman A. G. (eds.), *The Pharmacological Basis of Therapeutics,* Macmillan, New York, 1980, pp. 668–681.
60. Hartviksen, K.: Discussion. *Acta Neurol. Scand.* [*Suppl.*] 42:180, 1966.
61. Raz, S.: Methyldopa in treatment of neurogenic bladder disorders. *Urology* 9:188, 1977.
62. Raz, S., and Smith, R.: External sphincter spasticity syndrome in female patients. *J. Urol.* 115:443, 1976.
63. Kleeman, F.: The physiology of the internal urinary sphincter. *J. Urol.* 104:549, 1970.
64. Krane, R., and Olsson, C.: Phenoxybenzamine in neurogenic bladder dysfunction. I. A theory of micturition. *J. Urol.* 110:650, 1973.
65. Krane, R., and Olsson, C.: Phenoxybenzamine in neurogenic bladder dysfunction. II. Clinical considerations. *J. Urol.* 110:653, 1973.
66. Abel, B., Jameson, R., Gibbon, N., and Krishnan, K.: The neuropathic urethra. Lancet 2:1229, 1974.
67. Johnston, J., and Farkas, A.: Congenital neuropathic bladder: Practicalities and possibilities of conservational management. *Urology* 5:719, 1975.
68. Stockamp, K.: Treatment with phenoxybenzamine of upper urinary tract complications caused by intravesical obstruction. *J. Urol.* 113:128, 1975.
69. Stockamp, K., and Schreiter, F.: Alpha adrenolytic treatment of the congenital neuropathic bladder. *Urol. Int.* 30:33, 1975.
70. Whitfield, H., Doyle, P., Mayo, M., and Poopalasingham, N.: The effect of adrenergic blocking drugs on outflow resistance. *Br. J. Urol.* 47:823, 1976.
71. Hachen, H.: Clinical and urodynamic assessment of alpha adrenolytic therapy in patients with neurogenic bladder function. *Paraplegia* 18:229, 1980.
72. Mobley, D.: Phenoxybenzamine in the management of neurogenic vesical dysfunction. *J. Urol.* 116:737, 1976.
73. Scott, M., and Morrow, J.: Phenoxybenzamine in neurogenic bladder dysfunction after spinal cord injury. I. Voiding dysfunction. *J. Urol.* 119:480, 1978.
74. Harrison, N., Whitfield, H., and Innes-Williams, D.: The place of alpha blocking drugs in the treatment of children with neuropathic bladders. *Urol. Int.* 32:224, 1977.
75. Elmer, M.: Stimulation of adrenergic nerve fibres to the urinary bladder of the rat. *Acta Physiol. Scand.* 94:517, 1975.
76. Norlen, L., Dahlstrom, A., Sundin, T., and Svedmyr, N.: The adrenergic innervation and adrenergic receptor activity of the feline urinary bladder and urethra in the normal state and after hypogastric and/or parasympathetic denervation. *Scand. J. Urol. Nephrol.* 10:177, 1976.

77. Sundin, T., Dahlstrom, A., Norlen, L., and Svedmyr, N.: The sympathetic innervation and adrenoreceptor function of the human lower urinary tract in the normal state and after parasympathetic denervation. *Invest. Urol.* 14:322, 1977.
78. Nordling, J., Christensen, B., and Gosling, J.: Noradrenergic innervation of the human bladder in neurogenic dysfunction. *Urol. Int.* 35:188, 1980.
79. Koyanagi, T.: Denervation supersensitivity of the urethra to alpha adrenergics in the chronic neurogenic bladder. *Urol. Res.* 6:89, 1978.
80. Koyanagi, T.: Further observation on the denervation supersensitivity of the urethra in patients with chronic neurogenic bladder. *J. Urol.* 122:348, 1979.
81. Parsons, K., and Turton, M.: Urethral supersensitivity and occult urethral neuropathy. *Br. J. Urol.* 52:131, 1980.
82. Nordling, J., Meyhoff, H., Hald, T., Gerstenberg, T., Walter, S., and Christensen, N.: Urethral denervation supersensitivity to noradrenaline after radical hysterectomy. *Scand. J. Urol. Nephrol.* 15:21, 1981.
83. Nanninga, J., Kaplan, P., and Lal, S.: Effect of phentolamine on perineal muscle EMG activity in paraplegia. *Br. J. Urol.* 49:537, 1977.
84. Wein, A., Benson, G., and Jacobowitz, D.: Lack of evidence for adrenergic innervation of the external urethral sphincter. *J. Urol.* 121:324, 1979.
85. Rossier, A., Fam, B., Lee, I., Sarkarati, M., and Evans, D.: Role of striated and smooth muscle components in the urethal pressure profile in traumatic neurogenic bladders: a neuropharmacological and urodynamic study: a preliminary report. *J. Urol.* 128:529, 1982.
86. Turner-Warwick, R., Whiteside, G., Worth, P., Milroy, E., and Bates, C.: A urodynamic view of the clinical problems associated with bladder neck dysfunction and its treatment by endoscopic incision and transtrigonal posterior prostatectomy. *Br. J. Urol.* 45:44, 1973.
87. Smey, P., King, L., and Firlitt, C.: Dysfunctional voiding in children secondary to internal sphincter dyssynergia: treatment with phenoxybenzamine. *Urol. Clin. North Am.* 7:337, 1980.
88. Kaneko, S., Minami, K., Yachiku, S., and Juritait: Bladder neck dysfunction: the effect of the alpha adrenergic blocking agent phentolamine on bladder neck dysfunction and a fluorescent histochemical study of bladder neck smooth muscle. *Invest. Urol.* 18:212, 1980.
89. Olsson, C., Siroky, M., and Krane, R.: The phentolamine test in neurogenic bladder dysfunction. *J. Urol.* 117:481, 1977.
90. McNally, C.: Smith Kline and French Laboratories: personal communication (letter).
91. Tannebaum, P.: Smith Kline and French Laboratories, personal communication.
92. Atkins, G., and Nicolosi, G.: Alpha adrenergic blocking activity of prazosin. *Biochem. Pharmacol.* 28:1233, 1979.
93. Graham, R., and Pettinger, W.: Prazosin. *N. Engl. J. Med.* 300:232, 1979.
94. Macgregor, R., and Diokno, A.: The alpha adrenergic blocking action of prazosin hydrochloride on the canine urethra. *Invest. Urol.* 18:426, 1981.
95. Andersson, K., Ed, A., Hedlund, H., and Mattiasson, A.: Effects of prazosin on isolated human urethra and in patients with lower motor neuron lesions. *Invest. Urol.* 19:39, 1981.
96. Blaschke, T., and Melmon, K.: Antihypertensive agents and drug therapy of hypertension. In Gilman, A. G., Goodman, L. S., and Gilman, A. (eds.), *The Pharmacological Basis of Therapeutics.* Macmillan, New York, 1980, pp. 793–818.
97. Raz, S., Kaufman, J., Ellison, G., and Mayers, L.: Methyldopa in treatment of neurogenic bladder disorders. *Urology* 9:188, 1977.
98. Vaidyanathan, S., Rao, M., Bapna, B., Chary, K., and Palaniswamy, R.: Beta adrenergic activity in human proximal urethra: a study with terbutaline. *J. Urol.* 124:869, 1980.
99. Bianchine, J.: Drugs for Parkinson's disease: centrally acting muscle relaxants. In Gilman, A. G., Goodman, L. S., and Gilman, A. (eds.), *The Pharmacological Basis of Therapeutics.* Macmillan, New York 1980, pp. 475–493.
100. Byck, R.: Drugs and the treatment of psychiatric disorders. In: Goodman, L. S., and Gilman, A. (eds.), *The Pharmacological Basis of Therapeutics,* 5th ed., Macmillan, New York, 1975, pp. 152–200.
101. Murdock, M., Sax, D., and Krane, R.: Use of dantrolene sodium in external sphincter spasm. *Urology* 8:133, 1976.
102. Hackler, R., Broecker, B., Klein, F., and Brady, A.: A clinical experience with dantrolene sodium for external urinary sphincter hypertonicity in spinal cord injured patients. *J. Urol.* 124:78, 1980.
103. Jones, R., Burke, D., Marosszeky, J., and Gillies, J.: A new agent for the control of spasticity. *J. Neurol. Neurosurg. Psychiatry* 33:464, 1970.
104. Duncan, G., Shahani, B., and Young, R.: An evaluation of baclofen treatment for certain symptoms in patients with spinal cord lesions. *Neurology* 26:441, 1976.
105. Roussan, M., Abramson, A., Levine, S., and Feibel, A.: Bladder training: its role in evaluating the effect of an antispasticity drug on voiding in patients with enurogenic bladder. *Arch. Phys. Med. Rehabil.* 56:463, 1975.
106. Abromowicz, A. (ed.): Baclofen (Lioresal). *Med. Lett. Drugs. Ther.* 20:43, 1975.
107. Florante, J., Leyson, J., Martin, B., and Sporer, A.: Baclofen in the treatment of detrusor-sphincter dyssynergy in spinal cord injury patients. *J. Urol.* 124:82, 1980.
108. Hachen, H., and Krucker, V.: Clinical and laboratory assessment of the efficacy of baclofen on urethral sphincter spasticity in patients with traumatic paraplegia. *Eur. Urol.* 3:237, 1977.
109. Pedersen, E., and Grynderup, V.: Clinical pharmacology of the neurogenic bladder. *Acta Neurol. Scand.* [*Suppl*] 42:111, 1966.
110. Diokno, A., Hyndman, C., Hardy, D., and Lapides, J.: Comparison of action of imipramine (Tofranil) and propantheline (Pro-Banthine) on detrusor contractions. *J. Urol.* 107:42, 1972.
111. Blaivas, J., Labib, K., Michalik, S., and Zayed, A.: Cystometric response to propantheline in detrusor hyperreflexia: therapeutic implications. *J. Urol.* 124:259, 1980.
112. Jensen, D., Jr.: Pharmacological studies of the uninhibited neurogenic bladder. *Acta Neurol. Scand.* 64:175, 1981.

113. Ulmsten, U., and Andersson, K.: The effects of emprone on intravesical and intraurethral pressures in women with urgency incontinence. *Scand. J. Urol. Nephrol.* 11:103, 1977.
114. Gibaldi, M., and Grundhofer, B.: Biopharmaceutic influences on the anticholinergic effects of propantheline. *Clin. Pharmacol. Ther.* 18:457, 1975.
115. Mirakhur, R., Dundee, J., and Jones, C.: Evaluation of the anticholinergic actions of glycopyrronium bromide. *Br. J. Clin. Pharmacol.* 5:77, 1978.
116. Mirakhur, R., and Dundee, J.: Comparison of the effects of atropine and glycopyrrolate on various end organs. *J. R. Soc. Med.* 73:727, 1980.
117. Levin, R., Staskin, D., and Wein, A.: The muscarinic cholinergic binding kinetics of the human urinary bladder. *Neurourol. Urodyn.* 1:221, 1982.
118. Lapides, J., and Dodson, A.: Observations on effect of methantheline bromide in urological disturbances. *AMA Arch. Surg.* 66:1, 1953.
119. Hebjorn, S.: Treatment of detrusor hyperreflexia in multiple sclerosis. *Urol. Int.* 32:209, 1977.
120. Stanton, S.: A comparison of emepronium bromide and flavoxate hydrochloride in the treatment of urinary incontinence. *J. Urol.* 110:529, 1973.
121. Hebjorn, S., and Walter, S.: Treatment of female incontinence with emepronium bromide. *Urol. Int.* 33:120, 1978.
122. Ekeland, A., and Sander, S.: An urodynamic study of emepronium bromide in bladder dysfunction. *Scand. J. Urol. Nephrol.* 10:195, 1976.
123. Meyhoff, H., and Nordling, J.: Different cystometric types of deficient micturition reflex control in female urinary incontinence with special reference to the effect of parasympatholytic treatment. *Br. J. Urol.* 53:129–133, 1981.
124. Ritch, A., George, C., Castleden, C., and Hall, M.: A second look at emepronium bromide in urinary incontinence. *Lancet* 1:504:1977.
125. Cardozo, L., and Stanton, S.: An objective comparison of the effects of parenterally administered drugs in patients suffering from detrusor instability. *J. Urol.* 122:58–59, 1979.
126. Perera, L., Ritch, A., and Hall, M.: The lack of effect of intramuscular emepronium bromide for urinary incontinence. *Br. J. Urol.* 54:259, 1982.
127. Hansen, W., Hansen, L., Maegaard, E., Mayhoff, H., and Nordling, J.: Urinary incontinence in old age: a controlled clinical trial of emepronium bromide. *Br. J. Urol.* 54:249, 1982.
128. Finkbeiner, A., Welch, L., and Bissada, N.: Uropharmacology. IX. Direct acting smooth muscle stimulants and depressents. *Urology* 12:231, 1978.
129. Lish, P., Labbude, J., Peters, E., and Robbins, S.: Oxybutynin: a musculotropic antispasmodic drug with moderate anticholinergic action. *Arch. Intern. Pharmacodyn.* 156:467, 1965.
130. Fredericks, C., Anderson, G., and Kreulen, D.: A study of the anticholinergic and antispasmodic activity of oxybutynin (Ditropan) on rabbit detrusor. *Invest. Urol.* 12:317, 1975.
131. Finkbeiner, A., Bissada, N., and Welch, L.: Uropharmacology. IV. Parasympathetic depressants. *Urology* 10:503, 1977.
132. Fredericks, C., Green, R., and Anderson, G.: Comparative in vitro effects of imipramine, oxybutynin and flavoxate on rabbit detrusor. *Urology* 12:487, 1978.
133. Diokno, A., and Lapides, J.: Oxybutynin: a new drug with analgesic and anticholinergic properties. *J. Urol.* 108:307, 1972.
134. Paulson, D.: Oxybutynin chloride in control of post transurethral vesical pain and spasm. *Urology* 11:237, 1978.
135. Thompson, I., and Lauvetz, R.: Oxybutynin in bladder spasm, neurogenic bladder and enuresis. *Urology* 8:452, 1976.
136. Moisey, C., Stephenson, T., and Brendler, C.: The urodynamic and subjective results of treatment of detrusor instability with oxybutynin chloride. *Br. J. Urol.* 52:472, 1980.
137. Johns, A., Tasker, J., Johnson, C., Theman, M., and Paton, D.: The mechanism of action of dicyclomine hydrochloride on rabbit detrusor muscle and vas deferens. *Arch. Int. Pharmacodyn.* 224:109, 1976.
138. Downie, J., Twiddy, D., and Awad, S.: Antimuscarinic and noncompetitive antagonist properties of dicyclomine hydrochloride in insolated human and rabbit bladder muscle. *J. Pharmacol. Exp. Ther.* 201:662, 1977.
139. Khanna, O., DiGregorio, C., Barbieri, E., McMichael, R., and Ruch, E.: In-vitro study of antispasmodic effects of dicyclomine hydrochloride on vesicourethral smooth muscle of guinea pig and rabbit. *Urology* 13:457, 1979.
140. Fischer, C., Diokno, A., and Lapides, J.: The anticholinergic effects of dicyclomine hydrochloride in uninhibited neurogenic bladder dysfunction. *J. Urol.* 120:328, 1978.
141, Kohler, R., and Morales, P.: Cystometric evaluation of flavoxate hydrochloride in normal and neurogenic bladder. *J. Urol.* 100:729, 1968.
142. Bradley, D., and Cazort, R.: Relief of bladder spasm by flavoxate: a comparative study. *J. Clin. Pharmacol.* 10:65, 1970.
143. Dalaere, K., Michiels, H., Debruyne, F., and Moonen, W.: Flavoxate hydrochloride in the treatment of detrusor instability. *Urol. Int.* 32:377, 1977.
144. Jonas, U., Petri, E., and Kissal, J.: Effect of flavoxate on hyperactive detrusor muscle. *Eur. Urol.* 5:106, 1979.
145. Briggs, R., Castleden, C., and Asher, M.: The effect of flavoxate on uninhibited detrusor contractions and urinary incontinence in the elderly. *J. Urol.* 123:665, 1980.
146. Benson, G., Sarshik, S., Raezer, D., and Wein, A.: Comparative effects and mechanisms of action of atropine, propantheline, flavoxate, and imipramine on bladder muscle contractility. *Urology* 9:31, 1977.
147. Larsen, J., and Mortensen, S.: Effect of ritodrine on the bladder capacity in unanaesthetized pigs. *Acta Pharmacol. Toxicol. (Copenh.)* 43:405, 1978.
148. Khanna, O., Barbieri, E., and McMichael, R.: The effects of adrenergic agonists and antagonists on vesicourethral smooth muscle of rabbits. *J. Pharmacol. Exp. Ther.* 216:95, 1981.
149. Norlen, L., Sundin, T., and Waagstein, F.: Beta-adrenoceptor stimulation of the human urinary

bladder in-vivo. *Acta Pharmacol. Toxicol (Copenh.)* 43:26, 1978.
150. Jensen, D., Jr.: Altered adrenergic innervation in the uninhibited neurogenic bladder. *Scand. J. Urol. Nephrol.* [*Suppl.*] 60:61, 1981.
151. Jensen, D., Jr.: Uninhibited neurogenic bladder treated with prazosin. *Scand. J. Urol. Nephrol.* 15:229, 1981.
152. Rohner, T., Hannigan, J., and Sanford, E.: Altered in-vitro adrenergic responses of dog detrusor muscle after chronic bladder outlet obstruction. *Urology* 11:357, 1978.
153. Perlberg, S., and Caine, M.: Adrenergic response of bladder muscle in prostatic obstruction: its relation to detrusor instability. *Urology* 20:524, 1982.
154. Cardozo, L., Stanton, S., Robinson, H., and Hole, D.: Evaluation of flurbiprofen in detrusor instability. *Br. Med. J.* 280:281, 1980.
155. Cardozo, L., and Stanton, S.: A comparison between bromocriptine and indomethacin in the treatment od detrusor instabililty. *J. Urol.* 123:399, 1980.
156. Forman, A., Andersson, K. Henriksson, L., Rud, T., and Ulmsten, U.: Effects of nifedipine on the smooth muscle of the human urinary tract in-vitro and in-vivo. *Acta Pharmacol. Toxicol. (Copenh.)* 43:111, 1978.
157. Sjogren, C., and Andersson, K.: Effects of chlinoceptor blocking drugs, adrenoceptor stimulants and calcium antagonists on the transmurally stimulated guinea pig urinary bladder in-vitro and in-vivo. *Acta Pharmacol. Toxicol. (Copenh.)* 44:228, 1979.
158. Husted, S., Andersson, K., Sommer, L., and Ostergaard, J.: Anticholinergic and calcium antagonistic effects of terodiline in rabbit urinary bladder. *Acta Pharmacol. Toxicol. (Copenh.)* 46:20, 1980.
159. Rud, T., Andersson, K., Boye, N., and Ulmsten, U.: Terodiline inhibition of human bladder contraction: effects in-vitro and in women with unstable bladder. *Acta Pharmacol. Toxicol.* (Copenh.) 46:31, 1980.
160. Ekman, G., Andersson, K., Rud, T., and Ulmsten, U.: A double-blind crossover study of the effects of terodiline in women with unstable bladder. *Acta Pharmacol. Toxicol. (Copenh.)* 46:39, 1980.
161. Palmer, J., Worth, P., and Exton-Smith, A.: Flunarizine: a once daily therapy for urinary incontinence. *Lancet* 2:279, 1981.
162. Ek, A., Andersson, K., and Ulmsten, U.: The effects of norephedrine and bethanechol on the human urethral closure pressure profile. *Scand. J. Urol. Nephrol.* 12:97, 1978.
163. Obrink, A., and Bunne, G.: The effect of alpha adrenergic stimulation in stress incontinence. *Scand. J. Urol. Nephrol.* 12:205, 1978.
164. Diokno, A., and Taub, M.: Ephedrine in treatment of urinary incontinence. *Urology* 5:624, 1975.
165. Awad, S., Downie, J., and Kiruluta, H.: Alpha adrenergic agents in urinary disorders of the proximal urethra. I. Stress incontinence. *Br. J. Urol.* 50:332, 1978.
166. Stewart, B., Banowsky, L., and Montague, D.: Stress incontinence: conservative therapy with sympathomimetic drugs. *J. Urol.* 115:558, 1976.
167. Montague, D., and Stewart, B.: Urethral pressure profiles before and after Ornade administration in patients with stress incontinence. *J. Urol.* 122:198, 1979.
168. Rees, D., and Ransley, P.: Eskornade in the treatment of diurnal incontinence in children. *Br. J. Urol.* 52:476, 1980.
169. Jonas, D., Linzbach, P., and Weber, W.: The use of midodrine in the treatment of ejaculation disorders following retroperitoneal lymphadenectomy. *Eur. Urol.* 5:184–187, 1979.
170. Kiesswetter, H., Hennrich, F., and Englisch, M.: Clinical and urodynamic assessment of pharmacologic therapy of stress incontinence. *Urol. Int.* 38:58, 1983.
171. Gleason, D., Reilly, R., Bottaccini, M., and Pierce, M.: The urethral continence zone and its relation to stress incontinence. *J. Urol.* 112:81, 1974.
172. Donker, P., and VanderSluis, C.: Action of beta adrenergic blocking agents on the urethral pressure profile. *Urol. Int.* 31:6, 1976.
173. Milner, G., and Hills, N.: A double-blind assessment of antidepressants in the treatment of 212 enuretic patients. *Med. J. Aust.* 1:943, 1968.
174. Petersen, K., Anderson, O., and Hansen, T.: Mode of action and relative value of imipramine and similar drugs in the treatment of nocturnal enuresis. *Eur. J. Clin. Pharmacol.* 7:187, 1974.
175. Raezer, D., Benson, G., Wein, A., and Duckett, J.: The functional approach to the management of the pediatric neuropathic bladder. *J. Urol.* 117:649, 1977.
176. Castleden, C., George, C., Renwick, A., and Asher, M.: Imipramine—a possible alternative to current therapy for urinary incontinence in the elderly. *J. Urol.* 125:218, 1981.
177. Hollister, L.: Tricyclic antidepressants. *N. Engl. J. Med.* 299:1106, 1978.
178. Rosenbaum, A., Maruta, T., and Richelson, E.: Drugs that alter mood: tricyclic agents and monoamine oxidase inhibitors. *Mayo Clin. Proc.* 54:335, 1979.
179. Baldessarini, R.: Drugs and the treatment of psychiatric disorders. In Gilman, A. G., Goodman, L. S., and Gilman, A. (eds.), *The Pharmacological Basis of Therapeutics*. Macmillan, New York, 1980, pp. 391–447.
180. Richelson, E.: Antimuscarinic and other receptor blocking properties of antidepressants. *Mayo Clin. Proc.* 58:40, 1983.
181. Crews, F., and Smith, C.: Presynaptic alpha receptor subsensitivity after long-term antidepressant treatment. *Science* 202:322, 1978.
182. Spyraki, C., and Fibiger, H.: Functional evidence for subsensitivity of noradrenergic α-2 receptors after chronic desipramine treatment. *Life Sci.* 27:1863, 1980.
183. Dhattiwalla, A.: The effect of imipramine on isolated innervated guinea pig and rat urinary bladder preparations. *J. Pharm. Pharmacol.* 28:453, 1976.
184. Olubadewo, J.: The effect of imipramine on rat detrusor muscle contractility. *Arch. Int. Pharmacodyn.* 245:84, 1980.
185. Tulloch, A., and Creed, K.: A comparison between propantheline and imipramine on bladder and salivary gland function. *Br. J. Urol.* 51:359, 1979.
186. Bigger, J., Giardino, E., Perel, J., Kantor, S., and

Glassman, A.: Cardiac antiarrhythmic effect of imipramine hydrochloride. *N. Engl. J. Med.* 296:206, 1977.
187. Cole, A., and Fried, F.: Favorable experiences with imipramine in the treatment of neurogenic bladder. *J. Urol.* 107:44, 1972.
188. Mahony, D., Laferte, R., and Mahoney, J.: Observations on sphincter augmenting effect of imipramine in children with urinary incontinence. *Urology* 2:317, 1973.
189. Noack, C.: Enuresis nocturia: a long-term study of 44 children treated with imipramine hydrochloride (Tofranil) and other drugs. *Med. J. Aust.* 1:191, 1964.
190. Woodhead, D., Hall, T., and Snodgrass, W.: An effective control of benign enuresis. *J. Urol.* 97:98, 1967.
191. Kunin, S., Limbert, D., Platzker, A., and McGinley, J.: The efficacy of imipramine in the management of enuresis. *J. Urol.* 104:612, 1970.
192. Korczyn, A., and Kish, I.: The mechanism of imipramine in enuresis nocturna. *Clin. Exp. Pharmacol. Physiol.* 6:31, 1979.
193. Burgess, C., and Turner, R.: Cardiotoxicity of antidepressant drugs. *Neuropharmacology* 19:1195, 1980.
194. Muller, J., and Schulze, S.: Imipramine cardiotoxicity: an electrocardiographic and hemodynamic study in rabbits. *Acta Pharmacol. Toxicol. (Copenh.)* 46:191, 1980.
195. Petti, T., and Law, W.: Abrupt cessation of high dose imipramine therapy treatment in children. *JAMA* 246:768, 1981.
196. Caine, M., and Raz, S.: The role of female hormones in stress incontinence. Presented at the 16th Congress of Societé International d'Urologie, Amsterdam, 1973.
197. Schreiter, F., Fuchs, P., and Stockamp, K.: Estrogenic sensitivity of alpha receptors in the urethral musculature. *Urol. Int.* 31:13, 1976.
198. Hodgson, B., Dumas, S., Bolling, D., and Heesch, D.: Effect of estrogen on sensitivity of rabbit bladder and urethra to phenylephrine. *Invest. Urol.* 16:67, 1978.
199. Rud, T.: The effects of estrogens and gestagens on the urethral pressure profile in urinary incontinent and stress incontinent women. *Acta Obstet. Gynecol. Scand.* 59:265, 1980.
200. Rud, T.: Urethral pressure profile in continent women from childhood to old age. *Acta Obstet. Gynecol. Scand.* 59:331, 1980.
201. Levin, R., Shofer, F., and Wein, A.: Estrogen induced alteration in the autonomic responses of the rabbit urinary bladder. *J. Pharmacol. Exp. Ther.* 215:614, 1980.

26

Behavioral Urology

GENE G. ABEL, M.D., AND DORIS BLENDINGER, Ph.D.

The urologist frequently encounters patients having urologic problems for which traditional surgical–medical interventions have been of limited value. These patients have a variety of symptoms (psychogenic urinary retention, dysfunctional bladder syndromes, incontinence, recurrent urinary tract infections, or enuresis) that appear to result from abnormal urination patterns. Traditional psychiatric treatment of these conditions has been problematic because (a) patients have seen their problem as organic in etiology and are reluctant to accept any psychiatric–psychological treatment intervention, and (b) classic psychoanalytic treatment of these conditions has been exceedingly time-consuming, unaffordable for most patients, and of limited effectiveness.

During the mid-1960s a different treatment approach called behavior therapy (behavior modification) was developed and applied to various medical problems. When applied to urologic disorders this assessment and treatment approach is called behavioral urology. Behavioral urology differs from many psychiatric–psychological treatment interventions because: (a) it relies on treatment methods that directly change behavior, rather than attempting to alter inferred unconscious, unobservable processes; (b) it is based on the principles of learning (*1*); (c) it does not focus on the patient's early life experiences as causing urologic symptoms but, instead, changes the behavioral antecedents and the behavioral consequences of those urologic symptoms to eliminate them; and (d) it emphasizes an empiric approach to treatment, quantification of treatment outcome, the use of appropriate experimental design, and what is termed the experimental analysis of behavior (*2*).

This chapter reviews the application of behavioral urology to various urologic syndromes and highlights the clinical application of its principles.

PSYCHOGENIC URINARY RETENTION

Individuals with psychogenic urinary retention present with an inability to urinate in specific environmental surroundings. Muellner (*3,4*) has described the various developmental stages in the acquisition of normal bladder functioning. By age 5 most individuals have learned to initiate and terminate urination irrespective of bladder fullness. Learning to inhibit involuntary detrusor contractions is necessary to prevent enuresis. Patients with psychogenic urinary retention appear to have overlearned this response primarily in specific environmental surroundings.

Case Report: Frank was 37 years of age when he started treatment because he was unable to urinate when standing next to other men in restrooms. History revealed that at age 18, while in college, he had attempted to urinate in the dormitory bathrooms near where individuals showered. As he was standing at the stall preparing to urinate a similarly aged, muscular man was drying off following his shower. Frank became intensely aware of this man's presence, was unable to urinate for the first time in his life, and became intensely anxious and frustrated. An avoidance pattern developed from then on. Each time he approached situations where he had to urinate in the presence of other men he became exceedingly anxious. He rapidly learned how to avoid that anxiety by avoiding restrooms with multiple urinals, so that he would never be in a situation where another man was standing next to him while he urinated. If he entered restrooms where other men were urinating, he used the sit-down, enclosed stalls, pretending to be having bowel movement and waited until they left. If another man came into the restroom while he was attempting to urinate, he would promptly pretend to have completed urination, flush the toilet, and leave with a full bladder.

Frank's case illustrates how learning theory can explain the development of urologic symptoms. The two-factor theory of the development of fear describes how Frank's fears were likely acquired and maintained. First, through classic conditioning, an act (urination) became paired or associated with extreme anxiety (his first anxiety experience at college). As a result, subsequent approaches to such feared surroundings or settings provoked further anxiety. Second, to avoid the intense anxiety associated with such approaches, the patient began to avoid these settings with a concomitant reduction of his fear and anxiety. Avoiding the fearful situation thus became rewarded (by the reduction of anxiety that follows avoidance of the feared situation) through the process of operant conditioning. In this fashion the patient's urologic symptoms continued over years, and indeed by the time Frank was seen at age 37 he had not urinated standing next to a man in 14 years and had a markedly disrupted work schedule because of his inability to urinate near other men when at work, professional meetings, sports events, shopping, etc. As a result of his failure to urinate in public restrooms or around others, he developed low self-esteem and viewed himself as a failure.

In addition to understanding how the patient behaves or acts because of his symptoms, it is also important to evaluate his inner thoughts and attitudes (cognitions) as well as the physiologic responses associated with his symptoms. Before entering restrooms Frank would ruminate about who might be in the restroom, that he probably would not be able to urinate, that if his urinary stream was not strong others would perceive that he was weird, that he was not a real man because he could not urinate properly. He also believed that if he were unable to urinate in a restroom he might in some way lose control, urinate all over himself, or carry out some other unspecified bizarre behavior. Physiologically he reported tachycardia and excessive sweating as he approached restrooms where others might be present.

A number of authors have reviewed treatment approaches for individuals with this "shy bladder" syndrome (*5–8*). The most effective behavioral treatment involves actual repeated exposure of the patient to the feared situations in order to extinguish the anxiety and fear associated with that situation.

Over the course of 1 month (a total of nine treatment sessions) Frank was taught that his symptoms were not due to intrapsychic conflicts but, rather, to a conditioned fear as explained by the two-factor theory of learned fears. Rapport was developed between Frank and his therapist as it was explained to him that effective treatment involved his approaching the fearful settings and remaining in them until his anxiety was dissipated. Frank was asked to examine all the restrooms in the therapist's office building and identify those that provoked the greatest anxiety and fear.

During his third through eighth sessions, while water-loaded (having drunk two quarts of fluid 1.5 hours prior to beginning each treatment session) and with strong urges to urinate, Frank was asked to go into these restrooms and carry out all the behaviors typically antecedent to urinating but not to urinate. While completing this task at various urinals (to ensure that treatment would extend to all urination settings) he was complimented by the therapist for carrying out the very behavior that frightened him.

He next went into restrooms accompanied (or followed) by the therapist who stood beside him or in back of him, making the noises and small talk that normally occur in such settings. As more urinals were entered Frank had less and less anxiety about the therapist's being in the restroom, as no negative experiences could occur because he had been prohibited from urinating.

Further treatment involved his entering restrooms where others (sometimes the therapist's co-workers) were already present or came in later. As his anxiety became minimal under these circumstances he was next asked to carry out all the behaviors as before, but now to just begin to urinate and then to immediately stop. Never being allowed to actually empty his bladder while being water-loaded allowed him to experience repeatedly the very feeling he had feared—being in a restroom with strong urges to urinate while others were near—without having the opportunity to fail to void. Being water-loaded ensured his having strong urges to urinate, and not voiding allowed those urges to persist over many treatment sessions. As he became less and less anxious in restrooms he was asked to extend his treatment into his own office environment and to approach office restrooms in a manner similar to his treatment with the therapist. In all stages of the treatment he was repeatedly encouraged for approaching these fearful situations, situations that to the average person might seem trivial but to him were initially highly anxiety-provoking.

To deal with Frank's faulty cognitions or beliefs about how others might perceive his difficulties urinating, the therapist and Frank approached a number of individuals working in a medical center to discuss a "research project" they were involved in that dealt with various ideas about how others might perceive their having difficulty urinating or urinating with a weak stream. None of these hospital workers were aware that Frank was the patient whose attitudes were being discussed. Prior to treatment Frank had maintained a number of false beliefs about how he might be perceived because he never validated these beliefs by discussing them with others. By discussing his faulty beliefs with others under the supervision of the therapist he learned that his fears about others, perceptions of his behavior were unfounded and subsequently changed these cognitive distortions.

His final treatment sessions emphasized his actual voiding in a variety of settings. He approached restrooms not only in the therapist's environment and at his own work site but all of the restrooms in the vicinity of his work site as well as public restrooms that were usually crowded, as in bus stations, restaurants, and hotels. Near the end of treatment, when he was able to begin urination standing next to others under crowded situations in public restrooms without anxiety, he was instructed to occasionally not only begin to urinate but to empty his bladder. As treatment ended Frank was actively seeking out new, crowded restrooms where he could practice urinating next to others. His self-esteem had improved immensely, and as he looked back on his urologic symptoms he wondered why he had ever believed he could not urinate around other men.

This case demonstrates the typical behavioral urology approach. Frank's urologic problem was viewed as a learned behavior, not as the result of some deep, unconscious conflict. Treatment focused on directly changing Frank's behavior by exposing him to the feared situations under conditions where he could not fail because he was not asked to attempt to urinate. Compliance with the treatment plan was ensured by the therapist's accompanying the patient to urinals, and generalization of the outcome was ensured by his going to multiple restrooms under various surroundings and conditions of crowding.

A urologist serves a critical role in the treatment of patients such as Frank with psychogenic urinary retention. Patients with these symptoms are exceedingly reluctant to approach psychiatrists or psychologists for treatment but, instead, seek urologic evaluations. The urologist should be able to diagnose this condition and teach the patient that brief, effective treatment is currently available. These patients also need encouragement and support for their compliance with the treatment regimen. The urologist by his or her training is able to legitimize behavioral treatment and to be a powerful rewarding force for the patient's compliance. A destructive aspect of patients' behavior is their conceptualizing themselves as weak or psychiatrically ill because of their urologic symptom. It is therapeutic for the urologist to label these symptoms not as psychiatric/psychological problems but as problems of learning improper physiologic functioning. The urologist's labeling of the disorder as nonpsychiatric/nonpsychological allows the patient to better accept entrance into treatment and subsequent treatment compliance. Labeling the disorder as a psychiatric/psychological problem is counterproductive as it stigmatizes the patient as a "weird" emotional cripple, rather than telling him how he can change his behavior to eliminate his urologic symptom.

PSYCHOGENIC ANURIA

Psychogenic anuria is diagnosed when the patient is unable to urinate in all settings and no organic disease can be identified. Because a number of organic factors can lead to anuria, a thorough urologic evaluation must be completed and there must be strong evidence establishing a definite relation between psychological anxiety factors and the onset and maintenance of the anuria. The most extensive assessment of patients with psychogenic anuria was completed by Larson *et al.* (*9*). Their data suggested that multiple factors may contribute to the development of psychogenic anuria. A high percentage of such patients have not only urologic symptoms but also multiple somatic complaints that have frequently led to operative procedures. Larson found that of those undergoing psychiatric evaluations, 68 percent were found to have neuroses, with 48 percent specifically having conversion reactions. The latter diagnosis is made when emotional stress closely precedes the development of anuria and patients model symptoms after others in their environment. Because of the latter characteristic it is important for the urologist to ask patients if they have been around others with similar symptoms (suggesting that they may have acquired some infectious disease) and if there are others in their families with this condition (suggesting that there may be some genetic contributors to the development of the symptom).

The hallmark of conversion symptoms is that they allow the patient to avoid some emotionally stressful situation, and the patient is inadvertently rewarded for the persistence of the symptom. Learning how such symptoms are being reinforced is elicited by explaining to patients that their symptoms must have severely interfered with their ability to function and to ask them to explain how their symptom has affected their lives. Talking with others in the patient's environment is also important, as patients with anuria not only show a casual disregard for their symptoms but frequently do not report emotional factors that are antecedent to their symptoms. Their family members, however, are likely to reveal the important, stressfull antecedents and describe how the symptom is being reinforced.

Only a few cases of treatment for psychogenic anuria are reported in the literature (*10,11*). Treatment has focused on reducing the stresses behind development of the symptom and altering the reward characteristics that maintain the symptom. Because the psychological or physical stressors precipitating the symptoms vary from patient to patient, they cannot be predicted for any one patient with psychogenic anuria. General factors that have been identified with anuria's onset include sexual difficulties, limited assertive skills, and physical and psychic stress (*9*).

In Larsen *et al.*'s experience 20 percent of such individuals were found to have schizophrenia and 12 percent were psychotically depressed (*9*). The high prevalence of neurotic complaints, schizophrenia, and psychotic depression indicate that psychiatric/psychological consultation is indicated in this population of patients. The urologist's role in obtaining such consultations is important because how such consultation is explained to the patient determines the patient's receptiveness to such evaluation and influences the patient's willingness to talk about emotional factors contributing to the symptoms. The urologist should avoid discussions with patients as to whether their symptoms are organic or psychogenic in origin. To focus on this dichotomy only places the urologist in an untenable situation. If forced to agree that the symptom is of an organic nature, the urologist is blocked from obtaining psychiatric/psychologic consultation. Forced to take the position that a major psychological component exists may sever the relationship between the patient and the urologist and cause the patient to leave treatment.

A better tactic is for the urologist to approach psychological assessment as one of many assessments that must be completed during the total evaluation. Psychological referral must be made early in the evaluation plan, along with neurologic, radiographic, medical, and other types of consultation. It is inappropriate to wait until organic assessments are completed and then report to the patient that because these organic work-ups have been negative, referral is being made to a psychiatrist/psychologist. The urologist would better approach the issue of psychiatric/psychological assessment "by the patient's side," that is, working with the patient to look at the results of various assessments to see if the urologist and the patient can arrive at a better understanding of what needs to be done to help eliminate the patient's symptoms.

FREQUENT PAINFUL URINATION

Frequent painful urination of no apparent organic etiology can be an extremely disruptive symptom for patients. The onset of their symptoms usually occurs in their mid-thirties; more than 75 percent have a history of urinary tract infection, and 65 percent have significant pain associated with their frequency. Nocturia occurs in more than 70 percent of cases, and more than 48 percent report a close correlation between sexual activities and worsening of their symptoms. Frewen (*12,13*), in a series of assessment and treatment studies of these patients (also referred to as the urethral syndrome), hypothesized that frequent urination by itself sensitizes or aggravates the detrusor muscle, causing an increased frequency of the urge to urinate. As patients subsequently urinate to relieve their urinary urge, the act of urination further sensitizes the detrusor muscle. Increased frequency follows as the cycle spirals into a progressively shorter frequency of urination. Frewen described a treatment for this condition involving "bladder drills" and medication. The bladder drills include teaching the patient to fully empty the bladder with each urination and to increase the intervoiding interval, thereby decreasing the frequency of urinating and decreasing sensitization of the detrusor muscle.

Abel and co-workers (*14*) described the treatment of 23 such individuals using the Frewen bladder drill technique plus the addition of a relaxation technique to assist patients in tolerating discomfort while prolonging their intervoiding interval. Treatment involved teaching the physiology of micturition and the causative relation that frequent urination itself plays in the development of increasing frequent urges to urinate. Patients next learned a standard behavioral technique for muscle relaxation to combat anxiety and painful urges to urinate.

Once patients could successfully reduce their anxiety/discomfort using muscle relaxation, they were asked to progressively increase their intervoiding interval by 15-minute increments. When successful in 80 percent of their attempts to tolerate one intervoiding interval, it was increased by an additional 15 minutes. Results showed that the median intervoiding interval increased from 45 minutes to 165 minutes as a result of treatment, with 87.5 percent of subjects able to increase their intervoiding interval to such an extent that they could once again function socially.

Unique to their findings was the ability to predict which patients would respond to treatment. When a strong, positive correlation was found between reported urges to urinate and the subsequent volume of urine voided, treatment was effective. When low correlations existed, treatment was less successful.

Case Report: Harvey was 68 years of age when seen for treatment of dysuria and frequency of urination that had been present since age 14. Although he was unable to recall the circumstances surrounding the initial onset of his symptoms, he reported dysuria disappearing shortly after urination, with the return of the urges to urinate and pain in the urethral area 10 minutes later. He subsequently urinated every 15 to 20 minutes in an attempt to relieve the burning sensation, only to have it return. The patient also reported a sleep disturbance associated with nocturia six to seven times per night.

Typical for such patients was his report that he had tried every way possible to control his frequent urination, but everything had failed. His life style had been molded around his frequent urination, as it required that he always be near a restroom. Shopping trips, social events, and his work were structured to include frequent breaks to urinate. In more than 30 years of marriage he and his wife had never been able to vacation because it would require knowing the whereabouts of restrooms in the area in which they were vacationing.

Treatment began by the patient's recording his intake and output over a 48-hour period. The correlation between the strength of his urge to urinate and his subsequent measured urine volume as high ($r = 0.79$). After being educated in the physiology of micturition and the necessity of increasing his intervoiding interval, the patient was taught progressive muscle relaxation, which he practiced on a daily basis. When particularly anxious or when having strong urges to urinate while waiting for his required intervoiding interval to pass, he would carry out progressive muscle relaxation as a means of reducing anxiety and tolerating his urinary discomfort. During 12 outpatient treatment session over an 11-month period, he gradually increased his intervoiding interval from 40 minutes to 3.5 hours.

Early in treatment Harvey insisted that his treatment would fail because of the longevity of his problem and his own inability to cure it. These negative cognitions were dealt with by asking the patient to approach his treatment as an experiment, an experiment to determine if this treatment regimen would be effective if applied with consistency. Clinically it is more effective to approach the patient's symptoms as something to be investigated, rather than by taking a strong, authoritative position that treatment would definitely help. As the patient's intervoiding interval increased, his pessimistic outlook toward therapy disappeared. By the end of treatment he and his wife were able to take a 3-week vacation because proximity to restrooms was no longer mandatory.

The urologist's role in the treatment of frequent painful urination includes: (a) legitimizing the therapy as the appropriate treatment for the patient's symptoms, (b) explaining the physiology of micturition and the necessity for the patient to increase his/her intervoiding interval, and (c) reinforcing the patient's attempts at treatment compliance. These functions may at first appear trite to a surgeon trained to perform complicated, intricate urologic surgery; but without the authoritative support from the patient's urologist, a therapist has a difficult time obtaining the necessary patient compliance to carry out treatment needed to ensure elimination of the symptoms.

NONNEUROGENIC–NEUROGENIC BLADDER

The nonneurogenic–neurogenic bladder syndrome involves symptoms of urinary retention and frequent diurnal dribbling. It is believed to result from a lack of coordination between detrusor contraction and external urethral sphincter relaxation. As intravesicular pressure increases, so does the external urethral sphincter muscle tension, preventing appropriate coordination for bladder emptying. No specific neurologic etiology can be identified.

Most of the reported treatment cases (*15–17*) describe urinary retraining that includes teaching the patient how to completely empty the bladder during voidings and the concomitant use of biofeedback training. To ensure the proper coordination of detrusor contraction and external sphincter relaxation biofeedback is advocated. This involves electrical recording abdominal muscle tension and external sphincter electromyographic (EMG) activity so that patients can observe directly when they are inappropriately having high external sphincter tension associated with detrusor contraction activity. Also important for improvement is teaching the patient how to relax the perineal musculature while maintaining a steady urinary stream, avoiding performance fears (by learning how to relax if fearful of not being able to urinate), and ensuring that the patient's practice of appropriate urinary habits is reinforced by family members.

Disruptive of effective treatment are an unsympathetic physician, poor therapist–patient communication, an unwillingness of the patient to practice appropriate voiding skills in his natural environment, and the absence of appropriate recording devices to display the necessary physiologic responses to be learned.

Biofeedback

Biofeedback is a relatively new treatment methodology that has considerable potential application for urologic conditions. Biofeedback training applies operant conditioning methods (a type of learning) so as to control physiologic responses. With the use of sophisticated electronic equipment a patient is placed in a closed feedback loop where normally unobservable, physiologic processes are made observable through auditory, visual, or tactile feedback (*18*). This new information provides the patients with a method to acquire volitional control over some bodily processes and thereby alleviate their symptoms. Using biofeedback, many physiologic processes, including those governed by the autonomic nervous system, can be brought under conscious awareness, including the contraction and relaxation of skeletal and smooth muscle, the alteration of cardiac rate, and the dilatation or contraction of blood vessels.

In recent years biofeedback has been used successfully with such urologic disorders as urinary frequency, urinary retention, incontinence, enuresis, and detrusor–sphincter dyssynergia (*19*–28). These symptoms may be produced by a wide spectrum of organic pathologies, including infections, urethral obstructions, and neurologic disorders. In the absence of organic involvement, urodynamic assessments may reveal an unstable bladder, reduced ability to sense bladder filling, poor control or coordination of the external urethral sphincter, or a pathologic urge to void with small bladder volumes. These disorders are good candidates for biofeedback training, as the primary objective is to enable patients to acquire an increased sensory awareness of their voiding patterns and train the muscles involved in contraction of the bladder and relaxation of the external urethral sphincter.

Several methods of biofeedback have been reported in the urologic literature, as indicated in Table 26–1. EMG biofeedback training has a twofold purpose: to increase the activity of weak muscle groups and to reduce the activity levels of spastic or tense muscles. Maizels *et al.* (*23*) and Sugar and Firlit (*27*) have treated a number of children with detrusor–sphincter dyssynergia, and Norgaard and Djurhuus (*25*) treated a young girl with enuresis using EMG biofeedback. The latter treatment began with a thorough explanation of the biofeedback procedures. The children were then hydrated to ensure frequent voidings and therefore the opportunity for trials of biofeedback training. EMG surface electrodes were placed perianally and connected to a recorder or an amplifier and loudspeaker. During voidings the patients received instructions to relax the urethral sphincter. Feedback was provided by either direct visual observations of the EMG activity of the urethral sphincter/pel-

Table 26–1. Biofeedback Training as Applied to Urologic Conditions

AUTHOR	UROLOGIC CONDITION	NO. OF SUBJECTS	TYPE OF BIOFEEDBACK	NO. OF TREATMENT SESSIONS	OUTCOME
Cardozo *et al.* (*19*)	Detrusor instability	6	Catheter	6–8	Cured 3/6 Improved 2/6
Ehrman (*20*)	Incontinence	22	Catheter	4–6	Cured 40% Improved 80%
Hafner (*21*)	Retention	1	Catheter	11	Cured
Maizels *et al.* (*23*)	Detrusor–sphincter dyssynergia	3	EMG, perianal	?	Cured 1/3 Improved 1/3
Myers *et al.* (*24*)	Urethral syndrome	5	Galvanic skin resistance	8–18	Cured 4/5
Norgaard & Djurhuus (*25*)	Enuresis	1	EMG, perianal	?	Cured
Pearne *et al.* (*26*)	Retention and incontinence	1	EMG, frontalis	28	Cured
Sugar & Firlit (*27*)	Vesical–sphincter dyssynergia	10	EMG, perianal	?	Cured 8/10 Improved 2/10
Wear *et al.* (*28*)	Retention and incontinence	8	Catheter, EMG	5	Cured 4/8

vic floor musculature or the intensity of sound reflecting the intensity of EMG activity. Recognition of the dyssynergic contractions was subsequently easily observed by the patients and in most cases corrected. Lasting results were achieved with many biofeedback sessions plus home practice to ensure maintenance of the learned response.

Wear *et al.* (*28*) used an intraurethral catheter with five surface electrodes for biofeedback training of eight adults with a history of urinary retention or incontinence. A carbon dioxide cystometer and sphincter EMG recorder were attached to an auditory unit for biofeedback. During the feedback sessions encouragement and support were provided to the patients for controlling their relevant muscle tensions. An average of eight sessions was required to obtain results.

Galvanic skin resistance (GSR), which measures changes in the electrical resistance of the skin to provide an indication of general anxiety or relaxation, has been another form of biofeedback training for treating urologic conditions. As summarized in Table 26–1, biofeedback has already been applied to a variety of urologic conditions, but controlled studies with larger subject populations and long follow-up intervals are needed before the effectiveness of biofeedback can be determined.

NEUROGENIC BLADDER

When gross evidence of organic disease is found concomitant with voiding symptoms, it is usually assumed that the urinary symptoms are of an organic etiology and therefore would be unresponsive to traditional treatment. However, the only reliable means of determining if symptoms are unchangeable with treatment is to carry out that treatment and then observe if the symptoms are eliminated. Consistent with this philosophy, a number of investigators have begun to retrain patients with neurogenic bladders using biofeedback and reeducation methodologies (*29,30*). Nergardh *et al.*, for example, treated 30 children with neurogenic bladders using the combined reeducation–biofeedback procedure described above (*29*). Using regular voiding intervals, procedures to decrease residual urine, medication, biofeedback, and reinforcement from the patient's parents for treatment compliance, 16 of 30 patients achieved social continence, and 13 of the remaining patients were much improved. These early findings confirmed that behavioral treatment can affect neurogenic bladder symptoms, symptoms traditionally believed to be of organic etiology and assumed to be unresponsive to treatment.

FUNCTIONAL NOCTURNAL ENURESIS

Functional nocturnal enuresis is diagnosed when the individual consistently wets the bed and organic work-ups fail to disclose an etiologic agent. Doleys *et al.* (*31*) in a review of the literature, reported that 20 percent of 5-year-olds, 5 percent of 10-year-olds, and 2 percent of 12- 14-year-olds meet the clinical criteria for the diagnosis of enuresis. Of these children, 80 percent have been continuously enuretic (primary enuresis) and 20 percent have been continent but later developed enuresis (secondary enuresis).

A variety of etiologic agents causing enuresis have been suggested including psychological stress, sleep disturbances or deficits in the ability to be aroused from sleep, genetic factors, and a reduced bladder capacity (*32–35*); but no empiric studies have been able to confirm these etiologic causes, and none has sufficiently explained all of the characteristics of the enuretic including response to treatment. Atthowe (*36*) has viewed enuresis as a learned disability in which a child fails to discriminate higher levels of bladder pressure, lacks training in how to appropriately empty the bladder, and has not been consistently encouraged by parents to acquire continence. A number of treatment approaches have originated from this behavioral model (*37,38*).

Drug intervention, daytime bladder expansion training, bell and pad urinating alarm devices, and dry-bed training have been attempted as treatment. Although the tricyclic antidepressant imipramine has been helpful with 85 percent of children (*39*), only 30 percent were able to achieve total continence; and relapse rates were exceedingly high, in the 60 to 95 percent range following discontinuation of imipramine. Daytime bladder expansion training (where the child learns to tolerate greater and greater bladder volumes during the day) has also failed to show consistent effectiveness.

The bell and pad alarm technique (*37*) has consistently produced good results (*40*). A small pad is placed under the child during sleeping hours. If enuresis occurs, an alarm is automatically tripped, awakening the child. Once awakened, the child, with the assistance of the parents, completes toileting. The major difficulty with this technique has been parental compliance with the treatment program (*35*). The urologist should therefore ensure that the parents are extensively involved in administering the treatment program and are made aware of their need to consistently apply it. The urologist should reinforce the attempts of the child and his parents to comply with the treatment.

Azrin *et al.* (*38,41,42*) described an equally effective treatment called dry-bed training that includes the parents training the child in urinary retention control and then rewarding the child for success during daytime awakenings (from naps) or administering negative reinforcement measures for enuresis. Especially promising has been the effectiveness of a manual (*42*) used by parents as a sole treatment for their enuretic children (*43*). Prior to the manual-administered treatment 68 percent of the treated children were extensively enuretic; after 1 week of treatment 27 percent; after 3 months of the treatment 10 percent; and after 6 months of treatment 7 percent. Parental compliance with, and proper understanding of, the treatment procedure were the major difficulties reported with this parent-controlled treatment.

Doleys *et al.* (*31*) strongly suggested that because treatments for enuresis are proving to be highly effective, it behooves the clinician to accurately diagnose these problems by obtaining a detailed description of the problem, elucidation of the family and medical history, questioning the parents about other nonenuretic problems in the family, identifying the surroundings in which enuresis occurs, and evaluating the child's daytime and nighttime urination pattern, current bladder capacity, and previous treatments undertaken for the enuresis. With proper evaluation and the application of either the bell and pad urine alarm of dry-bed training, it appears that a number of children can be effectively treated with current behavioral urology approaches.

INCONTINENCE IN ADULTS

Incontinence in adults is an infrequent problem until older age when a variety of organic factors impinge on the patient's ability to properly toilet. Willington has extensively reviewed this problem, especially in hospitalized patients, where more than 30 percent of individuals are incontinent at the time of hospitalization and 14 percent remain incontinent after discharge (*44*). Incontinence in the elderly is not only problematic for the patient (who suffers the embarrassment of incontinence) but is a labor-intensive process for caregivers in nursing homes and hospitals where bedding and clothing changes can be a time-consuming process.

A number of behavioral factors contributing to the development of incontinence can be altered by the health delivery system. Because the older patient has less mobility, greater efforts need to be taken to (a) provide appropriate privacy; (b) make toilets, bed pans, and urinals readily available and accessible to the patient; (c) reinforce regular voiding patterns and complete emptying of the bladder; (d) maintain normal fluid intake; and especially (e) motivate the care-giving staff to appreciate how effective these environmental changes can be (*44,45*).

The major problem when establishing an environment conducive to continence in institutional settings centers around the attitude of the care-givers. As many as 20 percent view incontinence in the older patient as strictly an organic problem requiring no behavioral treatment (*46*). So long as these incorrect attitude prevail, the health provider staff will not carry out the various behavioral changes necessary to reduce the incidence of incontinence. Education of the staff and demonstrating to them the effectiveness of treatment interventions appears critical.

PREVENTION OF URINARY TRACT INFECTIONS

Our current medical care system emphasizes the treatment of disease after it has been acquired, with little emphasis on preventing the causes of disease. Treating acquired diseases is a costly business, especially in our current medical system with its spiraling costs. A few studies have examined factors contributing to the development of urinary tract infections primarily in female populations (*47,48*). Decreased fluid intake and longer intervoiding intervals appear to be causative factors leading to urinary tract infections. An equally important finding has been that a number of factors such as sexual behavior, cleanliness of the perineal area, the use of tampons, or frequent douching are not associated with an increased frequency of urinary tract infections.

Case reports evaluating multicomponent treatment packages to reduce the incidence of urinary tract infections have produced significant reductions in new cases of infection (*47*). The next step is to carry out controlled studies applying these same methodologies to demonstrate quantitatively the impact of patient education methods on the development of urinary tract infections.

CONCLUSIONS

Behavioral urology is a new field that has already demonstrated itself to be effective with a number of specific urologic conditions. Because it focuses on changing specific behaviors antecedent to and following urologic symptoms that effectively eliminate the patient's symptoms, it can be easily applied to a variety of urologic conditions. A strength of behavioral urology is its focus on elimination of the patient's symptoms without becoming extensively entangled in whether the symptom is organically or psychologically caused. These mind–body controversies are of theoretical interest but are not productive in terms of helping the patient, as they divert the patient's and physician's attention away from the issue of treatment.

Although behavioral urology's goal is to be empiric and based on observable behavior, the current studies using behavioral approaches still lack rigorous empiricism. The cornerstone of the empiric approach involves developing valid dependent measures to assess the need for treatment and if the patient's symptoms have responded to treatment. As Doleys *et al.* (*31*) have suggested, developing objective assessment methods appears to be the first task when applying behavioral principles to urologic disorders. Although initial behavioral treatments of some urologic conditions show considerable promise, further empiric research is necessary to quantify just how effective behavioral interventions are with urologic disorders.

REFERENCES

1. Agras, W. S. (ed.): *Behavior Modification: Principles and Clinical Application.* 2nd ed. Little, Brown, Boston, 1978.
2. Hersen, M., and Barlow, D. H.: *Single Case Experimental Designs: Strategies for Studying Behavior Change.* Pergamon, New York, 1976.
3. Muellner, S. R.: Development of urinary control in children: a new concept in cause, prevention and treatment of primary enuresis. *J. Urol.* 84:714–716, 1960.
4. Muellner, S. R.: Development of urinary control in children. *JAMA* 172:1256–1261, 1960.
5. Ciminero, A. R., and Doleys, D. M.: Childhood enuresis: considerations in assessment. *J. Pediatr. Psychol.* 4:17–20, 1976.
6. Lamontagne, Y., and Marks, I. M.: Psychogenic urinary retention: treatment by prolonged exposure. *Behav. Ther.* 4:581–585, 1973.
7. Shelton, J. L.: Using systematic behavioral assignments for the treatment of conditioned urinary retention. Paper presented at the Association for Advancement of Behavior Therapy Convention. San Francisco, November 1978.
8. Wilson, G. T.: Innovations in the modification of phobic behaviors. *Behav. Ther.* 4:426–430, 1973.
9. Larson, J. W., Swenson, W. M., Utz, D. C., and Steinhilber, R. M.: Psychogenic urinary retention in women. *JAMA* 184:697–700, 1963.
10. Cooper, A. J.: Conditioning therapy in hysterical retention of urine. *Br. J. Psychiatry* 111:575–577, 1965.
11. Campbell, D., and Latimer, P.: Biofeedback in the treatment of urinary retention. *Behav. Ther. Exp. Psychiatry* 11:27–30, 1980.
12. Frewen, W. K.: The management of urgency and frequency of micturition. *Br. J. Urol.* 52:367–369, 1980.
13. Frewen, W. K.: A reassessment of bladder training in detrusor dysfunction in the female. *Br. J. Urol.* 54:372–373, 1982.
14. Abel, G. G., Blaivas, J., and Blendinger, D.: Treatment of frequent-painful urination. Presented at the 4th Scientific Session of the Society of Behavioral Medicine, Baltimore, March 4, 1983.
15. Maizels, M., King, L. R., and Firlit, C. F.: Urodynamic biofeedback: a new approach to treat vesical sphincter dyssynergia. *J. Urol.* 122:205–209, 1979.
16. Wear, J. B., Wear, R. B., and Cleeland, C.: Biofeedback in urology using urodynamics: preliminary observations. *J. Urol.* 119:464–468, 1979.

17. Allen, T. D.: The non-neurogenic neurogenic bladder. *J. Urol.* 117:232–238, 1977.
18. Andrasik, F., Coleman, D., and Epstein, L. H.: Biofeedback: clinical and research considerations. In Doleys, D. M., Meredith, R. L., and Ciminero, A. R., (eds.), *Behavioral Medicine: Assessment and Treatment Strategies.* Plenum Press, New York, 1982.
19. Cardozo, L., Stanton, S. L., Hafner, J., and Allan V.: Biofeedback in the treatment of detrusor instability. *Br. J. Urol.* 50:150–254, 1979.
20. Ehrman, J. S.: Use of biofeedback to treat incontinence. *J. Am. Geriatr. Soc.* 31:182–184, 1983.
21. Hafner, R. J.: Biofeedback treatment of intermittent urinary retention. *Br. J. Urol.* 53:125–128, 1981.
22. Huisman, A. B., Dantuma, R., and Salome, A. J.: A new method for electromyography of the female urethra. *J. Urol.* 121:209–211, 1979.
23. Maizels, M., King, L. R., and Firlit, C. F.: Urodynamic biofeedback: a new approach to treat vesical sphincter dyssynergia. *J. Urol.* 122:205–209, 1979.
24. Myers, H. K., MacKinnon, K. J., and Corson, J. A.: Biobehavioral treatment of excessive micturition. *Biofeedback Self Regul.* 7:467–477, 1982.
25. Norgaard, J. P., and Djurhuus, J. C.: Treatment of detrusor-sphincter dyssynergia by biofeedback. Urol. Int. 37:236–239, 1982.
26. Pearne, D. H., Zigelbaum, S. D., and Peyser, W. P.: Biofeedback-assisted EMG relaxation for urinary retention and incontinence; a case report, *Biofeedback Self Regul.* 2:213–217, 1977.
27. Sugar, E. C., and Firlit, C. G.: Urodynamic biofeedback: a new approach for childhood incontinence/infection (vesical voluntary sphincter dyssynergia). *J. Urol.* 128:1253–1258, 1982.
28. Wear, J. B., Wear, R. B., and Cleeland, C.: Biofeedback in urology using urodynamics: preliminary observations. *J. Urol.* 121:464–468, 1979.
29. Nergardh, A., von Hedenberg, C., Hellstrom, B., and Ericssen, N.: Continence training of children with neurogenic bladder dysfunction. *Dev. Med. Child Neurol.* 16:47–52, 1974.
30. Schneider, R. D., and Westendorf, K.: Adjuvant bladder-pressure biofeedback in treating neurogenic bladder dysfunction: a case report. *Behav. Therapist* 2:29–31, 1979.
31. Doleys, D. M., Meredith, R. L., and Ciminero, A. R. (eds.): *Behavioral Medicine: Assessment and Treatment Strategies.* Plenum Press, New York, 1982.
32. Doleys, D. M.: Behavioral treatments for nocturnal enuresis in children: a review of the recent literature. *Psychol. Bull.* 84:30–54, 1977.
33. Doleys, D. M.: Assessment and treatment of enuresis and encopresis in children. In Hersen, M., Eisler, R., and Miller, P. (eds.), *Progress in Behavior Modification.* Academic Press, New York, 1978.
34. Doleys, D. M.: Assessment and treatment of childhood enuresis. In Finch, A. J., and Kendall, P. C. (eds.), *Treatment and Research in Child Psychopathology.* Spectrum, New York, 1979.
35. Doleys, D. M., Schwartz, M., and Ciminero, A. R.: Elimination problems. In March, E. J., and Terdal, L. G., (eds.), *Behavioral Assessment of Childhood Disorders.* Guilford Press, New York, 1981.
36. Atthowe, J. M.: Controlling nocturnal enuresis in severely disabled and chronic patients. *Behav. Ther.* 3:232–239, 1972.
37. Mowrer, O. H., and Mowrer, W. M.: Enuresis—a method for its study and treatment. *Am. J. Orthopsychiatry* 8:436–459, 1938.
38. Azrin, N. H., Sneed, T. J., and Foxx, R. M.: Drybed: a rapid method of eliminating bedwetting (enuresis) of the retarded. *Behav. Res. Ther.* 11:427–434, 1973.
39. Shaffer, D.: Enuresis. In Rutter, M., and Hersov, L., (eds.), *Child Psychiatry, Modern Approaches.* Blackwell, Philadelphia, 1977.
40. Turner, R. K.: Conditioning treatment of nocturnal enuresis: present status. In Kolvin, I., MacKeith, R. C., and Meadow, S. R., (eds.), *Bladder Control and Enuresis.* Lippincott, Philadelphia, 1973.
41. Azrin, N. H., Sneed, T. J., and Foxx, R. M.: Drybed training: rapid elimination of childhood enuresis. *Behav. Res. Ther.* 12:147–156, 1974.
42. Azrin, N. H., and Besalel, V. A.: *Parent's Guide to Bedwetting Control: A Step-by-Step Method.* Simon & Schuster, New York, 1979.
43. Basalel, V. A., Azrin, N. H., Thienes-Honton, P., and McMorrow, M.: Evaluation of a parent's manual for training enuretic children. *Behav. Res. Ther.* 18:358–360, 1980.
44. Willington, F. L. (ed.), *Incontinence in the Elderly.* Academic Press, New York, 1976.
45. Mandelstam, D.: *Incontinence: A Guide to the Understanding and Management of a Very Common Complaint.* Heinemann, London, 1977.
46. Corp, M., and Turner, K.: A survey of nurse attitudes to incontinence: a summary of findings. Unpublished manuscript, Towers Hospital, London, 1978.
47. Adatto, K., Doebele, K. G., Galland, L., and Granowetter, L.: Behavioral factors and urinary tract infection. *JAMA* 241:2525–2526, 1979.
48. Ervin, C., Kamaroff, A. L., and Pass, T. M.: Behavioral factors and urinary tract infection. *JAMA* 243:330–331, 1980.

27

Clean Intermittent Self-Catheterization

ANANIAS C. DIOKNO, M.D.

Clean intermittent catheterization is now an accepted form of therapy for patients with bladder emptying dysfunction. Sir Ludwig Guttmann in 1966 demonstrated the value of intermittent urethral catheterization using sterile technique in the early management of traumatic paraplegia and tetraplegia (*1*). Guttmann and Frankel have shown that repeated urethral instrumentation using a urethral catheter in men and women is safe. The major drawback to their regimen was the expense and limitation, since the aseptic technique called for involved physicians and registered nurses to perform each and every sterile catheterization on the patient. In addition, this technique is not possible to conduct outside a medical facility.

In 1972 Lapides *et al.* introduced clean intermittent self-catheterization as a temporary or permanent means of emptying the urinary bladder in partial or complete urinary retention (*2*). This technique was first used in 1970 on a 30-year-old woman with multiple sclerosis. She had urge incontinence, incomplete bladder emptying and recurrent urinary tract infection. She was successfully taught self-catheterization. To alleviate urge incontinence, an anticholinergic agent was used. This successful experience led us to apply the same techniques not only to patients suffering from neurogenic bladder dysfunction but also to patients with no neurogenic problems.

Clean intermittent self-catheterization has become popular because of the belief that infection is the result of interaction between invading microorganisms and host resistance, and the bacteria cannot invade tissues if the host has sufficient immunity. Most cases of urinary infection are due to some underlying structural or functional abnormality of the urogenital tract that leads to decreased tissue resistance and bacterial invasion. Obvious causes such as inlying catheters, urinary calculi, and traumatic instrumentation also can lead to urinary infection. In the case of anatomic or functional outlet obstruction or chronic bladder overdistension, the patient is believed to be susceptible to infection because of increased intravesical pressure or overdistension causing decreased blood flow to the tissue. The resulting ischemic wall is susceptible to infections. It is important, therefore, to avoid high intraluminal pressures and overdistension by frequent, and complete bladder emptying. Although bacteria are necessary in the causation of infection, they cannot invade normal healthy tissues.

INDICATIONS

The main objective in caring for a patient with complete or partial urinary retention is to help him/her regain the ability to initiate and complete the act of voiding voluntarily. If this goal cannot be attained and retention persists, clean intermittent self-catheterization should be considered whenever possible.

Intermittent catheterization can be used as

a temporary or permanent form of bladder emptying. Temporary uses include urinary retention observed in patients following certain surgical procedures such as suprapubic or vaginal bladder suspension, anterior colporrhaphy, hemorrhoidectomy, laminectomy, hysterectomy, and other pelvic or abdominal surgery. Transient retention may also occur during the postpartum period as well as in cases of psychogenic urinary retention. Permanent urinary retention is usually encountered in patients with severe spinal cord lesions such as transverse myelitis, multiple sclerosis, myelodysplasia, peripheral neuropathy, and other disorders, including hypotonic or acontractile bladder due to chronic obstruction or infrequent voiding.

Patients who are being managed with suprapubic tubes or indwelling catheters for voiding difficulties should be considered as candidates for periodic self-catheterization. Most of these patients have neuropathic bladder, prostatism for which they refuse or are not candidates for operation, or acontractile bladders. These patients should be evaluated to determine their fitness for the intermittent urethral catheterization program.

Contraindications for the use of intermittent catheterization include mental incompetence, blindness, inability to use the hands, a small-capacity bladder, and intractable incontinence. Calling upon another person to perform clean intermittent catheterization in a patient must be considered carefully, as it would tie this person to the patient considerably. The relationship between husband and wife and their perception of what the program entails should be explored before starting it. Children who are dependent on unreliable parents for performance of the regimen are excluded from the program.

Innovative operative procedures have been introduced to overcome problems that may contraindicate intermittent urethral catheterization. By creating a continent vesicostomy stoma into the abdomen and bypassing the urethra, intermittent catheterization can easily be performed through the new bladder port (*3*). This method is helpful to those who have weak and/or poorly coordinated hands as well as in cases of difficult urethral catheterization. In patients with small bladder capacity, the bladder can be enlarged by augmentation with a segment of bowel, which may be done in conjunction with creation of a new continent abdominal stoma (*4*).

Another technique of improving the chance of using the intermittent catheterization program is the use of mechanical devices for quadriplegics to aid in the catheterization program (*5*). On occasion, hand motion can be improved with arthroplasty procedures.

EVALUATION

Prospective patients for clean intermittent self-catheterization are evaluated prior to the teaching session. Knowledge of the cause of urinary retention and the status of the bladder and urethra is important for the success of intermittent catheterization program. The physician taking care of the patient must be aware of the need for supplemental therapy in patients with hyperreflexia and urethral incompetence; otherwise incontinence will persist. One must also make sure that no preexisting calculus is present in the bladder, especially in patients who are on indwelling catheters prior to conversion to intermittent catheterization. These stones may continue to grow inside the bladder. The instructor of the regimen must also be sure that the urethra is intact and free of strictures and false passages.

As mentioned earlier, the patient and his helper are screened for willingness to comply with the program. Compliance is improved when the patient and the family are instructed the concept and the basis for the intermittent catheterization program. They should be informed of the rationale for the rigid catheterization schedule and the need for long-term surveillance. It is also important for them to be aware of the alternatives to intermittent catheterization, so that they are well informed and confident of the choice of therapy. Once a decision is reached that the patient and his/her helper will be taught intermittent catheterization, an arrangement is made for them to view the technique on teaching videotapes or slide presentations which are usually available at medical centers. Such viewing is extremely helpful to the individuals concerned and makes learning the technique much easier.

INSTRUCTION

The instructor should be someone who is knowledgeable of the basic principles of the method and has had considerable experience. In our institution, the teachers have been nurses, enterostomal therapists, physicians, and physician's assistants.

The patients are requested to report for their catheterization lesson with a full bladder if possible. The female subject sits on the examining table with feet on the table, lower limbs flexed and knees held apart, to expose the introitus and urethral meatus. The head of the table is elevated to allow the patient to visualize the perineum in a mirror at the footend of the table. The labia are separated, and the introital anatomy such as the clitoris, urethral meatus, and vaginal outlet are shown to the patient. A 14F plastic or rubber catheter is introduced to the patient, who is allowed to inspect the catheter to alleviate any fears about the catheter. The patient is then instructed to insert the catheter through the urethral meatus into the bladder. The patient is directed to hold the catheter about 1.0 to 1.5 in. from the tip with the dominant hand, and with the fingers of the other hand to hold the labia apart with the index and fourth finger while pressing on the meatus with the third finger (Fig. 27–1). The third finger is then lifted off the meatus and the catheter passed into the urethra. The patient is advised to partially empty the bladder, withdraw the catheter completely, and recatheterize herself. Thereafter she is taken to the bathroom, where she either sits on the toilet seat or stands facing the toilet with one foot on the toilet seat. She catheterizes herself several times again until she feels confident about the procedure.

The teaching of self-catheterization to the male subject is simple. It is accomplished with the patient in the sitting position initially and then standing if possible. It is necessary to apply a water-soluble surgical lubricant in generous fashion to the outer terminal portion of the catheter in order to avoid traumatic urethritis. The patient is instructed to hold the penis up on both sides just behind the glans penis. He is further instructed to apply steady pressure during the catheter insertion, and that resistance may be encountered as the catheter passes the area of the membranous urethra and external sphincter.

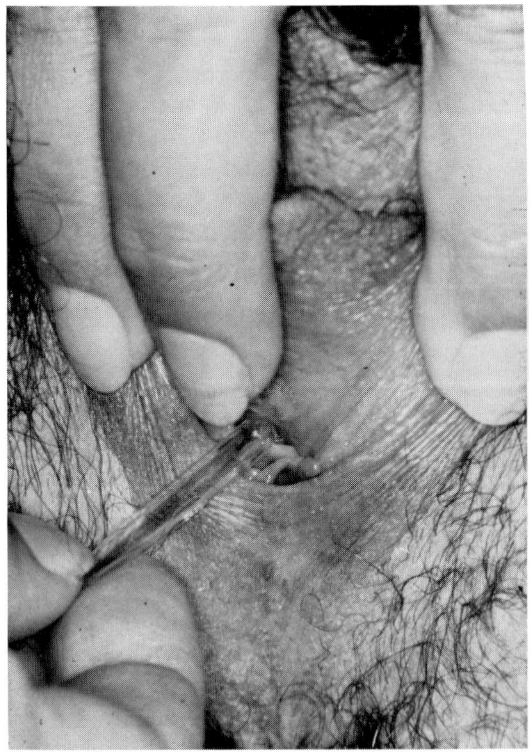

Figure 27–1. Technique of self-catheterization using urethral meatal palpation. The dominant hand holds the plastic catheter 1.5 in. from the tip. The fingers of the other hand hold the labia apart with the index and fourth finger, and the middle finger is used to palpate the meatus.

At this point, continuous, gentle but firm pressure on the catheter is needed to advance the catheter into the bladder cavity.

Upon completion of the catheterization lesson, the pupil is given an instruction sheet reiterating the principles and methods involved and a list of necessary materials. The catheter can be carried in a dry state in a plastic bag, paper towel, or something comparable. No sterilizing solution is used, and no lubricant is needed for the female subject. For the sake of cleanliness and prevention of malodor, the patient, whenever possible washes his or her hands and the outer surface of the catheter with the same soapy lather, then rinses both inside and outside of the catheter with clear water. The patient is warned never to forego catheterization when soap and water are not available but to catheterize at the prescribed time regardless of circumstances.

In the wheelchair-borne patient, urine disposal is accomplished in one of two ways. A catheter extension can be used to drain the urine directly into the toilet bowl or other appropriate receptacle, or a clear plastic liquid detergent container with a hanger is used as a temporary receptacle.

The frequency of catheterization varies from patient to patient; however, we generally recommend that regular and complete bladder emptying be done every 3 to 4 hours during the waking hours and once at night. In an adult patient the goal is to remove no more than 300 to 400 ml of urine from the bladder with each catheterization. The maximum catheterized volume is 150 ml in 1- to 5-year olds, 250 ml in 6- to 9-year olds, and 300 ml for those children 9 years and older.

It is also important to sterilize the urine or place the patient on an antimicrobial agent at least 1 day prior to teaching intermittent catheterization. It is our practice to continue the antimicrobial agent for at least 2 to 3 weeks following initiation of the program. Long-term antimicrobial prophylaxis is determined by the subsequent clinical course of the patient.

POTENTIAL COMPLICATIONS

Bacteriuria and Urinary Sepsis

It is predictable that whenever clean or unsterile intermittent self-catheterization is introduced to a medical community or a hospital for the first time, resistance will be strong from many nursing and medical personnel because of the fear that urinary tract infection is the inevitable consequence of unsterile bladder instrumentation. However, since its first introduction by Lapides *et al.* in 1972 (*2*), this procedure has become a widely accepted technique, mainly because people who have tried it over the years have found it to be safe and efficacious. The long-term experience with this technique has supported the beliefs of Lapides (*6*) and Hinman and Cox (*7*) that a bacterial inoculum introduced into a bladder causes little harm so long as frequent and complete bladder emptying is accomplished.

Asymptomatic bacteriuria is a constant finding in most patients placed on clean intermittent catheterization. The study of Kass *et al.* reported a 56 percent incidence of bacilluria in 255 children treated with clean intermittent catheterization (*8*). Only 5 percent of the patients had a single episode of bacteriuria during the entire follow-up period. The most common organisms cultured were *Escherichia coli* (in 50%), *Pseudomonas* (in 20%), *Proteus* species (in 12%), and *Klebsiella* (in 9%). Kass reported febrile urinary tract infections in 37 percent of 65 children with vesicoureteral reflux but only 3 percent of 190 patients without reflux following the start of clean intermittent catheterization.

Plunkett and Braren reported a 52 percent incidence of bacteriuria among 34 pediatric patients treated by intermittent catheterization (*9*). They reported that 7 of 34 patients maintained persistently sterile urine. Despite these numbers, only two cases of acute pyelonephritis developed, and both occurred in patients with massive vesicoureteral reflux.

McGuire and Savastano reported the incidence of bacteriuria among 41 spinal cord injured patients treated by intermittent self-catheterization for a mean follow-up period of 4.6 years (*10*). Their data on quarterly bacteriologic studies revealed abacteriuria in 32 percent, occasional bacteriuria in 32 percent, and chronic bacteriuria in 36 percent. During the entire follow-up, only three patients developed febrile urinary tract infection.

A report from Michigan on 27 patients who were placed on the catheterization program followed for at least 10 years revealed a 74 percent incidence of bacteriuria (*11*). In this group only two patients developed acute pyelonephritis, and both had vesicoureteral reflux.

Complications from genital infection is rare and occurs only in men. Acute epididymitis has been reported in association with self catheterization. Maynard and Diokno reported that 4 of 50 spinal cord injured men developed epididymitis (*12*). In their analysis, the epididymal infection was linked to a previous inlying urethral catheter and infected penile prosthesis. All infections were cleared with appropriate antibiotic therapy.

The experience to date with long-term intermittent catheterization suggests that chronic bacteriuria does not produce any urinary sepsis provided that vesicoureteral reflux does not exist and bladder over distension and trauma are avoided. Many patients on long-term catheterization have persistent bacteriuria without apparent implication. Such tolerance of the procedure is consistent with our observations on chronic bacteriuria among vesicostomy patients followed for 20 years (*13*).

Urinary Incontinence

Clean intermittent catheterization is ideal in the patient with overflow urinary incontinence due to a neurogenic areflexic bladder. In patients with detrusor–sphincter dyssynergia or patients with detrusor areflexia and reduced urethral resistance from partial sphincter dysfunction, adjunctive pharmacologic agents are needed to maintain continence. For detrusor hyperreflexia, oral anticholinergic-antispasmodic agents such as oxybutynin (Ditropan) 5 mg b.i.d. or t.i.d., propantheline (Pro-Banthine) 15 mg t.i.d. or q.i.d. and dicyclomine (Bentyl) 20 mg t.i.d. or q.i.d. are the agents commonly used. The major advantage of these drugs is that they reduce detrusor hyperreflexia and urge incontince but also permit longer intervals between catheterizations because of the increased bladder capacity. When the incontinence is due in part to weakness of the sphincteric mechanism, benefit may be obtained with the use of an alpha-adrenergic agent such as ephedrine sulfate 25 to 50 mg q.i.d. or phenylpropanolamine 50 to 75 mg b.i.d.

Preteaching evaluation should also identify incontinence on the basis of a small, noncompliant bladder. In the presence of a relatively normal urethra, augmentation cystoplasty may be performed to creat a low-pressure reservoir that can be emptied at reasonable intervals. If the urethral resistance is poor or the urethral abnormality prevents intermittent urethral catheterization, various urethral reconstructions or continent diversions may be carried out.

The experience to date with use of intermittent catheterization to alleviate or reduce urinary incontinence is favorable. Hilwa and Perlmutter reported their experience in 39 children who wer predominantly myelodysplastic (*14*). Of the 24 girls, 5 achieved total continence without drugs, and 15 became continent with adjunctive pharmacologic agents (79%). Of 13 boys, 2 became dry without drugs and 8 were continent with medication (77%). Our experience with 43 myelodysplastic patients screened for and assigned to our clean intermittent catheterization program showed that 38 (88%) maintained satisfactory continence (*15*).

In 60 patients who were placed on the catheterization program 10 years ago, only one patient terminated the program because of persistent incontinence. Of 27 patients who were followed for 10 years or more, there were 10 whose initial major problem was urinary incontinence. In this group four became continent on catheterization alone and six with the aid of pharmacologic agents (*11*). Maynard and Diokno reported 63 patients with spinal cord injury who were treated by intermittent catheterization (*12*). In this group, five patients discontinued the catheterization program because of persistent incontinence between catheterizations.

Renal Deterioration

Renal function and renal architecture are probably two of the most important factors on which the program of intermittent catheterization can base its success or failure. Over the years intermittent catheterization has proved to be safe in terms of preserving renal function and architecture. In some cases dramatic improvement has taken place (Fig. 27–2). Occasional cases of renal deterioration have been seen but usually in patients with vesicoureteral reflux or other preexistent renal lesions.

Lyons and his associates reported no instances of renal function loss during a 3-year period of follow-up of his pediatric patients with catheterization (*16*). Hilwa and Perlmutter reported stabilization or improvement of the upper tracts following the use of the intermittent catheterization regimen (*14*). In their series, 7 of 10 patients with hydronephrosis improved and none regressed. Kass *et al.* also noted no deterioration of renal function as measured by serum creatinine and blood urea nitrogen in all of their 255 children (*8*). Progressive hydronephrosis, however, was observed in 13 of 96 kidneys (12%) but only in patients with grade 2B to 4 reflux.

Maynard and Diokno reported that spinal

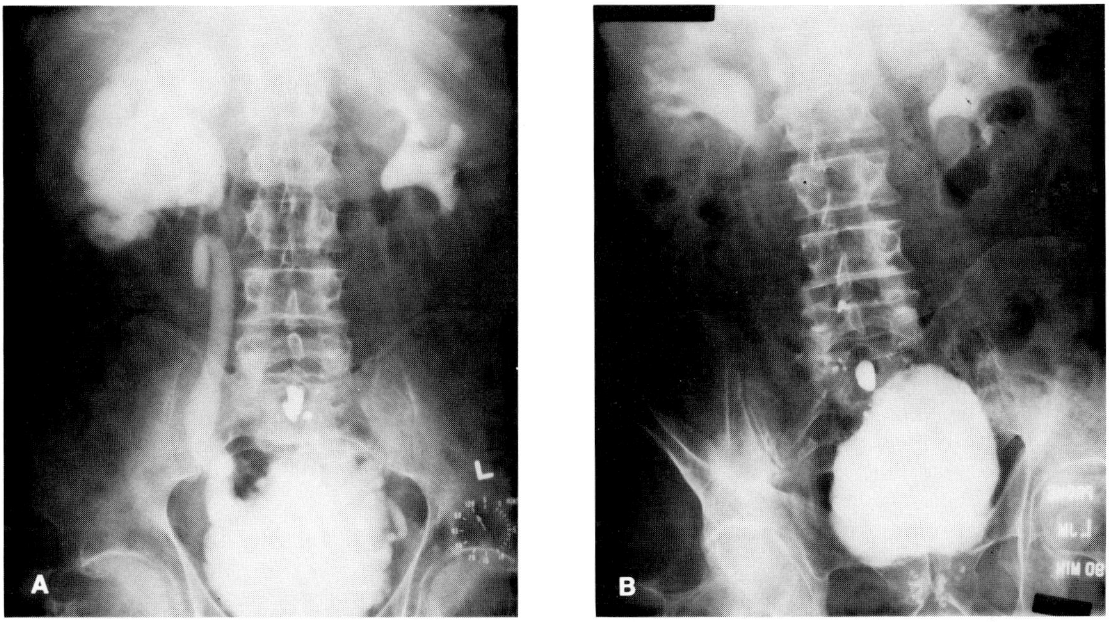

Figure 27–2. **A.** Urogram before intermittent self-catheterization demonstrating severe right hydroureteronephrosis and bladder trabeculations. **B.** Follow-up urogram showing resolution of the hydroureteronephrosis and reduction of bladder trabeculations.

cord injured patients treated with intermittent catheterization showed no evidence of hydronephrosis, hydroureter, or radiographic evidence of pyelonephritis (*12*). Similar experience was reported by McGuire and Savastano among their 41 patients with neurogenic bladder dysfunction (*10*).

In another series of 60 patients placed on the catheterization program for 10 years, no deterioration of renal function or change in renal parenchymal architecture was noted (*10*). To date, the only factor that seems to cause deterioration of the upper tracts is high-grade vesicoureteral reflux. If it does not improve with catheterization, serious consideration should be given to reimplant the ureters.

Urolithiasis

The mechanism of stone formation in the urinary tract is still not fully understood. Several factors, however, are known to contribute to stone formation. Among these are hypercalciuria and urinary infection by urea-splitting organisms. Patients who are candidates for intermittent catheterization program such as patients with spinal cord injury and other neurologic diseases causing neuropathic bladder are also likely to have these factors. Despite these factors urolithiasis is rare in patients on the clean intermittent catheterization program.

To date, no patient in the pediatric age group treated with intermittent catheterization has been reported to develop a renal calculus. Bladder calculi have been reported in adult and pediatric patients while on intermittent catheterization. The only known report of nephrolithiasis following intermittent catheterization was by Maynard and Diokno in 3 of 63 patients with spinal cord injury (*12*). All of the stones were small and were passed spontaneously without surgical treatment. Hypercalciuria and immobilization were suspected to be major factors in the development of those upper tract calculi. Solomon *et al.* presented four male patients with bladder calculi as a complication of intermittent catheterization (*17*). All of these were found to have a pubic hair as the nidus. It is believed that the hair was introduced into the bladder by the catheter. On this basis, all patients should be reminded to wipe the meatus free of pubic hair to avoid its introduction into the bladder.

During our early experience with clean catheterization, several patients with vesicolithiasis were discovered several weeks or months after initiation of the therapy. Review of these stones and pretreatment x-rays revealed that the stones were preexistent.

Urethral Trauma

One of the major surprises in application of clean intermittent catheterization program is the lack of significant urethral trauma despite multiple self-instrumentation. Plunkett and Braren reported three cases of transient urethritis: one boy developed cystourethritis and two girls hematuria (*9*). All these patients were able to reinstitute the program later. In the same report, two patients with preexisting problems, a urethral stricture and a vesical neck contracture, had difficulty with the catheterization.

In 1974 Lapides *et al.* reported two cases of urethritis in a series of 100 patients (34 men) treated with intermittent catheterization (*18*). One case was gonorrheal in origin, and the other was due to trauma from using a larger catheter than was prescribed. Maynard and Diokno reported one case of urethral trauma with persistent urethritis among 63 patients with spinal cord injury treated with intermittent urethral catheterization (*12*).

All these experiences suggest that patients with normal sensation as well as those with impaired sensation can successfully catheterize at frequent intervals for many years without urethral trauma. Care must be taken to use the appropriate catheter and avoid excessive force when introducing the catheter. Male patients very often complain difficulty passing the catheter through the external urinary sphincter region. These patients are cautioned to apply continuous gentle pressure, to overcome resistance due to sphincter muscle spasm. In men who have had previous prostatectomy or intractable sphincter spasticity or women with previous bladder suspension procedures, straight catheters may be difficult if not impossible to insert. In these cases, rubber of plastic Coude catheter are recommended.

REFERENCES

1. Guttmann, L., and Frankel, H.: The value of intermittent catheterization in the early management of traumatic paraplegia and tetraplegia. *Paraplegia* 4:63, 1966.
2. Lapides, J., Diokno, A. C., Silber, S. J., and Lowe, B. S.: Clean, intermittent self-catheterization in the treatment of urinary tract disease. *J. Urol.* 107:458–461, 1972.
3. Schneider, K. M., Reid, R. E., and Fruchtman, B.: The continent vesicostomy: clinical experiences in the adult. *J. Urol.* 117:571, 1977.
4. Green, D., Mitcheson, J. D., and McGuire, E. J.: Management of bladder by augmentation ileocecocystoplasty. *J. Urol.* 180:133–134, 1983.
5. Dailey, J., and Michael, R.: Nonsterile self intermittent catheterization for male quadriplegic patients. *Am. J. Occup. Ther.* 31:86–89, 1977.
6. Lapides, J.: Pathophysiology of urinary tract infection. *Univ. Mich. Med. Center. J.* 39:103–112, 1973.
7. Hinman, F., and Cox, C.: The voiding vesical defense mechanism: the mathematical effect of residual urine, voiding interval and volume on bacteriuria. *J. Urol.* 91:491–498, 1966.
8. Kass, E. J., Koff, S. A., Diokno, A. C., and Lapides, J.: The significance of persistent bacilluria in children on long term intermittent catheterization. *J. Urol.* 126:223–225, 1981.
9. Plunkett, J. M., and Braren, V.: Clean intermittent catheterization in children. *J. Urol.* 121:469–471, 1979.
10. McGuire, E. J., and Savastano, J. A.: Long term follow-up of spinal cord injury patients managed by intermittent catheterization. *J. Urol.* 129:775–776, 1983.
11. Diokno, A. C., Sonda, L. P., Hollander, J., and Lapides, J.: Fate of patients started on clean intermittent self-catheterization therapy ten years ago. *J. Urol.* 129:1120–1122, 1983.
12. Maynard, F., and Diokno, A. C.: Clean intermittent catheterization for spinal cord patients. *J. Urol.* 128:477–480, 1982.
13. Sonda, L. P., and Solomon, M. H.: Twenty year outcome of cutaneous vesicostomy. *J. Urol.* 124:326, 1980.
14. Hilwa, N., and Perlmutter, A. D.: The role of adjunctive drug therapy for intermittent catheterization and self catheterization in children with vesical dysfunction. *J. Urol.* 119:551–554, 1978.
15. Diokno, A. C., Kass, E., and Lapides, J.: New approach to myelodysplasia. *J. Urol.* 117:646–648, 1976.
16. Lyon, R. P., Scott, M. P., and Marshall, S.: Intermittent catheterization rather than urinary diversion in children with myelomeningocele. *J. Urol.* 113:409–417, 1975.
17. Solomon, M. H., Koff, S. A., and Diokno, A. C.: Bladder calculi complicating intermittent catheterization. *J. Urol.* 124:140–141, 1980.
18. Lapides, J., Diokno, A. C., Lowe, B. A., and Kalish, M. D.: Followup on unsterile, intermittent self-catheterization. *J. Urol.* 111:184–187, 1974.

28

Functional Electrical Stimulation of the Lower Urinary Tract

ANDREW TALALLA, M.D., AND JOSEPH W. BLOOM, Ph.D.

When any neural structure, whether the brain, spinal cord, or a peripheral nerve, is subjected to an electrical stimulus, axonal action potentials indistinguishable from the naturally occurring signals are propagated to any effector organ within its neural control or influence. This fact has been exploited for clinical application by coupling electrodes and implanted radioreceivers to appropriate neural targets. The effector system can then be activated by radiofrequency signals passed through the skin from a patient-controlled, hand-held transmitter. Thus influenced the end-organ responds in a manner of varying clinical usefulness.

The phenomenon of "functional electrical stimulation" of the nervous system (FES) has assumed a clinical status of multidisciplinary dimensions for an increasing number of therapeutic applications. These established FES techniques range from such relatively simple systems as peroneal nerve stimulation for gait disorders due to footdrop (*1,2*) to more exotic neurophysiologic manipulations such as periaqueductal gray matter stimulation, which by activating an endogenous endorphin-mediated pain-modulating system offers relief to many patients whose pain syndromes have defied management by other means (*3,4*). Not least among the organ systems that have been considered for FES is the genitourinary tract.

Compromise of neural control of the urinary bladder leads to a series of disturbances caused by failure of the two cardinal functions of this organ: the storage and periodic controlled expulsion of urine. These functions normally result from a complex series of reflex mechanisms that include interaction among sacral parasympathetic and somatic micturition nuclei, the thoracolumbar sympathetics, and the brainstem micturition center (*5–7*).

Failure of the sacral parasympathetic neurons leads to a lower motor neuron pattern of vesicourethral dysfunction with a hypotonic, hyporeflexic bladder. By contrast, the so-called upper motor neuron type of bladder dysfunction is due to a spinal cord or brain lesion that leaves the sacral parasympathetic neurons intact. With bladder dysfunction due to such a suprasacral lesion, the act of micturition is deprived of descending excitatory and inhibitory influences and is thereby demoted to a spinal reflex of poor discrimination and of diminished hydrodynamic efficiency. Furthermore, the normal coordination of bladder contraction with sphincter relaxation is lost, and the role of this reflex inhibition is replaced by a dyssynergia between the detrusor and the urethral striated sphincter. At present there is no completely acceptable method of dealing with this condition of detrusor hyperreflexia and detrusor–sphincter dyssynergia.

Functional electrical stimulation is of little avail in the atonic hyporeflexic bladder. On the other hand, the hyperreflexic bladder, which retains its neural connections to the sacral micturition centers, is amenable to a variety of potentially useful electrophysiologic manipulations.

FES TECHNIQUES

The rationale underlying FES for the neurologically disabled lower urinary tract is to supplement or replace the abnormal motor outflow to the bladder and its outlet with a more efficient but artificially patterned signal. This signal ideally promotes complete emptying of the bladder by detrusor contraction while eliminating or circumventing dyssynergic sphincteric contractions.

Attempts to electrically induce bladder emptying by neural stimulation have centered mainly on three techniques: spinal cord surface stimulation, intra-axial stimulation of the conus medullaris, and stimulation of the sacral outflow from the spinal cord.

Spinal Cord Stimulation

The gate theory of pain (*8*) led to the development of electrical stimulation of peripheral nerves as a useful treatment modality for selected pain syndromes. Its application by transcutaneous nerve stimulation was taken to the logical next step of spinal cord stimulation (SCS) to activate the dorsal columns (*9*). The fortuitous observation that SCS for pain in a multiple sclerosis (MS) patient also improved other neurologic functions (*10*), especially spasticity, and led to widespread use of SCS in patients suffering from MS and from other spinal cord disturbances (*11–13*).

These initial reports of SCS were uniformly encouraging but were based mostly on subjective evaluation. Later, carefully conducted studies by quantitative measurements of neurologic function showed that the earlier reports could not be corroborated (*14–17*). However, some of these later studies showed improvement in bladder function in those patients in whom paraparesis was accompanied by a variety of disturbances of micturition. Thus urinary flow studies, voiding cystourethrograms, and sphincter electromyography (EMG) showed convincing evidence of improvement. It has been suggested that the improvement in bladder function results from an increased descending inhibition of the centers in the conus medullaris (*16*). In this regard it has been shown in the rhesus monkey that at the stimulus parameters used in clinical SCS the electrical charge spreads beyond the dorsal columns and activates most ascending and descending systems in the cord (*18*).

Although a more accurate evaluation of SCS in MS patients is difficult because of the relapsing nature of the disease and its diurnal symptomatic variation, SCS in MS is now indicated predominantly for the relief of bladder dysfunctions.

Conus Medullaris Stimulation

Since it was first demonstrated that contraction of the detrusor occurred in response to electrical stimulation of the sacral spinal cord, several studies have led to a clearer understanding of micturition centers in the conus medullaris. With the use of both degeneration and tracer techniques, the locations of groups of sacral motor neurons innervating the detrusor muscle and the periurethral striated muscle have been established (*19–26*). These groups of neurons, which are separate, are located in the intermediolateral columns and in the ventromedial gray matter of the anterior horns, respectively.

Penetrating electrodes have been used to activate the spinal micturition centers. The latest published clinical report of this technique summarizes a multicenter experience of 28 paraplegic patients. Neurologic and urodynamic details are not reported, but 55.6 percent of the patients had "good results" with some instances of stimulation systems functioning for periods of up to 10 years (*27*). However, unpredictable and disadvantageous expressions of stimulus current spread, e.g., involuntary muscle contractions in the lower limbs, sweating, piloerection, paroxysmal hypertension, and other features of autonomic dysreflexia, were experienced by some patients (*28,29*). This technique fails to resolve the problem of dyssynergia between the detrusor and external sphincter because of the proximity of their respective neuron pools. Current spread remains a significant problem with this technique until the technology is clinically established for the focal stimulation of selected small populations of neurons.

Sacral Outflow Stimulation

Of all FES techniques for detrusor hyperreflexia, sacral outflow stimulation merits special interest. For this technique to succeed, the survival and integrity of neural connections between the sacral cord neurons and the periphery is obligatory.

All experiences with sacral stimulation have shown that it is relatively easy to generate substantial intravesical pressures. The major impediment to success lies in the fact that electrical stimulation of the sacral neural system is expected to cause co-contraction of detrusor and striated sphincter (Fig. 28–1). To circumvent the co-contraction of the striated urethral sphincter, a number of surgical and electrophysiologic strategies have been proposed.

The most obvious approach is surgical section of somatic efferents by pudendal neurectomy. Such techniques have been effective in dogs (*30,31*), but objections to their clinical application include their irreversibility and the possible interference with sexual function in men. In addition, this applicability of pudendal neurectomy to humans may be questioned, as the innervation of some of the somatic sphincteric mechanisms may be partly nonpudendal in transit (*32,33*).

Clearly, reversible means of blocking sphincteric mechanisms are preferred to any permanent interruptions. Electrophysiologic block of action potential conduction is a potentially useful and reversible technique for this application. The technique of anode block has been considered, but it has not been clinically useful (*34,35*). High-frequency currents have been variously described as a useful means of achieving conduction failure (*36–39*), but the method has not been clinically successful in our hands (*40*). The electrophysiologic technique of action potential collision is another strategy to consider, but this technique is at a preclinical stage of development and will not be available for clinical FES for some time (*41–43*). Several attempts have been made to generate fatigue of the striated sphincter (*44,45*). These strategies have not, as yet, been clinically useful (*35*).

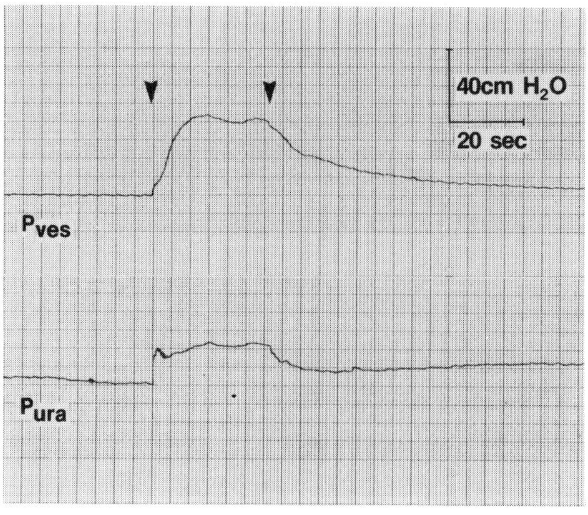

Figure 28–1. Urodynamic study of the effect of stimulation of bilateral S_3 nerves in their intraspinal, extradural course. The effect of co-contraction of detrusor and striated sphincter is clearly seen. Arrowheads mark the period of stimulation.

Intermittent electrical stimulation is a technique that takes advantage of the differences in duration of the contraction and relaxation phases of the detrusor and urethral striated sphincter. If the sacral nerve roots are activated with appropriately timed trains of electric stimuli, both detrusor and striated sphincter contract during stimulation, but only the striated sphincter relaxes during the intertrain interval (Fig. 28–2). This type of intermittent stimulation can result in spurts of voiding during the period when the stimulation is shut off (*44*). This technique has been clinically effective in inducing interrupted micturition by sacral anterior root stimulation (*35*) and sacral mixed nerve stimulation (Fig. 28–3).

The artificial stimulation of a mixed spinal nerve by an electrical impulse induces volleys of action potentials propagated in opposite directions from the point of stimulus application. Afferent volleys thus set up can induce uncontrolled and unpredictable reverberations within the intact portion of the spinal cord (Fig. 28—4). It has often triggered reflex voiding but without sufficient reliability and effectiveness to consider it a definitive technique (Fig. 28–5).

Stimulation of the sacral peripheral neural system has been attempted both experimentally and clinically at three sites. Each has advantages that are offset by either physiologic or surgical considerations when applied in humans.

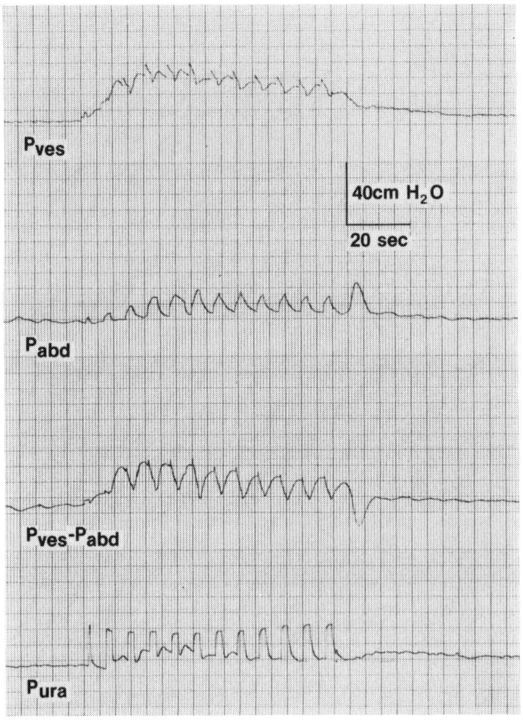

Figure 28–2. Urodynamic study of intermittent stimulation of bilateral S_3 nerves in their intraspinal extradural course. The well sustained intravesical pressure contrasts with the abrupt fall in intraurethral pressure at each stimulus train off-set.

Sacral Anterior Root. Extensive experimental and preclinical studies suggested the feasibility of sacral nerve or anterior root stimulation as a useful clinical technique in chronic detrusor hyperreflexic states (*30,31,44,46*). The first clinical report of sacral anterior root stimulation was on 11 patients with traumatic spinal cord lesions. Electrodes within the cerebrospinal fluid (CSF) compartment selectively enclosed the S_2 and S_3 anterior roots and the S_4 anterior and posterior roots. Postoperatively, the electrodes were activated by radiofrequency-coupled stimulation. In most but not all patients, S_3 stimulation provided the principal detrusor activation. Intermittent stimulation was necessary to achieve voiding. Of the first 50 patients treated by sacral anterior root stimulation, 43 are using their stimulations to successfully empty their bladders, with a follow up period of up to 8 years (*48*). Voiding pressures in this group were less than 80 cms. H_2O and residual urine volumes are less than 60 ml. 31 patients are continent both day and night and 5 have achieved nocturnal continence only. It is further reported that increase in bladder capacity in all, and alleviation of vesicoureteral reflux in 4 of the patients, was observed. Penile erection could be achieved in 26 of the 38 patients by the use of appropriate stimulus parameters. These erections could be sustained and are of sufficient quality for sexual intercourse in 20 patients (*48*).

Intraspinal Extradural Sacral Nerve. Stimulation of sacral spinal nerves (mixed) in their extradural course has produced a short term, successful result (*40*). To achieve better results and a long term success, additional surgical intervention—dorsal sacral (sensory) rhizotomies are probably needed.

Pelvic Nerve. The sacral nerves leave the spinal canal by way of the anterior foramina of the sacrum and enter the retroperitoneal space of the pelvis. (Reference to the mixed spinal nerve emerging from the anterior sacral foramen as the anterior *root* has led to unnecessary confusion.

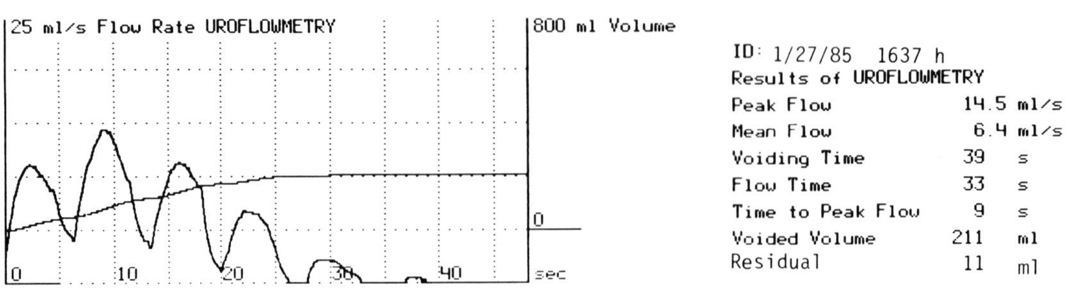

Figure 28–3. Study from the same patient as in Figure 28–2. It shows the episodic character of flow in response to intermittent stimulation of bilateral S_3 nerves.

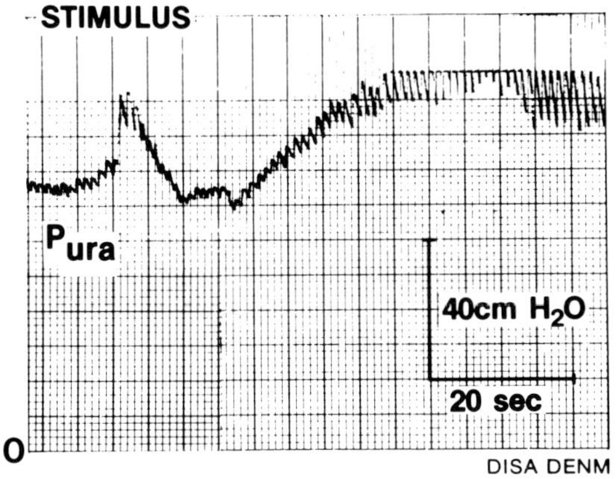

Figure 28–4. Lingering effect on the urethral pressure of a brief stimulus applied to the right S_3 nerve in its extradural course. Note also that this patient has a high resting intraurethral pressure.

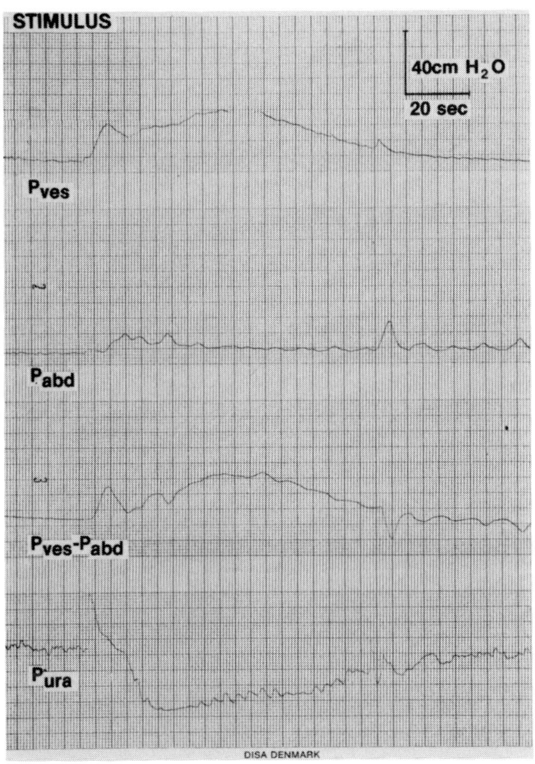

Figure 28–5. Effect of sacral nerve stimulation on triggering reflex relaxation of the urethra, which leads to incomplete voiding.

The anterior and posterior roots of each spinal nerve are both intraspinal and intradural.) After a short segment, approximately 2.0 cm, each nerve divides into a predominantly parasympathetic component (pelvic nerve, nervus erigente) and a somatic component (pudendal nerve). Until that division, the sacral nerve is a continuation of the intraspinal mixed nerve.

In 1967 successful sacral spinal nerve stimulation was reported in two patients (*49*). The trunk of the third sacral spinal nerve in one patient and the fourth sacral spinal nerve in the other was selected for electrode coupling. The surgical approach was transabdominal and retroperitoneal to the sacral spinal nerves at their exit from the anterior sacral foramina. No details were given of the exact site of electrode attachment in relation to the takeoff of the pelvic nerve branches. One presumes that stimulation was at one point proximal to the origin of the pelvic nerves, as the report clearly described co-activation of the somatic efferents to the striated sphincters. Both patients voided effectively by electrical stimulation, with urinary continence between each stimulation. The follow-up period was 4 and 5 months, respectively, after which the stimulation was discontinued owing to infection along the electrical cables, which with the technique used emerged from the abdominal wall.

Burghele *et al.* appear to be the first to report successful experimental micturition by stimulation of the pelvic nerves (*50,51*). Their clinical experiences, reported in English translation, do not give much detail and appear to have ceased after 1973 (*52*). Kaekenbeeck in 1970 treated four paraplegic patients with the "technique de Brughele;Ichim-Demetrescu" by coupling electrodes to the pelvic branches of S_2 and S_3 as they emerged from the anterior sacral foramina. Three of the patients achieved "excellent" stimulus-induced voiding. In 1978 a further 12 patients were similarly treated, with eight "excellent" and two "average" results. Some patients in this series of 16 also had hypogastric nerve section, but no details, neurologic or urodynamic, were given (*53*).

Choice of Site. The selection of the site for electrode coupling to the sacral outflow depends on several factors. Chief among these factors are the electrophysiologic advantage afforded by any one site and the extent of the surgical manipulations necessary to expose it.

Sacral Anterior Root. The advantage of anterior root stimulation is great, for it neatly circumvents the unsettling sensory bombardment of the intact spinal cord below the lesion. Such afferent bombardment of the cord can lead to lasting activation of bladder outlet mechanisms (Fig. 28–4). Anterior roots of sacral and other spinal nerves carry a population of afferent axons (*54, 55*). Some of these afferents convey nociceptive impulses from abdominal viscera including the bladder (*56*). It is possible that the afferents conveyed in the sacral anterior roots subserve as yet unknown neurologic mechanisms that may facilitate the micturition reflex. The disadvantages of the anterior root technique are the obligatory invasion of the CSF compartment by the electrode array and the egress of the electrode cables through the dura to the implanted devices. It is not possible without prohibitive damage, if at all, to surgically separate the motor from the sensory root once they have joined to form the mixed sacral nerve just outside the dura. A 30-year history of a variety of CSF diversions for the treatment of hydrocephalic states suggests that even in competent hands a foreign-body invasion of the CSF compartment is associated with significant risk.

Intraspinal Extradural Sacral Nerve. The main advantages of the intraspinal extradural site for electrode application are the ease of access and the protection from stimulus-induced injury afforded by investment of the nerves with a sleeve of dura. The drawback of the extradural technique is that the sacral nerve at this site has a mixed composition, carrying both afferent and efferent parasympathetic and somatic axons. Stimulation at this site therefore causes co-activation of the detrusor and striated urethral sphincter as well as afferent bombardment of the cord.

The intraspinal extradural technique is relatively simple and has much to commend it if preliminary reports of success can be substantiated by additional clinical experience.

Pelvic Nerve. The selective coupling of electrodes to the pelvic nerves may largely avoid the major impediment to successful FES of the urinary system, and the co-activation of outlet continence mechanisms that annuls otherwise effective detrusor contractions. The disadvantage of the technique is the considerable surgical procedure required for it, as the approach to the pelvic nerves is transabdominal and retroperitoneal. Evidence has accrued for a sacral sympathetic outflow to the bladder neck conveyed by the pelvic nerves (*57,58*). The functional implication of this outflow in FES of the pelvic nerves remains to be evaluated.

OUTSTANDING PROBLEMS

With the pioneering work of Barrington and others, neurourology has assumed the status of its own speciality (*59*). Even though a vast body of experimental and clinical data has accrued, much remains elusive for a comprehensive understanding of micturition mechanisms. The application of FES techniques to the neurologically disabled lower urinary tract thus faces particular difficulties in addition to the general problems associated with electrical stimulation of the nervous system.

Urethral Innervation

Despite several reports on urethral innervation and urethral anatomy, the understanding in relation to human striated sphincter remains unclear (*32,33,60*). It is suggested that the striated sphincter is innervated by nonpudendal somatic axons (*32,33*), which have motor neurons serving them in the ventral gray matter (*25*). The implication here for pudendal neurectomy as a means of overcoming striated sphincter co-activation is obvious.

Neural Tissue Damage

Any discussion of chronic electrical stimulation of peripheral nerves must take into consideration the possibility of neural damage to by the techniques and apparatus of stimulation. Such damage may result from two sources: the effects of the physical presence of the electrodes and their surgical implantation, and the effects of passage of current through the nerves from the implanted electrodes.

Information on the adverse effects of chronic stimulation on peripheral nerves, including spinal nerves, is limited. The studies that address this issue attribute most observed neural damage to the physical presence of the electrodes. Sources of nerve injury include direct surgical manipulation (*35,44,61*), pressure or tension on the nerve due to the design of the nerve cuff (*61–63*), or postoperative movement of the cuff (*44,61*). A buildup of dense connective tissue within and around the cuff is in some cases associated with the nerve damage (*63,64*). Of particular importance is the need for a loose fit of the cuff around the nerve. Snugly fitting cuffs have been associated with severe neural damage in animals (*63*) and with a reduction of the effectiveness of stimulation in patients (Fig. 28–6). In both animals and patients, reduction in the effectiveness of stimulation due to electrode-related injury recovered after several months (*35,44*) (Fig. 28–6). The relation of histologic nerve damage to functional damage is unclear, as in dogs (*63*) and humans (*61*) a substantial response to electrical stimulation persisted in nerves that proved to be significantly injured at the histologic level. Another potential source of damage in chronic peripheral nerve stimulation is chemical irritation of the nerve, either by use of nonbiocompatible materials for fabrication of the electrode array (*65*) or from the residues of improper sterilization (*66*). In the transfer of electrical charge from the electrode to the biologic fluid interface at the nerve, any incomplete reversal of a faradic reaction can lead to a net chemical change that may cause neural damage and even electrode failure (*67*).

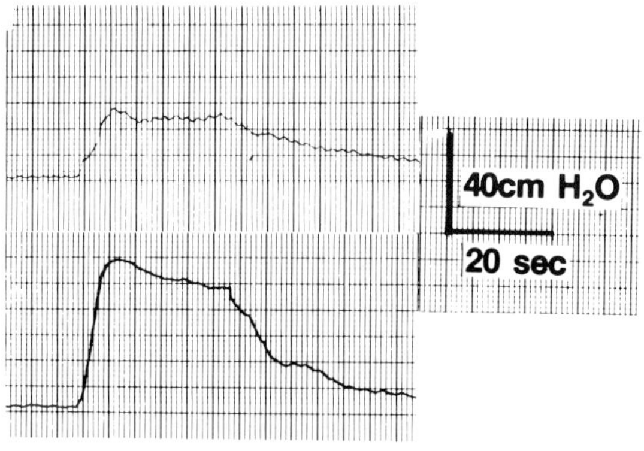

Figure 28–6. Pressure studies from the same patient using near-identical parameters of stimulation of bilateral S_3 nerves, showing improvement of function over time. *Upper trace:* 63 days after surgical electrode coupling. *Lower trace:* 332 days later. Scale bar applies to both traces.

In contrast to a sizable literature on the effects of electrical stimulation on the central nervous system (CNS) tissues (*68–75*), systematic studies of electrical damage to peripheral nerves are few (*61–64,76*). Acute studies with direct-current stimulation show it to be the most damaging of stimulus waveforms (*77,78*). Nonetheless, at clinically effective levels of stimulation no stimulus-related damage has been reported and sacral nerves have remained electrically excitable and stimulators clinically functional for up to 6 years (*48*). Studies establishing safe limits for chronic electrical activation of peripheral nerves are greatly needed.

Plasticity

It is now generally believed that the adult CNS is not as static and is capable or reorganization after injury (*79,80*). Specifically, the changes in reflex organization of the micturition centers, isolated after spinal cord injury, may reflect not just the loss of supraspinal influences but also changes in the structural organization and pharmacologic characteristics of the spinal neural centers themselves (*81*). It has been shown that skeletal muscle responds to artificial modification of its pattern of activation with structural (*82*), chemical (*83*), and functional changes (*84*). These changes have been observed in the urethral striated musculature of the dog in response to sacral nerve stimulation (*85*), and similar changes may occur in patients subjected to chronic electrical stimulation. The effects of long-term electrostimulation on the physiologic and possibly the pharmacologic characteristics of micturition in spinal cord-damaged patients remain unknown.

CONCLUSION

Functional electrical stimulation is a promising option for treatment of patients disabled by detrusor hyperreflexia. Several matters await resolution before the definitive technique is identified. Criteria for success and acceptability of FES of the lower urinary tract include the fulfillment of strict urologic requirements, the use of effective but safe stimulus parameters, and a surgical technique that is acceptable to the informed patient. FES requires a multidisciplinary team for its development, implementation, and evaluation. Such team must include skills and resources that may not ordinarily reside within a single institution, and therefore, collaborative efforts across institutional borders are encouraged. Advantage can thereby be taken of special talents and interests without the need for duplication of resources. This approach should accelerate progress in the development of a potentially powerful tool for the rehabilitation of paraplegic and quadriplegic patients in whom disturbances of bladder function can seriously undermine the quality of their lives.

ACKNOWLEDGMENTS

Our work, which is part of the NIH Neural Prosthesis Program under the facilitating direction of F. Terry Hambrecht, is supported by contract NO1-NS-2-2396 and NO1-NS-52378. It is a pleasure to acknowledge the participation of Leo Bullara, Quang Nguyen, Markad Kamath, and Robert Pudenz in some of the original work herein reported.

REFERENCES

1. Liberson, W. T., Holmquest, H. J., Scott, D., and Dow, M.: Functional electrotherapy: stimulation of the peroneal nerve synchronized with the swing phase of the gait of hemiplegic patients. *Arch. Phys. Med.* 42:101–105, 1961.
2. Waters, R. L., McNeal, D. R., and Perry, J.: Experimental correction of footdrop by electrical stimulation of the peroneal nerve. *J. Bone Joint Surg.* 57-A:1047–1054, 1975.
3. Hosobuchi, Y.: Periaqueductal gray stimulation (PAGS) for pain suppression. In Bonica, J. J., Liebeskind, J. C., and Albe-Fessard, D. (eds.), *Advances in Pain Research and Therapy*, Vol. 3, Raven Press, New York, 1979, pp. 515–524.
4. Hosobuchi, Y., Adams, J. E., and Linchitz, R.: Pain relief by electrical stimulation of the central gray matter in humans and its reversal by naloxone. *Science* 197:183–185, 1977.
5. Blaivas, J. G.: T he neurophysiology of micturition: a clinical study of 550 patients. *J. Urol.* 127:958–963, 1982.
6. Bradley, W. E., Timm, G. W., and Scott, F. B.: Innervation of the detrusor muscle and urethra. *Urol. Clin. North Am.* 1:3–27, 1974.
7. DeGroat, W. C.: Nervous control of the urinary bladder of the cat. *Brain Res.* 87:201–211, 1975.
8. Melzack, R., and Wall, P. D.: Pain mechanisms: a new theory. *Science* 150:971–979, 1965.
9. Shealy, C. N., Mortimer, J. T., and Hagfors, N. R.: Dorsal column electroanalgesia. *J. Neurosurg.* 32:560–564, 1970.
10. Cook, A. W., and Weinstein, S. P.: Chronic dorsal column stimulation in multiple sclerosis: preliminary report. *N.Y. State J. Med.* 73:2826, 1973.
11. Campos, R. J., Dimitrejevic, M. M., and Sharkey, P. C.: Clinical evaluation of the effects of spinal cord stimulation on motor performance in patients with upper motor neuron lesions. In *Proceedings 6th International Symposium on the External Control of Human Extremities.* Yugoslav Committee for Electronics and Automation, Belgrade, 1978, pp. 569–574.
12. Richardson, R. R., Cerullo, L. J., McLone, D. G., Gutierrez, F. A., and Lewis, V.: Percutaneous epidural neurostimulation in modulation of paraplegic spasticity. *Acta Neurochir. (Wein)* 49:235–243, 1979.
13. Waltz, J. M., and Pani, K. C.: Spinal cord stimulation in disorders of the motor system. In *Proceedings 6th International Symposium on the External Control of Human Extremities.* Yugoslav Committee for Electronics and Automation, Belgrade, 1978, pp. 545–556.
14. Hawkes, C. H., Wyke, M., Desmond, A., Bultitude, M. I., and Kanegaonkar, G. S.: Stimulation of dorsal column in multiple sclerosis. *Br. Med. J.* 280:889–891, 1980.
15. Illis, L. S., Sedgwick, E. M., and Tallis, R. C.: Spinal cord stimulation in multiple sclerosis: clinical results. *J. Neurol. Neurosurg. Psychiatry* 43:1–14, 1980.
16. Read, D. J., Matthews, W. B., and Higson, R. H.: The effect of spinal cord stimulation on function in patients with multiple sclerosis. *Brain* 103:803–833, 1980.
17. Tallis, R. C., Illis, L. S., and Sedgwick, E. M.: The quantitative assessment of the influence of spinal cord stimulation on motor function in patients with multiple sclerosis. *Int. Rehabil. Med.* 5:10–16, 1983.
18. Bantli, H., Bloedel, J. R., Long, D. M., and Thienprasit, P.: Distribution of activity in spinal pathways evoked by experimental dorsal column stimulation. *J. Neurosurg.* 42:290–295, 1975.
19. Kuzuhara, S., Kanazawa, I., and Nakanishi, T.: Topographical localization of the Onuf's nuclear neurons innervating the rectal and vesical striated sphincter muscles: a retrograde fluorescent double labelling in cat and dog. *Neurosci. Lett.* 16:125–130, 1980.
20. Morgan, C., Nadelhaft, I., and DeGroat, W. C.: Location of bladder preganglionic neurons within the sacral parasympathetic nucleus of the cat. *Neurosci. Lett.* 14:189–194, 1979.
21. Nadelhaft, I., DeGroat, W. C., and Morgan, C.: Location and morphology of parasympathetic pre-

ganglionic neurons in the sacral cord of the cat revealed by retrograde axonal transport of horseradish peroxidase. *J. Comp. Neurol.* 193:265–281, 1980.
22. Nadelhaft, I., Roppolo, J., Morgan, C., and DeGroat, W. C.: Parasympathetic preganglionic neurons and visceral primary afferents in monkey sacral spinal cord revealed following application of horseradish peroxidase to pelvic nerve.. *J. Comp. Neurol.* 216:36–52, 1983.
23. Oliver, J. E., Bradley, W. E., and Fletcher, T. F.: Identification of preganglionic parasympathetic neurons in the sacral spinal cord of the cat. *J. Comp. Neurol.* 137:321–328, 1969.
24. Oliver, J., Bradley, W., and Fletcher, T.: Spinal cord distribution of the somatic innervation of the external urethral sphincter of the cat. *J. Neurol. Sci.* 10:11–23, 1970.
25. Schroder, H. D.: Onuf's nucleus. X. A morphological study of human spinal nucleus. *Anat. Embryol.* 162:443–453, 1981.
26. Thüroff, J. W., Bazeed, M.A., Schmidt, R. A., Luu, D. H., and Tanagho, E. A.: Regional topography of spinal cord neurons innervating pelvic floor muscles and bladder neck in the dog: a study by combined horseradish peroxidase histochemistry and autoradiography. *Urol. Int.* 37:110–120, 1982.
27. Nashold, B. S., Friedman, H., and Grimes, J.: Electrical stimulation of the conus medullaris to control bladder emptying in paraplegia; a ten-year review. *Appl. Neurophysiol.* 45:40–43, 1982.
28. Friedman, H., Nashold, B. S., Jr., and Grimes, J.: Electrical stimulation of the conus medullaris in the paraplegic—a five year review. In Hambrecht, F. T., and Reswick, J. B., (eds.), *Functional Electrical Stimulation.* Marcel Dekker, New York, 1977, pp. 173–184.
29. Nashold, B. S., Friedman, H., Glenn, J. H., Grimes, J. H., Barry, W. F., and Avery, R.: Electromicturition in paraplegia. *Arch. Surg.* 104:195–202, 1972.
30. Schmidt, R. A., Bruschini, H., and Tanagho, E. A.: Sacral root stimulation in controlled micturition: peripheral somatic neurotomy and stimulated voiding. *Invest. Urol.* 17:130–134, 1979.
31. Schmidt, R. A., and Tanagho, E. A.: Feasibility of controlled micturition through electric stimulation. *Urol. Int.* 34:199–230, 1979.
32. Donker, P. J., Droes, J. Th. P. M., and Van Ulden, B.M.: Anatomy of the musculature and innervation of the bladder and the urethra. In Williams, D. I., and Chisholm, G. M. (ed), *Scientific Foundations of Urology.* Vol. II. Heinemann, London, 1976. pp. 32–39.
33. Gil Vernet, S.: Innervation somatique et vegetative des organes genito-urinaires. *J. Urol. Nephrol.* 70:45–56, 1964.
34. Brndley, G. S., and Craggs, M.D.: A technique for anodally blocking large nerve fibres through chronically implanted electrodes. *J. Neurol. Neurosurg. Psychiatry* 43:1083–1090, 1980.
35. Brindley, G. S., Polkey, C. E., and Rushton, D. N.: Sacral anterior root stimulators for bladder control in paraplegia. *Paraplegia* 20:365–381, 1982.
36. McNeal, D. R., Bowman, B. R., and Momsen, W. L.: Peripheral block of motor activity. In Gavrilovic, M., and Wilson, A. B., (eds.), *Advances in External Control of Human Extremities.* Belgrade, 1973, pp. 35–46.
37. Pudenz, R.: Personal communication.
38. Solomonow, M., Foster, J., Eldred, E., and Lyman, J.: Proportional control of paralyzed muscle. *Fed. Proc.* 37:215, 1978.
39. Tanner, J. A.: Reversible blocking of nerve conduction by alternating-current excitation. *Nature* 195:712–713, 1962.
40. Talalla, A., Bloom, J. W., and Nguyen, Q.: Successful intraspinal extradural sacral nerve stimulation for bladder emptying in a victim of traumatic spinal cord transection. *Neurosurgery* 19:955–961, 1986.
41. Sweeney, J. D., and Mortimer, J. T.: A modified bipolar cuff electrode for collision block of peripheral nerve. *Neurosci. Abstr.* 9:1038, 1983.
42. Van den Honert, C., and Mortimer, J. T.: A technique for collision block of peripheral nerve: single stimulus analysis. *IEEE Trans. BME* 28:373–378, 1981.
43. Van den Honert, C., and Mortimer, J. T.: A technique for collision block of peripheral nerve: frequency dependence. *IEEE Trans. BME* 28:379–382, 1981.
44. Brindley, G. S.: An implant to empty the bladder or close the urethra. *J. Neurol. Neurosurg. Psychiatry* 40:358–369, 1977.
45. Thüroff, J. W., Bazeed, M. A., Schmidt, R. A., Wiggin, D. M., and Tanagho, E. A.: Functional pattern of sacral root stimulation in dogs. I. Micturition. *J. Urol.* 127:1031–1033, 1982.
46. Schmidt, R. A., Bruschini, H., and Tanagho, E. A.: Urinary bladder and sphincter responses to stimulation of dorsal and ventral sacral roots. *Invest. Urol.* 16:300–304, 1979.
47. Cardozo, L., Krishnan, K. R., Polkey, C. E., Rushton, D. N., and Brindley, G. S.: Urodynamic observations on patients with sacral anterior root stimulators. *Paraplegia* 22:201–209, 1984.
48. Brindley, G. S., Polkey, C. E., Rushton, D. N., and Cardozo, L.: Sacral anterior root stimulators for bladder control in paraplegia: the first 50 cases. *J. Neurol. Neurosurg and Psychiat.* 49: 1104–1114, 1986.
49. Habib, H. N.: Experience and recent contributions in sacral nerve stimulation for voiding in both human and animal. *Br. J. Urol.* 39:73–83, 1967.
50. Burghele, Th., Ichim, V., and Demetrescu, M.: L'electroexcitation de la vessie medullaire: etude experimentale. *J. Urol.* 64:317–329, 1958.
51. Burghele, Th., Ichim, V., and Demetrescu, M.: Experimental studies on the physiology of micturition and the emptying of the urinary bladder in patients with lesions of the spinal cord. *Romanian Med. Rev.* 3:48–51, 1959.
52. Burghele, Th.: Electrostimulation of the neurogenic urinary bladder. In Lutzmeyer, W., and Melchior, H. (eds.), *Urodynamics. Upper and Lower Urinary Tract.* Springer-Verlag, New York, 1973, pp. 319–322.
53. Kaeckenbeeck, B.: Electrostimulation de la vessie des paraplegiques: technique de Burghele-Ichim-Demetrescu. *Acta Urol. Belg.* 47:139–140, 1979.
54. Applebaum, M. L., Clifton, G. L., Coggeshall, R. E., Coulter, J. D., Vance, W. H., and Willis, W. D.: Unmyelinated fibres in the sacral 3 and caudal 1

ventral roots of the cat. *J. Physiol. (Lond.)* 256:557–572, 1976.
55. Coggeshall, R. E., Applebaum, M. L., Fazen, M., Stubbs, T. B., and Sykes, M. T.: Unmyelinated axons in human ventral roots, a possible explanation for the failure of dorsal rhizotomy to relieve pain. *Brain* 98:157–166, 1975.
56. Coggeshall, R. E.: Law of separation of function of the spinal roots. *Physiol. Rev.* 60:716–755, 1980.
57. Downie, J. W., Pillay, D., Nance, D. M., and Champion, J. A.: Influence of the sacral sympathetic chain on urethral function in the cat. *Neurosci. Abstract.* 9:111, 1983.
58. Kuo, D. C., Hitsamitsu, T., and DeGroat, W. D.: A sympathetic projection from sacral paravertebral ganglia to the pelvic nerve and to postganglionic nerves on the surface of the urinary bladder and large intestine of the cat. *J. Comp. Neurol.* 226:76–86, 1984.
59. Hald, T., and Bradley, W. E.: *The Urinary Bladder. Neurology and Dynamics.* Williams & Wilkins, Baltimore, 1982.
60. Gosling, J. A., Dixon, J. S., Critchley, H. O. D., and Thompson, S. A.: A comparative study of the human external sphincter and periurethral levator ani muscles. *Br. J. Urol.* 53:35–41, 1981.
61. Kim, J. H., Manuelidis, E. E., Glenn, W. W. L., and Kaneyuki, T.: Diaphragm pacing: histopathological changes in the phrenic nerve following long-term electrical stimulation. *J. Thorac. Cardiovasc. Surg.* 72:602–608, 1976.
62. Hershberg, P. I., Sohn, D., Agrawal, G. P., and Kantrowitz, A.: Histologic changes in continuous, long-term electrical stimulation of a peripheral nerve. *IEEE Trans. BME* 14:109–114, 1967.
63. Yuen, T. G. H., Agnew, W. F., and Bullara, L. A.: Histopathological evaluation of dog sacral nerve after chronic electrical stimulation for micturition. *Neurosurgery* 14:449–455, 1984.
64. Kim, J. H., Manuelidis, E. E., Glenn, W. W. L., Fukuda, Y., Cole, D. S., and Hogan, J. F.: Light and electron microscopic studies of phrenic nerves after long-term electrical stimulation. *J. Neurosurg.* 58:84–91, 1983.
65. Hambrecht, F. T.: Neural prostheses. *Annu. Rev. Biophys. Bioeng.* 8:239–267, 1979.
66. Bullara, L.: Personal communication.
67. Brummer, S. B., and McHardy, J.: Current problems in electrode development. In Hambrecht, F. T., and Reswick, J. B., (eds.), Marcel Dekker, New York, 1977, pp. 499–514.
68. Agnew, W. F., Yuen, T. G. H., Pudenz, R. H., and Bullara, L. A.: Electrical stimulation of brain. IV. Ultrastructural studies. *Surg. Neurol.* 4:438–448, 1975.
69. Agnew, W. F., Yuen, T. G. H., Bullara, L. A., Jacques, D., and Pudenz, R. H.: Intracellular calcium deposition in brain following electrical stimulation. *Neurol. Res.* 1:187–202, 1979.
70. Brown, W. J., Babb, T. L., Soper, H. V., Lieb, J. P., Ottino, C. A., and Crandall, P. H.: Tissue reactions to long-term electrical stimulation of the cerebellum in monkeys. *J. Neurosurg.* 47:366–379, 1977.
71. Pudenz, R. H., Bullara, L. A., Dru, D., and Talalla, A.: Electrical stimulation of the brain. II. Effects on the blood-brain barrier. *Surg. Neurol.* 4:265–270, 1975.
72. Pudenz, R. H., Bullara, L. A., Jacques, S., and Hambrecht, F. T.: Electrical stimulation of the brain. III. The neural damage model. *Surg. Neurol.* 4:389–400, 1975.
73. Pudenz, R. H., Agnew, W. F., and Bullara, L. A.: Effects of electrical stimulation of brain: light and electron-microscope studies. *Brain Behav. Evol.* 14:103–125, 1977.
74. Pudenz, R. H., Agnew, W. F., Yuen, T. G. H., and Bullara, L. A.: Electrical stimulation of the brain: light and electron microscopy studies. In Hambrecht, F. T., and Reswick, J. B. (eds.), *Functional Electrical Stimulation.* Marcel Dekker, New York, 1977, pp. 437–456.
75. Yuen, T. G. H., Agnew, W. F., Bullara, L. A., Jacques, S., and McCreery, D. B.: Histological evaluation of neural damage from electrical stimulation: considerations for the selection of parameters for clinical application. *Neurosurgery* 9:292–299, 1981.
76. Bowman, B. R.: Acute and chronic implantation of coiled wire intraneural electrodes. In *Proceedings 6th Annual Conference on Rehabilitation Engineering,* San Diego, June 1983.
77. Hughes, G. B., Bottomy, M. B., Dickins, J. R. E., Jackson, C. G., Sismanis, A., and Glasscock, M. E.: A comparative study of neuropathologic changes following pulsed and direct current stimulation of the mouse sciatic nerve. *Am. J. Otolaryngol.* 1:378–384, 1980.
78. Hughes, G. B., Bottomy, M. B., Jackson, C. G., Glasscock, M. E., and Sismanis, A.: Myelin and axon degeneration following direct current peripheral nerve stimulation: a prospective controlled experimental study. *Otolaryngol. Head Neck Surg.* 89:767–775, 1981.
79. Schultzberg, M.: The peripheral nervous system. In Emson, P. C. (ed.), *Chemical Neuroanatomy.* Raven Press, New York, 1983, pp. 1–51.
80. Devor, M.: Plasticity in the adult nervous system. In Illis, L. S., Sedgwick, E.M., and Glanville, H. J. (eds.), *Rehabilitation of the Neurological Patient.* Blackwell, Oxford, 1982, pp. 44–84.
81. Thor, K. B., Kawatani, M., Roppolo, J. R., Erdman, S. L., and DeGroat, W. C.: Altered spinal distribution of leucine enkephalin, somatostatin, vasoactive intestinal polypeptide, and substance P immunoreactivity in chronic spinal cats. *Neurosci. Abstr.* 10:25.5, 1984.
82. Ciesielski, T. E., Fukuda, Y., Glenn, W. W., Gorfien, J., Jeffery, K., and Hogan, J. F.: Response of the diaphragm muscle to electrical stimulation of the phrenic nerve. *J. Neurosurg.* 58:92–100, 1983.
83. Pette, D., and Tyler, K. R.: Response of succinate dehydrogenase activity in fibres of rabbit tibialis anterior muscle to chronic nerve stimulation. *J. Physiol. (Lond.)*338:1–9, 1983.
84. Salmons, S., and Vrbova, G.: The influence of activity on some contractile characteristics of mammalian fast and slow muscles. *J. Physiol. (Lond.)* 201:535–549, 1969.
85. Bazeed, M. A., Thüroff, J. W., Schmidt, R. A., Wiggin, D. M., and Tanagho, E. A.: Effects of chronic electrostimulation of the sacral roots on the striated urethral sphincter. *J. Urol.* 128:1357–1362, 1982.

29

Neural Prostheses and Bladder Control

RICHARD A. SCHMIDT, M.D.

Several million people in the United States suffer from various forms of neurogenic muscular dysfunction; paraplegics and quadriplegics alone number more than 500,000, and about 10,000 new cases are added to this pool yearly (*1*). It is virtually axiomatic that any injury or disease associated with paralysis of the lower limbs affects the behavior of the urinary bladder, which, more than anything else, can dramatically alter the quality of life and threaten to shorten life expectancy.

In addition to spinal injury, a multitude of other neurologic disorders commonly involve the bladder: multiple sclerosis, stroke, Parkinson's disease, tumors of the spine or central nervous system (CNS), and congenital spinal abnormalities. Approximately 1.5 million such patients have developed a significant disturbance in bladder function (*1*). In addition, thousands become socially and professionally disabled from symptoms of urinary leakage and frequency as well as from pelvic discomfort in the absence of any easily definable organic disease.

For these people, life is filled with frustration. Incontinence, the risk of urinary infection, and renal complications render a satisfactory professional career and personal life almost impossible. The cost of treatment is also a major consideration. For the paraplegic, physician visits, hospitalization, medications, and catheters may total as much as $10,000 per year. The cost to the nation for the care of the paralyzed approximates $6 billion per year.

Therapy for the disabled bladder is limited and generally follows a few selected options, depending on the specific problem (*2–5*). Whereas drugs may effectively relax a spastic bladder and improve storage, they are of little use for enhancing sphincter tone. For evacuation, drugs may be able to improve tonus, but they cannot restore bladder contractility or significantly decrease resistance within the urethral sphincter (*4*). The failure of drugs to influence the urinary sphincter has led to the development of surgical approaches to the problem, among which are neural ablation (*6*), the artificial sphincter (*7*), and sphincteric incisions to eliminate urinary retention from spasticity (*8*). Because these techniques cannot restore bladder function to normal, the result is a tenuous compromise —a fragile protection of renal function in return for permanent incontinence or dependence on some form of catheter drainage.

There is a possible alternative, i.e., a neuroprosthetic device. Electrostimulation can potentially rehabilitate the neurogenically compromised bladder without risking the complications that accompany the other treatments (*9*).

NEUROPROSTHETIC CONTROL OF THE BLADDER

During the 1960s electrical control of the bladder was widely attempted (*10–15*). The spinal center for micturition control was used as the site of stimulation, as were the pelvic nerves and the bladder muscle itself. Although these techniques met with some success, they were gradually abandoned because of major difficulties. Chief among them was the inability to separate bladder contraction from a simultaneous sphincter response. Voiding occurred only as a result of the differential in relaxation time between the bladder muscle and the voluntary muscle of the urinary sphincter (*14*) (Fig. 29–1): Because the bladder muscle relaxes slowly, pressure within its cavity exceeds that of the urethral outlet for several seconds after a stimulus, forcing a few milliliters of urine out of the bladder. This technique works quite well in animals (*14*) and humans (*15*). However, it does not address the complex interplay that normally exists between the detrusor and the urethral sphincter. Indeed, although the technique of poststimulus voiding can be used for bladder evacuation, it diverges from a basic principle, i.e., for neuroprosthesis to be effective over several years, or even decades, it should duplicate normal bladder behavior.

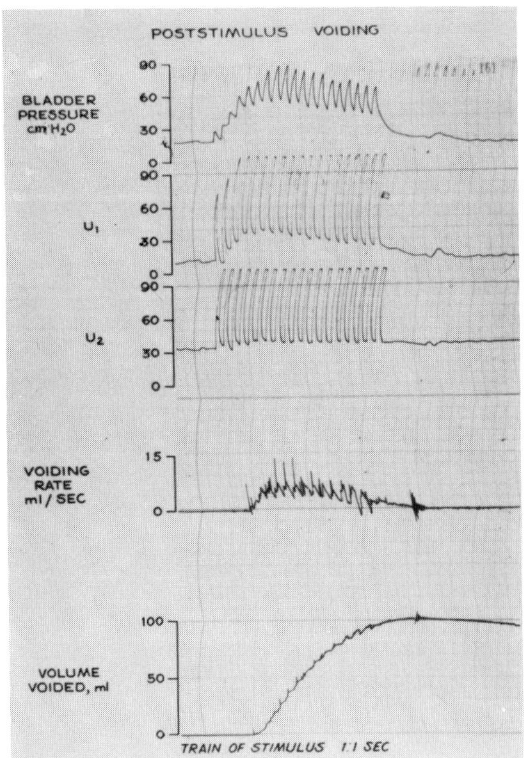

Figure 29–1. Effect of a train of electrical stimulation of the micturition center after high cord transection. The duration of electrical stimulation is 1 second; the interval between stimulations is also 1 second (ratio of 1:1). Complete emptying was achieved. (From Jonas, U., *et al.*: *Invest. Urol.* 13:151, 1975. © 1975, The Williams & Wilkins Co., Baltimore.)

Recent years have seen greatly increased understanding of the clinical effects and biologic consequences of stimulation (*16*), the physiology of the bladder in normal (*17–19*) and disease (*20,21*) states, and the nerve pathways that may be utilized to restore normal function of the urinary bladder (*9*). We are now on the verge of applying this information to patients. Our experience with implants supports the hopeful prospect that neural prostheses will dramatically improve the quality of life for patients disabled by a poorly functioning bladder.

Sacral Nerves as the Site for Electrical Control of Bladder Function

One may exercise control over the urinary bladder from four potential sites: the spinal cord, the bladder wall itself, the pelvic nerves between the spine and the bladder, and the sacral nerves within the vertebral column before they enter the pelvis. All were evaluated thoroughly in animal studies, and the sacral nerves were found to be the most appropriate (*22*). Their anatomy is such that bladder and pelvic floor activity can be distinguished from a host of other muscular responses; situated within the bony canal of the spine, they are easily accessible for surgical implantation of electrodes.

Stimulation of Dorsal and Ventral Roots

Stimulation of the dorsal roots elicits reflex activity mediated by the spinal cord and other nerves (*23*). The extent of the reflex response is broad and goes beyond sphincter contraction. With the exception of pain, many of these responses are not understood; they include hormonal and vascular changes within the body. With regard to neuroevacuation of the bladder, reflex sphincter contraction is the most undesirable of these responses (Fig. 29–2) and in the human seems to trigger other reflexes. For example, in the human quadriplegic, au-

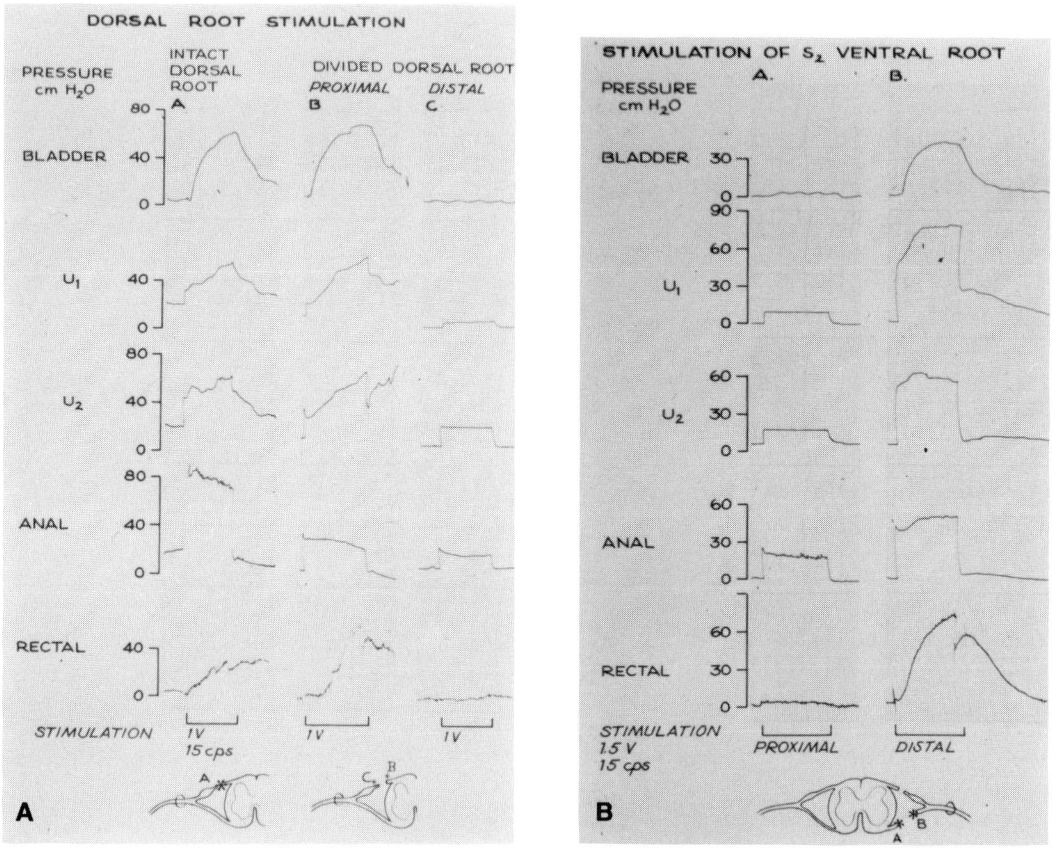

Figure 29–2. Peripheral and spinal reflex responses obtained with stimulation of dorsal and ventral sacral roots. **A.** Responses to stimulation of the intact (*A*) and divided (*B* and *C*) dorsal root of S_2. Bladder and sphincter responses were seen with stimulation of the proximal end (*B*), whereas sphincter responses mainly were seen with stimulation of the distal end (*C*). (From Schmidt, R. A., *et al.*: *Invest. Urol.* 16:300, 1979 © 1979, The Williams & Wilkins Co., Baltimore.)

tonomic dysreflexia does not result from stimulation of a dorsal root per se but from contraction of the striated sphincter simultaneously with the bladder. In the quadriplegic, any sphincter contraction coupled with detrusor contraction, whether spontaneous or induced, may risk dangerously elevating the systolic blood pressure. Stimulation of intact sacral nerves or the dorsal or ventral roots after a complete pudendal block does not trigger dysreflexia because of the absence of outlet resistance.

Another important point about stimulation of the dorsal roots is that a reflex facilitation or inhibition of detrusor behavior can result. Inhibition of the bladder, with improvement of storage is fortunately or unfortunately the response obtained with stimulation. Whether it results from closure of the striated sphincter or from a direct afferent inhibitory signal fed into the spinal cord is unknown, but the former seems most probable. The bladder response seen with stimulation in the paraplegic or quadriplegic can be improved after a pudendal block as opposed to that seen with simultaneous contraction of the urethral sphincter. This finding is true regardless of whether both dorsal and ventral roots or the ventral root alone are stimulated, suggesting that the inhibition results intrinsically from the closure tone of the urethral sphincter. However, this observation does not negate the role of higher centers in controlling the bladder but reinforces the hypothesis that higher centers influence bladder behavior via the striated sphincter mechanism.

From our animal work, as well as from observation in spinal injury patients, we concluded that electrodes should be implanted around the ventral component of individual sacral roots to achieve direct and predictable muscular responses within the pelvis. The dorsal roots are eliminated from the stimulus field to avoid unwanted reflex activity. Whether they should simply be separated from the ventral root or divided is as yet undetermined.

Selective Division of Somatic Sphincter Nerves

As each sacral nerve enters the pelvis, it divides into two major ramifications, the pelvic autonomics traveling to the urinary bladder and the pudendal somatics to the urinary sphincter (Fig. 29–3). It is possible to expose the nerves selectively and then separate the contribution of each to the pelvic and pudendal nerves (*23*). In animals it can be done by microsurgical techniques without jeopardizing the motor nerves to either the bladder or the pelvic viscera. An implanted electrode can then be used to stimulate the bladder selectively. The voiding produced is approximately 90 percent efficient because only one side of the bladder wall is activated. The voiding stream is continuous, with low pressures generated in the bladder, in contrast to the intermittent, high-pressure type of voiding produced by intermittent repeated stimulation (*15*). Although human anatomy is much more complex, it is also possible to trace the ramifications of the sacral nerve surgically for selective division of the individual contributions to pudendal innervation of the urinary sphincter.

Voiding and Sphincter Fatigue

Another type of voiding produced in animal experiments is that which follows intentional fatigue of the striated muscles of the urethra (*24*). All muscles fatigue after being stimulated to contraction for varying lengths of time. This fatigue is more rapid in striated (voluntary) muscles with a 100-Hz stimulus than it is at lower frequencies. Thus by allowing the striated muscles to fatigue, a good urinary stream (90 percent efficient) can be produced in animals (Fig. 29–4). Our experience with this technique suggested that it is not directly applicable to humans because the fatigue involves only an evoked muscle contraction. It does not alter the basal (preexisting) tension within the sphincter; in other words, the net effect is neither a drop nor an increase in sphincter tone. Thus if basal sphincter tone is low (as in the dog), voiding occurs; but if it is high (as in humans), high bladder pressures are required. In addition, the technique is less efficient in humans because of the reflex inhibition of the detrusor that results from stimulation of the pelvic muscles.

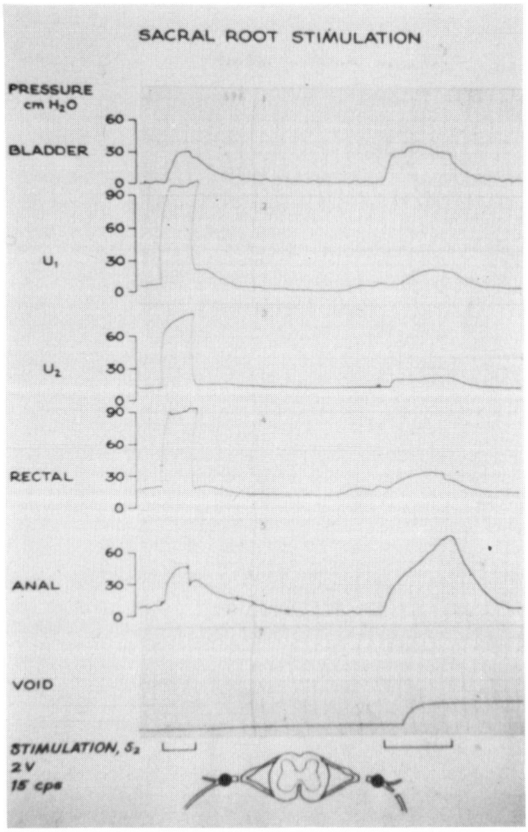

Figure 29–3. Comparing the responses of a divided canine S_2 nerve to stimulation with and without division of somatic nerves to the sphincter. Note the absence of urethral resistance and void seen on the side on which somatic fibers are divided. (From Schmidt, R. A.: *Eng. Med. Biol.* 2:2, 1983. © 1983, IEEE.)

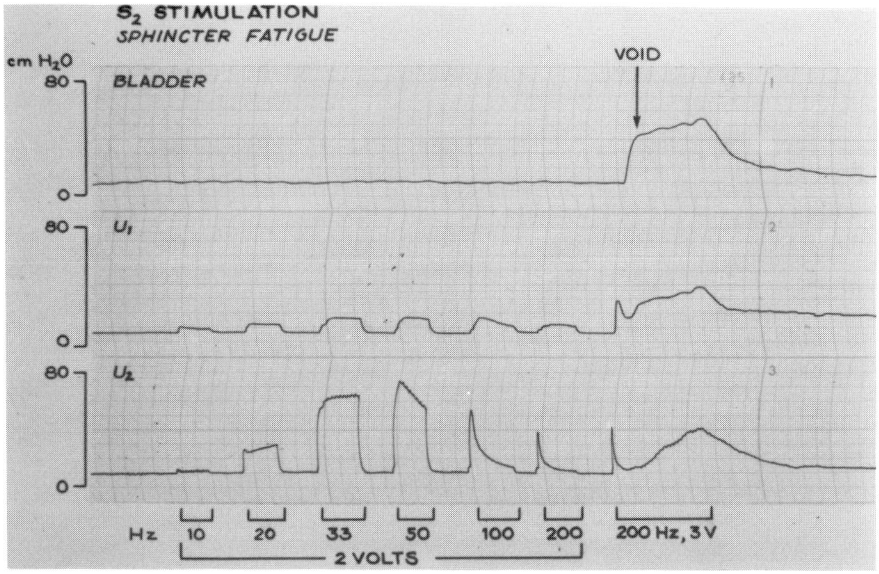

Figure 29–4. S_2 stimulation with increasing frequency in a paraplegic dog. With continuous stimulation at constant voltage (1 V), sphincteric fatigability is proportional to the frequency of stimulation. With 200-Hz stimulation above the threshold of the bladder, micturition is induced after sphincter fatigue. (From Schmidt, R. A.: *Eng. Med. Biol.* 2:2, 1983. © 1983, IEEE.)

Human Application of the Above Principles

In humans pelvic autonomic (smooth muscle) behavior is largely controlled and influenced by the S_3 nerve (Fig. 29–5), which is also a principal contributor to innervation of somatic muscles of the foot and pelvic sphincters. S_2 also contributes significantly to control of the pelvic sphincters and to pelvic sensation but little to the bladder; S_4 has not been shown to be significant in any of the humans tested intraoperatively, although slight sphincteric and bladder contractions are occasionally produced by its stimulation.

With stimulation of intact sacral nerves, one must consider the responses obtained via both the sensory afferents and the motor efferents. The efferent response is predictable and controllable, and it affects urinary storage and evacuation. The afferent response, which is highly variable and unpredictable, is associated with reflex amplification of sphincter tone and can thus result in detrusor inhibition.

All peripheral nerves have a mixture of nerve fiber types (*25*). Selective stimulation of the bladder cannot be achieved with intact sacral nerves because of the difference in threshold between large somatic axons and smaller autonomic axons. This threshold difference is much larger in humans than in animals, resulting in much higher stimulation levels for the bladder than for the sphincter. However, this principle makes independent

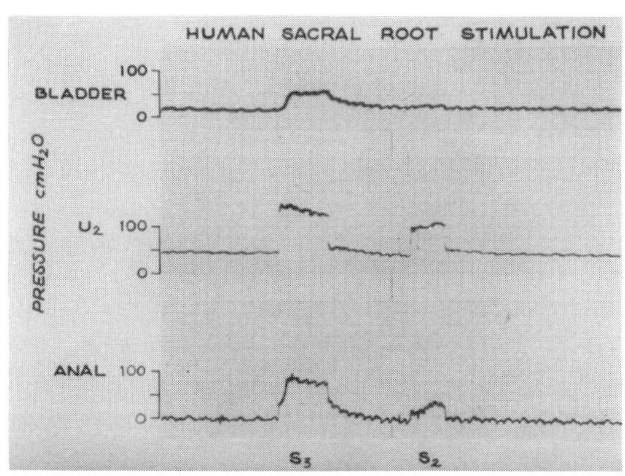

Figure 29–5. Intraoperative responses to stimulation of the human S_2 and S_3 nerve roots. Bladder activity is seen almost exclusively at the S_3 level. Stimulation of the S_2 nerve produces considerable sphincteric activity but no significant bladder activity.

stimulation of the sphincter possible, which is important because neurostimulation is extremely effective in suppressing sphincter spasticity. Stimulation of striated muscle groups in the pelvis of patients with intact spinal cords can also be achieved without discomfort because of a narrower but still significant difference between the threshold for pain and that for exciting muscle activity. This difference is important because it allows application of neurostimulation of sacral nerves to be used effectively as a therapy for mild forms of voiding dyssynergia.

Stimulation of the Human Neuropathic Bladder

Thus far we have implanted electrode arrays in six patients: three quadriplegics and three paraplegics. The electrode arrays were implanted in a variety of patterns in these six patients, including intact sacral roots, ventral roots after separation from their dorsal components, and ventral roots after dorsal rhizotomy. These patterns were carried out in both the S_2 and S_3 nerves; in all patients electrodes were implanted on at least one S_3 and at least one S_2. Subsequently, a unilateral complete or selective pudendal neurectomy was performed. Evaluation of these patients revealed the following basic principles of bladder control via neurostimulation.

1. Voiding occurred only in situations where sphincter tone was greatly weakened, usually as a result of selective somatic section or pharmacologic block of the pudendal nerves, or both (Fig. 29–6).
2. Unilateral pudendal neurectomy in highly spastic patients was not sufficient to allow voiding; even minimal degrees of pelvic tone elicited with stimulation continued to be highly obstructive to bladder evacuation.
3. No changes occurred in lower extremity spasticity, bowel or bladder continence, or reflex erections as a result of any of the electrode implants or the unilateral pudendal neurectomy.
4. Reflex voiding could be triggered by the sphincteric activity resulting from stimulation (Fig. 29–7); this response was sporadic and unpredictable.

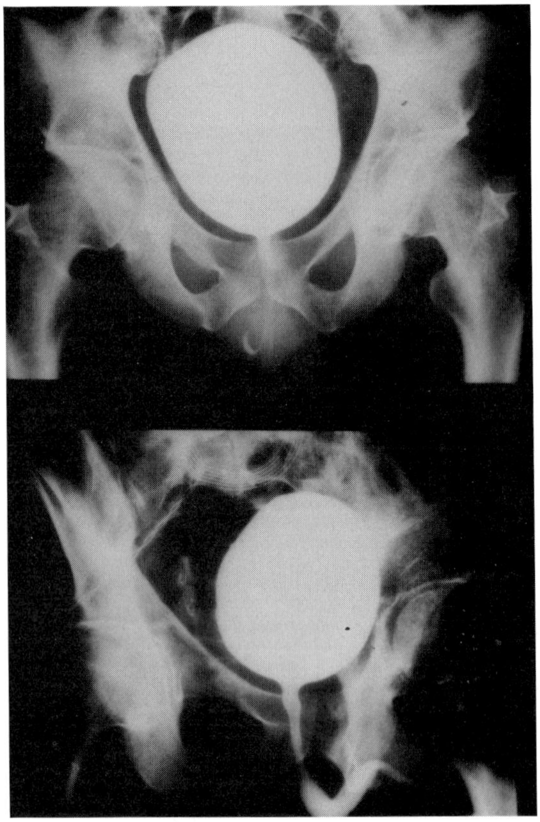

Figure 29–6. Radiologic views of the bladder before and during neuromicturition. Stimulation of S_3 nerves bilaterally was accomplished via a surgically implanted electrode. In addition, a bilateral selective somatic nerve section was performed. Evacuation of the bladder with this technique is complete, and voiding pressure within the bladder remains low. This response persisted for 4 months before failing (due to the return of sphincteric activity).

It seems clear now that bilateral surgical manipulation of the pudendal nerves is required to minimize the inhibitory effect of the urethral outlet during electrode micturition. Future alternatives may avoid actual cutting of nerve fibers. Reversible nerve blocks with drug-delivery devices or sophisticated stimulation techniques (anodal block) may permit temporary weakening of the urethral outlet and protect erections and continence. Thus far, unilateral pudendal neurectomy or bilateral selective pudendal neurectomy has not affected spontaneous reflex erections or continence. Notably, the bladder does tend to become less spastic and

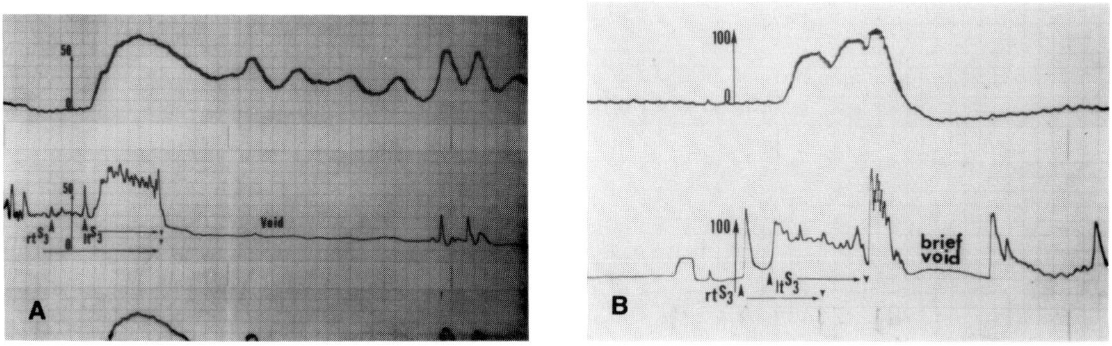

Figure 29–7. **A.** Voiding triggered by stimulation of the S_3 sacral root. During the interval of actual stimulation, no voiding occurred. Upon withdrawal of the stimulus, sphincteric relaxation was sustained along with persisting detrusor contraction, resulting in a void. **B.** More often, however, a small poststimulus void was all that was seen. Repetitive on–off patterns of stimulation did not produce the same degree of successful voiding seen in the animal experiments.

more controllable because of decreased facilitation of the afferent input to the micturition center.

Preoperative Evaluation. Fortunately, because of the anatomy of the sacrum, one has easy access to various sacral nerves traveling through the sacral canal. An insulated needle or electrode can easily be inserted into various sacral foramina for test stimulation of individual sacral roots; bladder and sphincter activity can be demonstrated, and one can use these responses to assess responsiveness to implanted electrodes. It is worth noting that a poor bladder contraction may be obtained with this test for one of two reasons. The first is technical: inefficient coupling of the electrodes to the sacral roots; in such cases a visibly poor response in the pelvic muscles and lower extremities results. The second reason is the inhibitory effect that contraction of the pelvic floor exerts on detrusor contraction; if this situation appears to be the case, a pudendal nerve block is attempted.

Initial testing is necessary to determine a candidate's suitability for electrode implantation and to gain insight into the sensory feelings and muscle responses achieved with stimulation of any particular nerve. One should not rely entirely on the responses seen at one setting, however, as the electrical coupling with the individual nerve can be unpredictable. Repeated testing is important in that it assesses viability of somatic and autonomic nerves, sensitivity to pain (because many spinal lesions are associated with mixed deficits), adverse blood pressure responses, and thresholds of stimulation required to produce the desired responses.

Spasticity. It is at this point that sacral nerve pacemakers have their most immediate application (*25*). Because electrical stimulation suppresses spontaneous neuronal activity, it can be used to modulate spastic behavior of both smooth and striated muscles. For instance, with paraplegia the spinal injury releases bladder control from the inhibitory influences of higher brain centers, resulting in spasticity of the bladder and urethral sphincter. Bladder capacity is greatly reduced, and the patient suffers from incontinence. Continuous stimulation of the sacral nerves can suppress this spasticity by replacing some of the inhibition normally provided by the higher brain centers. As more benefits are obtained with each nerve stimulated, there is a better chance of suppressing spasticity by stimulating as many of the sacral nerves dealing with bladder control as possible. Bladder evacuation may still need to be performed by catheter, but it is also possible that voiding might occur spontaneously when the stimulator is turned off.

Given the erratic performance of the neurogenic bladder in any individual, predictable restoration of a free and continuous urinary flow in all cases seems at present to be unrealistic. However, those patients with coordinated reflex voiding will do well with the added storage achieved by neural stimulation. In time, others will be helped through continued evaluation of other techniques.

CONCLUSIONS

Neurostimulation attempts to restore, to as near normal as possible, the storage and evacuation functions of the urinary bladder. Many patients without spinal injury have already benefited from careful observation and documentation of its effects on bladder and sphincter function. There does not appear to be any risk from or adverse effect of neurostimulation—a major consideration, as surgical therapy can cause permanent, undesirable side effects if not completely successful.

For the neuromicturition pacemaker to have a chance of success, the bladder must have reflex contractility. Fortunately, most injuries of the nervous system are at or above the mid-thoracic level of the spinal cord, leaving intact the spinal nuclei for control of micturition, located below that level.

Remember, however, that events triggered in the body through electrical stimulation of a major nerve cannot be considered to parallel those occurring normally. The intact biologic event is modulated through selective firing of thousands of individual nerve axons. The sequence of axonal firing responsible for a smooth bladder contraction simply cannot be duplicated by neurostimulation. What can be achieved is simultaneous firing of most of the axons within a sacral nerve that influence either bladder or sphincter contraction, which is a major leap toward restoring continence and eliminating urinary retention.

REFERENCES

1. *Public Health Bulletin 1426*. National Institutes of health, Bethesda, 1978.
2. Bors, E., and Comarr, A. E.: *Neurological Urology. Physiology of Micturition: Its Neurological Disorders and Sequelae*. University Park Press, Baltimore, 1971.
3. McLellan, F. C.: *The Neurogenic Bladder*. Charles C Thomas, Springfield, IL, 1939.
4. Caine, M.: Pharmacology of the lower urinary tract musculature. In *Scientific Foundations of Urology*, Yearbook Medical Publishers, Chicago, 1982, p. 433.
5. Raz, S., and Bradley, W. E.: Neuromuscular dysfunction of the lower urinary tract. In Harrison, J. H., Gittes, R. F., Perlmutter, A. D., Stamey, T. A., and Walsh, P. C. (eds.), *Campbell's Urology*, 4th ed. Saunders, Philadelphia, 1979, p. 1215.
6. Torrens, M., and Hald, T.: Bladder denervation procedures. *Urol. Clin. North Am.* 6:283, 1979.
7. Scott, F. B., Bradley, W. E., and Timm, G. W.: Treatment of urinary incontinence by implantable prosthetic sphincter. *Urology* 1:252, 1973.
8. Golji, H.: Urethral sphincterotomy for chronic spinal cord injury. *J. Urol.* 123:204, 1980.
9. Schmidt, R. A., and Tanagho, E. A.: Feasibility of controlled micturition through electrical stimulation. *Urol. Int.* 34:199, 1979.
10. Nashold, B. S., Friedman, H., Glenn, J. F., Grimes, J. H., Barry, W. F., and Avery, R.: Electromicturition in paraplegia. *Arch. Surg.* 104:195, 1972.
11. Habib, H. N.: Experience and recent contributions in sacral nerve stimulation for voiding in both humans and animals. *Br. J. Urol.* 39:73, 1967.
12. Holmquist, B.: Electromicturition by pelvic nerve stimulation in paraplegia. *Scand. J. Urol. Nephrol.* 2(Suppl.):2, 1968.
13. Merrill, D. C.: Clinical experience with the Mentor bladder stimulator. III. Patients with urinary vesical hypotonia. *J. Urol.* 113:335, 1975.
14. Jonas, U., Heine, J. P., and Tanagho, E. A.: Studies on the feasibility of urinary bladder evacuation by direct spinal cord stimulation. II. Poststimulus voiding: a way to overcome outflow resistance. *Invest. Urol.* 13:151, 1975.
15. Brindley, G. S.: An implant to empty the bladder or close the urethra. *J. Neurol. Neurosurg. Psychiatry* 40:358, 1977.
16. Pudenz, R., Bullara, L., and Agnew, W.: Adverse effects of electrical energy applied to the nervous system. *Appl. Neurophysiol.* 40:72–87, 1977.
17. De Groat, W. C., Booth, A. M., Milne, R. J., and Roppolo, J. R.: Parasympathetic preganglionic neurons in the sacral cord. *J. Auton. Nerv. Syst.* 5:23, 1982.
18. Kuffler, S. W., and Nichols, J. G.: *From Neuron to Brain*. Sinauer Associates, Sunderland, MA, 1976.
19. Gosling, J. A.: Structure of the bladder and urethra in relation to function. *Urol. Clin. North Am.* 6:3, 1979.
20. Thomas, D. G.: The urinary tract following spinal cord injury. In *Scientific Foundations of Urology*, Yearbook Medical Publishers, Chicago, 1982, p. 421.
21. Murowsky, A. M., Scheibert, C. D., and Hrinchez, T. R.: Studies in the sacral reflex arcs in paraplegia. II. Differential sacral neurotomy—an operative method. *J. Neurosurg.* 7:39, 1950.
22. Schmidt, R. A., Bruschini, H., and Tanagho, E. A.: Urinary bladder and sphincter responses to stimulation of dorsal and ventral sacral roots. *Invest. Urol.* 16:300, 1979.
23. Schmidt, R. A., Bruschini, H., and Tanagho, E. A.: Sacral root stimulation in controlled micturition: peripheral somatic neurotomy and stimulated voiding. *Invest. Urol.* 17:130, 1979.
24. Thüroff, J. W., Bazeed, M. A., Schmidt, R. A., Wiggin, D. M., and Tanagho, E. A.: Functional pattern of sacral root stimulation in dogs. II. Urethral closure. *J. Urol.* 127:1034, 1982.
25. Schmidt, R.A.: Neural prosthesis and bladder control. *Eng. Med. Biol.* 2:2, 1983.

30

Surgery for Urethral Sphincter Reconstruction

EMIL A. TANAGHO, M.D.

Urinary sphincteric function is still controversial. Everyone, however, agrees that there is no anatomic entity that can definitively be called the sphincter and can be isolated and dissected (*1–4*). Indeed, what we know as the sphincteric mechanism is nothing more than a muscular tube with abundant circular fibers. It is easier to study in women than in men, but it is similar in both. In women the entire urethra, which is about 4 cm long, acts as the sphincteric unit, providing enough outlet resistance to maintain urinary continence. This urethral muscular tube has two coats, an inner longitudinal coat and an outer semicircular coat (Fig. 30–1); the latter provides the sphincteric function (*5*). The muscular elements are embedded in dense collagen, which provides firmness and minimal stretchability. In men the prostate gland is interposed between the two coats, incorporating within it the outer semicircular coat, which constitutes the prostatic stroma with partial condensation around the urethral lumen, especially at the level of the internal meatus and toward the apex of the prostate. Myogenically, neurologically, and histologically, the muscular urethral sphincteric unit is the same as the detrusor and is directly continuous with it. Its sphincteric function is attributed to the abundance of circular fibers, which generate sufficient centrally oriented forces to maintain closure of the bladder outlet.

Correction of urinary incontinence remains a surgical challenge for which several procedures have been used with varied success. Anatomic stress incontinence, frequently encountered in women as a result of pelvic floor weakness, can easily be corrected by proper suspension to the vesicourethral segment. Complete loss of urinary sphincteric function is a much more challenging problem. Congenital incontinence, as commonly seen with complete epispadias, does not result from a simple defect in the roof of the urethra in the region of the sphincteric segment, which could be corrected by trimming the edges and forming a tube; rather, there is a lack of proper musculature in this segment that fails to offer sufficient sphincteric function. The defect in the urogenital diaphragm aggravates the condition. Postoperative incontinence is best exemplified by postprostatectomy incontinence, which is most commonly seen after transurethral resection of the prostate. To remove the obstruction, the surgeon might encroach on the musculature of the bladder neck as well as on the inframontanal prostatic segment and the abundant smooth musculature in this critical location, which normally provides adequate sphincteric tone postoperatively. This encroachment, compounded by the weakness of the compressed prostatic tissue and the surgical capsule, enfeebles the sphincteric mechanism. If the weakness is significant, the patient is left with a patulous segment, the prostatic fossa, which is functionless despite its location, as normally it should be guarding the bladder outlet. The membranous urethra, by itself, with its voluntary sphincteric intrinsic mus-

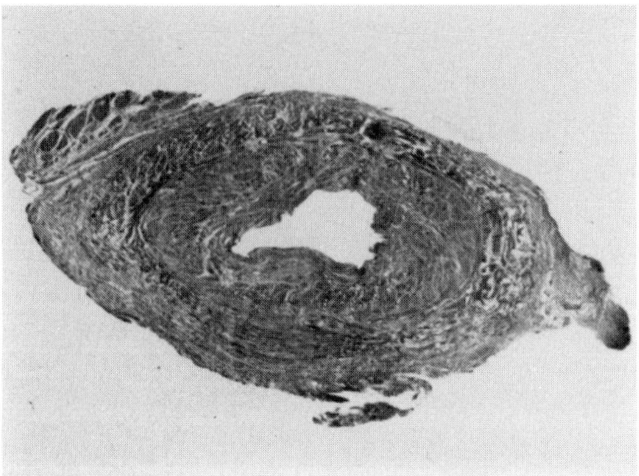

Figure 30–1. Cross section of the female urethra showing the muscular arrangement of the sphincteric unit distributed along the entire length. Abundant circularly oriented fibers form the outer coat surrounding the inner longitudinal coat embedded in dense collagen tissue. (From Tanagho, E. A.: *J. Urol.* 125:321, 1981. Copyright © 1981, The Williams & Wilkins Co., Baltimore.)

culature, is not adequate to maintain continence in such patients.

Traumatic incontinence, most often seen with severe pelvic injury, results in women from disruption and irreparable laceration of the urethrovesical segment. In men, if the same severe damage involves the bladder neck and prostatomembranous urethra, the patient is left without a functioning sphincteric unit.

Iatrogenic complete urinary incontinence in women is encountered after repeated surgical attempts to correct what was initially stress urinary incontinence. Ill-advised techniques, resulting in marked scarring and fibrosis of the delicate urethral musculature, can damage the intrinsic sphincteric mechanism completely. Iatrogenic urinary incontinence is also seen occasionally after repair of extensive urethrovaginal fistulas or excision of multiple urethral diverticula if the surgeon was not careful to preserve urethral sphincteric musculature.

Neurogenic incontinence is a totally different and more complicated problem that does not lie within the scope of this presentation. However, the same principles discussed below can be applied to sphincteric reconstruction in some cases of neurogenic bladder to generate enough outlet resistance and maintain reservoir function of the bladder, so that the patient can then rely on intermittent catheterization. If the neurogenic deficit is partial, a functional result from sphincteric reconstruction may be obtained.

Techniques using modifications of slings from fascia or muscles, or a more distal approach designed to create compression on the bulbous urethra, have been tried, but the long-term results have not been completely satisfactory (*6–10*). Revising the prostatic cavity by reducing its size and reversing the YV-plasty technique to obtain a narrow tube distal to the internal meatus has more often been a failure than a success, because of the use of damaged and scarred tissue for reconstruction of the tube.

Rationale for Techniques of Sphincteric Reconstruction

Lessons learned from cases of postprostatectomy incontinence are probably the most valuable in identifying the objectives and rationale of sphincteric reconstruction. Urinary incontinence after transurethral resection results from damage to the tissue from the level of the vesical outlet to the urogenital diaphragm, which consequently is unable to provide sphincteric action. Surprisingly, after radical prostatectomy (in which the entire prostatic urethra is excised, from the level of the internal meatus down to the urogenital diaphragm with all its sphincteric muscular elements), 90 to 95 percent of patients are completely continent. The main difference anatomically is that, in the first group, a worthless structure is left between the vesical neck and the urogenital diaphragm, whereas in the second group direct anastomosis of the musculature around the internal meatus to the membranous urethra enables it to provide a certain sphincteric action, attain a tubular formation of variable length, and preserve continence.

Sphincteric reconstruction should take advantage of the sphincteric potential of the muscular element around the internal meatus. The surgical techniques described below do just that, i.e., tubularize this musculature to give it the opportunity to provide the desired sphincteric action (*5*) (Fig. 30–2).

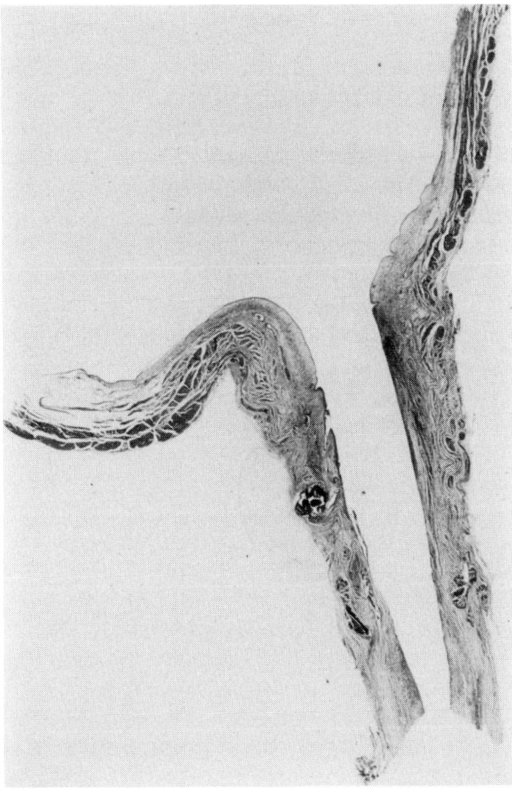

Figure 30–2. Sagittal section of the reconstructed bladder neck in an experimental animal model. Note the close similarity to normal bladder outlet configuration and the heavy musculature in the proximal reconstructed tube now acting as the sphincter. (From Tanagho, E. A.: *J. Urol.* 125:321, 1981. Copyright © 1981, The Williams & Wilkins Co., Baltimore.)

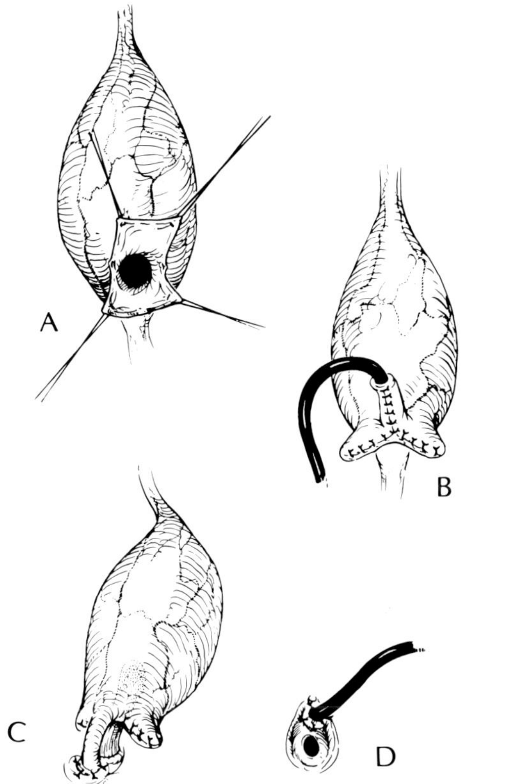

Figure 30–3. Principles of the anterior bladder flap technique as applied in the woman. After the bladder neck is isolated from the urethra (**A**), the anterior flap is raised and formed into a tube around a 12F catheter (**B**). The bladder outlet is reconstructed (**C**), and the tube is anastomosed to the distal urethra or brought out to the vaginal vestibule if there is no remnant of urethra (**D**). (From Tanagho, E. A.: Neourethra: rationale, surgical technique, and indications. In *Surgery of Female Incontinence*. Stanton, S. L., and Tanagho, E. A. [eds.]. Springer-Verlag, Berlin, 1980.)

SURGICAL TECHNIQUES

There are two basic techniques of sphincteric reconstruction based on the above rationale of utilizing the musculature around the bladder neck to provide the lost sphincteric action. The following sections describe each technique as performed in women.

Anterior Bladder Flap

Tanagho's technique (*11,12*) (Fig. 30–3) utilizes an anterior bladder flap. Fortunately, a segment of the bladder wall just above the internal meatus anteriorly possesses a muscular arrangement that is essentially the same as the sphincteric unit (*5*) (Fig. 30–4). Our previous anatomic studies revealed a heavy ventral condensation of the middle circular fibers just above the internal meatus concentrated over a 2.5-cm segment (*2,3*). These fibers are arranged in an arc that fans out and becomes less dense as it is followed laterally and dorsally; the fibers also fan out appreciably about 1 in. above the level of the internal meatus. The flap fashioned from this segment and turned into a tube includes an appreciable amount of these circular fibers with some longitudinal fibers on either side.

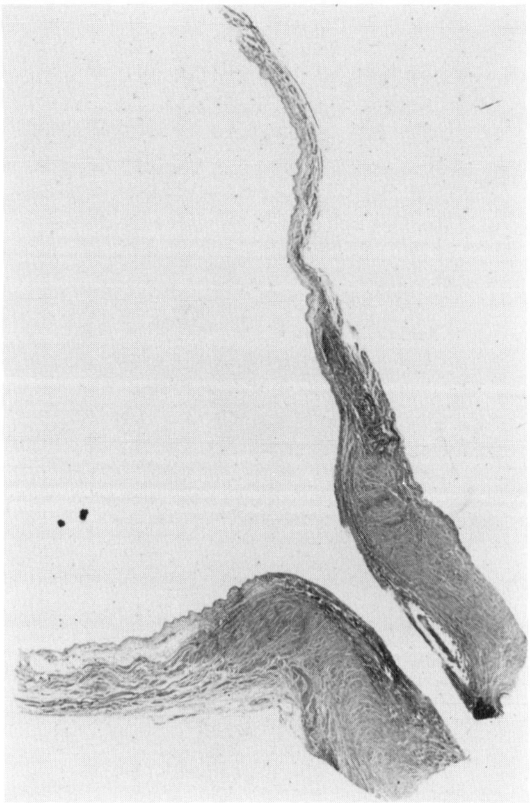

Figure 30–4. Sagittal section of the female bladder neck showing heavy condensation of circular fibers of the ventral bladder wall just above the internal meatus. Morphologic features of this segment are similar to those of the urethral musculature below. (From Tanagho, E. A.: *J. Urol.* 125:321, 1981. Copyright © 1981, The Williams & Wilkins Co., Baltimore.)

This tube possesses enough tone with perfect muscular arrangement to offer adequate closure (*12,13*). When positioned to replace an excised or damaged prostatic segment, a scarred female urethra, or a congenitally absent urethral sphincteric tube, it offers a sphincteric mechanism in the exact anatomic location of the normal sphincteric segment (*11,12,14*).

The surgical procedure is relatively simple; its main feature is transection of the bladder wall at the exact level of the internal meatus, separating the bladder on one side from the urethra on the other. Before this transection is attempted, the bladder is half-distended, and the outlines of the flap to be raised from its anterior wall are marked by four stay sutures, 2.5 cm apart, in either direction. The result is a 2.5 × 2.5 cm flap that is still attached to the anterior bladder wall by its base. After the flap is outlined, the anterior bladder wall is cut at the level of the internal meatus until the lumen of the proximal urethra is entered. This incision is then continued from inside to complete separating the bladder from the distal urethra. After the bladder is completely isolated, it is slightly dissected around its base. Two lateral incisions to complete the development of the flap are made. A 12F or 14F Foley catheter is passed through the urethra and pulled in the wound; the flap is then folded around it, incorporating the heavily condensed circular fibers of the anterior bladder wall. An interrupted 3-0 Dexon suture at the base of the tube and another at its apex, together with a one-layer closure, are used. To reconstitute the normal anatomic relation between the bladder cavity and the neourethra, the apex of the trigone is secured by a mattress suture to the base of the flap, which results in a V-shaped incision in the base of the bladder. Each side of this incision is now closed by interrupted 3-0 Dexon sutures. Usually the bladder is drained by a suprapubic tube, and the neourethra is supported by the urethral catheter, which is used as a stent. After complete closure of the bladder base, the reconstructed tube is anastomosed by four or five interrupted 3-0 Dexon sutures to the cut end of the urethra. If there is no urethral canal, that end of the tube can be brought out to the vaginal vestibule just below the pubic arch. This will either establish direct continuity between the bladder and the residual segment of the urethra or create a completely new urethra with its outside opening in the vaginal vestibule. Both ways have been tried, and both have been successful.

Upon completion of reconstruction and establishment of the anastomosis, it is advisable to support the new vesicourethral junction to avoid collapse of the neourethra under the weight of the mobilized bladder. Two sutures are used to attach the vesicourethral junction to the back of the rectus muscles, providing minimum stretch with no tension.

Posterior or Trigonal Tube

With Leadbetter's technique (*8,9*) (Fig. 30–5), a posterior or trigonal tube is created.

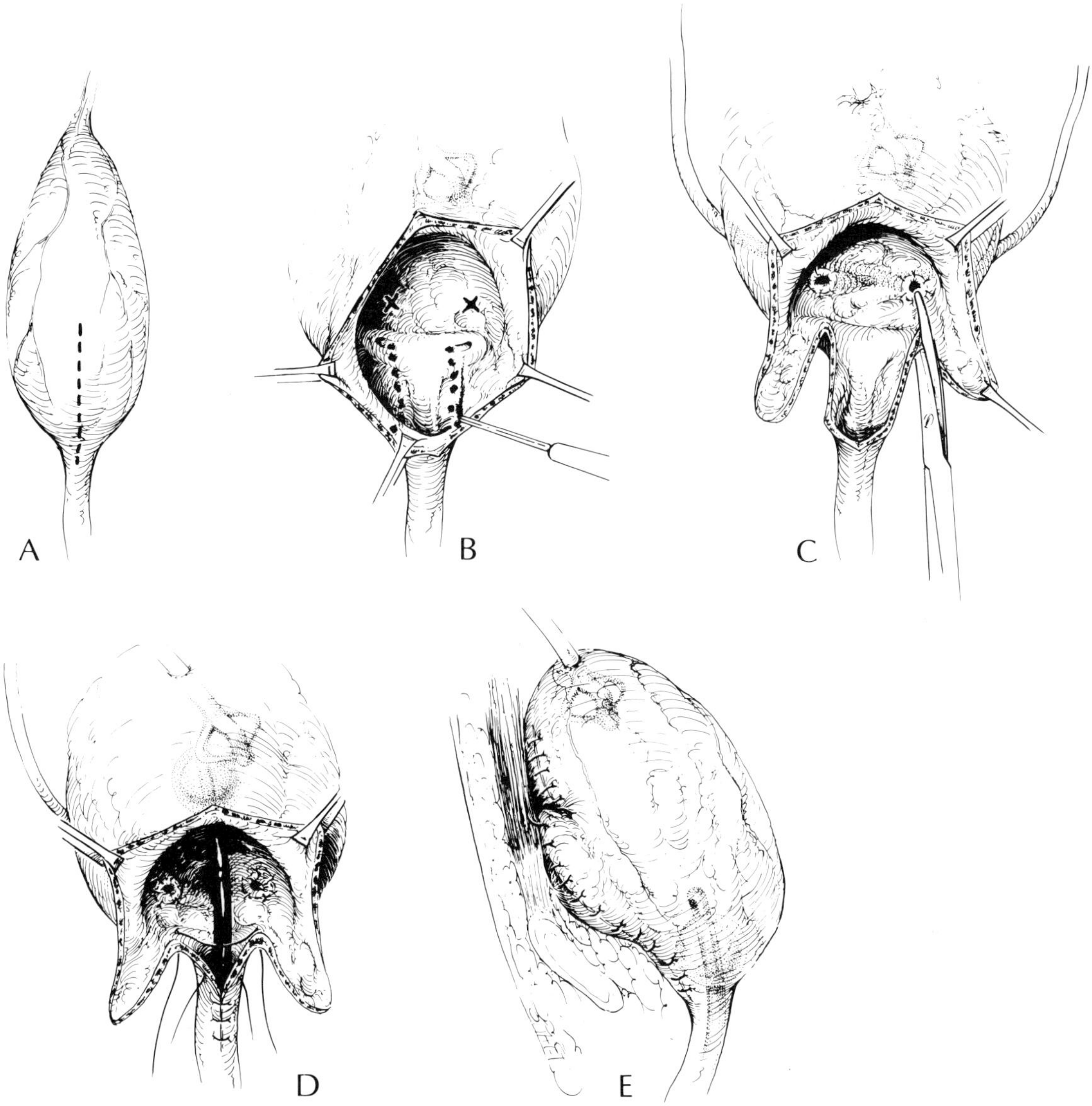

Figure 30–5. Stages of posterior bladder flap (Leadbetter's) technique: **A.** Midline incision, anterior bladder wall, extending to internal meatus. **B.** Marking of the posterior trigonal flap using cautery. **C.** Bilateral ureteral implantation at a higher level and cutting of premarked edges of the trigonal flap. **D.** Beginning of closure of the trigonal tube. **E.** Final stage with fixation of the bladder to the anterior abdominal wall.

Posteriorly, just above the level of the internal meatus, lie the superficial and deep trigone with detrusor musculature behind it. Again, there is an abundance of circular and longitudinal fibers leading into the bladder base, which, if turned around into a tube, would lengthen the urethra and provides a tubular muscular structure with sphincteric function. It is effective inasmuch as it maintains continuity between the urethral canal and the bladder base. However, it lacks the mobility, elasticity, and versatility of a neourethra fashioned from an anterior bladder flap. In addition, this technique requires bilateral reimplantation of the ureter at a higher point in the bladder base so as to have adequate space below the ureteral orifices, incorporating the entire trigone, which can be fashioned into a tube to form the sphincteric unit.

After complete mobilization of the bladder neck and urethra, a midline incision is made down to the internal meatus. After bilateral ureteral reimplantation at a higher level from inside the bladder is completed, the intended posterior flap is outlined by stay sutures, which are usually placed up to the level of the interureteric ridge and down to the apex of the trigone. They form a 1.0 to 1.5 cm wide strip of trigonal and detrusor musculature in the bladder base. The midline incision is then curved downward around the internal meatus and directed posteriorly to be extended along the marked stay sutures in the base of the bladder. The full segment of the bladder is cut, leaving behind another 1.5 cm wide strip attached to the anterior vaginal wall and the urethral vaginal septum. These two lateral flaps with the anterior bladder wall are raised, and then the posterior trigone and flap are shaped into a tube wrapped around a small catheter or stent of 8F or 10F caliber. This step is done in either one or two layers, but we usually find it difficult to use two layers; we are satisfied with a one-layer interrupted closure with 3-0 Dexon sutures. The most proximal end of the tube is the new site of the internal meatus. The two flaps of the bladder wall are then sutured in the midline in a continuous line with the anterior incision in the bladder wall. Suprapubic drainage is established, and the urethral catheter is left as a stent. After this operation, a certain degree of support should be provided, as is done in vesicourethral colpopexy.

This procedure lends itself well to reconstruction in women because the urethra itself can easily be molded around to flow into the reconstructed tube, maintaining its continuity with the base of the bladder. It does require, however, the existence of a urethral tube and bilateral ureteral reimplantation, adding to its magnitude and concomitantly introducing potential complications and morbidity. Nevertheless, when a case requires both reimplantation and a neourethra, this technique is ideal.

We have applied both techniques of neourethral construction for congenital anomalies, as well as in iatrogenic cases and a variety of other indications, with a high rate of success (approximately 80 percent).

POSTOPERATIVE MANAGEMENT

With both techniques we rely on suprapubic drainage for at least 3 weeks and maintain a urethral stent for about the same time. Immediately after surgery, excessive bladder spasm frequently occurs, which is controlled by anticholinergic drugs and muscle relaxants. Usually we remove the urethral stent first and plug the suprapubic tube to test for voiding as well as for residual urine. Patients may remain completely incontinent immediately postoperatively, but this has no real prognostic significance; in this situation we pull the suprapubic tube and wait for the functional result of the reconstruction to develop. Occasionally, there is complete obstruction from surgical edema at the site of reconstruction, and in these patients we maintain suprapubic drainage, intermittently plugging the tube and testing for voiding. The suprapubic tube is never removed until there is no significant residual urine and the bladder is completely empty. It is not uncommon for some patients, immediately after surgical repair, to be capable of both retaining urine and emptying the bladder completely and freely; in such cases the suprapubic tube can be removed.

COMPLICATIONS

The potential for complications must not be underestimated because the procedures for bladder neck reconstruction are not technically easy. They require experience and skill and present various pitfalls. The surgeon who is unfamiliar with them should observe several times, on video tape if necessary. It is also advisable to practice them at least once on an animal model. The procedures should never be undertaken for less than complete urinary incontinence.

From a technical point of view, bladder neck reconstruction is easiest on the postprostatectomy patient because the bladder neck is usually rather high and one can readily visualize the prostatovesical junction and make the transection there without too much difficulty. The most complicated cases are those with congenital anomalies because the anatomic defects are not standard and much dissection is necessary. Every case must be approached individually; applying the same principles, whatever is needed should be done.

The most common postoperative complication is functional bladder outlet obstruction, which may remain for several months in varying degrees but usually resolves spontaneously. Occasionally, a stricture forms at the site of anastomosis between the tube and the prostatic fossa; once detected with direct endoscopic visualization, this segment should be dilated early, before subjecting the reconstructed tube to the high voiding pressure against this distal obstruction. If the obstruction persists, a limited internal urethrotomy may be indicated. Other potential complications include fistulas, usually at the site of anastomosis because of poor healing, or along the suture line, especially if integrity of the tissue is not optimal. Complete sloughing or loss of the tube has been reported, but we have never encountered it ourselves. Meticulous care to preserve the blood supply of the flap is essential for proper healing. Bilateral ureteral obstruction is something to look for, especially in the trigonal tube. This situation is not uncommon but usually has no clinical significance. However, in an occasional case it can become significant, leading to increased residual urine and progressive back-pressure on the upper urinary tract.

All current techniques to achieve continence present an element of functional obstruction. The decrease in urethral pressure that immediately precedes or is simultaneous with bladder contraction in the normal voiding act does not occur exactly in the same manner after bladder neck reconstruction. The fine synchronicity and harmony between the bladder musculature and the natural sphincter are lacking. In a urodynamic study after reconstruction (mainly for epispadias, since, catheterization is difficult in the postprostatectomy patient), we found that at the initiation of voiding urethral pressure remained stable and bladder contraction exceeded it, after which pressure in the urethra decreased and voiding proceeded; or there was some increase in pressure in the reconstructed tube until it was pulled open by contraction of the bladder wall, funneling it out so that its pressure decreased and voiding could occur. This element of functional obstruction fortunately disappears completely as soon as voiding continues. Some patients have as good a flow rate after bladder neck reconstruction as before, whereas in others it is somewhat reduced.

OVERALL RESULTS

We reported our results in 81 patients (25 women, 56 men) with complete urinary incontinence elsewhere (*5*) (Table 30–1). Of these 81 patients, 25 were managed by the posterior bladder tube (Leadbetter) technique (*8*) and 56 by the anterior tube reconstruction (Tanagho) technique (*11*). Four years later, our series exceeded 105 patients, but the breakdown and analysis of our results remained essentially the same.

We categorized the outcome of reconstruction as excellent, good, fair, and failed. In some of the failures, incontinence was corrected and some patients became completely dry; however, they remained unable to void spontaneously and had to rely on intermittent catheterization. We therefore counted these patients as failures because the procedure was intended to reinstate functional control. Results were considered fair in those patients who showed improvement but who remained incontinent and had to rely on protective measures or an external apparatus. Patients with good results showed significant improvement; they might lose a few drops of urine with overdistension or stress but required no protection most of the

Table 30–1. Results of Sphincteric Reconstruction by the Tanagho and Leadbetter Techniques

RESULT	ANTERIOR TUBE (NO.)		POSTERIOR TUBE (NO.)	
Excellent	23	71.5%	4	52%
Good	17		9	
Fair	9	28.5%	6	48%
Failed	7		6	
Total	56		25	

*From Tanagho, E. A.: Bladder neck reconstruction for total urinary incontinence. J. Urol. 125:321, 1981. © 1981. The Williams & Wilkins Co., Baltimore.

Table 30–2. Indications for Sphincteric Reconstruction and Postoperative Results

INDICATION	EXCELLENT	GOOD	FAIR	FAILED
Postprostatectomy incontinence	17	16	6	5
Trauma	–	3	2	2
Epispadias	2	4	4	2
Other congenital anomalies	2	1	1	1
Internal urethrotomy	2	2	1	
Operation	1	2	1	2
Urethral excision		1		1
Total	24	29	15	13
	53 (65.4%)		28 (34.6%)	

* From Tanagho, E. A.: Bladder neck reconstruction for total urinary incontinence. *J. Urol.* 125:321, 1981. © 1981, The Williams & Wilkins Co., Baltimore.

time. The excellent results denoted those patients with an overall superior outcome: no obstruction, leakage, residual urine, or urge incontinence. Our classification of 81 patients, as related to the indications for reconstruction, is summarized in Table 30–2. In properly selected patients, with meticulous technique, an acceptable outcome is easily achievable.

REFERENCES

1. Elbadawi, A.: Ultrastructure of vesicourethral innervation. I. Neuroeffector and cell junctions in the male internal sphincter. *J. Urol.* 128:180, 1982.
2. Tanagho, E. A.: Anatomy and physiology of the urethra. In Caldwell, K. P. S. (ed.), *Urinary Incontinence.* Sector, London, 1978, p. 27.
3. Tanagho, E. A.: The anatomy and physiology of micturition. In Inglis, D. S. B. (ed.), *Clinics in Obstetrics and Gynaecology.* Saunders, London, 1978, p. 3.
4. Tanagho, E. A., and Smith, D. R.: Mechanism of urinary continence. I. Embryologic, anatomic and pathologic considerations. *J. Urol.* 100:640, 1968.
5. Tanagho, E. A.: Bladder neck reconstruction for total urinary incontinence: ten years of experience. *J. Urol.* 125:321, 1981.
6. Berry, J. L.: A new procedure for correction of urinary incontinence: preliminary report. *J. Urol.* 85:771, 1961.
7. Girgis, A. S., and Veenema, R. J.: Perineal urethroplasty: a new operation for correction of urinary incontinence in the male patient. *J. Urol.* 93:703, 1965.
8. Leadbetter, G. W., Jr.: Surgical correction of total urinary incontinence. *J. Urol.* 91:261, 1964.
9. Leadbetter, G. W., Jr., and Fraley, E. E.: Surgical correction for total urinary incontinence: five years later. *J. Urol.* 97:869, 1968.
10. Young, H. H.: An operation for the cure of incontinence of urine. *Surg. Gynecol. Obstet.* 28:84, 1919.
11. Tanagho, E. A.: Neourethra: rationale, surgical technique, and indications. In Stanton, S. L., and Tanagho, E. A. (eds.), *Surgery of Female Incontinence.* Springer-Verlag, Berlin, 1980, p. 111.
12. Beck, P. H., McAninch, J. W., and Stutzman, R. E.: Anterior bladder tube flap reconstruction of the urethrovesical neck after radical retropubic prostatectomy. *J. Urol.* 121:379, 1979.
13. Tanagho, E. A., and Smith, D. R.: Clinical evaluation of a surgical technique for the correction of complete urinary incontinence. *J. Urol.* 107:402, 1972.
14. Tanagho, E. A.: Urethrosphincteric reconstruction for congenitally absent urethra. *J. Urol.* 116:237, 1976.

31

Surgical Treatment of Urinary Incontinence

ROGER HADLEY, M.D., PHILIPPE E. ZIMMERN, M.D., AND SHLOMO RAZ, M.D.

This chapter outlines the various operative procedures available for the treatment of urinary incontinence. Operative intervention is indicated only after the previously discussed conservative methods of treatment have failed. The operative treatments are divided into several categories: (a) operative correction of female urethral incompetence, (b) operative treatment for detrusor instability in both men and women, (c) operative treatment of male urethral incompetence, and (d) continent urinary diversion.

FEMALE INCONTINENCE

Bladder Neck Suspension

Why Bladder Neck Suspension Works. Regardless of the surgical approach, bladder neck suspension is designed to restore and fix (without obstruction) the bladder neck and proximal urethra to their normal intraabdominal retropubic position. This maneuver cures incontinence in 85 to 95 percent of cases. The reason for such cure is not known, but some consistent objective observations in cured patients are as follows: (a) a well-supported and nonmobile urethra and bladder neck on physical examination; (b) an elevated and closed bladder neck on cystoscopic examination; (c) lateral cystourethrogram showing the urethral catheter in place, which demonstrates that the urethra is in a high fixed (nonmobile) retropubic position; (d) restoration of normal functional urethral length on the urethral closure pressure profile (UCPP) with or without an increase in urethral closing pressure; of (e) change of negative pressure gradients to positive pressure gradients on the stress UCPP.

One explanation is that it places the urethra in a position where an increase in intraabdominal pressure is reflected in a simultaneous increase in intraurethral pressure as a result of reflex pelvic floor contraction. Such a fixed support of the urethra offers a "backboard" on which intraabdominal pressure is exerted to compress it, instead of the pressure being absorbed by a downward motion of the urethra, preoperatively. Another explanation is that bladder neck suspension may transpose the internal urethral orifice away from the most dependent location in the bladder, so that maximal downward forces no longer are exerted on that orifice. It is indeed possible that the bladder base is rotated posteriorly and downward toward the newly restored and fixed bladder neck, which in effect creates a valve-like mechanism that closes off the urethra during stress (*1*) (Fig. 31–1).

Why Bladder Neck Suspension Fails. Persistent incontinence after bladder neck suspension is due to either technical failure or improper preoperative indications. Failure to restore the urethra and bladder neck to a high fixed retropubic position is the most frequent cause of persistent stress urinary incontinence following bladder neck suspen-

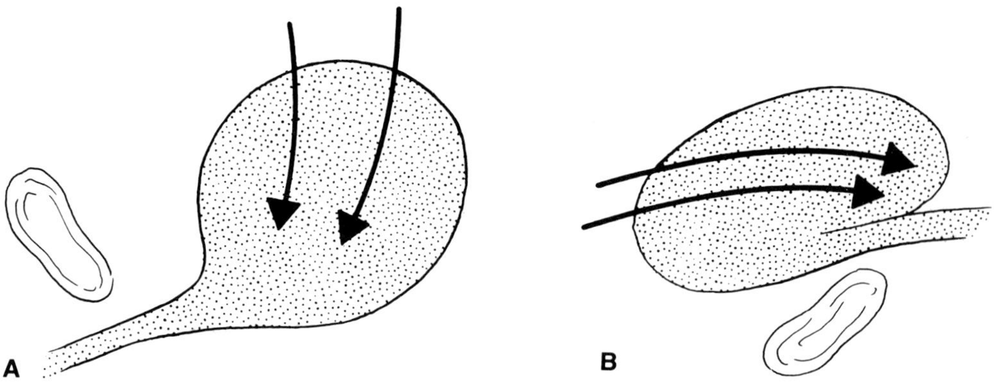

Figure 31–1. A. Forces that result in stress urinary incontinence in the descended and hypermobile urethra (Note that the urethra is not in the normal retropubic position). **B.** Urethra and bladder neck placed in a retropubic position. The intraabdominal forces are no longer directed at the bladder neck and indeed may cause a "valve-like" mechanism that shuts off the proximal urethra.

sion. It may be due to: (a) inadequate mobilization of the urethra and bladder neck during the operative procedure; (b) placement of sutures either proximal or distal to the level of the bladder neck; (c) suture failure (catgut sutures may absorb before adequate retropubic adhesions have formed); or (d) poor tissue integrity.

Persistent incontinence despite good fixation of the bladder neck in the retropubic position may be due to an overactive bladder or to impairment of intrinsic sphincter mechanisms. In retrospective studies detrusor instability has been implicated in as many as 70 percent of the patients who have failed bladder neck suspension (*2–6*). Cordoza *et al.* studied 92 patients with preoperative and postoperative cystometry and discovered that 18.5 percent of patients whose bladders were stable prior to colpocystourethropexy demonstrated bladder instability postoperatively (*7*). Others, however, believe that detrusor instability is an uncommon cause of operative failure (*8*).

Damage to the intrinsic urethral mechanisms or insufficient functional urethral length may be caused by multiple operations, sutures placed too close to the urethra, or periurethral scarring, as well as by neurologic conditions such as myelodysplasia. These complications are likely to occur during operations that place the suspending sutures in the paraurethral fascia. These patients are the most challenging to the surgeon. The treatment options are to improve the closing pressure by pharmacologic therapy, urethropexy, Polytef injection (see below), urethral fascial slings, or (rarely) artificial sphincter. A decrease in functional urethral length may be corrected by anterior vaginal wall urethropexy or proximal urethral reconstruction as described by Tanagho, Leadbetter, and Dees (see Chapter 30).

Selection of Patients. Proper selection of the patient is crucial to the success of a bladder neck suspension. Management of the patient who has symptoms of stress urinary incontinence depends on the presence or absence of other urinary complaints. Whereas many patients require no evaluation beyond the history and physical examination, others require complete urodynamic and radiographic evaluations to predict favorable results.

Patients who do not require full urodynamic and radiographic studies are those who: (a) have not had previous urethral or bladder neck surgery; (b) manifest symptoms of urinary incontinence only with stress; (c) have no urinary symptoms of urgency, frequency or obstruction; (d) are dry in the supine resting position; (e) demonstrate stress urinary incontinence during the physical examination; and (f) have a positive Marshall-Bonney test. In all other patients, urodynamic and radiographic studies may be indicated prior to operative intervention.

As many as 50 percent of patients with stress urinary incontinence also suffer from irritative voiding symptoms suggestive of an overactive bladder (urgency and frequency). Such patients are managed as follows. If the patient has genuine stress incontinence as witnessed by the physician, and if a filling cystometrogram (CMG; supine and standing) reveals a stable bladder, bladder neck suspension may be done. If the patient has both genuine stress incontinence and urodynamic evidence of an overactive bladder, an initial trial of medical therapy may be indicated. If stress incontinence persists after successful medical treatment has cured the urgency and frequency, bladder neck suspension is indicated. If the patient has a medically intractable overactive bladder and continues to suffer from a combination of stress and urgency incontinence, operative intervention may be contemplated primarily to cure the symptoms of stress urinary incontinence. It is not uncommon, therefore, that bladder neck suspension not only cures the patient's stress urinary incontinence but also may alleviate the associated urgency and frequency (9). If the patient continues to have a medically intractable overactive bladder after bladder neck suspension, the surgeon must then consider an operative alternative to improve bladder stability.

Techniques of Bladder Neck Suspension. When treating stress urinary incontinence operatively, the surgeon's goal is to restore the bladder neck and urethra to a high fixed retropubic (intraabdominal) position. During the procedure it is imperative to avoid damage to the delicate intrinsic urethral sphincter mechanisms. Sutures placed too close to the urethra may not only result in urethral fibrosis and obstruction but may tend to "hold open" the urethra and compromise sphincteric function.

Anterior Colporrhaphy

For many years anterior colporrhaphy has been popular among gynecologists for the treatment of cystocele and urethrocele. The operation is performed through a midline vaginal incision. For repair of a cystocele the bladder is imbricated with interrupted sutures placed in the perivesical fascia or the surrounding pubocervical fascia. If urethral suspension is required, the dissection is extended distally toward the external urethral meatus. One or two (Kelly) sutures are placed at the bladder neck and proximal urethra to ensure elevation and compression. Additional sutures are placed more superficially in the pubocervical fascia to add further support to the bladder neck and urethra. Some surgeons have modified the procedure by locating the edges of the pubococcygeus muscle and coapting the edges at the midline (*10*).

Anterior colporrhaphy may offer sufficient urethral support to cure stress urinary incontinence in the patient with mild urethral hypermobility. In the patient with moderate to severe urethral hypermobility, however, anterior colporrhaphy cannot move the urethra away from the most dependent portion of the bladder or effectively elevate the bladder neck or urethra in a high fixed intraabdominal position without causing bladder outlet obstruction. Most of the 40 to 60 percent of stress incontinent patients cured by anterior colporrhaphy had minimal preoperative symptoms (*11*). Because of the generally unsatisfactory results of anterior colporrhaphy, transabdominal bladder neck suspension or transvaginal needle suspension procedures have been designed to provide better support to the urethra and bladder neck.

Abdominal Approach

Marshall–Marchetti–Krantz Cystourethropexy. In 1949 Marshall, Marchetti, and Krantz described transabdominal vesicourethral suspension for treatment of stress urinary incontinence. They used three No. 1 chromic catgut sutures placed through the lateral wall of the urethra and deeply into the adjacent vaginal wall, with similar sutures subsequently placed on either side of the vesical outlet (Fig. 31–2). While the surgeon maintains upward traction on the sutures, the assistant places two fingers in the vagina to confirm that good elevation of the anterior vaginal wall has been obtained. The sutures are secured to the periosteum of the symphysis pubis and then tied so as to move the urethra upward to a high retropubic position. Additional sutures are then placed in

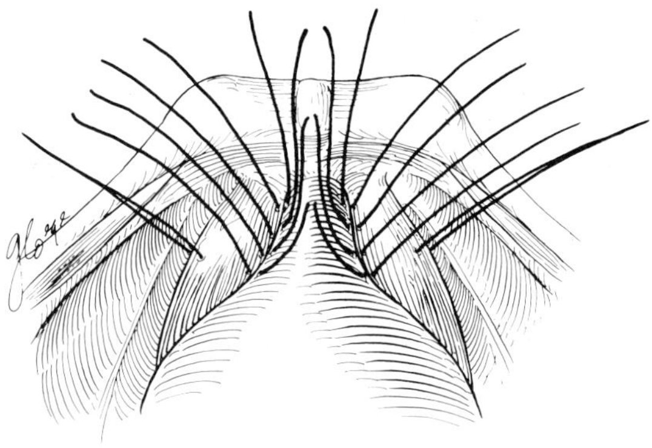

Figure 31–2. Marshal-Marchetti-Krantz cystourethropexy. Anteroposterior view of the bladder neck, urethra, and anterior vaginal wall depicts the location of the periurethral sutures used in this procedure. In addition to these sutures, there is one lateral suture placed in the vagina at the level of the bladder neck. Not included here are the three sutures that are placed in the anterior bladder wall.

the musculature of the lower anterior and lateral portions of the bladder. The long ends of these sutures are sewn into the posterior rectus fascia and tied in order to pull the bladder more anteriorly into the space of Retzius (*12*).

In 1982 Parnell, Marshall, and Vaughan reported a 46-month follow-up study of 140 patients who underwent this procedure as a first attempt to cure stress urinary incontinence. Their results were 90 percent cure, 9 percent improvement and 1 percent failure. Although there were no deaths, there was a 11.4 percent incidence of significant complications; osteitis pubis occurred in 10 percent and prolonged urinary retention in 10 percent of the patients (*13*). The latter may have been because the periurethral sutures did not allow the urethra to properly open and become funneled during voiding. Other authors reported similar results (*14,15*).

Colpocystourethropexy (Burch). Colpocystourethropexy, with a transabdominal approach, supports the bladder neck and urethra in the retropubic space by suspending the anterior vaginal wall to the overlying ligament of Cooper. Since Burch first described this procedure in 1961 (*16*), several modifications have been reported (*17–19*). We prefer to do the Burch colpocystourethropexy in the following way.

The patient is placed in the supine position with the hips slightly flexed and abducted ("frog leg" position) to allow easy access to the vagina. A urethral catheter is inserted and kept on the sterile field. The retropubic space is then entered through a low transverse or midline incision. The urethra is easily identified because of the presence of the catheter. Exposure of the lateral aspect of the anterior vaginal wall is facilitated by placing a finger or a "stick sponge" in the vagina. At a point lateral to the bladder neck, two sutures of No. 1 Dexon (polyglycolic acid) are placed in the anterior vaginal wall, exercising caution to avoid damage to the urethra. Each of the four sutures are placed twice in the vaginal wall and then secured to the overlying Cooper's ligament (Fig. 31–3.). Because a small hiatus between these structures does not affect the overall operative result it is not necessary to place the vaginal wall in juxtaposition to Cooper's ligament. If the patient has a concomitant cystocele, further support in the region of the bladder may be obtained by suspending the vagina with additional sutures proximal to the bladder neck. A retention catheter is removed on the third to fifth postoperative day. If the patient is unable to void, she is treated with "intermittent self-catheterization." Patients rarely continue to have significant postvoid residual urine for more than a few weeks postoperatively.

Needle Urethral Vesical Suspension Procedures

Pereyra first described the use of a long needle to pass sutures from the vagina to the

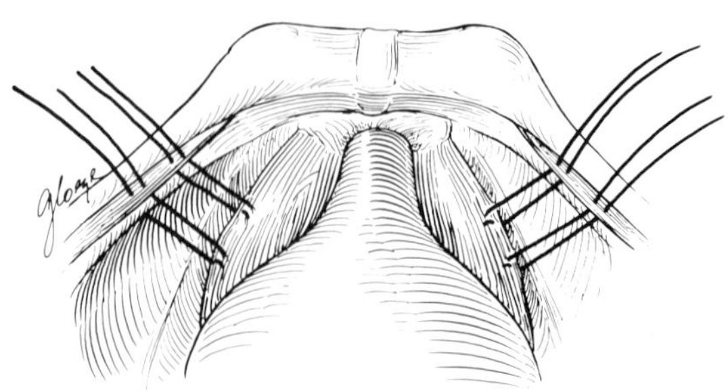

Figure 31–3. Anteroposterior view of a modification of the Burch colpocystourethropexy. Figure-of-eight sutures are placed in the anterior vaginal wall lateral to the urethra and at the level of the bladder neck.

abdominal wall in order to suspend the bladder neck and urethra in a fixed retropubic position. Many subsequent modifications of his technique have been reported.

Original Pereyra Procedure (1959). With the patient in a dorsal lithotomy position, a small transverse incision is made just above the symphysis pubis. Without making an incision in the vagina, Pereyra's specially designed needle is passed through this small abdominal incision, lateral to the bladder neck, and through the anterior wall of the vagina. The ends of a No. 30 stainless steel wire are placed in the needle and its trocar. When the trocar and needle are withdrawn to the abdominal wound, the wire loops around and catches the anterior vaginal wall. A similar maneuver is done on the opposite side of the urethra. The bladder neck and urethra are then fixed into a high retropubic position by uniting the two left and the two right wires in the abdominal incision. Of 31 patients so treated and followed for 14 months, 90 percent were cured. Two of the three failures reported were cured after a second operation (*20*).

Modifications of the Pereyra Needle Suspension. In 1965 Harer and Gunther reported on their experience using a modification of Pereyra's technique. Their modifications included the following: (a) the use of No. 1 chromic catgut instead of wire; (b) the use of a vertical vaginal incision in order to mobilize the urethra and bladder neck, to perform a Kelly urethral plication when indicated, and to cover the suspending sutures; and (c) use of a continuous suture extending from the right periurethral tissue over the rectus fascia down to the left periurethral tissue, then returning to the rectus fascia. Of 30 patients so treated, 25 were considered to have an excellent result on follow-up for 2 to 36 months (*21*).

In 1967 Tauber and Wapner reported their modification of needle suspension, which is similar to that of Harer and Gunther. Rather than depending on the suture to "hook" the anterior vaginal wall, they secured the pubocervical fascia with a nonabsorbable No. 0 stitch with an attached needle. With one stitch on each side of the bladder neck, the urethrovesical junction was fixed in the retropubic position by lifting each stitch and securing all in the small suprapubic incision. The operation was performed on four patients with no results reported (*22*).

In 1967 Pereyra and Lebherz reported yet another modification (*23*). The urethra and bladder neck are well mobilized through a vaginal incision. The long needle is passed under with fingertip control. With the same technique as described in the original Pereyra procedures, a No. 1 chromic suture is transferred to the suprapubic space. A Kelly paraurethral plication of the tissues beneath the bladder neck and urethra is then completed. During a follow-up of 12 to 89 months the cure rate was 92 percent in 172 patients. Among the 8 percent (*11*) who were initially considered failures, five were cured after a second operation (*23*).

Stamey's Endoscopic Vesical Neck Suspension. In 1973 Stamey described a technique for needle suspension of the vesical neck (*24*). In a modified lithotomy position, two 1-in. transverse incisions are made above the symphysis pubis just lateral to the midline. A "T" incision is made in the anterior vaginal wall at the level of the mid-urethra (Fig. 31–4). A vaginal flap is raised down to the level of the vesical neck. A long, special needle is passed through the anterior rectus fascia toward the undersurface of the symphysis pubis and into the vaginal incision just lateral to the bladder neck (Fig. 31–5). While observing cystoscopically, the surgeon moves the needle medially and laterally to insure that the needle is indeed in the periurethral tissue at the level of the bladder neck. Once cystoscopy has confirmed that the needle not only is in the correct position but also that no damage to the urethra or bladder has resulted, a No. 2 monofilament nylon suture is threaded through the eye of the needle and then withdrawn to the suprapubic incision. The needle is next passed 1 cm lateral to the previous puncture site in the rectus fascia and guided into the vaginal incision 1 cm distal to the previous periurethral site. The other end of the same monofilament suture is placed in the eye of the needle after it has been threaded through a 1-cm segment of a 5-mm Dacron arterial graft. The needle is again withdrawn to the suprapubic incision. The Dacron acts as a buttress in the periurethral tissue when the suture is secured over the rectus fascia (Fig. 31–6). The procedure is repeated on the opposite side. The endoscopist observes closure of the bladder neck during upward traction on both sutures. A punch suprapubic tube is placed after the procedure has been completed.

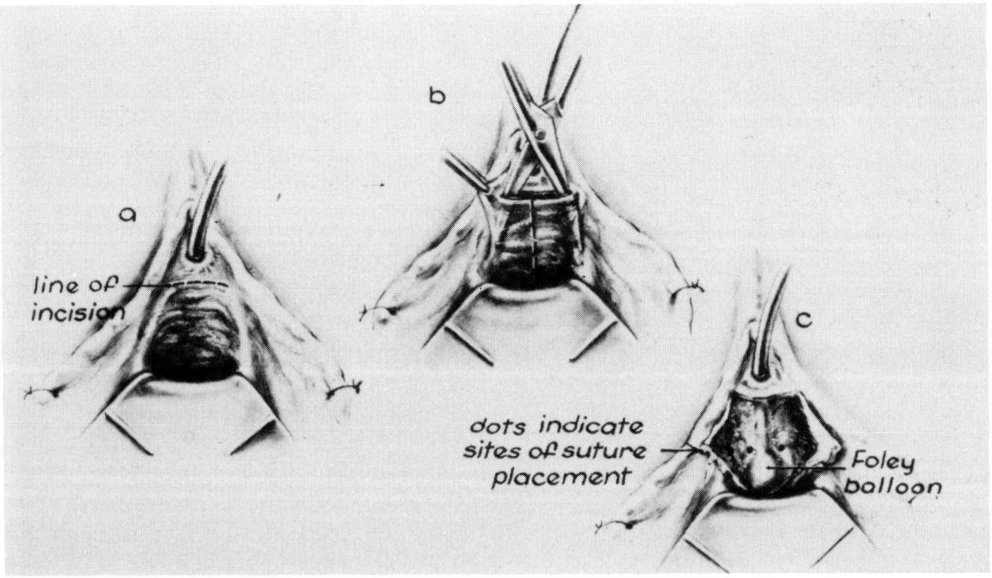

Figure 31–4. Stamey needle bladder neck suspension. A "T" incision is made in the anterior vaginal wall. The underlying periurethral fascia is exposed. (From Stamey, T. A.: *Surg. Gynecol. Obstet.* 136:547, 1973.)

After the vaginal incision is closed, the nylon sutures are tied firmly to each other with considerable tension. The vaginal incision is closed prior to tying the nylon sutures because the anterior vaginal wall is difficult to visualize after the suspension sutures have been secured.

In 1980 Stamey reported an overall cure rate of 91 percent with minimal complications in 203 consecutive patients treated by this procedures (*25*).

Needle Suspension of Raz. This modification of Pereyra's original procedure includes the following features: (a) An inverted "U"

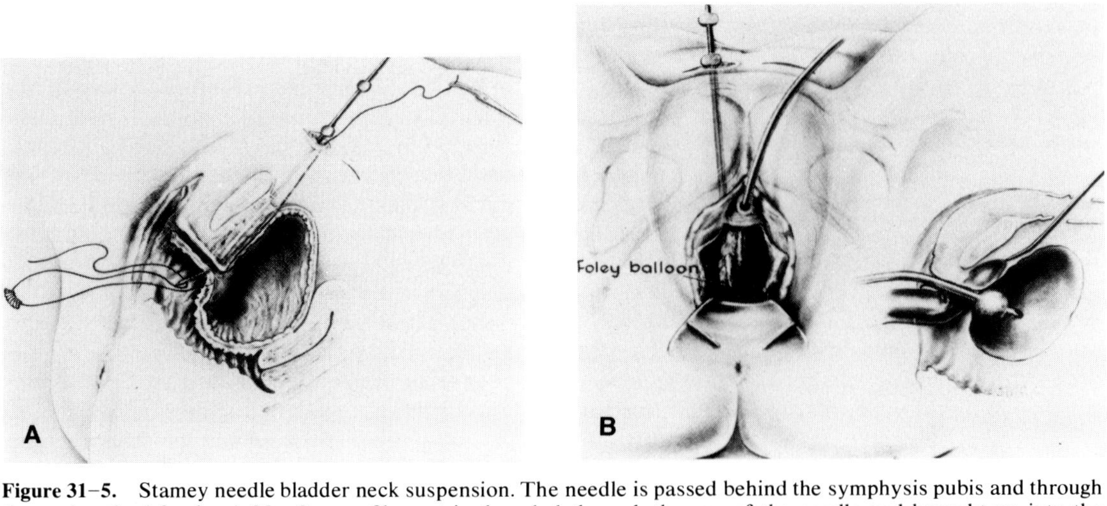

Figure 31–5. Stamey needle bladder neck suspension. The needle is passed behind the symphysis pubis and through the periurethral fascia. A No. 2 monofilament is threaded through the eye of the needle and brought up into the suprapubic incisions. (From Stamey, T. A.: *Surg. Gynecol. Obstet.* 136:547, 1973.)

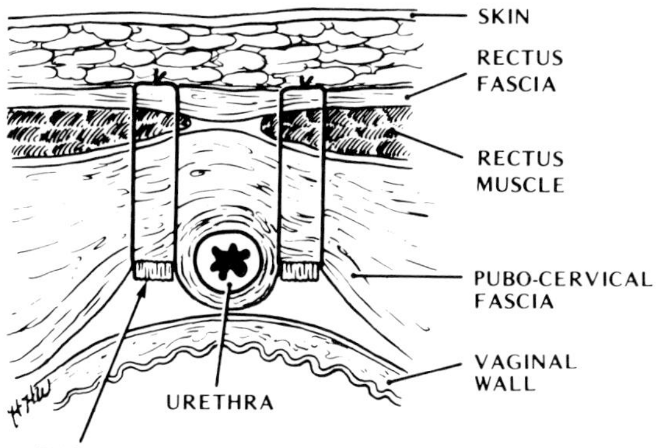

Figure 31–6. Stamey needle bladder neck suspension. This cross section of the urethra demonstrates the suspending suture and its Dacron buttress in the paraurethral fascia. When secured to the rectus fascia, the urethra is lifted into the retropubic space. (From STAMEY, T.A.: *Ann. Surg.* 192:465, 1980.

incision is made to allow vaginal dissection to be lateral to the urethra and bladder neck. (b) The retropubic space is entered to sufficiently mobilize the urethra and bladder neck; this step is especially important in the patient whose urethra is fixed by scar tissue due to a previous operation(s). (c) The suspension needle is passed under fingertip control to avoid injury to either the urethra or the bladder. (d) The monofilament suspension sutures are anchored in the full thickness of the vaginal wall (excluding the mucosa). (e) The suspension sutures are placed in the vaginal wall lateral to the bladder neck, so that they do not interfere with dynamic responses of the urethra that normally occur during voiding. (f) Cystoscopy is done to verify adequate bladder neck elevation and absence of injury to the urethra, bladder, or ureters (*26*)

On the night before surgery the patient is started on a course of parenteral antibiotics (an aminoglycoside and ampicillin) and given a Betadine douche to minimize bacterial contamination from vaginal flora. At operation the patient is placed in the dorsal lithotomy position and then cleansed from the umbilicus to the perineum, including the vagina. A Foley catheter is inserted to empty the bladder. A posterior vaginal retractor is placed in the vagina to expose the anterior wall. Traction on the Foley catheter facilitates identification of the level of the bladder neck. A semicircular inverted "U" incision is made in the anterior wall of the vagina (Fig. 31–7A). The apex of the incision should cross at the level of the mid-urethra where the distinctive glistening, white paraurethral fascia is identified. At the level of the bladder neck the dissection under the anterior vaginal wall is advanced laterally toward the pubic bone (Fig. 31–7B). The retropubic space is then entered, either bluntly or sharply, between the pubic bone and the endopelvic fascia. A finger is inserted through this incision to gently free the endopelvic fascia from its lateral attachment to the pubic bone (Fig. 31–7C). If the retropubic space is entered in this plane, bleeding should not be troublesome, and injury to the bladder or the ureter is unlikely. The mobilization is extended down to the level of the ischial tuberosity in order to create adequate mobility of the vaginal wall, bladder neck, and urethra. If the patient has had a previous urethral suspension, sufficient mobilization may require sharp dissection of the resultant paraurethral and perivaginal scar tissue. A No. 6 Mayo needle is used to secure a No. 1 Prolene suture in the vaginal wall at a point lateral to the bladder neck. This suture should include at least three separate passes through the whole vaginal wall, excluding the mucosa, in order to form a helical suture line (Fig. 31–7D). After each pass of the needle, traction is placed on the suture to test the integrity of the tissue and to ensure that sufficient bulk of the vaginal wall has been secured. The endopelvic (pubocervical) fascia is incorporated in this continuous suture. A second continuous suture is placed similarly on the contralateral side. The anterior fascia of the rectus abdominus is next exposed through a 3-cm transverse suprapubic incision. The surgeon's finger is then placed in the retropubic space to guide the suspension needle from the rectus fascia into the retropubic space and out of the vaginal introitus (Fig. 31–7E). With finger guidance, penetration of the bladder by the suspension needle should not occur. The two free ends of each Prolene suture are threaded through the eye of the needle and withdrawn into the suprapubic incision (Fig. 31–7F). The needle is then passed through the contralateral side so that 4 to 5 cm of rectus fascia lies between the Prolene sutures in the suprapubic incision.

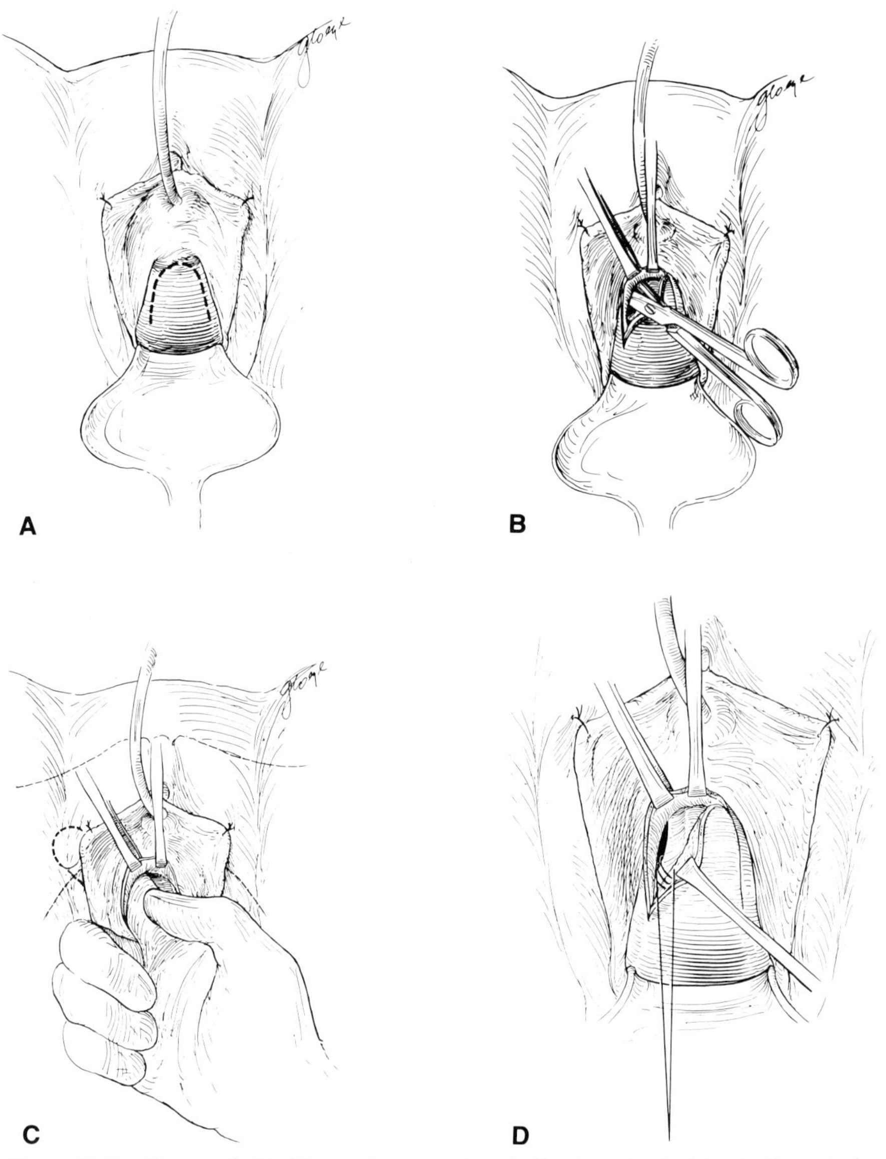

Figure 31–7. Raz needle bladder neck suspension. **A.** Semicircular incision in the anterior vaginal wall, which extends from the level of the bladder neck to the level of the mid-urethra. **B.** Dissection is directed laterally toward the symphysis pubis. **C.** Retropubic space is entered with the index finger. **D.** Prolene suture is placed in the anterior vaginal wall and the endopelvic fascia.

Upon completion of the procedure, cystoscopy is performed to confirm that there has been no penetration of the bladder or urethra. Blue efflux from both ureteral orifices after intravenous indigo carmine administration indicates that the ureters have not been injured. When the cystoscope is withdrawn to the level of the mid-urethra, the bladder neck should become elevated and should close with upward traction on the Prolene sutures. Such elevation of the bladder neck should not require more than minimal tension on the sutures. If considerable force is necessary to elevate the bladder neck, further mobilization of the vagina is required. Whereas cystoscopy is crucial to placement of the sutures and needles during Stamey's procedure, it is used only to con-

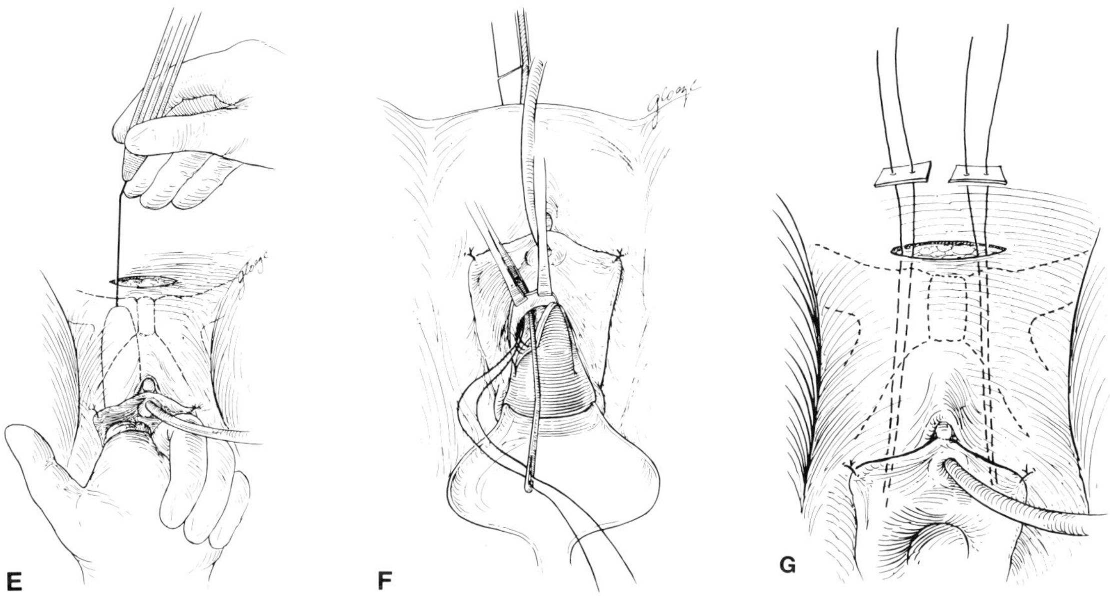

Figure 31–7. (*Cont.*) **E.** With finger guidance, the suspension needle is passed into the vaginal incision. **F.** Prolene suture is transferred from the vaginal incision to the suprapubic incision. **G.** Prolene sutures are tied over a small Teflon pledget and then tied across the rectus fascia to each other.

firm adequate bladder neck elevation and the absence of urinary tract injury during Raz's procedure.

Following cystoscopy the vaginal incision is closed with a running absorbable suture. The two ends of each Prolene suture are threaded through a 2 × 1 Teflon pledget and then tied to each other (Fig. 31–7G). Tying the ends of each suture over the pledget fixes the anterior vaginal wall and urethra in a high fixed retropubic position. Because each suture is secured individually, failure or breakage of one suture does not compromise the integrity of the contralateral suture. Preservation of one suture commonly is sufficient for achieving continence. When the Prolene sutures are being secured, only minimal tension is required to elevate the bladder neck sufficiently. Because the suspension sutures are placed in the vaginal wall lateral to the urethra, it is unlikely that urethral compression will occur; therefore urinary retention by overzealous traction on the sutures is unusual. After the Prolene sutures have been secured over the Teflon pledgets, the free ends are tied over the midline.

The Foley catheter and vaginal pack are removed 12 to 24 hours after operation. Intravenous antibiotics are continued for 24 hours postoperatively, followed by a 5-day course of oral antibiotics. If the patient is unable to void, she is instructed to perform clean intermittent self-catheterization. Hospitalization averages 3 to 4 days. Ninety percent of the patients are able to void without significant residual urine during the first week after the operation.

In 100 consecutive patients undergoing the Raz needle bladder neck suspension, 96 patients were classified as having an excellent result. It had been reported that 52 of 55 (94%) patients who were considered failures from one or more previous operative attempts to cure stress urinary incontinence were cured after being treated with this technique (*27*). In general, perioperative morbidity with this procedure was minimal; one patient had significant postoperative bleeding due to anterior wall varices, two developed superficial suprapubic wound infections, and none had a retropubic infection.

The difference between this suspension and the above described Stamey suspension is similar to the difference between MMK cystourethropexy and the Burch colpocystourethropexy. The sutures in Raz's suspension are anchored in the anterior vaginal wall lateral to the bladder neck to avoid damage to or obstruction of the urethra, whereas Stamey's needle suspension utilizes periurethral tissues to anchor the sutures and support the urethra and bladder neck. On the other hand, Raz entered the retropubic space and guided the needle from the rectus fascia to the vagina under fingertip control. Stamey did not enter the retropubic space but elected to observe the urethra endoscopically during the passage of the needle. In the patient who has had multiple vaginal and urethral operations, we believe that entering the retropubic space is necessary to adequately mobilize the urethra and anterior vaginal wall and to be sure the needle is guided to the proper position without damaging adjacent tissues. It is important that we remember that no suspension procedure can be successful if the urethra and bladder neck are not adequately mobilized and then fixed in a high retropubic position.

Sling Procedures

The first sling procedure was described by Goebell in 1910 (*28*). Similar techniques have subsequently been described to provide good support to the proximal urethra in a high fixed retropubic position. Although it has been recommended by some to reserve fascial slings for patients who have failed other types of suspension procedures, there are many medical centers throughout the world who use slings as the primary operative treatment of genuine stress urinary incontinence.

Muscle, fascia, and synthetic fabrics have been advocated for sling operations. In general, muscular slings have been abandoned because of technical problems that include poor blood supply; moreover, the inadequate length and bulk of the muscle sling provides inadequate urethral support. Synthetic materials such as Marlex mesh and Mersilene strips (*29*) prevailed for some time. Being foreign bodies, however, these materials may induce infection and excessive scar tissue reaction (*30*). Most surgeons now prefer to use an autologous fascial strip obtained from the fascia lata or rectus sheath.

Fascia Lata (Oxford Sling) Procedure. With the patient in the low lithotomy position, the lower abdominal wall, vagina and one thigh are appropriately prepared and cleansed. A 1 × 18 cm strip of fascia lata is harvested from that thigh and placed in normal saline. Through a transverse suprapubic incision, the bladder neck and urethra are adequately mobilized, and an inverted "V" incision is made in the anterior vaginal wall. Through the latter incision, the vaginal flap is separated from the underlying pubocervical fascia and is extended to a point slightly beyond the bladder neck. After one end of the fascial strip has been fixed to the anterior rectus sheath, the other end is transferred from the abdominal incision to the vaginal incision. Through the vaginal incision, the sling is grasped, positioned correctly under the urethra, and inserted back into the retropubic space on the opposite side. With the anterior vaginal wall supported by the surgeon's fingers, the fascia is secured to the contralateral rectus sheath with sufficient tension to provide an eventual high fixed retropubic position of the urethra and bladder neck. Through the vaginal incision, the fascial strip is secured to the pubocervical fascia to avoid distal migration of the sling. Postoperative care of the leg wound includes loose bandages, early mobilization, and late removal of sutures. A transurethral or suprapubic catheter is left in place until the postvoid residual urine becomes less than 50 ml. The most common postoperative complications are delayed voiding (over 4 to 6 weeks) and urinary tract infection. Occasionally, patients with normal detrusor function prior to the operation develop a postoperative overactive bladder, which is best treated with medications. Most series report an overall cure rate of 85 to 90 percent (*31,32*).

Another commonly employed pubovaginal sling is the Goebell-Stoeckel procedure, which uses a strip of fascia from the rectus sheath. Procurement of the fascia is also done before the vaginal portion of the sling operation. With this procedure a midline incision is made from the umbilicus to the symphysis, and the rectus sheath is separated from overlying subcutaneous tissues for 1 to 2 cm on either side of the midline. A strip of rectus sheath (1 cm in width) is mobilized craniocaudally in the midline and is left attached at its caudal end. This long fascial strip is passed through the rectus muscle, delivered into the vaginal incision, passed beneath the urethra, brought up through the space of Retzius, and attached to the contralateral rectus fascia with the appropriate tension, leaving the strip exposed in the vagina (*33*).

Modifications of the above procedure have been reported. With Aldridge's technique (*34*) a broader strip from the symphysis to the umbilicus is freed and divided longitudinally; each end is brought down on either side of the urethra where it is reunited and secured through a vaginal incision.

Ridley's technique (*35*) is recommended when a mid-vaginal incision or dissection is not feasible (previous closure of a urethrovaginal fistula or construction of a neourethra). For this modification the fascial strip is split in two portions, each portion being sutured on either side of the urethra.

Paraurethral and Transurethral Polytef Injection

Polytef (polytetrafluoroethylene, Teflon), an inert plastic, reportedly adds bulk to the urethra when injected into the urethral and paraurethral layers. In women it is best used in patients who suffer mild urinary incontinence due to poor urethral luminal coaptation. The added "tissue" bulk may result in continence because of improved urethral resistance and urethral coaptation.

Polytef may be injected transperineally or transurethrally into the wall of the urethra. The former technique utilizes a 10 cm long 17-gauge needle attached to a Lewy syringe filled with Polytef. The needle is inserted near the external urethral meatus and is advanced toward the bladder neck. Repeated injection of Polytef is made at the 3, 6, and 9 o'clock positions. During these injections the urologist observes their effects cystoscopically to ascertain they do not extend beyond the bladder neck into the bladder. The latter technique utilizes a cystoscope equipped with a special needle and an injector. After the cystoscope is placed in the mid-urethra, the needle is advanced to and then under the urethral mucosa. Polytef is repeatedly injected until bulk has been added at the 3, 6, 9, and 12 o'clock positions (Fig. 31–8A, B). The transurethral technique requires less Polytef than the paraurethral technique because it allows more specific and accurate placement of the paste.

Between 1964 and 1980, Politano treated 54 incontinent women with paraurethral injection of Polytef. There were 51 percent excellent and 20 percent good results. On the average, these patients were injected 1.8 times. Although many patients may remain incontinent immediately after the injections, urinary control can be obtained over a period of several weeks. It is recommended, therefore, to wait 4 to 6 months before repeating the injections (*36*).

The above technique is attractive to the urologist because of its simplicity, the short hospitalization required, and the option of repeating injections. Although the Food and Drug Administration (FDA) has not yet approved Polytef for urethral use, intracordal injection of the paste has been used for many years, without known complications, by the otolaryngologist for the treatment of paralytic vocal dysphonia. Other studies, however, have demonstrated widespread migration of the Teflon particles to lymph nodes, lungs, and other sites. The long-term effects of this phenomenon are unknown (*37*).

Urethral Lengthening Procedures

If inadequate urethral length is a significant contributor to urinary incontinence, a transvesical or transvaginal urethroplasty may be indicated.

Transvaginal Urethral Lengthening. The vaginal wall may be used to lengthen the urethra in the patient who has a congenitally absent or short urethra, a short urethra due to trauma or excision of a distal urethral diverticulum, or a urethrovaginal fistula, or if there is an inaccessible urethra in a patient who needs intermittent catheterization.

Two techniques have been used to create a neourethra. The first technique creates the neourethra by raising a flap of anterior vaginal wall. A "U" incision is made in the anterior vaginal wall, the open end of the incision being near the urethral meatus. The convex portion of the "U" extends posteriorly toward the apex of the vagina; after the vaginal flap has been raised, it is reflected toward the vaginal introitus. The lumen of the neourethra therefore is lined by vaginal

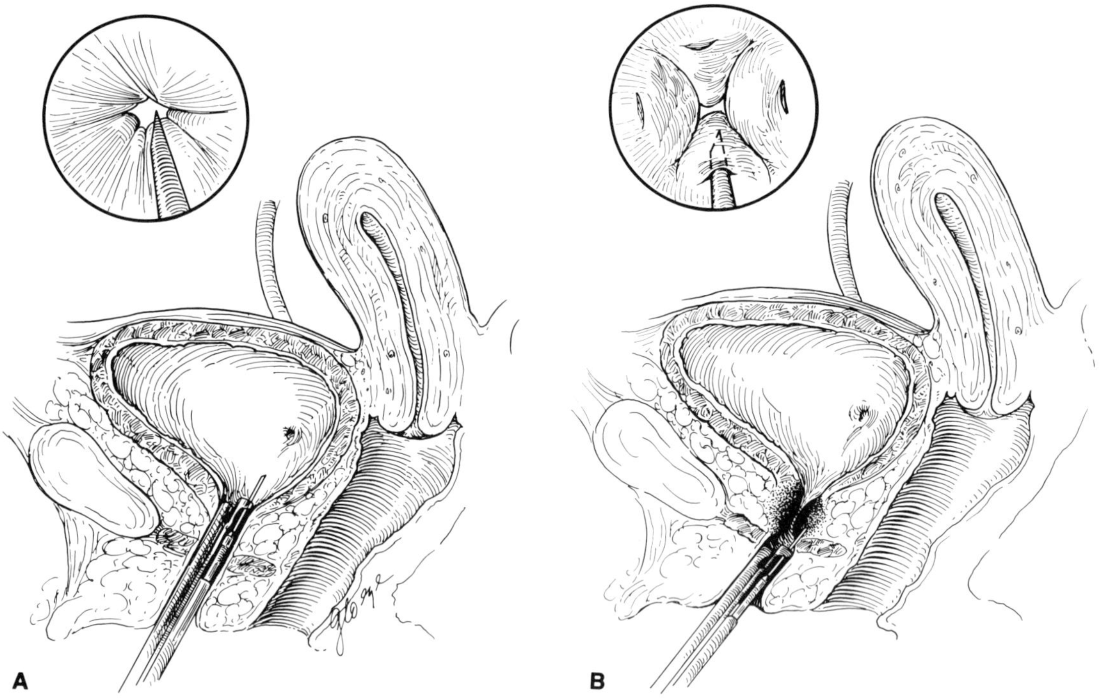

Figure 31–8. Transurethral Polytef injection. **A.** Cystoscope and cystoscopic needle used for transurethral injection of Polytef into the urethra. **B.** The needle is placed in the paraurethral tissue. The effect of the paraurethral Polytef injection is seen.

mucosa. All denuded surfaces are covered by mobilized lateral vaginal wall tissues that are approximated over the neourethra and the vaginal sites where the original flap was raised.

Another technique is to make two parallel vertical incisions in the vaginal wall that extend from the old urethral opening to the location of the new urethral opening. The medial aspect of each incision is mobilized and then tubularized over an 8F to 10F catheter. The lateral aspect of one incision is then undermined so it can be secured to the opposite side. By undermining only one side, an overlapping suture line is avoided (*38*) (Fig. 31–9). A suprapubic tube and a urethral catheter remain in place for 3 weeks. If an outpatient cystogram demonstrates no extravasation, the catheters may be removed.

If the surgeon is concerned about tissue tension, poor blood supply to tissues, or the lack of sufficient coverage of the neourethra, operative failure may be prevented by using the fibrofatty tissue of the labia or a pedicle skin flap from the perineum (*38,39*). The labial fibrofatty pad is mobilized through a separate vertical incision in the labia majora, brought through the vaginal incision and interposed between the suture lines. A pedicle flap of perineum may be used as definitive coverage of the neourethra, thereby obviating the need for extensive vaginal wall mobilization. The flap should be full thickness and from a nonhairy region. Several weeks after the flap is well healed, it can be transected at an appropriate point, which repositions the labia and replaces the base of the flap in its original position (Fig. 31–10).

Operative Treatment for the Unstable Bladder

Urinary incontinence due to an overactive bladder can usually be treated nonoperatively. Among such treatments are behavioral modification, pharmacologic therapy,

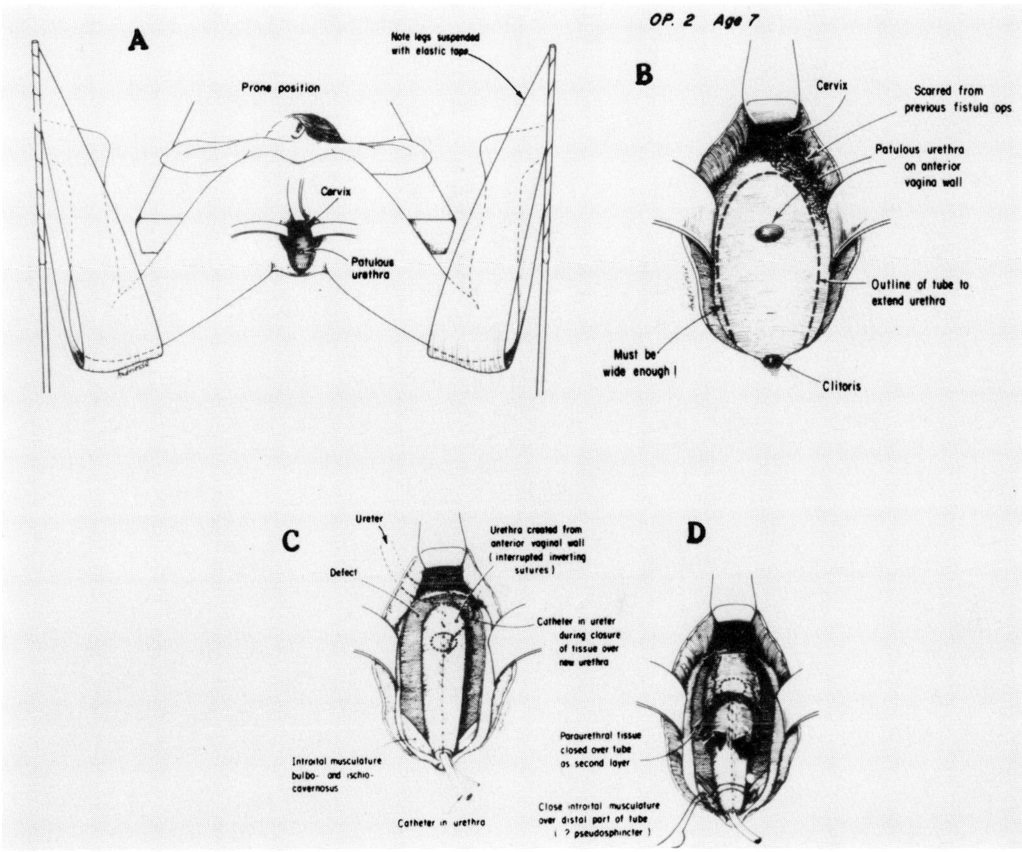

Figure 31–9. Creation of a distal urethra by tubularizing the anterior vaginal wall. **A.** Prone position, which affords much easier access for the operation than the dorsal lithotomy position. **B.** Outline of the vaginal incision to lengthen the urethra. **C, D.** Neourethra is closed and covered with available paraurethral tissue. (From Hendren, H. W.: *J. Urol.* 123:662, 1980. Copyright © 1980, The Williams & Wilkins Co., Baltimore.)

and electrostimulation. If the conservative methods fail to successfully treat incontinence that is due to an overactive bladder and that has forced a significant change in the patient's life style, the physician may consider operative therapy. The operative options available include cystolysis, bladder transection, peripheral bladder denervation, and augmentation enterocystoplasty.

Cystolysis, Bladder Transection, and Peripheral Bladder Denervation. *Cystolysis* or denervation of the supratrigonal bladder was described in 1967 by Turner-Warwick and Ashken (*40*). The rationale was to interrupt the motor and sensory innervation of the bladder above the trigone, reducing both afferent and efferent supplies of the overactive bladder. Cystolysis, as originally described by Turner-Warwick and Ashken, involved dividing the perivesical attachments above the superior vesical arteries.

Bladder transection has also been described as treatment for the overactive bladder. It is performed through a lower abdominal incision. A transverse cystotomy is made just above the bladder neck; and after entering the bladder, a circumferential incision separates the body of the bladder from the trigone. A catheter placed in each ureter allows their easier identification when dividing the posterior wall of the bladder. The bladder is then reattached to the trigone with an absorbable suture. The bladder is drained with a suprapubic tube and a urethral catheter for 7 to 10 days. After removal of the catheter frequency and urgency are usually

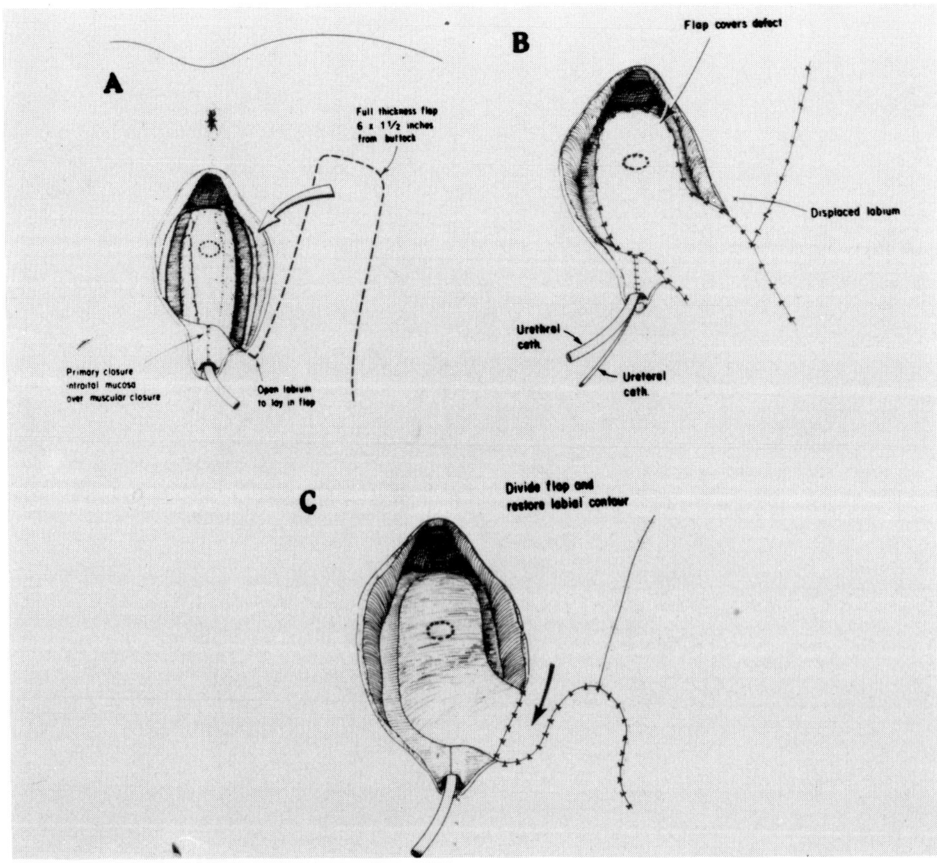

Figure 31–10. **A, B.** A perineal pedicle flap may be used to cover a tenuous neourethra. **C.** After the flap has healed, it is divided to restore the labia to a normal contour. (From Hendren, H.W.: *J. Urol.* 123:662, 1980. Copyright © 1980, The Williams & Wilkins Co., Baltimore.)

present for the first 24 to 48 hours, but they rapidly disappear thereafter (*41*). During follow-up that ranged between 6 months and 7 years, 53 percent of 45 patients with incapacitating symptoms secondary to an overactive bladder were asymptomatic following bladder transection (*42*).

Parsons *et al.* modified the above technique by adding parallel transverse detrusor myotomy above the transection; 81 percent of 28 patients followed for up to 4 years were improved by this technique (*43*). Mundy modified the transection by dividing only the anterior aspect of the bladder just above the bladder neck. He reported 44 consecutive patients with severe urge incontinence treated by this technique. During a follow-up of 6 to 28 months, 77 percent were considered to have an excellent result (*44*).

The following is a description of how we prefer to perform *perivesical bladder denervation.* On the night before surgery the patient is given a Betadine douche and preoperative parenteral prophylactic antibiotics. With the patient in the "frog leg" position and the lower abdomen and vagina appropriately cleansed, a low transverse extraperitoneal incision is made. The peritoneum is separated from the anterosuperior aspect of the bladder and apex of the vagina. A plane is developed between the anterior wall of the vagina and the base of the bladder and then extended to the vesical neck. The peritoneum is next reflected off the lateral aspect of the bladder and vagina, exposing the endopelvic fascia, urethra, and both ureters. A gauze grasped by a kidney pedicle clamp may be placed in the vagina to facilitate exposure of its anterolateral walls. The bladder is now held by its lateral pedicles, which contain the ureters and inferior vesical vessels. These pedicles are meticulously thinned in order to divide as many nerves as possible without damaging the ureters or their blood supply (*45*). Following the denervation we routinely do a colpocystourethropexy (Burch) to fix the bladder neck and urethra in their normal retropubic position (see previous section on bladder neck suspension).

Peripheral denervation by the above described technique has been used to treat 22 patients with a hyperreflexic bladder. Eight of these subjects had permanent indwelling catheters, but their severe hyperreflexia caused leakage around the catheter despite appropriate pharmacologic therapy. Seven of the eight patients responded with cessation of leakage. The other 14 patients had disabling frequency and urgency incontinence. Following bladder denervation, 10 of these 14 patients were able to void spontaneously: four urinated every 4 to 6 hours, and four every 2 to 4 hours; two patients continued to experience frequency and urgency incontinence, and four developed permanent urinary retention who were treated by intermittent self-catheterization.

Bladder Augmentation (Enterocystoplasty). Bladder augmentation by enterocystoplasty (cecocystoplasty, ileocystoplasty, or sigmoidocystoplasty) has generally been employed for the patient with a pharmacologically intractable overactive bladder or a bladder with a limited functional capacity. The procedure is performed with the intent of increasing the intravesical volume and decreasing bladder wall tension. Bladder augmentation may also be performed in combination with a perivesical denervation procedure with the goal of simultaneously ablating the detrusor instability and providing an adequate "holding" capacity to minimize urinary incontinence.

Prior to surgery the patient's bowels are appropriately cleansed with cathartics, enemas, and nonabsorbable oral antibiotics active against bowel flora. The dome of the bladder is resected through an abdominal incision to allow a wide area of anastomosis to the bowel segment. Although we prefer the cecum, the choice of bowel used for the augmentation depends on the surgeon's experience. The cecum is carefully mobilized up to the hepatic flexure, preserving the ileocecal artery. Whereas most surgeons rotate the ascending colon down to the bladder for the cecovesical anastomosis, we prefer to open the entire cecum and ascending colon along their antimesenteric border. We then sew a cecocolonic "cap" to the open bladder with a running single layer of 2-0 Dexon suture. We believe that opening the entire antimesenteric border interrupts the powerful circular fibers of the colon, preventing coordinated high-pressure contractions and allowing greater distension of the cecal segment. A suprapubic tube, a urethral catheter, and perivesical drains are placed at the time of the operation. The urethral catheter is removed on the fifth postoperative day. If a cystogram demonstrates no extravasation on the tenth postoperative day, the suprapubic catheter and perivesical drains are removed.

Results of bladder augmentation for the overactive bladder are generally good. Linder *et al.* reported excellent results in 82 percent of 17 patients with follow-up of 12 to 120 months. After a follow-up of 6 months to 5 years, Bramble reported satisfactory results in 13 to 15 patients who were treated with augmentation enterocystoplasty for urge incontinence (*46–48*).

Transvaginal Closure of the Urethra and Bladder Neck. Long-term urethral catheterization may be complicated by urethral necrosis and leakage around the catheter. In the high risk patient, transvaginal closure of the bladder neck and permanent suprapubic catheterization may be the most appropriate therapeutic alternative. Through a vaginal approach the urethra and bladder neck are mobilized sufficiently dividing the pubic bone and perivesical attachments. The bladder neck is closed vertically in one layer. A second layer of deep endopelvic fascia and full thickness of bladder wall is apposed to cover the underlying suture line perpendicularly. A third layer consists of a rotational vaginal flap, which allows adequate vaginal closure without overlapping of the suture lines. Feneley has reported a technique of urethral invagination into the bladder by means of three purse-string sutures (*49*).

POSTPROSTATECTOMY INCONTINENCE

Because postprostatectomy incontinence (PPI) is the most common cause of nonelderly male urinary incontinence, it is important to recognize preoperatively the patient at high risk for this complication and to understand how to avoid the technical errors that may result in incontinence.

Prevention of PPI

For the purpose of discussion in this chapter, we arbitrarily divide the distal urethral sphincter (DUS) into three longitudinal zones of continence: the verumontanum to the apex of the prostate; the apex of the prostate; and apex of the prostate to the bulbous urethra. This zonal approach is helpful to our understanding of mechanisms participating in postprostatectomy continence and incontinence (*50*).

Because the proximal urethral sphincter (PUS) is removed during prostatectomy, postoperative continence essentially depends on the DUS. This dependence is demonstrated by a urethral pressure profile that shows no increase in pressure at the level of the bladder neck (prostatic fossa) but sufficient pressure increase in the region of the DUS. Removal of the proximal third of the DUS (i.e., verumontanum to prostatic apex) during simple prostatectomy (transurethral resection of the prostate or open prostatectomy) is not followed by incontinence. Radical prostatectomy removes the proximal two-thirds of the DUS (i.e., verumontanum to and including the prostatic apex), leaving the remaining distal one-third to maintain continence. Preservation of the latter (apex to the bulbous urethra) therefore is essential for maintaining passive continence after prostatectomy.

Transurethral Resection of the Prostate

During transurethral resection of the prostate (TURP) limitation of the resection to the level of the verumontanum is the classic and most reliable way to ensure future continence. The verumontanum is only a landmark and serves no physiologic function in continence. As the prostate gland enlarges, however, the distance between the verumontanum and the apex of the prostate increases. In a patient with a large prostate gland, therefore, a transurethral resection restricted to above the verumontanum may leave a significant amount of obstructive tissue proximal to the apex of the prostate. Surgeons are justifiably reticent to resect this residual tissue because of the increased probability of postoperative incontinence secondary to DUS damage. So long as the surgeon does not stray too distal from the verumontanum and resects only the characteristically white prostatic tissue, the DUS should remain sufficiently intact to allow passive continence. When there is significant damage to the DUS, it is most frequently located anteriorly between the 10 and 2 o'clock positions (*51*). It may be prevented by the use of a zero degree lens and a nonbeaked resectoscope that allows good vision of the verumontanum during this delicate anterior phase of the procedure.

Excessive coagulation in the region of the DUS may destroy the soft inner layer of the distal urethra. It may result in the loss of urethral suppleness, which is important for closure and sealing of the urethral lumen. Because the subsequent fibrotic scar may not properly coapt, sufficient urethral occlusive seal does not develop, and the patient is incontinent. In addition, this scarred tissue may cause a significant stricture, which explains the paradox of obstructive voiding symptoms concurrent with urinary incontinence.

Open Simple Retropubic Prostatectomy

During a properly performed simple retropubic prostatectomy, the verumontanum and the apex (of the true prostate) are left *in situ*. To prevent damage to the DUS, it is recommended to first divide the adenoma on its anterior surface before mobilizing its lateral aspects. This step ensures proper visualization of the verumontanum and the DUS when the adenoma is sharply divided from the apex of the true prostate. Second, upward traction on the adenoma is avoided because this maneuver may "tent up" the DUS, making it more susceptible to injury during dissection of the apex.

Radical Retropubic Prostatectomy

The extrinsic skeletal portion of the DUS is rarely damaged during radical retropubic prostatectomy, demonstrated by the fact that active (voluntary) continence is maintained in most patients with post-radical-prostatectomy incontinence (*52*). By contrast, this extrinsic skeletal sphincter may be damaged during radical perineal prostatectomy. Because of preservation of the anatomy and autonomic innervation of the passive continence mechanism (intrinsic skeletal and smooth muscle portions of the DUS), a pudendal block does not render incontinent a continent postprostatectomy patient, whereas postprostatectomy incontinent patients are worse after such a block (*53*). At the time of radical retropubic prostatectomy, the verumontanum and apex of the prostate are removed. Continence therefore depends on the distal portion of the DUS (region from the apex to the membranous urethra). Because 90 to 95 percent of patients undergoing this operation are continent after surgery, we may conclude that this portion of the DUS is sufficient to maintain passive continence. Any compromise of this short, delicate portion of the DUS, however, may result in an unhappy and wet patient. Continence is best preserved by avoidance of: (a) excessive coagulation and dissection of the membranous urethra in order to preserve the delicate inner layer of the membranous urethra and the innervation of the DUS that courses along the posterolateral aspect of the prostate; (b) tension on the urethra during its transection; and (c) anastomotic leaks that may lead to fibrosis.

Despite meticulous surgical technique, postprostatectomy incontinence may occur because of preoperative unrecognized DUS insufficiency. It is prudent therefore that these conditions are searched for prior to prostate surgery. These patients may have a history of radical pelvic surgery (abdominoperineal resection) previous inlay urethroplasty, neuropathy (diabetic, alcoholic), fractured pelvis (with prostatomembranous urethral disruption), cancer of the prostate, or pelvic irradiation.

Patients after abdominoperineal resection may suffer from either urinary retention or urinary incontinence. Urinary retention may be due to an acontractile bladder secondary to detrusor denervation. Urinary incontinence may be due to a denervated DUS associated with proximal urethral sphincter insufficiency. If, after the abdominoperineal resection the patient has urinary retention, he should be placed on a program of intermittent catheterization for 6 to 12 months or until residual urine is minimal. A urodynamic investigation is indicated if the patient continues to have urinary retention. A detrusor–flow study that demonstrates high detrusor pressure with a poor urinary flow may indicate bladder outlet obstruction secondary to an enlarged prostate. Prior to prostatectomy, however, it is important to assess the functional capabilities of the DUS. If the DUS is functional, a urethral pressure profile should show an increase in pressure in the region of the membranous urethra. A pelvic floor electromyogram (EMG) that demonstrates normal activity of the pelvic floor muscles reflects an intact pudendal nerve. Unfortunately, it may not correlate with the status of the pelvic nerve supply to the DUS.

A patient with a previous inlay urethroplasty may have an inadequate inner layer of intrinsic muscle at the level of the DUS. Prior to prostatectomy these patients should also have a careful urodynamic evaluation to assess the ability of the DUS to maintain passive continence. This evaluation may include videourodynamics to demonstrate the radiographic location of the pressure transducer catheter while it is being withdrawn from the bladder to the bulbous urethra. An inadequate rise of urethral closing pressure in the region of the DUS would indicate DUS insuffciency.

Patients with spinal root lesions or peripheral neuropathy may have a denervated DUS secondary to damage of the pelvic nerves. This situation may occur with autonomic neuropathy, herpes zoster, cauda equina tumors, protruded lumbar disc, etc.

Continence in patients who have suffered traumatic prostatomembranous urethral disruption may be entirely dependent on the proximal urethral sphincter. Again, prostatectomy in these patients will likely be complicated by incontinence.

Cancer of the prostate also demands careful attention. Incontinence may result from invasion of the sphincters or TUR of the proximal urethral sphincter with tumor invasion in the DUS. Previous radiotherapy for the carcinoma may damage sphincteric function, placing the patient at high risk for incontinence after a TURP.

Another cause of postprostatectomy incontinence is a combination of urethral insufficiency and failure to empty the bladder ("overflow incontinence"). It may result from an outlet obstruction (urethral stricture or bladder neck stenosis) or a chronic and acontractile distended bladder secondary to benign prostatic hypertrophy (BPH) or due to a preexisting neuropathy (diabetes).

Finally, one of the more common causes of postprostatectomy incontinence is an overactive bladder, even if the DUS is competent. Only 60 percent of patients who were suffering from preoperative detrusor instability associated with obstructive symptoms were cured after prostatectomy (*54*). A persistently overactive bladder may be explained by permanent residual damage of the bladder wall (compensatory hypertrophy of the detrusor secondary to chronic urinary retention) (*55*), a normal decrease in cortical inhibitory stimuli in an otherwise neurologically intact elderly individual (*56,57*), or underlying subclinical neurologic disorders such as parkinsonism or multiple sclerosis.

In many cases the patient's incontinence is due to more than one cause. The most common combination is that of sphincter weakness and detrusor instability (*58,59*). It is for this reason that a complete evaluation by urodynamic studies is indispensable for detecting the mechanism responsible for postprostatectomy incontinence.

EVALUATION OF MALE URINARY INCONTINENCE

Evaluation of the incontinent male patient may include the history, physical examination, cystourethroscopy, radiographs of the bladder and urethra, and urodynamic studies. This information assists in determining the type of incontinence (urethral insufficiency, overactivity of the bladder), the severity of the incontinence, the presence of strictures, and any associated conditions.

OPERATIVE PROCEDURES FOR THE TREATMENT OF MALE INCONTINENCE

The history of the treatment of male urinary incontinence is characterized by trial, error, early rejoicing, and late frustration (*60*). There has been a wide range of treatment modalities reported since the turn of this century.

Operations in the Region of the Bladder Neck and the Proximal Urethra

Use of the bladder wall to construct a neourethra (neosphincter) has been applied to patients with a nonfunctioning urethra due to an operation, trauma, or congenital anomalies. In 1969 Tanagho reported a technique that created a neourethra from the anterior bladder wall for correction of complete urinary incontinence. The rationale for this technique was based on his observation that the anterior bladder wall above the proximal sphincter has abundant transverse fibers similar to those seen in the bladder neck. These fibers, when tubularized, became circularly oriented and thus capable of exerting sufficient urethral resistance to maintain continence. Although the operation has most often been used for postprostatectomy incontinence, other indications have included trauma, congenital anomalies (epispadias, congenital absence of the urethra, etc.), extensive deep internal urethrotomy, and urethral excision for carcinoma. (See Chapter 30 for description of operative technique.)

Free autogenous muscle transplantation has been used to increase urethral resistance. In children, Gierup and Hakelius used a segment of skeletal muscle (usually the extensor hallucis brevis) that had been denervated 2 to 3 weeks prior to surgery. This muscle is then transplanted to the posterior urethra, close to the normally innervated muscles of continence. The latter acts as a reinnervating source for the transplanted muscle. During the following 6 months, the patient gradually gains continence. The overall results were considered good (i.e., increased functional bladder capacity with no need for protective pads during the day) in 10 of 16 patients (*61*). Others did not obtain comparably good results (*62*).

Operations in the Region of the Bulbous Urethra

In the presence of normal detrusor and abdominal muscle function, passive compression of the bulbous urethra can provide continence for patients in whom bladder neck and proximal urethral sphincteric activity has been compromised. Numerous procedures have been devised to increase urethral resistance by providing permanent passive compression on the bulbous urethra. The Kaufman I (crura detached and crossed) and its modification, the Kaufman II (crura approximated and secured in the midline), procedures were introduced during the early 1970s to achieve compression of the bulbous urethra (*63*). After a minimum of 6 months' follow-up, 50 to 60 percent of the patients were markedly improved or cured by the Kaufman II procedure (*64*).

In an attempt to obtain a longer length of urethral compression, others have mobilized the bulbous urethra from the triangular ligament to 2 cm beyond the penoscrotal junction. The surrounding corpora are separated along their length and reapproximated over the bulbous urethra. The central tendon is incised and a noninterrupted "U" suture is placed over the lateral margin of the bulbous urethra. This suture is then anchored distally to the lower margins of the corpora in order to compress and push forward the bulbous urethra. During a follow-up ranging from 4 months to 7 years, 75 percent of 34 patients were considered to have an excellent result; in the same series 15 percent were improved and 10 percent failed (*65*).

Another operation used to treat DUS insufficiency is the telescoping of a dismembered bulb into the prostatomembranous urethra. A small suprapubic incision is made over a Lowsley retractor that has been passed transurethrally. A 14F Foley catheter is grasped by the jaws of the retractor and brought out the external urethral meatus; a large suture is secured to the catheter. The catheter is withdrawn back into the urethra so that its tip is near the penoscrotal junction (Fig. 31–11A). The bulbous urethra is mobilized through a perineal incision from the urogenital diaphragm to 2 cm beyond the penoscrotal junction. After the 14F Foley catheter is pulled back into the bladder, the bulbous urethra is transected 1 cm distal to the membranous urethra. With Hegar dilators the prostatomembranous urethra is dilated to a 2.0 cm diameter (Fig. 31–11B). By pulling on the attached suture the 14F Foley catheter is again brought from the bladder into the perineal wound and subsequently back into the dismembered bulbous urethra (Fig. 31–11C). The tip of the catheter is secured to the bulbous urethra with 3.0 plain catgut sutures (Fig. 31–11D). The catheter is again withdrawn into the bladder, pulling with it the dismembered and well mobilized bulbous urethra (Fig. 31–11F). This maneuver telescopes the bulbous urethra into the prostatomembranous urethra. (Fig. 31–11F), increasing urethral resistance sufficiently to maintain continence in 55 percent of the cases (*66*). Another advantage of this telescoping manuever is that it provides a relatively easy means of urethral reconstruction in the patient with a seemingly irreparable posterior urethra.

Nonpressure-Regulated Prosthetic Devices

Berry (*67*) proposed the first operation in which an acrylic prosthesis was implanted in the perineum. This procedure fell into disuse because of difficulties such as migration of the prosthesis and urethral erosion, as well as its inconsistent results.

Kaufman and Raz compressed the bulbous urethra by implanting a silicone gel pillow into the perineum (*68*). Its position was secured by four or six straps placed around the penile crura (Fig. 31–12). In a more recent version, the two lower straps are placed around staples previously inserted into the pubic rami. The gel prosthesis is designed so that percutaneous postoperative needle injection of the pillow can add further compression on the underlying urethra. Of 184 cases reported, 61 percent had an excellent or good result. There were 20 (11%) major complications, including 12 urethral or perineal skin erosions. Eight patients had infections that required surgical removal of the prosthesis (*68*). In other reports the success rate ranged from 30 to 82 percent (*69,70*). After reviewing the results and complications of the silicone gel prosthesis, the following conclusions were drawn. (a) The silicone gel prosthesis should not be used in patients who have had previous pelvic radiotherapy (*70*). (b) Concomitant penile prostheses significantly increase the risk of implantation. (c) Success is likely only if preoperative manual perineal compression significantly increases urethral closing pressure

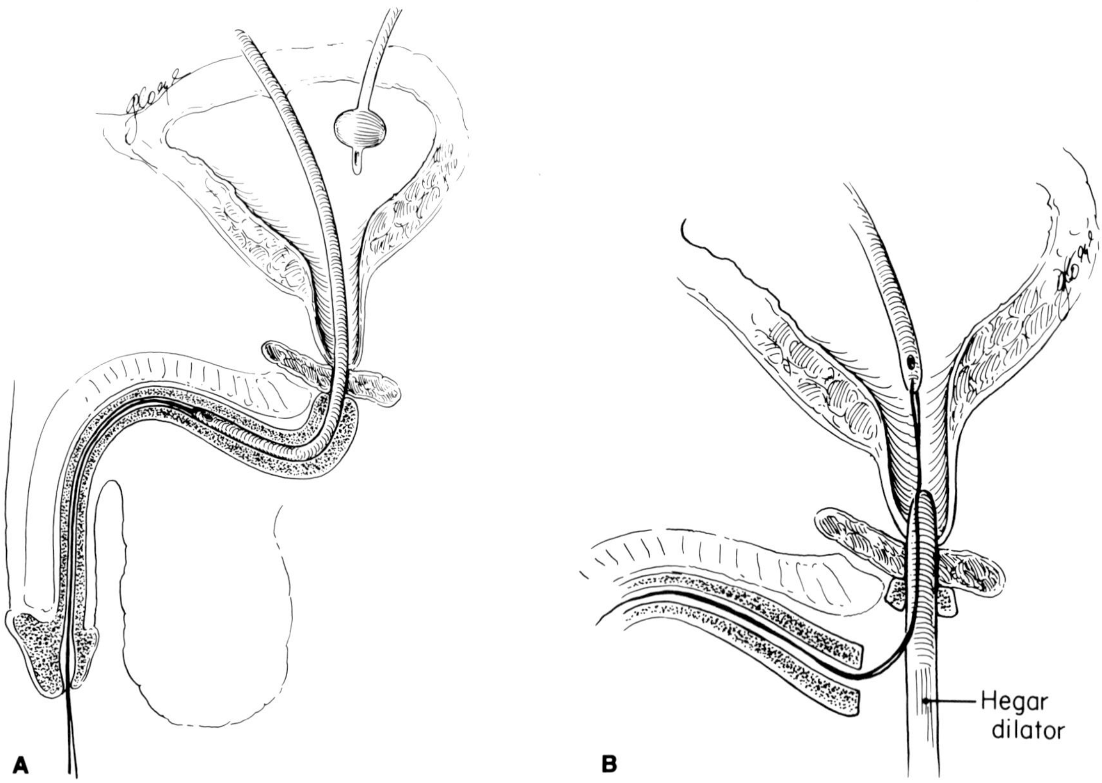

Figure 31–11. **A.** Suprapubic catheter is advanced to the bulbar urethra. **B.** Membranous urethra is dilated with Hegar dilators.

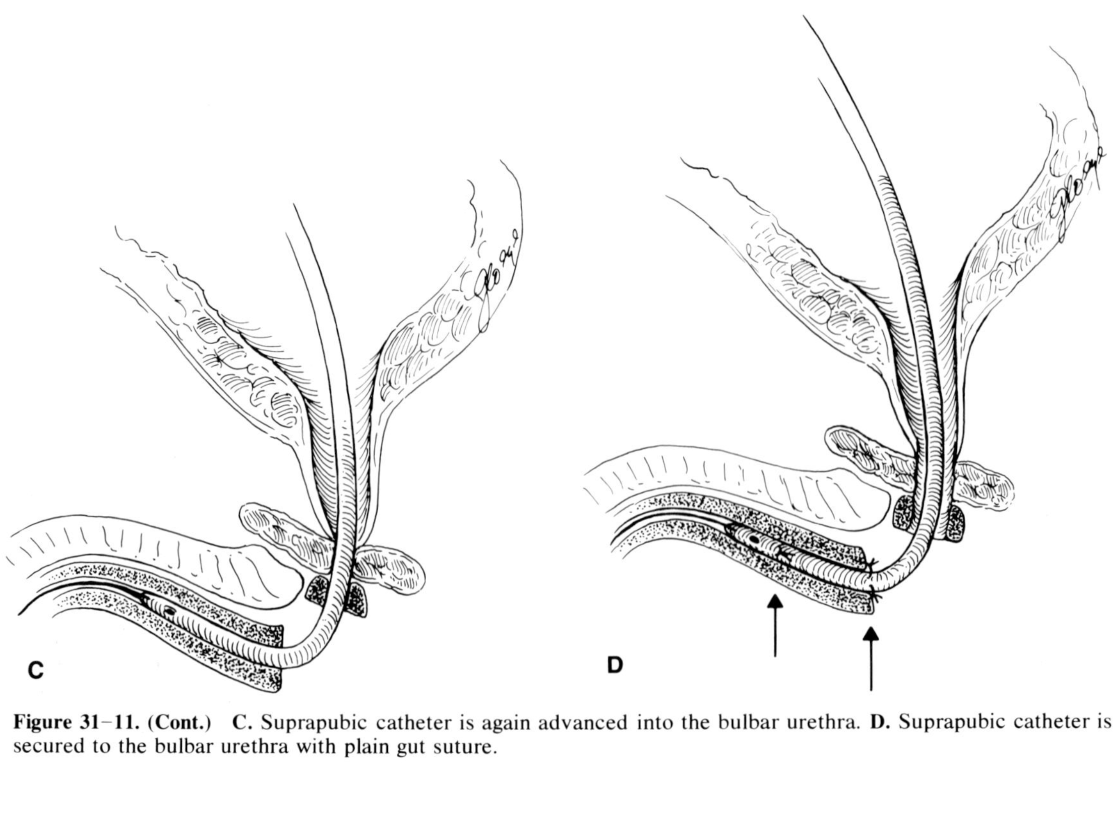

Figure 31–11. (Cont.) **C.** Suprapubic catheter is again advanced into the bulbar urethra. **D.** Suprapubic catheter is secured to the bulbar urethra with plain gut suture.

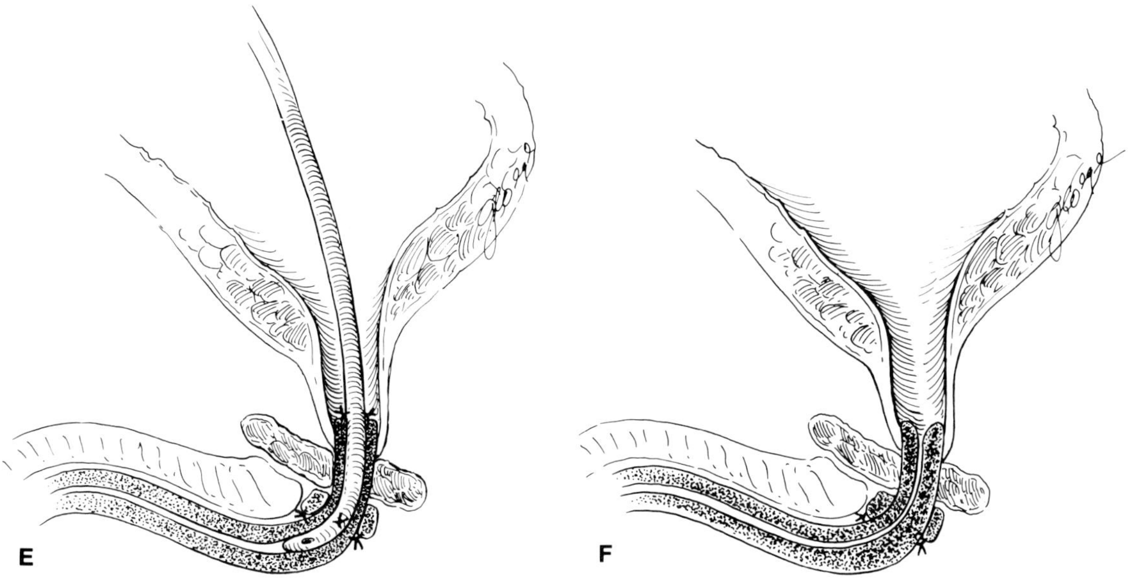

Figure 31–11. (*Cont.*) **E.** The well-mobilized bulbar urethra is advanced into the membranous urethra and secured with Dexon sutures. **F.** After 3 weeks the suprapubic catheter is removed.

(*71*). (d) If intraurethral pressure exceeds 90 cm H_2O as a result, erosion is likely to occur.

Periurethral and Transurethral Teflon Injections

The technique of Polytef injection is similar to that described in women earlier in this chapter. Injection in men may be either transperineal or transurethral. We now prefer the transurethral route because less paste is required to obtain adequate urethral coaptation. Politano reported a 6-month to 16-year follow-up of 103 male patients who had undergone transperineal Polytef injection. Seventy-five percent had a good to excellent result. Each patient had an average of 1.8 injections (*72*). Transurethral Polytef injection in incontinent patients after TURP and simple open prostatectomy have been successful in 85 percent and 75 percent, respectively. Whereas in incontinent patients with a neurogenic bladder 40 to 50 percent had an excellent result from transurethral injection, only 25 percent of patients with a combination of prostatic surgery and radiotherapy were cured (*73*). The obvious advantages of this procedure are that the hospital

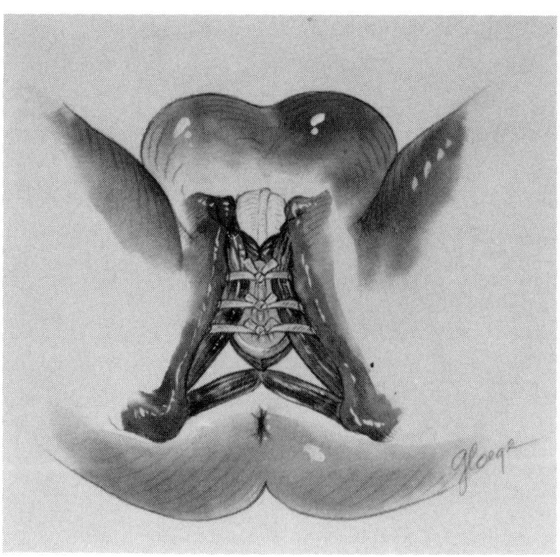

Figure 31–12. Silicone gel prosthesis after it has been secured in the perineum. The prosthesis is held in place by straps that have been passed around the crura of the penis.

stay is only 1 to 2 days; there are few (and only minor) complications (occasional urethritis, temporary retention, and one case of abscess formation), and injections can be repeated.

Operative Procedures for Detrusor Instability

The reader is referred to an earlier section of this chapter that discusses bladder denervation, bladder transection, and augmentation enterocystoplasty.

Urinary Diversion

In patients in whom the bladder and urethra are not capable of storing and transporting urine, respectively, despite all treatment measures, the most appropriate option may be supravesical urinary diversion. It may be either incontinent or continent. Incontinent diversions include an ileal conduit, a colonic conduit, cutaneous ureterostomy, vesicostomy with bladder neck closure, and nephrostomy. Only techniques for continent supravesical urinary diversion are reviewed here.

the ileum, ileocecal, and sigmoid colon have been used to create continent pouches. Kock *et al.*, who had encouraging results from a continent ileostomy made in post-proctocolectomy patients, applied their technique to create a urinary reservoir. Approximately 75 cm of small bowel is required to make a reservoir and two nonrefluxing valves. The nonrefluxing valves prevent ureteral reflux (afferent limb) and continence (efferent limb). The valves are constructed by intussuscepting the two limbs into the reservoir (Fig. 31–13). To prevent reduction of the intussuscepted segment, three or four rows of staples are inserted over the mucosa covering the protruding nipple. The two ureters are anastomosed to the afferent limb, and the efferent limb is brought through the rectus fascia to the skin. The pouch capacity grows to 500 to 600 ml and is drained intermittently with self-catheterization. Because the stoma is flush with the skin, only a small dressing is required for coverage. Kock *et al.* reported excellent results (*74,75*) in 16 patients.

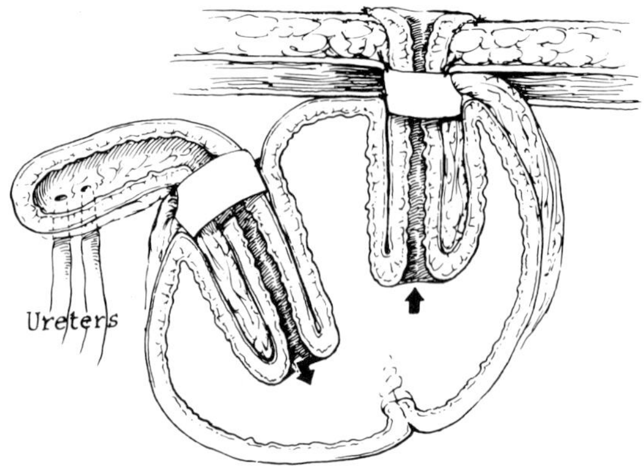

Figure 31–13. Completed ileal urinary reservoir (Kock pouch). The ureters are attached to the afferent limb, which has been intussuscepted to prevent ureteral reflux. The afferent limb is brought out to the skin as a flush stoma. It is intussuscepted in order to maintain continence of the reservoir. (From Kock, N. G., *et al.: J. Urol.* 128:469, 1982. Copyright © 1982, The Williams & Wilkins Co., Baltimore.)

Some patients are best treated by closure of the bladder neck and placement of a suprapubic catheter or the development of a continent vesicostomy. Simple ligation around the bladder neck rarely cures urethral incontinence; rather, the bladder neck must be well mobilized, denuded from the inside, and then closed with opposing concentric sutures. Only with good drainage and healing of the denuded tissues does the bladder neck remain closed. Reid *et al.* performed a continent vesicostomy on 24 patients with neurogenic bladder. The procedure utilizes a tubularized bladder flap brought through the lower abdominal wall, and intermittent catheterization is done through this stoma (*76,77*).

Zingg and Tscholl's continent reservoir intussuscepts the terminal ileum into the cecum, which has been removed from the fecal stream. The proximal portion of this ileal segment is brought to the skin as a stoma, which is intubated intermittently. Antirefluxing ureterocecostomies are placed on the antimesenteric border. Two of four patients were dry without reflux 5 to 14 months after surgery (*78,79*).

REFERENCES

1. Hertogs, K., and Stanton, S. L.: The mechanism of successful colposuspension: a new model. In *Proceedings of the International Continence Society*, Aachen, 1983, p. 152.
2. Stanton, S. L., Cardozo, L., Williams, J. E., Ritchie, D., and Allan, V.: Clinical and urodynamic features of failed incontinence surgery in the female. *Obstet. Gynecol.* 51:515, 1978.
3. Hodgkinson, C. P.: Stress urinary incontinence in the female. *Surg. Obstet. Gynecol.* 120:595, 1965.
4. Turner-Warwick, R. J.: Some clinical aspects of detrusor dysfunction. *J. Urol.* 113:539, 1975.
5. Kaufman, J. M.: Urodynamics in stress urinary incontinence. *J. Urol.* 122:778, 1979.
6. Bates, C. P., Loose, H., and Stanton, S. L.: The objective study of incontinence after repair operations. *Surg. Gynecol. Obstet.* 136:17, 1973.
7. Cardozo, L. D., Stanton, S. L., and Williams, J. E.: Detrusor instability following surgery for genuine stress incontinence. *Br. J. Urol.* 51:204, 1979.
8. McGuire, E. J., Lytton, B., Pepe, V., and Kohorn, E. T.: Stress urinary incontinence. *Obstet. Gynecol.* 47:255, 1976.
9. McGuire, E. J., Lytton, B., Kollorn, E. I., and Pepe, V.: The value of urodynamic testing in stress urinary incontinence. *J. Urol.* 124:256, 1980.
10. Pacey, K.: Pathology and repair of genital prolapse. *J. Obstet. Gynaecol. Br. Emp.* 56:1, 1949.
11. Low, J. A.: Management of anatomic urinary incontinence by vaginal repair. *Am. J. Obstet. Gynecol.* 97:308, 1967.
12. Marshall, V. F., Marchetti, A. A., and Krantz, K. E.: The correction of stress incontinence by simple vesico-urethral suspension. *Surg. Gynecol. Obstet.* 88:509, 1949.
13. Parnell, J. P., Marshall, V. F., and Vaughan, E. D.: Primary management of urinary stress incontinence by the Marshall-Marchetti-Krantz vesicourethropexy. *J. Urol.* 127:679, 1982.
14. Uhle, C. A. W., Bradley, R. H., and MacKinney, C. C.: Suprapubic vesicourethral suspension for stress incontinence in women. *J. Urol.* 81:749, 1959.
15. Mcduffie, R. W., Litin, R. B., and Blundon, K. E.: Urethrovesical suspension (Marshall-Marchetti-Krantz): experience with 204 cases. *Am. J. Surg.* 141:297, 1981.
16. Burch, J. C.: Urethrovaginal fixation to Cooper's ligament for correction of stress incontinence, cystocele and prolapse. *Am. J. Obstet. Gynecol.* 81:281, 1961.
17. Tanagho, E. A.: Colpocystourethropexy: the way we do it. *J. Urol.* 116:751, 1976.
18. Cowan, W., and Morgan, H. R.: A simplified retropubic urethropexy in the treatment of primary and recurrent urinary stress incontinence in the female. *Am. J. Obstet. Gynecol.* 133:295, 1979.
19. Stanton, S. L., Williams, J. E., and Ritchie, D.: The colposuspension operation for urinary incontinence. *Br. J. Obstet. Gynaecol.* 83:890, 1976.
20. Pereyra, A. J.: A simplified surgical procedure for the correction of stress incontinence in women. *West. J. Surg.* 67:223, 1959.
21. Harer, W. B., and Gunther, R. E.: Simplified urethral vesical suspension and urethroplasty. *Am. J. Obstet. Gynecol.* 91:1017, 1965.
22. Tauber, R., and Wapner, P. M.: Surgical repair of severe and recurrent urinary incontinence. *Obstet. Gynecol.* 30:741, 1967.
23. Pereyra, A. J., and Lebherz, T. B.: Combined urethral vesical suspension vaginal urethroplasty for correction of urinary stress incontinence. *Obstet. Gynecol.* 30:37, 1967.
24. Stamey, T. A.: Cystoscopic suspension of the vesical neck for urinary incontinence. *Surg. Gynecol. Obstet.* 136:547, 1973.
25. Stamey, T. A.: Endoscopic suspension of the vesical neck for urinary incontinence in females: report on 203 consecutive patients. *Ann. Surg.* 192: 465, 1980.
26. Raz, S.: Modified bladder neck suspension for female stress incontinence. *Urology* 18:82, 1981.
27. Leach, G. E., O'Donnel, P., and Raz, S.: Needle vesicourethral suspension procedures. In Raz, S. (ed.), *Female Urology*. Saunders, Philadelphia, 1983, p. 267.
28. Goebell, R.: Zur Operativen Beseiligung der Angeharenen Incontinentia Vesicae. *A. Gynak, Urol.* 2:187, 1910.
29. MacFarlane, K. T.: Discussion of a sling operation using Marlex polypropylene mesh for treatment of recurrent stress incontinence. *Am. J. Obstet. Gynecol.* 106:376, 1970.
30. Cukier, J., Mangin, P., Cabane, H., Ruarte, A., and Pascal, B.: Traitement de l'incontinence des urines à l'effort de la femme par soutenement du col vesical à l'aide d'un greffon aponevrotique libre. *Chirurgie* 107:67–73, 1981.
31. Beck, R. P., and Lai, A. R.: Results in treating 88 cases of recurrent urinary stress incontinence with the Oxford fascia lata sling procedure. *Am. J. Obstet. Gynecol.* 142:649, 1982.
32. McGuire, E. J., and Lytton, B.: Pubovaginal sling procedure for stress incontinence. *J. Urol.* 119:82–84, 1978.
33. Te Linde, R. W., and ;Mattingly, R. F.: *Operative Gynecology*, 4th ed. Lippincott, Philadelphia, 1970, p. 555.
34. Aldridge, A. H.: Transplantation of fascia for relief of urinary stress incontinence. *Am. J. Obstet. Gynecol.* 44:398, 1942.
35. Ridley, J. H.: Surgery for stress urinary incontinence. In *Gynecologic Surgery, Errors, Safeguards, Salvage*. Williams & Wilkins, Baltimore, 1974, pp. 132–146.
36. Carrion, H. M., and Politano, V. A.: Periurethral 'polytef' injection for urinary incontinence. In Raz, S. (ed.), *Female Urology*. Saunders, Philadelphia, 1983, p. 293.
37. Malizia, A. A., Reiman, H. M., Myers, R. P., Sande, J. A., Barham, S. S., Benson, R. C., Dewanjee, M., and Otz, J.: Teflon injected periurethrally: migration and granulomatous reaction. In *Proceedings of 79th Annual Meeting of the American Urological Association*, New Orleans, May 1984, p. 222A.
38. Hendren, H. W.: Construction of female urethra from vaginal wall and perineal flap. *J. Urol.* 123:657, 1980.

39. Davis, R. S., Linke, C. A., and Kraemer, G. K.: Use of labial tissue in repair of urethrovaginal fistula and injury. *Arch. Surg.* 115:628, 1980.
40. Turner-Warwick, R. T., and Ashken, M. H.: The functional results of partial, subtotal and total cystoplasty with special reference to ureterocaecocystoplasty, selective sphincterotomy and cystocystoplasty. *Br. J. Urol.* 39:3, 1967.
41. Essenhigh, D. M., and Yeates, W. K.: Transection of the bladder with particular reference to enuresis. *Br. J. Urol.* 45:299, 1973.
42. Hindmarsh, J. R., Essenhigh, D. M., and Yeates, W. K.: Bladder transection for adult enuresis. *Br. J. Urol.* 49:515, 1977.
43. Parsons, K. F., O'Boyle, P. J., and Gibbon, N. O. K.: A further assessment of bladder transection in the management of adult enuresis and allied conditions. *Br. J. Urol.* 49:509, 1977.
44. Mundy, A. R.: The surgical treatment of urge incontinence of urine. *J. Urol.* 128:481, 1982.
45. Leach, G. E., Goldman, D., and Raz, S.: Surgical treatment of detrusor hyperreflexia. In Raz, S. (ed.), *Female Urology*. Saunders, Philadelphia, 1983, p. 326.
46. Smith, R. B., Van Cangh, P., Skinner, D. G., Kaufman, J. J., and Goodwin, W. E.: Augmentation enterocystoplasty: a critical review. *J. Urol.* 118:35, 1977.
47. Linder, A., Leach, G. E., and Raz, S.: Augmentation cystoplasty in the treatment of neurogenic bladder dysfunction. *J. Urol.* 129:491, 1983.
48. Bramble, F. J.: The treatment of adult enuresis and urge incontinence by enterocystoplasty. *Br. J. Urol.* 54:693, 1982.
49. Feneley, R. C. L.: The management of female incontinence by suprapubic catheterisation, with or without urethral closure. *Br. J. Urol.* 55:203, 1983.
50. Turner-Warwick, R. T.: The sphincter mechanisms: Their relation to prostatic enlargement and its treatment. In *Benign Prostatic Hypertrophy*. Springer-Verlag, New York, 1983, pp. 809–828.
51. Turner-Warwick, R. T.: Sphincter mechanism and prostatic enlargement. In Hinman, F. (ed.), *Benign Prostatic Hypertrophy*. Springer-Verlag, New York, 1983, p. 815.
52. Tanagho, E. A.: Post-prostatectomy incontinence. I. Physiology and pathophysiology of micturition. In Weber, D., and Jonas, D. (eds.), *Postoperative Urinary Incontinence*. Georg Thieme Verlag, Stuttgart, 1981, p. 1.
53. Raz, S.: Symposium on male incontinence. *Urol. Clin. North Am.* 5:298, 1978.
54. Abrams, P. H.: The urodynamic changes following prostatectomy. *Urol. Int.* 33:181, 1978.
55. Bors, E. H., and Comarr, A. E.: *Neurological Urology: Physiology of Micturition: Its Neurological Disorders and Sequelae*. University Park Press, Baltimore, 1971.
56. Isaacs, B., and Walkey, F. A.: A survey of incontinence in the elderly. *Gerontol. Clin.* 6:367, 1964.
57. Milne, J. S., Williamson, J., Maule, M. M. *et al.*: Urinary symptoms in older people. *Mod. Geriatr.* 2:198, 1972.
58. Fitzpatrick, J. M., Gardiner, R. A., and Worth, P. H. L.: The evaluation of 68 patients with postprostatectomy incontinence. *Br. J. Urol.* 51:552–555, 1979.
59. Mayo, M. E., and Ansell, J. S.: Urodynamic assessment of incontinence after prostatectomy. *J. Urol.* 122:60–62, 1979.
60. Kaufman, J. J.: Symposium on male incontinence. *Urol. Clin. North Am.* 5:265, 1978.
61. Gierup, H. J. W., and Hakelius, L.: Further experience of free muscle transplantation in children with urinary incontinence. *Br. J. Urol.* 55:211–216, 1983.
62. Medgyese, S., Mortensen, S., and Nerstrom, B.: The failure of free muscle transplants in the treatment of urinary incontinence. *Br. J. Plastic Surg.* 32:336–338, 1979.
63. Kaufman, J. J.: A new operation for male incontinence. *Surg. Gynecol. Obstet.* 131:295, 1970.
64. Furlow, W.: *Second Urodynamic Workshop*. Mayo Clinic, Rochester, MN, 1976.
65. Lenzi, R., Barbagli, G., Stomaci, N., and Selli, C.: Surgical treatment of male urinary incontinence. *J. Urol.* 130:463, 1983.
66. Guzman, J. M.: Personal communication, 1983.
67. Berry, J. L.: A new procedure for correction of urinary incontinence: Preliminary report. *J. Urol.* 85:771, 1961.
68. Kaufman, J. J., and Raz, S.: Urethral compression procedure for the treatment of male urinary incontinence. *J. Urol.* 121:605, 1979.
69. Graham, S. D., Culley, C. C., and Anderson, E. E.: Long-term results with the Kaufman prosthesis. *J. Urol.* 128:328, 1982.
70. Confer, D. J., Beall, M. E.: Evolved improvements in placement of silicone gel prosthesis for post-prostatectomy incontinence. *J. Urol.* 126:605, 1981.
71. Kaufman, J. J.: The silicone-gel prosthesis for the treatment of male urinary incontinence: symposium on male incontinence. *Urol. Clin. of North Am.* 5:393, 1978.
72. Politano, V. A.: Periurethral polytetrafluoroethylene injection for urinary incontinence. *J. Urol.* 127:439, 1982.
73. Politano, V. A.: Personal communication, 1983.
74. Kock, N. G., Nilson, A. E., Nilsso, L. O., Norlen, L. J., and Philipson, B. M.: Urinary diversion via a continent ileal reservoir: clinical results in 12 patients. *J. Urol.* 128:469, 1982.
75. Kock, N. G., and Philipson, A. E.: Urinary diversion via a continent reservoir. In *Proceedings of the International Continence Society*, Aachen, 1983, p. 503.
76. Reid, R., Schneider, K., and Fruchtman, B.: Closure of the bladder neck in patients undergoing continent vesicostomy for urinary incontinence. *J. Urol.* 120:40, 1978.
77. Schneider, K. M., Ewing, R. S., and Signer, R. D.: Continent vesicostomy. *Urology* 3:654, 1974.
78. Zingg, E., and Tscholl, R.: Continent cecoileal conduit: preliminary report. *J. Urol.* 118:724, 1977.
79. Benchekroun, A.: Continent caecal bladder. *Br. J. Urol.* 54:505, 1982.

32

Infection With Neuropathic Bladder

INDER PERKASH, M.D., AND JANET A. GIROUX, R.N.

Neurologic bladder dysfunction secondary to spinal cord injury (SCI) causes disturbances in the normal micturition process, which leads to chronic bacteriuria and increased risk of renal disease. The causes of renal parenchymal damage in these patients are complex but usually can be attributed to: (a) vesicoureteral reflux, (b) hydronephrosis, (c) pyelonephritis, and (d) urinary tract stone disease (*1*). Despite progress in bladder retraining methods to develop reflex voiding, a high percentage still lack voiding control and therefore have significant urinary obstruction due to detrusor–sphincter dyssynergia (*2*). This inadequate voiding, leading to persistently high residual urine volumes, can be remedied by transurethral sphincterotomy (TURS), which surgically eliminates obstruction due to dyssynergia. However, it necessitates dependence on external condom drainage appliances, which increase the incidence of significant asymptomatic bacteriuria ($>10^5$ colonies/ml).

Because symptoms of dysuria, frequency, and fever are generally absent in an SCI population, significant bacteriuria poses a therapeutic dilemma. Is this bacteriuria truly tissue invasion eliciting a systemic response or simply colonization from exogenous sources? This lack of clarity concerning the definition of bacteriuria and its relevance to SCI patients continues to complicate the treatment and management picture.

In this chapter, we explore the pathogenesis of urinary tract infections (UTIs) and the definition and diagnostic indicators of bacteriuria. Finally, we propose management and prevention strategies for patients with neurogenic bladders.

PATHOGENESIS

Bladder emptying, a major urinary tract defense mechanism, is a precisely controlled neurophysiologic mechanism. Disruption of this mechanism by injury to the spinal cord and subsequent attempts to establish drainage leads to an increased incidence of UTIs. Breakdown of intrinsic host defenses such as (a) lack of effective mechanical washout, (b) reduction of the effectiveness of bladder wall antibacterial activity, and (c) changes in antibacterial activity of the urine itself through pH or osmotic changes have been implicated in the pathogenesis of chronic bacteriuria (*3,4*). Virulence of the pathogen and subsequent infection are thought to be influenced to a great extent not only by the host's ability to retard bacterial attachment but also by the bacteria's pili binding capacity to adhere to certain receptor sites (*5–7*) (Fig. 32–1).

Because of their dependence on alternate methods of urinary drainage, SCI patients are at great risk for developing bacteriuria. Indwelling catheter-associated UTIs continue to be widespread despite the advent of aseptic technique and closed drainage systems (*8*). Warren *et al.* reported a 98.4 percent incidence of bacteriuria ($\geq 10^5$ colonies/ml urine) in a group of 20 chronically catheterized patients. New episodes of bacteriuria were calculated at 56 per 100 patient-weeks (*9*). Complications such as acute and chronic pyelonephritis, urethral abscesses, bladder and renal stones, and renal failure have also been cited (*10*).

Intermittent catheterization (IC) provides an alternative to chronic indwelling catheterization during the early postinjury period.

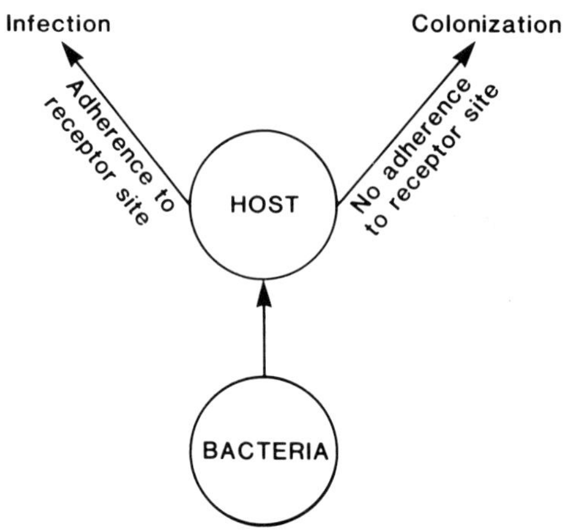

Figure 32–1. Pathogenesis: host and bacterial attributes.

As a short-term modality to effect a balanced bladder, the incidence of bacteriuria is significantly reduced compared to that seen with chronic catheterization (*11,12*). We documented an overall rate of 10.3 urinary tract infections per 1000 patient-days of intermittent catheterization (*13*). In the study by Donovan *et al.*, where an antimicrobial irrigant was not used, the respective rates of infection due to presumptively irrigant-sensitive organisms and presumptively irrigant-resistant organisms were, respectively, 22.8 and 11.8 infections per 1000 patient days (*12*). Corresponding rates in our patients were, respectively, 1.8 and 8.5 infections per 1000 patient days (*13*). However, use of IC on a long-term basis poses additional problems. An increase in UTI 15 months after rehabilitation was documented. (*14*). Upper tract deterioration with long-term IC has also been cited (*15*). Using transrectal sonography we have demonstrated the development of a significant (0.5–2.0 cm) lip at the bladder neck posteriorly in about 20 percent of SCI patients on IC from 2 months to 2.5 years (*16*).

External condom drainage is the preferred method of urinary drainage for most patients who void reflexly and are unobstructed. Complications such as stones, pyelonephritis, and penoscrotal abscesses are reduced. However, chronic recurrent bacteriuria continues to be a problem. Colonization of the perineum and urethra is facilitated by contaminated external drainage appliances, fecal incontinence, prolonged sitting, sweating, and soiled wheelchair cushions (*17,18*). These exogenous routes play critical roles in the occurrence of bacteriuria. Other causative factors influencing pathogenesis include inadequate intermittent voiding patterns and increased residual urine due to detrusor-sphincter dyssynergia. Vesicoureteral reflux, stone disease, and chronic pyelonephritis usually lead to persistent bacteriuria (*19,20*). Also, overzealous use of broad-spectrum antibiotics for suppressive purposes and treatment of asymptomatic bacteriuria have led to the emergence of drug-resistant organisms (*21*).

DIAGNOSIS

Because of complicating factors such as altered urodynamics and frequently associated asymptomatic bacteriuria, diagnosis of true UTI in a neurogenic bladder remains a perplexing issue for the practitioner. In the non-SCI woman a voided urine of 10^5 colonies/ml of urine was used as a reliable indicator for the presence of true bacteriuria for many years (*22,23*). However, this criterion as a sole indicator for infection in neurogenic bladders is questionable. Also, there is a lack of symptomatology in most of these patients even with significant bacteriuria. In a group of 110 SCI patients undergoing bladder localization, symptoms were documented in only 3 percent of the patients presenting with significant bacteriuria of more than 10^5 colonies/ml (*17*). To assist in clinical definition of UTI, quantitation of urine pyuria has proved helpful (*24*). Musher *et al.* reported that the presence of 10^4 (or more) white blood cells (WBCs) per milliliter of urine correlated with the presence of a UTI in a general hospital population (*24*).

We investigated the quantitative determination of pyuria in predicting the presence of bladder bacteriuria in an SCI population (*25*). The sample consisted of 43 SCI catheter-free men. Quantitative pyuria on 70 clean voided midstream (CVMS) specimens and suprapubic aspirate (SPA) was determined by hemocytometer. Results showed that pyuria ($\geq 10^4$ WBCs/ml urine) was an excellent predictor of UTI in 37 of 38 (97.4%) patients. However, 40.6 percent of the samples with a WBC count of fewer than 10^4/ml were also culture-positive ($\geq 10^4$ colonies/ml urine). Thus the absence of pyuria did not necessarily exclude infection. Overall, the consideration of the presence or absence of pyuria in relation to the presence of bacteriuria provided a sensitivity of 74.0 percent, specificity of 95.9 percent, and predictive value of a positive test of 97.4 percent. The predictive value of a negative test ($<10^4$ WBCs/ml urine), however, was only 57.4 percent. In summary, whereas WBC counts of fewer than 10^4/ml of urine were not predictive or urine culture results, counts of more than 10^4 WBCs/ml urine were found to be highly predictive of the presence of bacteriuria. Thus pyuria may reflect an inflammatory response and assist in distinguishing true tissue invasion from simple colonization.

Various invasive techniques have been utilized to define and localize the site of infection in normal voiders and those with neurogenic dysfunction, with differing results (*26–32*). Our studies with 100 SCI patients using the Fairley technique in conjunction with a prostatic localization procedure to determine the site of the UTI demonstrated both single and double sites of localization (*17*). Single sites of localization involved the following: upper tract 21 of 92 (23%), bladder 15 of 92 (16%), and prostate 8 of 92 (9%); 48 of 92 (52%) were undetermined. In eight cases, a double UTI site was documented: prostate and upper tract, six of eight (75%); prostate and bladder, one of eight (12%); and prostate and undetermined, one of eight (12%). Eighty-seven patients were followed after localization with urine cultures on the fourth or tenth day after the procedure; 31 percent had sterile urine cultures, 63 percent remained infected ($\geq 10^4$ colonies/ml), and 6 percent had fewer than 10^4 colonies/ml. The high percentage of sterile follow-up cultures in the face of upper tract and prostatic site of localization (28% and 29%, respectively) leads us to question the reliability of this test for patients with neurogenic bladders.

Limitations of the Fairley procedure may be attributed to the following: difficulty of sterilizing large, atonic and trabeculated bladders, transurethral sphincterotomy with widely open bladder neck, and heavy urethral colonization from use of external urinary collecting devices. Our experience with this combined procedure therefore revealed it to be an unreliable indicator of localization of UTIs. As a mechanical washout, however, it was shown to clear the bladder and urethra of bacteria in 31 percent of our patients for either 4 or 10 days after localization. With our additional modification of a urethral irrigation segment prior to the actual bladder washout, we hope to improve the reliability of this test for use in SCI patients.

The evolution of noninvasive markers such as antibody-coated bacteria (ACB), lactic acid levels, and urinary lactic dehydrogenase has given the practitioner additional help in the differential diagnosis of kidney and bladder infections. These noninvasive markers, however, have been tested almost exclusively in pediatric and non-SCI female populations (*33–37*). The use of ACB in populations with neurogenic bladder dysfunction had demonstrated varying degrees of accuracy (*38,39*). Two negative aspects are cited: (a) The presence of ACB in the urine cannot differentiate between renal, vesical, and prostatic site of infection; and (b) the ACB test cannot indicate which species is responsible for the tissue invasion in a urine specimen if there is more than one bacterial isolate (*40*). The clinical application of these noninvasive markers in a SCI population therefore has yet to be substantiated.

MANAGEMENT

Our main impetus throughout our investigative and diagnostic studies has been to formulate specific parameters in the treatment and management of UTIs in the neurologically compromised patient. The foremost measure is to ensure adequate bladder drainage. Effective voiding after TURS and relieving obstruction due to detrusor–sphincter dyssynergia seems critical for the prevention and treatment of recurrent symptomatic infection (*19*). Urodynamic evaluation is mandatory when assessing the degree of adequate drainage. Cystometrogram (CMG) with simultaneous periurethral electromyography (EMG) and voiding cystourethrography are recommended for all acute injuries as baseline data and for chronic injuries in order to update urologic evaluation. With these essential

Table 32–1. Chemical Disinfection of Leg Bags: *In vitro* Study*

	TAP WATER		0.25% ACETIC ACID		3% HYDROGEN PEROXIDE		1:16 SPORICIDIN†		0.06% SODIUM HYPOCHLORITE	
ORGANISM	*0 hr*	*24 hr*	*0 hr*	*24 hr*	*0 hr*	*24 hr*	*0 hr*	*24 hr*	*0 hr*	*24 hr*
Proteus mirabilis	$>10^5$	$>10^5$	$10/10^4$	$40/10^4$	0	0	0	0	0	0
Providencia stuartii	$>10^5$	$>10^5$	5×10^3	0	0	0	0	0	0	0
Pseudomonas aeruginosa	$>10^5$	$>10^5$	0/120	0/360	0	0	0	0	0	0
Klebsiella pneumoniae	$>10^5$	$>10^5$	2000/7000	40/620	0/60	0	0	0	0	0
Serratia marcescens	$>10^5$	$>10^5$	10^5	$10^3/1200$	$>10^5$	$60/10^3$	0	0	0	0
Herellea	$>10^5$	$>10^5$	6000/8000	420/1600	20/200	0/40	0	0	0	0
Enterococcus	$>10^5$	$>10^5$	$>10^4$	10^4	$>10^4$	0	0	0	0	0

*Two plates were inoculated at both 0 and 24 hours.

†Sporicidin is marketed by the Sporicidin Company, 400 Massachusetts Avenue N.W., Washington, D.C. It contains 0.13% alkaline glutaraldehyde and 0.52% alkaline phenate at 1:16 dilution.

From Giroux, J., and Perkash, I.: *J. Am. Paraplegia Soc.* 8:13–15, 1985.

data in hand, rational management can be planned. Appropriate alpha-blockers (i.e., prazosin), transurethral resection of the sphincter or prostate (TURS/TURP), or a combination of the two have proved effective for remedying detrusor–sphincter dyssynergia (*2*). To effectively decrease the residual urine volume, stimulation of the bladder through periodic suprapubic tapping or the Valsalva/Credé maneuver in cauda equina lesions is recommended. It also facilitates mechanical washout of the urethra and clearance of bladder bacteriuria. In reflex bladders, tapping externally over the bladder assists in relaxation of the bladder neck and external sphincter. However, an areflexic bladder due to a cauda equina lesion can be emptied by the Valsalva or Credé maneuvers. The effectiveness of these bladder-emptying techniques have been dramatically demonstrated by our use of transrectal sonography as an adjunct to urodynamic evaluation (*41*). Patients are educated about their particular type of neurogenic bladder function and the bladder-emptying technique that is most appropriate for them. By viewing a video monitor during transrectal sonography, patients learn to tap the bladder appropriately so that voiding occurs at acceptable pressures.

Colonization of gram-negative organisms in the perineum and urethra from use of external urinary appliances as well as contamination from bowel to bladder make prevention through proper hygiene imperative. From our localization data, it was observed that 84 percent of the patients studied had the infecting bladder organism simultaneously cultured from their external condom, drainage bag, perineum, or urethral swab (*17*). Therefore daily thorough perineal washing with plain soap and water, condom change, along with proper laundering of clothes, bedding, and soiled cushions are stressed. Finally, an effective leg bag cleaning procedure is recommended.

We performed an *in vitro* study investigating the bactericidal ability of five common cleaning agents for leg bags against organisms frequently causing UTI in SCI patients (*42*). The five agents were evaluated for effectiveness after an initial rinsing procedure and then 24 hours later after 15 ml of the solution had been left in the bag. The results, displayed in Table 32–1, demonstrated that Sporicidin, a cold sterilizing solution, and 0.06% sodium hypochlorite exhibited complete bactericidal ability. We believe that 0.06% sodium hypochlorite is most cost-efficient and is easily available to the patient for daily drainage bag cleaning.

In an effort to rationalize our clinical treatment procedures, we have outlined the following guidelines for intervention: We suggest treating the symptomatic patient who presents clinically with fever, chills, signs of dysreflexia, or evidence of reflux, acute pyelonephritis, or epididymoorchitis. After an appropriate course of antibiotic treatment, if obstruction appears to be a complicating factor, prompt correction through surgery, alpha-blockers, or a combination of the two is required. If the offending organism is a urea-splitter, i.e., *Proteus* or *Povidencia* species, antibiotic therapy is indicated because of the risk of stone formation. However, repeated use of broad-spectrum antibiotics to eradicate *Providencia* species has invariably resulted in the emergence of resistant strains. Treatment of the asymptomatic hospitalized patient is influenced by evidence of an inflammatory response as indicated by an elevated WBC response ($>10^4$ WBCs/ml urine). We suggest judicious use of broad-spectrum antibiotics and aminoglycosides because of the possible development of resistant bacterial strains from altered bowel flora. Lastly, treatment of asymptomatic bacteriuria with fewer than 10^4 WBCs/ml of urine in nonhospitalized patients may not be warranted. Without evidence of an inflammatory response, this type of bacteriuria could simply be colonization or contamination from the patient's own perineum or urinary drainage bag (*43*). Maintenance of adequate drainage, proper hygiene, and optimal fluid intake might be the key measures required to reduce or control the incidence of asymptomatic bacteriuria in this group of patients.

REFERENCES

1. Tribe, C. R.: Causes of death in the early and late stages of paraplegia. *Paraplegia* 1:19–47, 1963.
2. Perkash, I: Intermittent catheterization failure and an approach to bladder rehabilitation in spinal cord injury patients. *Arch. Phys. Med. Rehabil.* 59:9–17, 1978.
3. Mulholland, S. G., Perez, J. R., and Gillenwater, J.

Y.: Antibacterial properties of urine. *Invest. Urol.* 6:569–581, 1969.

4. Norden, C. W., Green, G. M., and Kass, E. H.: Antibacterial mechanisms of urinary bladder. *J. Clin. Invest.* 47:2689–2700, 1968.
5. Parsons, C. L., Shrom, S. H., Hanno, P. M., *et al.* : Bladder surface mucin, examination of possible mechanisms for its antibacterial effect. *Invest. Urol.* 16:196–200, 1978.
6. Svanborg-Eden, C., and Hansson, L. A.: Escherichia coli pili as possible mediators of attachment to human urinary epithelial cells. *Infect. Immun.* 21:229–237, 1978.
7. Weinstein, R., and Silverblatt, F. J.: Antibacterial mechanisms of antibody to mannose-sensitive pili of Escherichia coli. *J. Infect. Dis.* 147:882–889, 1983.
8. Garibaldi, R. A., Burke, J. P., Dickman, M. L., *et al.*: Factors predisposing to bacteriuria during indwelling urethral catheterization. *N. Engl. J. Med.* 211:215–219, 1974.
9. Warren, J. W., Tenney, J. H., Hoopes, J. M., *et al.*: A prospective microbiologic study of bacteriuria in patients with chronic indwelling urethral catheters. *J. Infect. Dis.* 146:719–723, 1982.
10. Warren, J. W., Muncie, H. L., Bergquist, E. J., and Hoopes, J. M.: Sequelae and management of urinary infection in the patient requiring chronic catheterization. *J. Urol.* 125:1–7, 1981.
11. Pearman, J. W., and England, E. J.: *The Urological Management of the Patient Following Spinal Cord Injury.* Charles C Thomas, Springfield, IL, 1973.
12. Donovan, W. H., Stolov, W. C., Clowers, D. E., *et al.*: Bacteriuria during intermittent catheterization following spinal cord injury. *Arch. Phys. Med. Rehabil.* 59:351–357, 1978.
13. Rhame, F. S., and Perkash, I.: Urinary tract infections occurring in recently injured spinal cord injury patients on intermittent catheterization. *J. Urol.* 122:669–673, 1979.
14. Erickson, R. P., Merritt, J. L., Opitz, J. L., and Ilstrup, D. M.: Bacteriuria during followup in patients with spinal cord injury. I. Rates of bacteriuria in various bladder-emptying methods. *Arch. Phys. Med. Rehabil.* 63:409–412, 1982.
15. Nanninga, J. B., Wu, J., and Hamilton, B.: Long-term intermittent catheterization in the spinal cord injured patient. *J. Urol.* 128:760–763, 1982.
16. Perkash, I., and Friedland, G.: Real-time gray-scale transrectal linear array ultrasonography in urodynamic evaluation. *Semin. Urol.* 3:49–59, 1985.
17. Giroux, J., and Perkash, I.: Limited value of the Fairley test in urologic infections in patients with neuropathic bladders. *J. Am. Paraplegia Soc.* 8:10–12, 1985.
18. Montgomerie, J. Z., and Morrow, J. W.: Pseudomonas colonization in patients with spinal cord injury. *J. Epidemiol.* 108:328–336, 1978.
19. O'Flynn, J. D.: Early and late management of the neuropathic bladder in spinal cord injury patients. *J. Urol.* 120:726–728, 1978.
20. Lapides, J., Diokno, A. C., Gould, F. R., and Lowe, B. S.: Further observations on self-catheterization. *J. Urol.* 116:169–172, 1976.
21. Turck, M.: Therapeutic principles in treatment of urinary tract infections and pyelonephritis. *Adv. Intern. Med.* 18:141–152, 1972.
22. Kass, E. H.: Asymptomatic infections of the urinary tract. *Trans. Assoc. Am. Physicians* 69:56–63, 1956.
23. Kass, E. H.: Bacteriuria and the diagnosis of infections of the urinary tract with observations on the use of methionine as a urinary antiseptic. *Arch. Intern. Med.* 100:709–714, 1957.
24. Musher, D. M., Thorsteinsson, S. B., and Airola, V. M. II: Quantitative urinalysis. *JAMA* 236:2069–2072, 1976.
25. Deresinski, S. C., and Perkash, I.: Urinary tract infection in male spinal cord injured patients. II. Diagnostic value of symptoms and quantitative urinalysis. *J. Am. Paraplegia Soc.* 8:7–10, 1985.
26. Stamey, T. A.: *Pathogenesis and Treatment of Urinary Tract Infections.* Williams & Wilkins, Baltimore, Maryland, 1980.
27. Fairley, K. F., Bond, A. G., Brown, R. B., *et al.*: Simple test to determine the site of urinary tract infection. *Lancet* 427–428, 1967.
28. Hellerstein, S., Duggan, E., Welchert, E., *et al.*: Localization of the site of urinary tract infections with the bladder washout test. *J. Pediatr.* 98:201–206, 1981.
29. Kuhlemeier, K. V., Lloyd, L. K., and Stover, S. L.: Failure of antibody-coated bacteria and bladder washout tests to localize infection in spinal cord injury patients. *J. Urol.* 130:729–732, 1983.
30. Merritt, J. L., and Keys, T. F.: Limitations of the antibody-coated bacteria test in patients with neurogenic bladders. *JAMA* 247:1723–1725, 1982.
31. Naso, F., and Ditunno, J. F.: The Fairley test: an aid in the diagnosis of pyelonephritis in paraplegia. *Arch. Phys. Med. Rehabil.* 55:279–281, 1974.
32. Stamey, T. A., and Meares, E. M.: Bacteriologic localization patterns in bacterial prostatitis and urethritis. *Invest. Urol.* 5:492–518, 1968.
33. Brook, I., Belman, B., and Controni, G.: Lactic acid in urine of children with lower and upper urinary tract infection and renal obstruction. *Am. Soc. Clin. Pathol.* 75:110–113, 1980.
34. Thomas, V., Shelokov, A., and Forland, M.: Antibody-coated bacteria in the urine and the site of urinary tract infection. *N. Engl. J. Med.* 290:588–590, 1974.
35. Carvajal, H. F., Passey, R. B., Berger, M., *et al.* Urinary lactic dehydrogenase isoenzyme 5 in the differential diagnosis of kidney and bladder infections. *Kidney Int.* 8:176–184, 1975.
36. Rumans, L. W., and Vosti, K. L.: The relationship of antibody-coated bacteria to clinical syndromes. *Arch. Intern. Med.* 138:1077–1081, 1978.
37. Devaskar, U., and Montgomery, W.: Urinary lactic dehydrogenase isoenzyme IV and V in the differential diagnosis of cystitis and pyelonephritis. *J. Pediatr.* 93:789–791, 1978.
38. Merritt, J. L., and Keys, T. F.: Limitations of the antibody-coated bacteria test in patients with neurogenic bladders. *JAMA* 247:1723–1725, 1982.
39. Newman, E., Price, M., and Ederer, G. M.: Urinary tract infection in patients with spinal cord lesions: antibody-coated bacteria tests as a diagnostic aid. *Arch. Phys. Med. Rehabil.* 61:406–409, 1980.
40. Jones, S., and Johnson, J.: Further evaluation of the test for detection of antibody-coated bacteria in urine sediment. *J. Clin. Microbiol.* 5:510–513, 1977.

41. Perkash, I., and Friedland, G. W.: Using transrectal sonography to teach patients with spinal cord injuries to retrain their bladders. *Radiology* 152:228–229, 1984.
42. Giroux, J., and Perkash, I.: In vitro evaluation of current disinfectants for leg bags. *J. Am. Paraplegia Soc.* 8:13–15, 1985.
43. Perkash, I., and Giroux, J.: Prevention, treatment and management of UTI in neuropathic bladders. *J. Am. Paraplegia. Soc.* 8:15–17, 1985.

33

Artificial Urinary Sphincter

DAVID M. BARRETT, M.D., WILLIAM L. FURLOW, M.D., AND BENAD GOLDWASSER, M.D.

Control of sphincteric urinary incontinence with implantable prosthetic devices has evolved rapidly (*1–3*). Clearly, the most significant contribution was the introduction in 1973 by Scott *et al.* (*4,5*) of a totally implantable artificial sphincter mechanism that could be used in adults and children of both sexes. This hydraulic device, composed of silicone rubber, allowed placement of an inflatable cuff around the bladder neck in male and female patients or around the bulbous urethra in men. The patient controlled the sphincter by small pumps placed in the subcutaneous tissue of the scrotum or labia. Unidirectional valves within the system directed the fluid from a reservoir to and from the inflatable cuff (Fig. 33–1). Pressure in the cuff was regulated by a bleed-off valve in the outflow tract.

Limited to placement around the bulbous urethra in male patients, the Rosen antiincontinence prosthesis was introduced in 1976 (*6*). This ingenious mechanism allowed the patient to titrate the degree of urethral closing pressure by pumping only the minimum amount of fluid required to maintain continence into the compression pillow. Unfortunately, many patients overinflated the device, and the unnecessarily high urethral closing pressure resulted in erosion of the urethra. Only limited clinical experience was gained with the Rosen device, and no modifications of the device have evolved.

DEVELOPMENTAL CONSIDERATIONS

Regardless of the type or model of sphincter device developed, it soon became apparent to implanting urologists that the magnitude of closing pressure created by the sphincter's occlusive mechanism was the crux to success or failure. Excessive occlusive pressure produced vascular ischemia of the underlying tissues of the urethra or bladder neck. The result was erosion of the occlusive mechanism into the lumen of the urinary tract and subsequent periprosthetic infection. Conversely, if occlusive pressure was insufficient, the patient's incontinence persisted.

The initial device developed by Scott *et al.* became commercially available in 1974 and was called the AS 721 sphincter (*4,5*). This device produced mixed results in patients with various types of sphincteric incontinence. Although many patients benefited from the device, the mechanical reliability and rate of erosion were unacceptably high.

In 1977, in conjunction with the manufacturer, several urologists began to work with a new sphincter design. The AS 742 and AS 761 devices created a new concept in implantable prosthetic sphincters. Subtly different in design, both used an elastic pressure-balloon reservoir to ensure constant, predetermined pressure within the hydraulic system of the sphincter. These balloon reser-

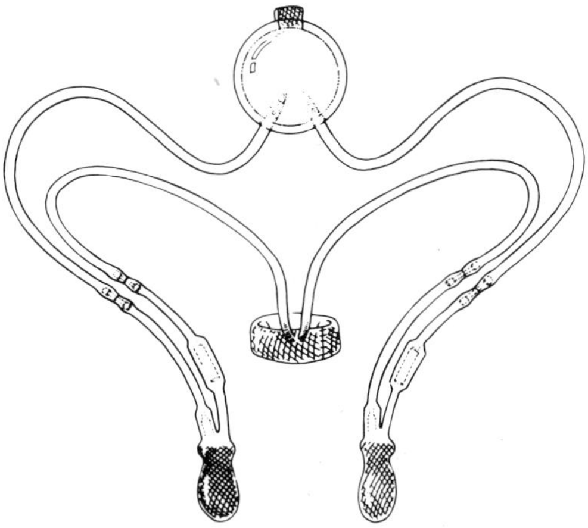

Figure 33–1. Scott AS 721 artificial sphincter.

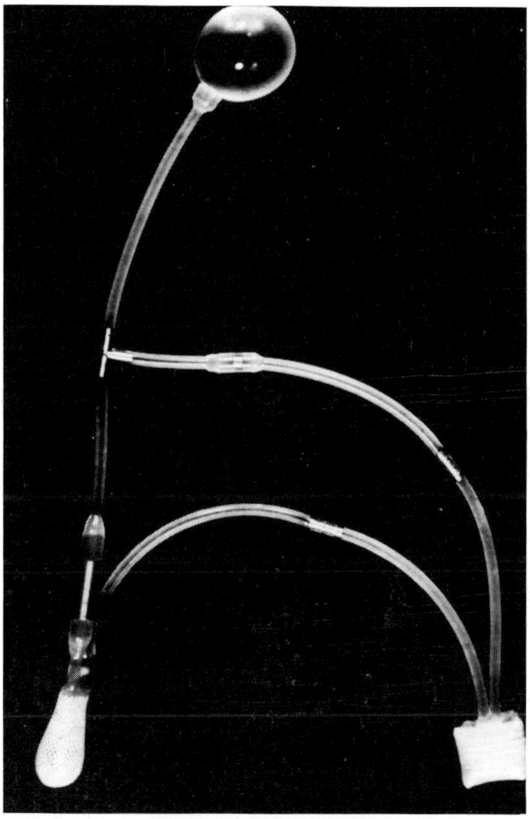

Figure 33–2. AS 742 artificial sphincter with pressure-balloon reservoir and flow resistor. (From Furlow, W. L.: Artificial sphincter. In Stanton, S. L., and Tanagho, E. A. [eds.]: *Surgery of Female Urinary Incontinence*, 2nd ed. Springer-Verlag, Berlin, 1986.)

voirs, by virtue of the elasticity inherent in their construction, exerted a given amount of intraluminal pressure depending on the volume of fluid in the balloon. The pressure-volume relation was linear only up to a given volume and then became predictable within a narrow range (Fig. 33–2). Balloon reservoirs were manufactured to deliver a range of preset pressures (51–60, 61–70, 71–80, and 81–90 cm H_2O). The urologist could select a pressure to fit the clinical situation and site of cuff placement. When pressurized, the cuff provided continuous closing pressure to the underlying urethra or bladder neck. The cuff was opened by compression of the pump until all of the cuff fluid was forced through a unidirectional valve into the balloon reservoir. Inherently, the fluid was directed back toward the cuff. However, its rate of refilling was regulated by a flow resistor that allowed the patient 3 to 5 minutes to urinate before repressurization was complete.

Because of the initial implanting success with the pressure-balloon reservoir concept, an artificial urinary sphincter research group was assembled in 1979 to evaluate a hybrid of the AS 742 device (*7*). Incorporating changes in the pump, cuff, and control assembly, the AS 791/792 sphincter proved to be mechanically reliable and afforded continence in most of the patients in whom it was implanted (Fig. 33–3). Several clinical series attested to the attributes of the device and its versatility. A distinct limitation, however, was lack of an external "on" and "off" capability. Once the sphincter had been implanted, constant pressure was delivered to the inflatable cuff except during the short period when the cuff was emptied to allow voiding. This function of the device, although easy to manage from the patient's standpoint, created several limiting and potentially complicated problems.

1. Cuff closing pressure began at the time of implantation without regard to the quality of the underlying tissues. Patients with previous urethral or bladder neck surgery, pelvic radiation therapy, or induced surgical trauma were at risk for vascular ischemia

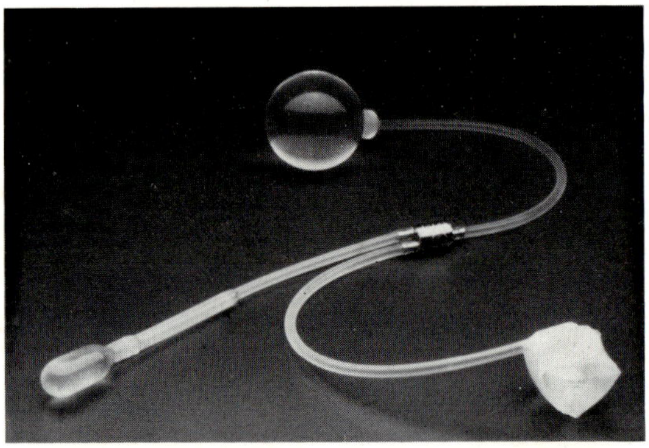

Figure 33–3. AS 791(A)/792 artificial sphincter.

and cuff erosion. The inability to limit this pressure during the early postoperative healing period led to the concept of primary deactivation. This technique allowed implantation of the sphincter cuff, balloon, and pump at one operation followed within 2 to 3 months by a second procedure to insert the control assembly and "activate" the sphincter mechanism (*8,9*).

2. For many patients, the implanted pump in the labia or scrotum produced extreme tenderness and edema in the overlying tissues during the early postoperative period. This reaction prohibited cuff decompression for voiding, so that a small-caliber catheter was necessary for bladder drainage until the swelling and tenderness resolved.

3. Long-term catheterization or instrumentation of the urethra or bladder was occasionally necessary in patients with implants. The inability to deactivate the cuff for prolonged periods predisposed the patient to cuff erosion because the inserted tube or instrument compressed the underlying tissues.

4. For the many incontinent patients who are wet only when upright or during physical activity, cuff compression ideally is necessary only during the "at risk" times. With the AS 791/792 concept, the patient endured cuff compression continuously even if the protection was not required. Urethral or bladder neck tissues were therefore at risk for erosion and atrophic deterioration more than necessary.

During late 1982 and early 1983, work began on a design alteration that provided for externally controlled cuff "on" and "off" capability. The result became commercially available in April 1983 and is known as the AS 800 artificial urinary sphincter (Fig. 33–4). The AS 800 control assembly contains unidirectional valves, a flow reservoir, an "on" and "off" button, and a deflate pump (Fig. 33–5). It allows nonsurgical delayed activation and complete control by physician and patient over periods of cuff compression (*10*).

Also included in the currently used AS 800 device is a vastly improved cuff, which, although it looks similar to its predecessors, has been contructed of silicone elastomer that is extremely resistant to excess wear and leakage.

PATIENT EVALUATION AND SELECTION

Not all patients with urinary incontinence are suitable for implantation of the artificial sphincter. Incontinence may be the result of a detrusor abnormality (e.g., detrusor hyperreflexia), a sphincteric abnormality (such as that after transurethral resection), or a combination of detrusor and sphincteric abnormalities. Ideally, the artificial sphincter is most appropriate for persons with pure sphincteric incompetence who have normal detrusor function. Evaluation of candidates for the artificial sphincter should therefore be designed to quantitate voiding

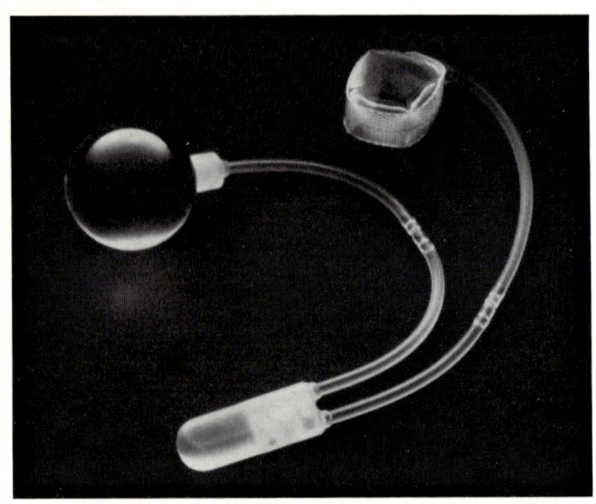

Figure 33–4. AS 800 artificial sphincter.

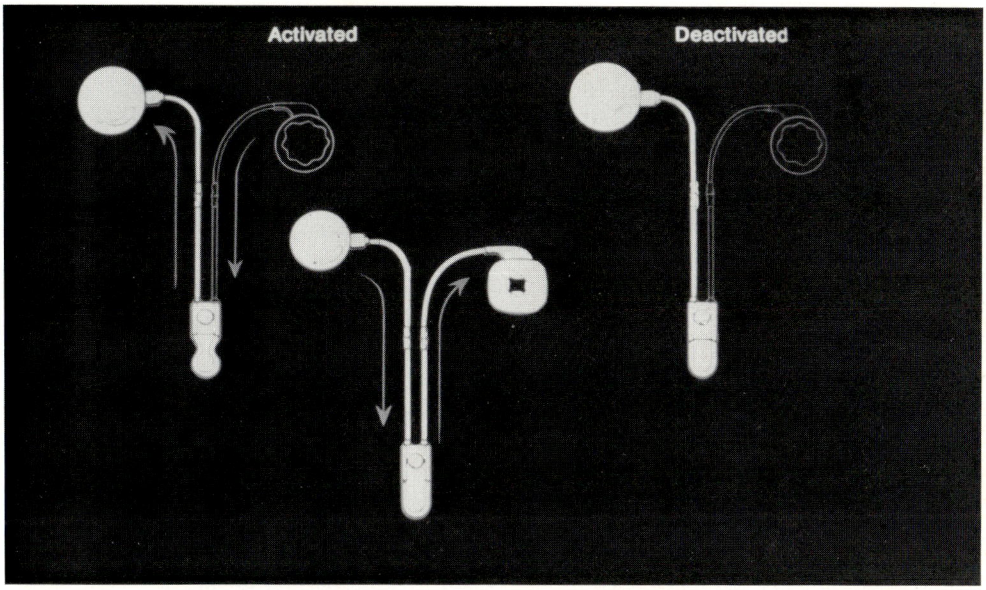

Figure 33–5. AS 800 artificial sphincter function.

function, usually through a combination of urodynamic, radiographic, and endoscopic tests. Even patients with an outwardly apparent cause for incontinence, e.g., previous radical prostatectomy, should be evaluated to exclude coincident abnormalities that may preclude success with an implanted sphincter.

An excretory urogram and voiding cystourethrogram are indicated to exclude upper tract or bladder structural abnormalities that would require repair before or during sphincter implantation. Vesicoureteral reflux, for example, may not be a problem for a totally incontinent patient because intravesical pressures do not usually exceed a critical level. With implantation of the artificial sphincter, continuous low intravesical, resting, and voiding pressures are likely to increase and to potentiate the problems inherent in vesicoureteral incompetence. Our policy has been to correct reflux of grade 2 or more either before or during sphincter implantation.

Cystourethroscopy is recommended to exclude urethral or bladder neck defects, e.g., false passages, stricture, diverticulum, contracture, and foreign body. All such abnormalities should be appropriately managed and considered stable before sphincter implantation. The location of urethral defects is also important. A stricture in the distal or mid-bulbous portion of the urethra may prevent implantation of the occlusive cuff at this level, and an alternative site is chosen.

Detrusor contractility and compliance are best evaluated by gas or water cystometry. Patients with low-volume detrusor hyperreflexia are poor candidates for sphincter implantation because contractile pressures override sphincteric resistance pressures or a dyssynergic pattern is created, inducing risk to the upper tracts. Similarly at risk are patients with decreased compliance and small functional bladder capacity. A combination of pharmacologic therapy may make such patients suitable candidates; however, most often such patients are best managed by either neurologic blockade or augmentation cystoplasty to decrease contractility or increase compliance and functional bladder capacity.

Persons with sphincteric incompetence and decreased detrusor contractility were formerly excluded from sphincter implantation because their residual volumes were too high to risk increasing outlet resistance for fear of potentiating urosepsis and frank retention. Since the acceptance of combined sphincter implantation and intermittent clean self-catheterization, we now consider this group of patients to be good candidates. As alternatives to intermittent catheterization, sphincterotomy in men and bladder flap urethroplasty in women may facilitate bladder emptying.

Table 33–1 lists the indications for implantation of AS 800 sphincters in 221 patients at the Mayo Clinic through January 1986. Radical prostatectomy, which is associated with a 5 percent rate of significant incontinence, remains the number one source of patients for implantation. Although many transurethral prostatectomies are performed annually, the incontinence rate is low; however, we still see patients with incontinence after transurethral prostatectomy who qualify for artificial sphincter implantation.

Patients with incontinence associated with congenital abnormalities such as myelomeningocele, exstrophy–epispadias, and sacral agenesis are good candidates for an artificial sphincter (*11,12*). Many patients in this group have incomplete emptying, and additional measures must be taken after the sphincter is implanted to ensure regular, complete voiding.

Selected patients with acquired injuries such as spinal cord trauma, pelvic fracture, and neurogenic bladder form a large group of candidates for implantation. Care must be taken in this group to adequately assess bladder contractility and compliance before and after implantation, as some authors have suggested that deterioration in the upper tracts results from a change in detrusor function after implantation.

Table 33–1. Causes of Incontinence in 221 Patients Who Had Implantation of the AS 800 Artificial Sphincter

CAUSE	NO. OF PATIENTS
Radical prostatectomy	95
Transurethral prostatectomy	45
Myelomeningocele, sacral agenesis	42
Spinal cord injury	11
Other causes	7
Neurogenic bladder	5
Stress incontinence	5
Urethral surgery	5
Exstrophy–epispadias	4
Pelvic fracture	2
Total	221

Patients with various other causes of incontinence may also benefit from artificial sphincter implantation. Noteworthy is the relative sparsity of female patients having had implants (*13–15*). In general, female stress incontinence is best managed by conventional methods to modify vesicourethral incompetence (*16,17*). Even techniques that create relative outlet obstruction, e.g., the sling procedure, may be better options than the artificial sphincter. Female patients with neurologic deficits such as those related to myelomeningocele, who have a poor response to conventional surgical procedures, are good candidates, and optimal results can be expected.

Before a patient can be considered an optimal candidate for AS 800 implantation, technical feasibility must be considered. The surgeon's ability to implant the inflatable cuff around the bulbous urethra or bladder neck is the key issue. Patients who have had multiple previous bladder neck or urethral procedures, pelvic trauma, or pelvic radiation therapy are difficult surgical challenges and must be considered high risks.

In men the cuff site that enhances the ease of implantation and provides the best chance of continence is selected. Ideally, the bladder neck is the most physiologic location for cuff placement. However, in patients who have undergone a radical prostatectomy, it is nearly impossible to circumferentially dissect the bladder neck without damaging the rectum or bladder (*18*). Thus it becomes necessary to choose the bulbous urethra for cuff placement. In children and women the bladder neck is the only site for cuff placement (*19*). Previous bladder neck tubularization makes the bladder neck dissection more difficult, but success is possible if the tubularization technique did not encroach on the vesicovaginal or vesicorectal plane (*20*). Patients with previous vesicovaginal fistula repair and rectal pull-through procedures should be cautioned that cuff placement may not be technically possible.

Aside from the physical characteristics of the patient's incontinence, the patient's expectations and motivation are assessed. Occasionally, patients have unrealistic expectations about the artificial sphincter. They must be told about the mechanical characteristics of the device and the likelihood of occasional stress incontinence. They must accept the possibility that additional surgery may be necessary in the future for adjustments or repairs, and that if the prosthesis becomes infected the components of the device must be removed.

PREOPERATIVE CONSIDERATIONS

Patients with urinary tract infection must be adequately treated before surgery, and all are given broad-spectrum parenteral antibiotics for prophylaxis. The bacterium most often associated with infected prostheses is *Staphylococcus epidermidis*, and prophylaxis should be designed to include this organism. Cephalosporins or aminoglycosides are the antimicrobials most often used. Administration of antibiotics is continued for at least 4 days after implantation.

Many patients with chronic urinary incontinence have various degrees of dermatitis on the lower abdomen and pelvis. It is best to insert a Foley catheter in these patients several days in advance of implantation to reduce the bacterial counts on the skin and promote healing.

Most patients scheduled for uncomplicated bulbous urethral cuff implantation are admitted to the hospital on the morning of the surgical procedure, whereas those having the bladder neck operation are admitted the evening before for a limited lower bowel preparation. All hair removal is done just before surgery to avoid bacterial colonization of the small scratches and nicks that may accompany shaving.

When placed on the operating table, patients receiving the bulbous urethral cuff are in the lithotomy position and those undergoing the bladder neck cuff operation are supine with their legs slightly spread.

Iodophors are preferred for skin preparation, and a full 10-minute scrubbing is used. All female patients have a vaginal preparation. A soft rectal tube is placed in male patients and children who will have bladder neck cuff placement. Draping is performed in such a way that there is access to the lower anterior abdominal wall and perineum. Urethral catheters are inserted after skin preparation and draping.

An antibiotic solution is prepared and used frequently for irrigation during the procedure. It is also best to irrigate the bladder with the solution before dissection of the urethra or bladder neck. Our formula consists of neomycin 0.1% and bacitracin 50,000 units in 1 liter of 0.9% sodium chloride solution.

Because of the infection risks in patients undergoing prosthetic implantation, all operating room personnel must wear hoods to ensure limited "fallout" in the operative field. Traffic in and out of the operating room is strictly limited.

OPERATIVE TECHNIQUE

Bulbous Urethral Cuff

A 12F or 14F Foley catheter is passed, and the bladder is emptied. Two incisions are made, one on the perineum in the midline over the bulbous urethra and another transversely on the lower anterior abdominal wall, to either the right or the left of the midline, depending on the site for pump placement. The bulbous urethra is circumferentially dissected through the perineal incision; the bulbocavernosus muscle is preserved if possible. The plane of dissection is about 2 cm wide and is as close as possible to the underlying tunica albuginea of the corporal bodies. The obvious concern is to avoid injury to the thin urethral tissues at the 12 o'clock position on the urethra, the point at which most urethral injuries occur.

If the urethra is injured, it may be possible to close the defect primarily with 4–0 or 5–0 absorbable suture. A different site on the urethra can then be selected for cuff placement. Unfortunately, some urethral injuries are not recognized and may result in early cuff erosion.

Once the urethral plane is established, the circumferential measurement is determined with a calibrated (1–12 cm) measuring strap. The properly sized cuff, which for the bulbous urethra is almost always 4.5, 5.0, or 5.5 cm in length, is passed tab-first under the urethra. The tab is passed under the urethra toward the side where the pump is to be placed. The tubing is passed through an opening in the tab, and the cuff is snapped in place while gentle opposing traction is placed on tab and tubing.

A long, curved forceps or similar instrument is used to create a tunnel in the subcutaneous tissues from the incision in the anterior abdominal wall down to the perineal incision. The cuff tubing is grasped and drawn into the upper incision through the subcutaneous tissues.

After the bulbous urethra is dissected and the quality of the urethral tissue is assessed, the balloon reservoir pressure may be selected. We have used the 61 to 70 cm H_2O reservoir in most patients with uncomplicated bulbous urethral cuffs. In high-risk patients, the 51 to 60 cm H_2O reservoir is selected to preserve tissue integrity.

A 1- to 2-cm incision is made in the rectus fascia, and the unfilled balloon is placed in a small pocket under the belly of the rectus muscle. The balloon tubing is passed through a separate puncture opening in the fascia, and the balloon is filled with 22 ml of isosmotic contrast medium (previously 18 ml).

The AS 800 pump-control assembly is placed in a subcutaneous tunnel most easily created with Hagar dilators in one side of the scrotum. The cuff tubing is attached to the control assembly tubing with a right-angle connector to prevent kinking. The balloon and the control assembly tubing are attached with a straight connector. Prolene suture, 2–0 or 3–0, is used to tie the connectors in place.

Various techniques have been used to evaluate cuff closing pressure and the degree of continence intraoperatively, but no perfect method exists. We have found that with urethral profilometry an increase of 40 cm H_2O in urethral closing pressure when the cuff is closed usually predicts continence. A less scientific but useful method is to fill the bladder with fluid and apply limited external pressure to the suprapubic area. Continence may be predicted if no urine escapes the urethra. Generally, no drains are necessary. The catheter remains in until the day after implantation. When the patient leaves the operating room, the cuff is pumped empty and the system deactivated (Fig. 33–6).

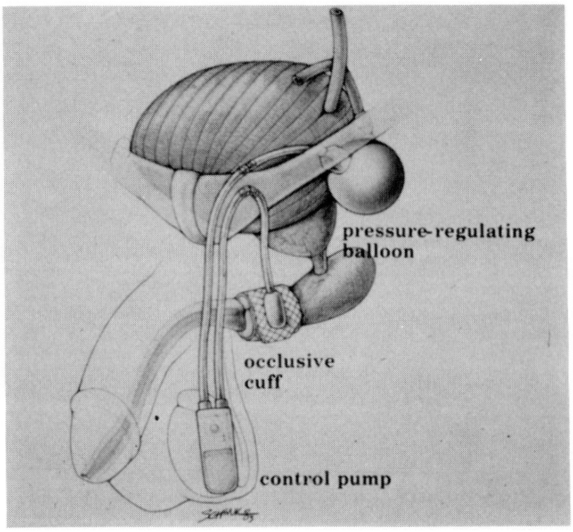

Figure 33–6. AS 800 sphincter with bulbous urethral cuff.

Bladder Neck Cuff Placement

A Foley catheter, the size appropriate to the age and sex of the patient, is passed. Larger Foley catheters (20F–24F) are used in female patients to more adequately assess the bladder neck urethral margins; catheters of smaller caliber (10F–14F) are used in children and male patients. A lower abdominal midline or transverse incision is used for bladder neck cuff implantation. There is no need to open the peritoneal cavity, and dissection is limited to the retroperitoneal space.

With a catheter in the bladder, the demarcation of the bladder neck and proximal portion of the urethra can be palpated. Care is taken during circumferential dissection of the bladder neck to avoid opening the endopelvic fascia. The plane between the posterior aspect of the bladder neck and the anterior surface of the underlying vagina or rectum must be established. A pack in the vagina assists in delineation of this area. Because of the difficulty of dissecting around the female bladder neck, some authorities prefer to open the bladder before beginning the dissection. Doing so provides for easier orientation during the dissection between bladder neck and vaginal wall and decreases the chance of perforating any of these organs. The opening in the bladder is made far above the bladder neck to prevent placement of the cuff over the suture line, which would increase the risk of erosion. Dissecting the plane between the bladder neck and the vagina through a vaginal approach was found to be associated with a high rate of infection. Therefore we do not recommend that approach. In the male patient, a rectal tube assists in demarcating the plane between the rectum and the bladder neck. The point of dissection is superior to the endopelvic fascia but far enough distal to avoid the areas where the ureters penetrate the posterior aspect of the bladder and trigone. Usually a combination of blunt and sharp dissection affords complete circumferential dissection.

Once this area has been completely opened, the width of the plane is approximately 2 cm so the cuff fits without crimping. A tape is passed around the bladder neck, and the bladder is filled with antibiotic solution to reveal small openings that may have been created during the dissection. If an opening is detected, it may be closed with 3–0 or 4–0 absorbable suture.

If a vaginal injury is created, it also may be closed primarily. Unfortunately, if a rectal injury is created, we would advise closing the rectal injury primarily and abandoning the procedure until another date.

As with the bulbous urethra, the bladder neck is circumferentially measured with the calibrated measuring strap. The catheter remains indwelling unless it is of large caliber. It is removed before measurement of the bladder neck area. Once the properly sized cuff has been passed underneath the bladder neck and snapped in place, the tubing from this sphincter component is passed through the belly of one rectus muscle and through the anterior abdominal wall fascia on the side of the patient where the pump will be placed. This tubing should penetrate the rectus muscle and fascia 3 to 4 inches above the pubic symphysis.

The pressure of the balloon reservoir is chosen on the basis of the quality of tissue and the size of cuff used. In most of our patients with bladder neck cuffs, a 71 to 80 cm H_2O pressure-balloon reservoir is chosen. In patients who have tissues of substandard quality, a 61 to 70 cm H_2O pressure-balloon reservoir is commonly used. In general, the larger the cuff, the higher the pressure-balloon reservoir selected.

Cuff sizes range up to 11 cm for placement around the bladder neck. In most children and women a 6- to 8-cm inflatable cuff is chosen, whereas in men an 8- to 14-cm cuff may be necessary.

The pressure balloon reservoir is placed in the prevesical space. Its tubing penetrates the rectus muscle next to the tubing of the cuff. Before the balloon is filled, the prevesical space is drained, and the anterior abdominal wall fascia is closed with absorbable suture. Once the closure is complete, the balloon is filled with 22 ml (previously 18 ml) of isosmotic contrast medium and the cuff is pressurized. Once the cuff is pressurized, the balloon is refilled to a maximum of 20 ml of fluid.

The cuff accommodates 0.5 to 1.5 ml of fluid, depending on the length of the cuff. The AS 800 control assembly is placed in a deep subcutaneous pocket in the scrotum or labia. Connections between the control assembly and balloon and the control assembly and cuff are established with straight connectors tied in place with Prolene suture (Fig. 33–7).

As before, the cuff is left in a deactivated configuration for 6 to 8 weeks. The patient's indwelling Foley catheter is removed the day after surgery; and, if necessary, bladder emp-

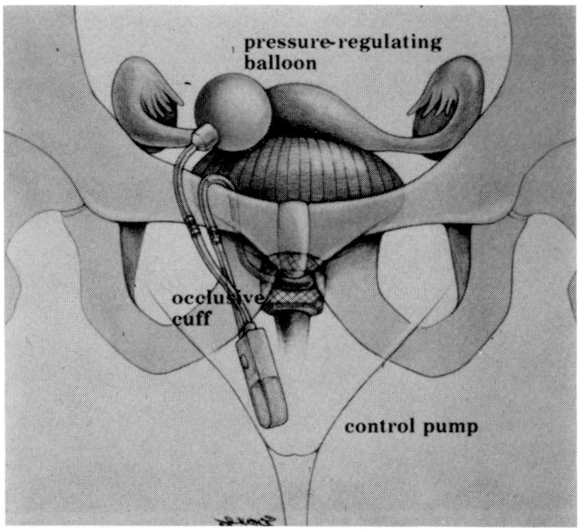

Figure 33–7. AS 800 sphincter with bladder neck cuff. (From Furlow, W. L.: Artificial sphincter. In Stanton, S. L., and Tanagho, E. A. [eds.]: *Surgery of Female Urinary Incontinence*, 2nd ed. Springer-Verlag, Berlin, 1986.)

tying is assisted by intermittent catheterization.

POSTOPERATIVE CARE AND ACTIVATION

The hospital stay for a patient with bulbous urethral cuff placement averages 3 or 4 days. Those with bladder neck placement are in the hospital 2 or 3 days longer. Postoperative discomfort is moderate; some swelling and edema occur at the pump site in the scrotum or labia. For the first 24 to 48 hours, ice packs are placed in the region of the pump to help reduce postoperative edema. Except in unusual circumstances, the urethral catheter is removed in the morning after implantation. Some patients report immediate improvement in their urinary control, which can be explained by increased resistance due to swelling and edema at the cuff site. In almost all patients, control is transient and incontinence is noted again in a few days. Rarely, the patient is unable to urinate, in which event intermittent catheterization with a small-caliber urethral catheter is necessary until spontaneous voiding develops. There is no question that prolonged intubation of the urethra or bladder neck through a recently implanted cuff enhances the risk of urethral cuff erosion.

Incontinence is expected to persist during the deactivation period, and some form of incontinence protection is worn until activation is undertaken. We have discouraged the use of clamps during this period and have advised most patients to use diapers or condom drainage devices.

Although ambulation is not limited after implantation, all patients are cautioned to avoid undue compression to their perineum and lower abdomen during the recovery period, with special consideration given to persons with bulbous urethral cuffs to avoid compression injury to the cuff area and the bulbous urethra. In our experience, patients are ready for activation in 6 to 8 weeks regardless of cuff site location. Scrotal or labial tenderness generally has subsided by that time, and the abdominal and perineal incisions are well healed. Activation is undertaken by firm compression of the pump. The deactivation pin "pops" into the activated configuration, allowing fluid to circulate through the control assembly. Activation can be monitored by deflation and inflation radiographs, which confirm filling of the cuff after activation.

Instruction of the patient about how the device functions generally begins before implantation. Most patients, however, require a direct demonstration of how to use the device after activation. Some patients are more nimble than others and learn to operate the sphincter pump easily (Fig. 33–8).

Many patients are dry at night and do not require cuff compression for continence. We instruct them about how to deactivate the device during the evening hours. Deactivation has the obvious benefit of reducing the risk of ischemia to the underlying urethra or bladder neck. Patients are told that after deflation of the cuff recompression requires 3 to 5 minutes; and that although bladder emptying was accomplished in less time, full continence can be expected only after the cuff is fully inflated. In patients with reduced flow rates, a second pumping may be required to adequately empty the bladder because cuff recompression occurs before voiding has been completed.

For patients unable to completely empty their bladders, intermittent self-catheterization is used (*21*). The patients are told to deflate the sphincter cuff before inserting the catheter into the bladder.

POSTOPERATIVE COMPLICATIONS

Hematoma

The most common minor complication of sphincter surgery is the formation of subcutaneous hematomas. Labial or scrotal hematomas cause the most concern, as they may displace the pump into an unfavorable location for external manipulation. Although most hematomas resolve spontaneously, occasionally a large hematoma is drained to prevent discomfort and enhance healing.

Retention

Another minor problem seen occasionally is incomplete voiding after implantation. The

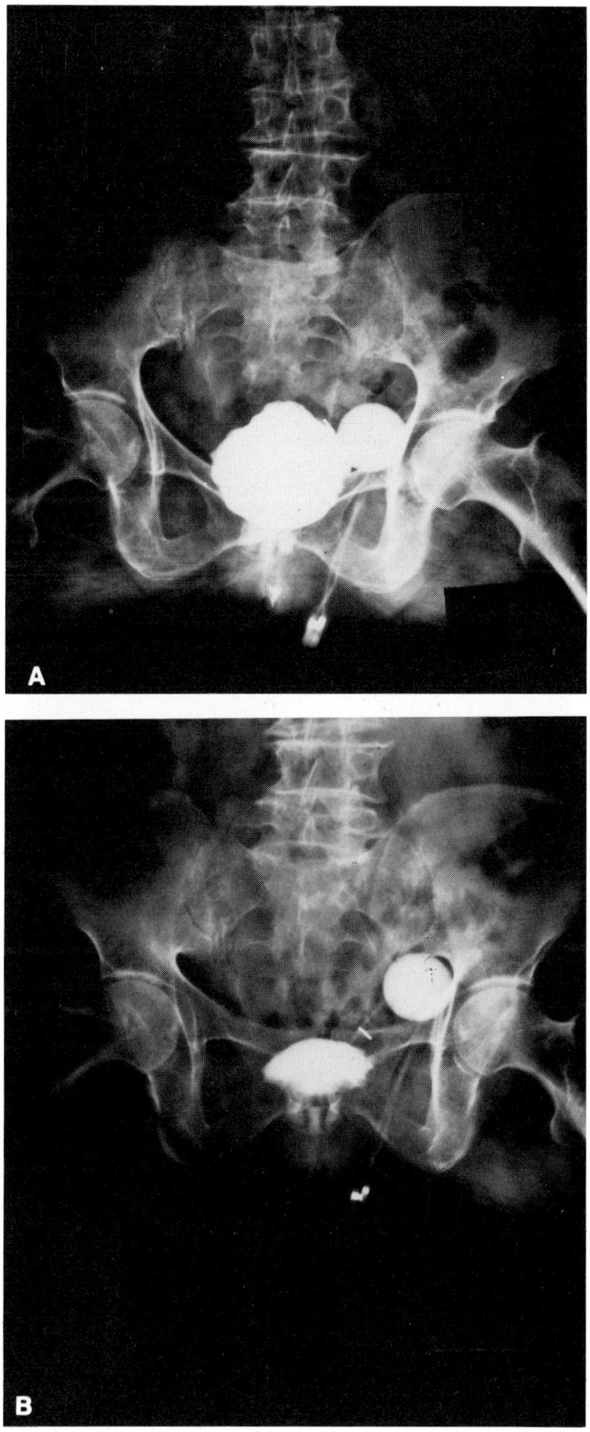

Figure 33–8. Cystograms before (**A**) and after (**B**) voiding in a female patient with an AS 800 sphincter.

initial assessment of the patient includes a check of the sphincter mechanism to confirm that the cuff is deactivated in the open position. Most patients, regardless of cuff location, begin to void after one or two in-and-out catheterizations with small-caliber catheters (10F or 12F). Those with bladder neck cuff placement may perform self-catheterization indefinitely, if necessary, without undue risk to the cuff and tissue. However, patients with bulbous urethral cuffs are at more risk for cuff-urethral injury from early repeated or prolonged catheterization.

Fortunately, incomplete voiding in patients with bulbous urethral cuffs is rare, but when it is a problem our policy has been to use a soft 10F or 12F catheter for self-catheterization. The patient is asked to deactivate the cuff in the open position before inserting the catheter. This maneuver ensures the minimum of external pressure on the urethra at the time of catheterization.

The same policy is followed if emergency medical problems mandate placement of an indwelling catheter. Should the need arise for elective prolonged bladder drainage, a suprapubic drainage system may be inserted with fluoroscopic monitoring to avoid the sphincter components.

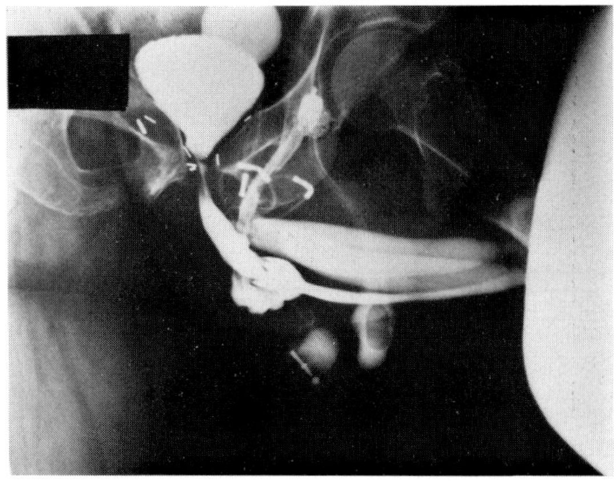

Figure 33–9. Urethrogram in a patient with an artificial sphincter and a penile prosthesis. Extravasation of contrast medium around the sphincter cuff is diagnostic of urethral cuff erosion.

Cuff Erosion

The most feared postoperative complications of sphincter surgery are cuff erosion and infection. Although cuff erosion has become uncommon since delayed activation has been used, this problem still implies at least temporary failure. Erosion can occur at any time, but it is most common during the first 3 to 4 months after implantation. Cuff erosions before activation usually imply unrecognized surgical injury to the urethra or bladder neck.

Clinically, patients with cuff erosion may have pain and swelling in the cuff or pump area, recurrent incontinence, and urosepsis. A urethrogram or urethroscopy confirms erosion (Fig. 33–9). Surgical removal of the cuff is mandatory; and if there is purulent drainage, the remaining sphincter components must also be removed. An 18F or 20F silicone Foley catheter is inserted and is retained for 3 to 4 weeks or until there is radiographic evidence of complete healing. Strictures are surprisingly rare after cuff erosion.

If the erosion is "clean" and uncomplicated, removing only the cuff and using a stainless steel tubing plug to temporarily occlude the tube leading to the pump sometimes are successful. Generous irrigation of the surrounding area with antibiotic solutions and drainage may prevent subsequent infection around the device components. Several weeks later, after complete healing with no evidence of infection, a new cuff may be inserted. In the case of the urethral cuff, another location around the bulbar portion is selected. For the bladder neck the same site may be selected, but because of technical difficulty placement of the cuff cannot be guaranteed.

We have used two techniques to facilitate replacement of a bladder neck cuff.

1. The eroded opening in the bladder neck is closed with absorbable suture. The area is generously irrigated with antibiotic solution. A thin strap of silicone about 2 cm wide is passed around the bladder neck in the cuff bed and is retained loosely. If infection is avoided, reoperation and cuff placement are facilitated by the plane maintained by the silicone strap.
2. The eroded bladder neck is closed and irrigated. The peritoneum is opened, and the omentum is tailored so a tongue of this structure can be placed under and around the bladder neck. Redissection of the plane around the bladder neck is thus facilitated.

Infection

Purulent infection of the implanted sphincter may appear as: (a) an abscess and drainage from the incisions; (b) pain, swelling, and induration of the pump or cuff site; (c) fever; (d) pump erosion through the skin; or (e) cuff erosion. It is not always clear whether cuff erosion is the result of an underlying infection or is caused by pressure necrosis. Treatment generally requires removal of the sphincter. Although drainage of the infected pyogenic process around a sphincter component can be attempted with drains and antibiotic solutions, most devices must be removed for ultimate resolution of the infection. Reimplantation can be done later with the same inherent risks as those in patients with previous cuff erosion.

Mechanical Malfunction

The mechanical reliability of the AS 800 sphincter is a remarkable tribute to biomechanical engineering. Compared with all other sphincter models, this device is relatively trouble-free. Potential risks are tubing kinks, system leaks, and control pump malfunction.

From December 1982 to January 1986, we implanted 221 AS 800 sphincters. The mechanical reliability is depicted in the life table (Fig. 33–10). To date, only six reoperations have been required: two cuff leaks, two tubing kinks, one pump malfunction, and one connector leak. All repairs were satisfactory. Although the exact longevity of this device cannot be predicted, it appears that the 5-year reliability rate will be more than 90 percent.

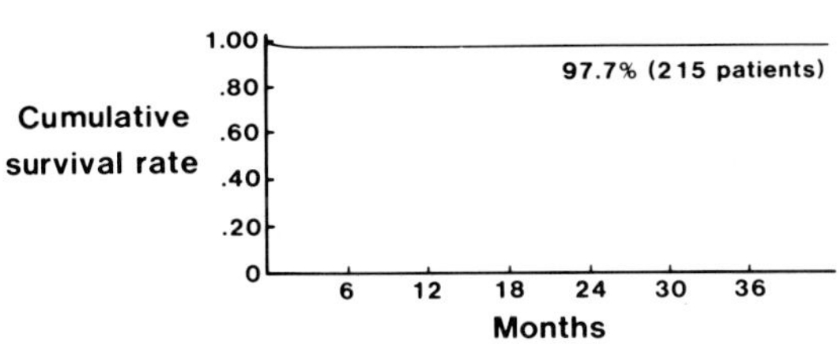

Figure 33–10. Mechanical reliability of the AS 800 artificial sphincter in 221 implantations.

Recurrent or Persistent Incontinence

Recurrent urinary incontinence after successful reimplantation requires a systematic means of defining the problem. An "inflate–deflate" radiograph confirms the hydraulic function of the device. If the radiopaque fluid is not present in the system a leak has occurred, but the exact location cannot be determined without surgical exploration (*22*).

In our experience, the most common site for leakage is the lower surface of the cuff. The leaking point may be small and not easily identifiable without removal of the cuff and close inspection. Because the cuff is the most difficult component to expose surgically, we recommend excluding leaks at the connector site and balloon stem before dissecting and removing the cuff. If fluid is present but the cuff fails to refill after pump compression, there may be a kink in the tubing or obstruction to the flow within the pump assembly. Again, surgical exploration is required to more adequately locate the obstruction. If radiography confirms normal deflation and inflation of the sphincter cuff, a urethrogram followed by direct-vision urethroscopy can exclude cuff erosion.

A urethral pressure profile of the cuff while inflated and deflated allows determination of the closing pressure differential. However, quantitating the closing pressure may be misleading. A pressure differential of 40 cm H_2O usually is associated with enough closing pressure to afford satisfactory continence. Unfortunately, this rule is not absolute; associated detrusor hyperreflexia and decreased detrusor compliance adversely influence differential pressure. If the differential pressure is low, an increase in balloon reservoir pressure may enhance urinary control.

Fourteen of 221 patients in our series underwent surgery for an increase in balloon pressure to enhance the degree of continence. Five of these patients were unsatisfactorily wet after initial activation of the first device. The other nine became insidiously incontinent some months after activation, presumably because of pressure atrophy of the tissue under the cuff, which ultimately results in reduced closing pressure.

Reduction in cuff size is another option to

be considered for compensation of recurrent or persistent incontinence in a patient with an otherwise normally functioning sphincter. The assumption is that because of erroneous measurement or underlying tissue atrophy the closed cuff cannot adequately compress the underlying urethra or bladder neck. Radiographs of this phenomenon are not helpful other than to confirm filling of the cuff. Differential closing pressure may be useful but, again, is misleading at times.

Our policy for persistent or recurrent incontinence in patients with bulbous urethral cuff placement is to increase balloon pressure to the next highest pressure category (e.g., from 51–60 cm H_2O to 61–70 cm H_2O) if the initial cuff size is 5.5 cm or less. If the cuff size is more than 5.5 cm, we change the balloon pressure upward, reexplore the cuff, and downgrade its size at least 0.5 cm.

Because the sizes of bladder neck cuffs vary much more and dissection of the implanted cuff is somewhat more difficult, we are inclined to increase the balloon pressure initially. An intraoperative urethral closing pressure differential may be useful in this situation. If the closing pressure is not increased appreciably with the new balloon pressurized in the system, exploration and down-sizing of the cuff are the next options.

Despite optimal sphincter function and closing pressure, unacceptable incontinence occasionally persists. Results may be improved by pharmacologic agents, e.g., propantheline and oxybutynin to decrease detrusor contractility or imipramine to enhance outlet resistance and decrease contractility.

SPECIAL CONSIDERATIONS

Inadequate detrusor compliance or hyperreflexia have historically excluded many patients from sphincter implantation. Bladder augmentation techniques have increased the need for sphincter implantation (Fig. 33–11). Reports of combined augmentation cystoplasty and sphincter implantation emphasize the need for caution in this select group of patients. Light and Engelmann (*23*), Light (*24*), and Light and Scott (*25*) mentioned the use of the sphincter around bowel segments used as total bladder replacements. We have had good short-term success in placing the sphincter cuff around a portion of bladder neck remnant while augmenting the bladder with split segments of colon or ileum. Our experience with the sphincter cuff around bowel has not been satisfactory to date.

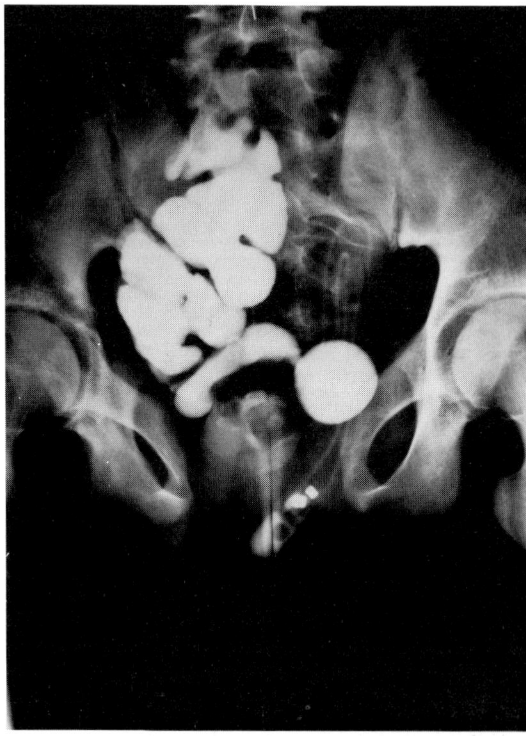

Figure 33–11. Cystogram showing cecocystoplasty and an AS 800 artificial sphincter with the cuff open.

RESULTS

What constitutes an optimal result in patients with an artificial sphincter depends on the continence afforded by the device, safety to the tissues of the urinary tract, preservation of sexual function, and mechanical reliability of the device.

Although there are reports of upper tract decompensation related to sphincter implantation, in our experience it has been uncommon. Failure to empty adequately predisposes the patient to relative ureterovesical obstruction or reflux with resulting hydronephrosis and urosepsis. Regular indefinite follow-up of the sphincter patient to ensure upper tract stability and adequate emptying is mandatory, and in doing so most upper tract problems can be avoided.

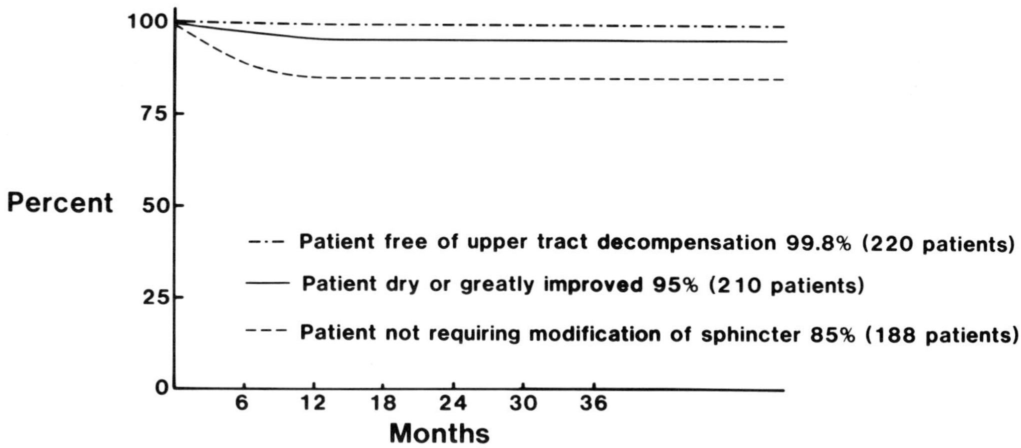

Figure 33–12. Successful implantation of an AS 800 artificial sphincter in 221 patients.

We have not noted a significant change in erectile function in men or problems with intromission in women after implantation. Two women achieved pregnancy, and the babies were delivered by cesarean section.

The percentage of successful implants in our series of 221 patients (203 men, 18 women) is reflected in Figure 33–12. Of the male group, 171 had implants at the bulbous urethra. Five devices were removed because of infection and three because of erosion (five from the bulbous urethra and three from the bladder neck). Four of these devices were successfully reimplanted.

Seven patients with functioning sphincter devices are somewhat improved but unacceptably wet and must wear multiple pads or diapers for protection. Thus, including successful reoperations, the acceptably dry rate is 95 percent (210 patients).

FUTURE CONSIDERATIONS

Prosthetic implants for the management of urinary incontinence have evolved rapidly. This progress is a tribute to biomedical engineering and the persistence of the clinician to constantly improve on the status quo. Our creativity with prosthetic materials and design concepts has many problem areas we must pursue. There is no doubt that the future will provide exciting new advances not only to combat incontinence and impotence but also in terms of replacements for the bladder, ureter, vas deferens, and urethra.

REFERENCES

1. Berry, J. L.: A new procedure for correction of urinary incontinence: preliminary report. *J. Urol.* 85:771–775, 1961.
2. Kaufman, J. J.: A new operation for male incontinence. *Surg. Gynecol. Obstet.* 131:295–299, 1970.
3. Foley, F. E. B.: An artificial sphincter: a new device and operation for control of enuresis and urinary incontinence. *J. Urol.* 58:250–259, 1947.
4. Scott, F. B., Bradley, W. E., Timm, G. W., and Kothari, D.: Treatment of incontinence secondary to myelodysplasia by an implantable prosthetic urinary sphincter. *South. Med. J.* 66:987–990, 1973.
5. Scott, F. B., Bradley, W. E., and Timm, G. W.: Treatment of urinary incontinence by an implantable prosthetic urinary sphincter. *J. Urol.* 112:75–80, 1974.
6. Rosen, M.: A simple artificial implantable sphincter. *Br. J. Urol.* 48:675–680, 1976.
7. *Artificial Urinary Sphincter Investigational Study Group.* American Medical Systems, Minnetonka, MN, 1980.
8. Furlow, W. L.: Implantation of a new semiautomatic artificial genitourinary sphincter: experience with primary activation and deactivation in 47 patients. *J. Urol.* 126:741–744, 1981.
9. Barrett, D. M., and Furlow, W. L.: Implantation of a new semi-automatic artificial genitourinary sphincter: experience with patients utilizing a new concept of primary and secondary activation. *Prog. Clin. Biol. Res.* 78:375–386, 1981.
10. Furlow, W. L., and Barrett, D. M.: The artificial urinary sphincter: experience with the AS 800 pump-control assembly for single-stage primary deactivation and activation—a preliminary report. *Mayo Clin. Proc.* 60:255–258, 1985.
11. Barrett, D. M., and Furlow, W. L.: The management of severe urinary incontinence in patients with myelodysplasia by implantation of the AS 791/792 urinary sphincter device. *J. Urol.* 128:484–486, 1982.

12. Mitchell, M. E., and Rink, R. C.: Experience with the artificial urinary sphincter in children and young adults. *J. Pediatr. Surg.* 18:700–705, 1983.
13. Light, J. K., and Scott, F. B.: Management of urinary incontinence in women with the artificial urinary sphincter. *J. Urol.* 134:476–478, 1985.
14. Donovan, M. G., Barrett, D. M., and Furlow, W. L.: Use of the artificial urinary sphincter in the management of severe incontinence in females. *Surg. Gynecol. Obstet.* 161:17–20, 1985.
15. Scott, F. B.: The use of the artificial sphincter in the treatment of urinary incontinence in the female patient. *Urol. Clin. North Am.* 12:305–315, 1985.
16. Barrett, D. M., and Furlow, W. L.: Artificial urinary sphincter in the management of female incontinence. In Raz, S. (ed.), *Female Urology.* Saunders, Philadelphia, 1983, pp. 284–292.
17. Barrett, D. M.: Female incontinence and the artificial urinary sphincter. In Kaufman, J. J. (ed.), *Current Urologic Therapy,* 2nd ed. Saunders, Philadelphia, 1986, pp. 273–275.
18. Barrett, D. M., and Furlow, W. L.: Radical prostatectomy incontinence and the AS791 artificial urinary sphincter. *J. Urol.* 129:528–530, 1983.
19. Barrett, D. M., and Furlow, W. L.: Artificial urinary sphincter in children. In Kelalis, P. P., King, L. R., and Belman, A. B. (eds.), *Clinical Pediatric Urology.* Saunders, Philadelphia, 1985, pp. 345–354.
20. Barrett, D. M.: Voiding dysfunction in children and the use of the artificial sphincter to correct sphincteric incontinence in the female child. In *Proceedings of the Symposium "Female Bladder Voiding Disburbances,"* December 1983, Milan.
21. Barrett, D. M., and Furlow, W. L.: Incontinence, intermittent self-catheterization and the artificial genitourinary sphincter. *J. Urol.* 132:268–269, 1984.
22. Webster, G. D., and Sihelnik, S. A.: Troubleshooting the malfunctioning Scott artificial urinary sphincter. *J. Urol.* 131:269–272, 1984.
23. Light, J. K., and Engelmann, U. H.: Reconstruction of the lower urinary tract: observations on bowel dynamics and the artificial urinary sphincter. *J. Urol.* 133:594–597, 1985.
24. Light, J. K.: The artificial urinary sphincter in children: experience with the AS 800 series and bowel reconstruction. *Urol. Clin. North Am.* 12:103–109, 1985.
25. Light, J. K., and Scott, F. B.: Total reconstruction of the lower urinary tract using bowel and the artificial urinary sphincter. *J. Urol.* 131:953–956, 1984.

Appendix
Use of Computers in Urodynamic Investigations

Appendix I
General Considerations

AUGUST E. J. L. KRAMER, Ph.D., AND UDO JONAS, M.D.

COMPUTERS IN URODYNAMICS: PAST

Computer applications in urodynamics began with the processing of huge amounts of data for statistical or other complex calculations or sorting. As is the case with most evolutionary steps, the actual beginnings are hidden in history. However, a trace can be found in 1964 when Scott *et al.* (*1*) coded their variables on punched cards for statistical analyses. The values found for various parameters in healthy men were compared to those obtained in patients grouped according to certain criteria (*2*). Gleason *et al.* (*3,4*) entered the digitized data from pressure, volume, and flow rate measurements by sampling the graphs manually every second and added clinical results from cystoscopy, cystography, urinalysis, and cultures. They created a composite micturition from the data of 269 patients and computed bladder wall tension and distal urethral diameter during voiding from the composed data. They also correlated the urodynamic findings with the clinical data in the patient groups assembled from the clinical diagnosis. Sundblad (*5*) followed a similar procedure.

Eyrick *et al.* (*6*) scrutinized the energy losses along the urethra during a period of steady flow from data derived from the urethrogram, and the pressure and the flow rate by rigorous application of the hydrodynamic equations. They digitized the two-dimensional geometry of the urethra from the urethrograms (*6*).

Cardus *et al.* (*7*) demonstrated the feasibility of a digitizing tablet for processing the urodynamic curves but also mentioned the need for a fully automatic digitizing process to circumvent this tedious task. Byrne *et al.* (*8*) used this last method to digitize measurements of flow rate, stream force, and bladder pressure in 0.2-second samples. The computer corrected for flow rate lag and calculated energy parameters.

Zinner *et al.* (*9*), with their drop spectrometer, presented an instrument that was essentially dependent on the availability of computer processing of the data. Coolsaet *et al.* (*10–12*) made extensive use of computer methods to develop their model of the bladder wall function *in vitro* and to apply the results to cystometry data. Schäfer (*13*) used the computer to represent the voiding data in curves that allow interpretation in physiologic parameters.

COMPUTERS IN URODYNAMICS: PRESENT

Computers now are regularly used in clinical fields for statistical procedures and for an easy check of existing data on the patient in the hospital's information system. In most of these cases it is not even specified that the data have been computer-processed. It must be appreciated, however, that much of the knowledge gained today would have become available much later, if at all, were it not for the speed and the reliability of the computer in processing the data.

Vast clinical drug trials, even multicentered ones, are performed according to standardized procedures and reported in standardized form to central computer institutes for evaluation. Ranges of normal values for various urodynamic parameters are defined from the collected material of single groups or from data in the literature. New clinically promising variables are found by the grouping of data and looking at decision boundaries, correlations, or interrelations, or by calculation from the measurement data to some value that has proved its worth in model studies. Types of studies are now being performed that would have been impossible without computer-aided analysis of the data.

Urodynamic Studies with Computer Evaluation

Susset *et al.* (*14*) analyzed several parameters of the flow rates of healthy men by computer using a specially designed protocol. They compared their data with those of patients with lower tract obstruction (*15*) and concluded that the maximal flow rate was the most sensitive single parameter. Their comparisons of the patient's flow curves to flow templates existing of the highest and lowest flow curves for the voided volume are illustrative but were not worked out. Their data were used later by Siroky *et al.* (*16,17*) to construct nomograms for maximal and average flow rate in dependence of volume voided and to judge the flow rates of obstructed men by these nomograms. These authors also concluded that the maximal flow rate is the most sensitive.

Jonas *et al.* (*18*) used a computer protocol (*19*) in an attempt to establish standards for cystometry, flowmetry, and urethral pressure profilometry. Although statistically significant differences were found between the data from their patient groups mutually and in comparison with "normal" values, the overlap was too great to reach decisive conclusions for an individual patient.

Donkervoort *et al.* (*20,21*) coded a number of clinical data, both subjective and objective, together with drop spectrometer criteria (*22,23*) to test drug effects versus placebo in double-blind noncrossover trials in patients with prostatic hypertrophy. They found no significant improvements either clinically or urodynamically in the drug groups.

Kondo *et al.* (*24*) used a digitizing tablet to feed 1-second samples of normal flow curves to the computer. Their results are presented in a number of regression lines with the voided volume. Rollema *et al.* (*25,26*) stored the flow rate trends on analog tapes that were afterward sampled and processed by computer. In our department Gallandat Huet *et al.* (*23*), Baldew (*27*), and Platenkamp (*28*) collected the data from drop spectrometer studies in digital form for computer processing. All these authors concluded that the flow rates are highly dependent on the voided volume and hardly on age, and that the concept of symmetrical distributions (*14*) in the definition of flow rate nomograms (*16*) is false (cf. *29*). They confirmed once again the great variability and overlap in data from urodynamic studies and consequently the vague decision boundaries between normal and patient values for urodynamic criteria.

Alternative ways of displaying the urodynamic data are proposed, e.g., by simply eliminating the time variable in two trend curves (*25,30–34*). These displays might be based on existing theoretical models or enhance the development of new ones (*34,35*). On the other hand, physiologic criteria that prove essential in model studies can be computed from clinical measurements to assess their clinical importance (*36–38*). Automated analysis of electromyographic (EMG) data (*39,40*) extends the basic analysis of the information contained in these signals. The computer averaging of electroencephalographic (EEG) signals even opens the possibility to study cerebral effects of urodynamic procedures (*41*).

Direct on-line processing of the urodynamic recordings has been performed (*42–48*), and an algorithm for computer-aided diagnosis has been developed (*49,50*). There exist various concepts that can be used to perform on-line computerized urodynamics, and those have been reviewed by Regnier (*50a*).

COMPUTERIZED URODYNAMIC INVESTIGATION

The system described here has been developed by the authors for application in their own department. It is presented as an example; and although details may be different, other investigators have developed their systems guided by the same concepts (*42,44,47,48*).

Hardware

This system (Fig. Ax–1) has been developed to function on a general-purpose microcomputer-based system (Digital Equipment Corporation, PDP 11/23). Four analog data channels are registered on-line. The four channels are sampled synchronously at a rate of 10 per second for each channel. This rate was considered adequate for the representation of urodynamic signals. The data are coded in eight-bit bytes (i.e., an accuracy of 1 in 256). The analog-to-digital converter is directly controlled by the central processing unit (CPU). The video terminal is used to control the program flow and to exchange messages with the CPU. The collected data are temporarily stored on floppy disks fitting 3.5 hours of continuous recording. Permanent storage is possible on these same diskettes, but they also can be read into the data base of a larger computer system. Hard copies of registrations are prepared on the printer/plotter.

The system can be easily adapted for implementation in other computer types comprising similar peripheral equipment.

Software

Pressure-flow studies or two types of urethral pressure profile studies have been programmed. During a cystometry and flow study, the intravesical and abdominal pressure, the flow rate, and the integrated EMG of the urethral sphincter are recorded. The urethral pressure studies accommodate intravesical pressure and up to three urethral pressure channels; the remaining channels are available for other variables, e.g., abdominal pressure and EMG.

The software is menu-based (Table Ax–1): After the system has been started up a program can be chosen from various possibilities. Some service programs, e.g., preparing the diskettes, are available, and the various sections in the urodynamics programs can be entered. From each section of

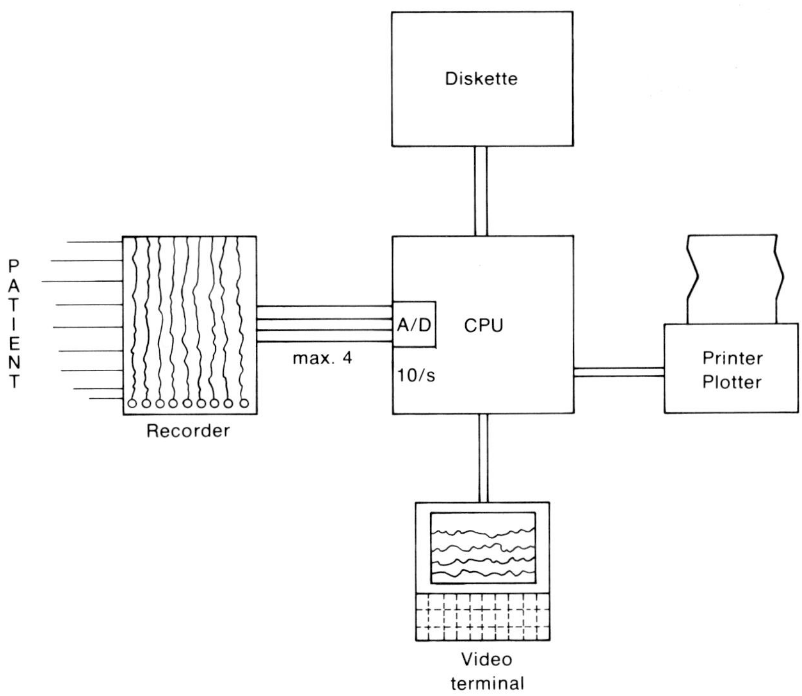

Figure Ax–1. Computer urodynamics block scheme.

Table Ax–1. Arrangement of the Urodynamics Software

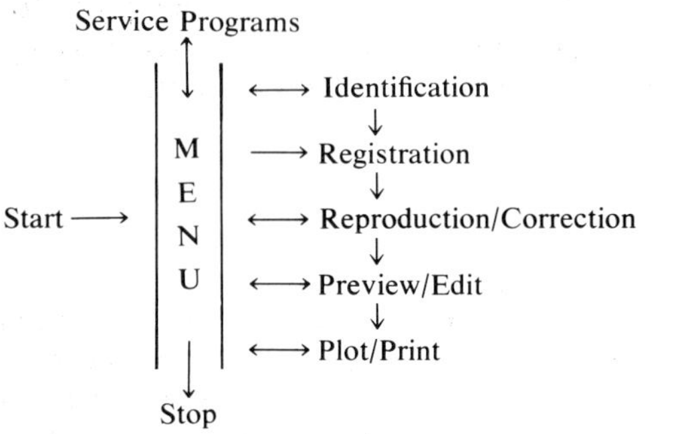

Table Ax–2. Variables to be Entered in Identification Section

1. Investigator name
2. Date of investigation (equals system date)
3. Patient name
4. Patient number
5. Date of birth
6. Sex
7. Height
8. Weight
9. Earlier urodynamics (Y/N: yes/no)
10. Position
    a. Supine
    b. Sitting
    c. Standing
    d. Telemetry
11. Type of investigation
    a. Cystometry and flow
    b. Urethral pressure profile
    c. Continuous urethral pressure

12–14. Sensitivities channels 1–4
15. Filling rate
16. Flow meter delay

Free text: 20 lines of 80 characters

the urodynamics programs the next can be entered directly. Returning to the menu is also possible except for the registration section, which is always followed directly by the reproduction/correction section. This measure was taken to ensure the validity of the data that are saved after the investigation. An example of a computerized cystometry and flow study is presented in the next sections to illustrate the practical use of this system.

Identification Section. The identification section is used for inclusion in the data files of patient and investigation identification and different preset parameters of the investigation, e.g., channel sensitivities and filling rate (Table Ax–2). Setting a channel sensitivity of 0 means the absence of recording in the particular channel.

Registration Section. In this example no EMG was recorded, and only three registration channels are reproduced: intravesical pressure, abdominal pressure, and flow rate. The registration section starts with definition of the reference levels for the various recorded variables. When the patient is fully prepared for the investigation, the four channels are sampled at a rate of 100 per second each. The samples are displayed on the video terminal as moving graphs. The transducers are leveled to their reference positions, and the average values of the offsets during 1 second are taken as the reference values.

Following this procedure the video terminal screen is put into the split screen mode and prepared for registration of the investigation. The channels now are sampled at 10 per second. Both parts of the screen are used to display the registrations as wrap-over graphs. One graph (Fig. Ax–2A) has a total length of 100 seconds of registration at 0.8-second intervals. For each curve the *highest* value of the eight preceding samples is plotted, as the highest value is thought to carry clinical importance. The other graph (Fig. Ax–2B) represents 30 minutes at 25.6-second intervals. Again the highest value from the preceding 256 is taken for each channel. The reference values are defined as zero for the various channels. In the pressure recordings, a negative deviation from this reference can be recorded up to one-fifth of the total pressure range; the flow rate can only be positive. In the present example, the sensitivities of the channels are such that $-56 \leftrightarrow +200$ cm H_2O pressures and a flow rate $0 \leftrightarrow 25.6$ ml/s can be reproduced. The eight-bit representation of the data thus implies an accuracy of, respectively, 1 cm H_2O and 0.1 ml/s. The flow rate recording is shifted backward in time to correct for the flowmeter's delay, 1 second in this example. This time shift is seen in Figure Ax–2A. All channels are jammed synchronously by electronic interference, which is displayed in the flow channel 1 second earlier.

During the investigation, events can be coded or other information entered by the investigator from the terminal keyboard. The events list recognized by the system is

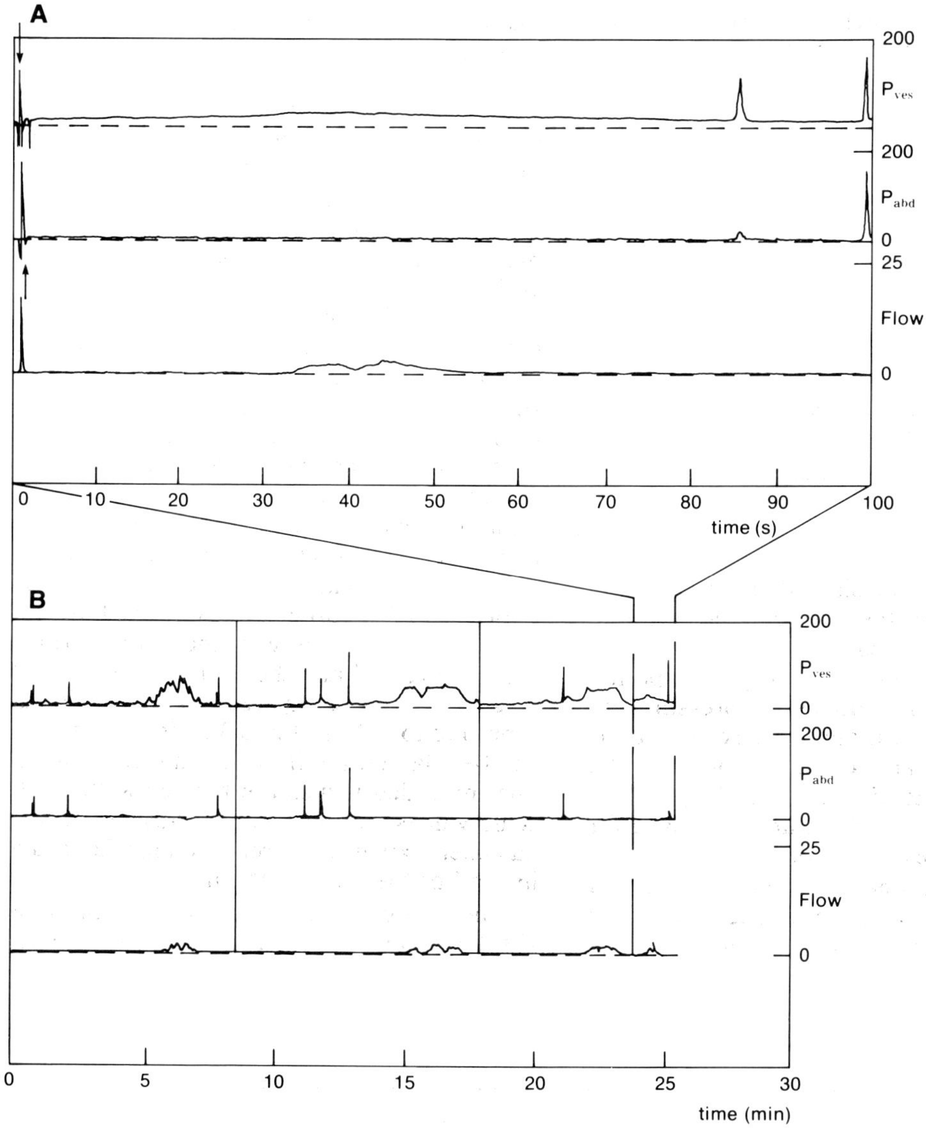

Figure Ax–2. Video terminal graphs during registration. **A.** A 100-second wrap-over graph. Note the flowmeter lag correction (*arrows*). **B.** A 30-minute wrap-over graph. Vertical scale: pressures are in centimeters of H_2O; flow rate is in milliliters per second.

shown in Table Ax–3. Events in this list imply certain preprogrammed actions on the data to be performed in a later stage. The event codes and the time of entering are stored in an event file. This file also keeps track of the start and stop times of, and any pauses during, the investigation.

Reproduction/Correction Section. After registration the raw data (Fig. Ax–3) may contain artifacts, erroneously recorded or timed event marks, or unrecorded events. In the reproduction/correction section the video terminal is used for interactive communication with the computer. The raw data are displayed in graphs using the full screen in steps of 10 minutes each (Fig. Ax.–4A). Artifacts can be eliminated by marking begin and end times with cursors and connecting the appropriate begin and end values by a straight line. It might affect only one (Fig. Ax–4B) or more (Fig. Ax–4C) channels at the same time. Any events that were incor-

Table Ax–3. List of Events Recognized by the Program

After contraction
Artifact
Capacity
Cough
Detrusor instability
End inhibition
Filling start/stop
First sensation
Incontinence
Inhibit
Lie down
Sit up
Stand up
Strain
Stop investigation (pause or end)
Stop voiding (voluntary)
Voiding

rectly entered can be discarded now from the files or shifted to the correct time position. The program automatically recognizes any flow that occurs during the displayed period or any change in intravesical pressure exceeding 5 cm H_2O. If any of these conditions was not marked already, it is brought to the investigator's attention by a flashing cursor at the appropriate position and a demand for the entry of an event code.

Preview/Edit Section. The corrected data now can be processed to produce parameters of interest. Depending on the type of investigation and the event code, various parameters are calculated. In this example maximal voiding pressure, maximal flow rate, voided volume, and residual volume are computed for each voiding. The presence of detrusor instability and the intermittency of micturition are recognized. No incontinence occurred during the investigation. These parameters are printed out later together with a graphic representation of the results to be included in the patient's hospital file. To obtain the graphic reproduction in a format that is easier to interpret than that given in Fig. Ax–3 and yet that is as compact as feasible, it was decided to abandon the linear time scale for a changing one (Fig. Ax–5). In principle, three paper speeds are used: 0.5 mm/s for fast events such as coughing, 0.1 mm/s for events such as voiding and detrusor contractions, and 1 mm/min for those periods in which no fast changes are found in any channel. In this way the latter periods are compressed and the first ones expanded (Fig. Ax–5A) compared to the original reproduction (Fig. Ax–5B). Vertical scales can be adapted too if, for instance, the maximal recorded values are far below the full-scale values. In this case the flow rate scale has been expanded to read 10 ml/s full scale instead of the normal 25 ml/s.

The recalculated graphic representation is displayed on the video terminal together with

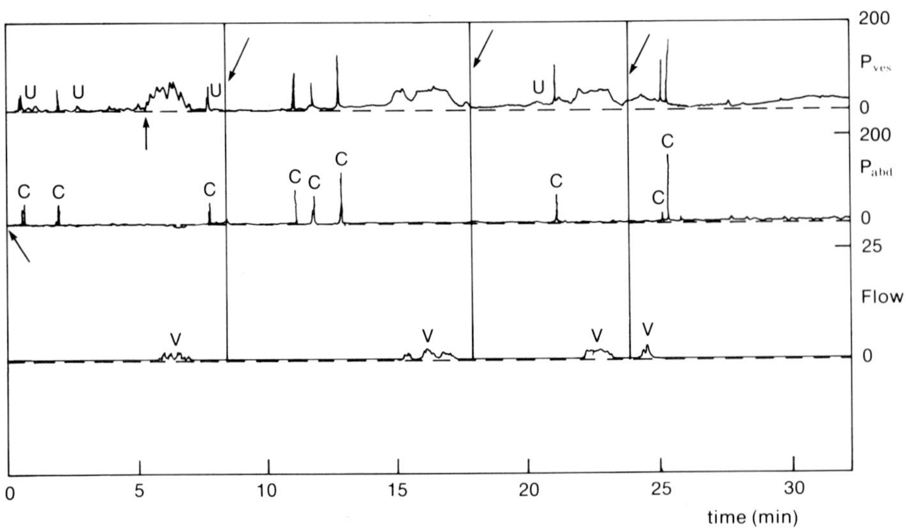

Figure Ax–3. Overview of raw data for a 32-minute recording. Vertical scale: pressures are in centimeters of H_2O; flow rate is in milliliters per second. *Arrows:* artifacts. *C* = coughing. *U* = unstable bladder. *V* = voiding.

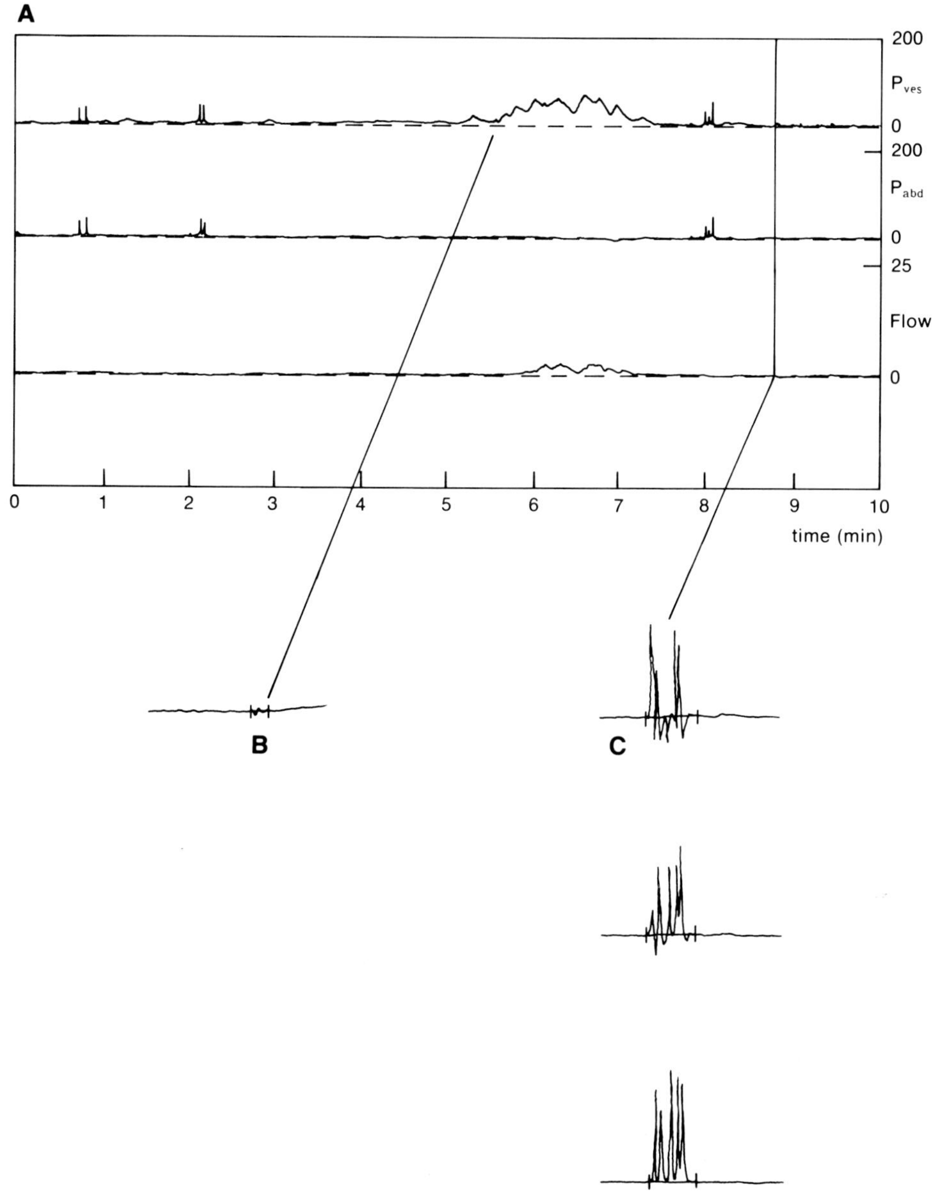

Figure Ax–4. **A.** A 10-minute episode in the reproduction/correction phase. Artifacts may affect only one channel (**B**) or all channels synchronously (**C**); they are corrected by enclosing them in markers and linearly connecting the begin and end points. Vertical scale: pressures are in centimeters of H_2O; flow rate is in milliliters per second. **B, C.** Time base × 10.

the parameters and forms a preview possibility for the final hard copy. Interactively again, the investigator may ask for changes in the display, e.g., scale changes either in time or in sensitivity.

A file is produced now for permanent storage. Data from compressed periods are skipped to reduce the size of this file, and the calculated parameters and identification data are added. This total information can be kept in a data bank for later statistics or reference use. Storage of the parameters only (*44*) would reduce the size even more drastically; however, this method was believed to impede the utility of the permanent file as a data bank, especially if in future new models

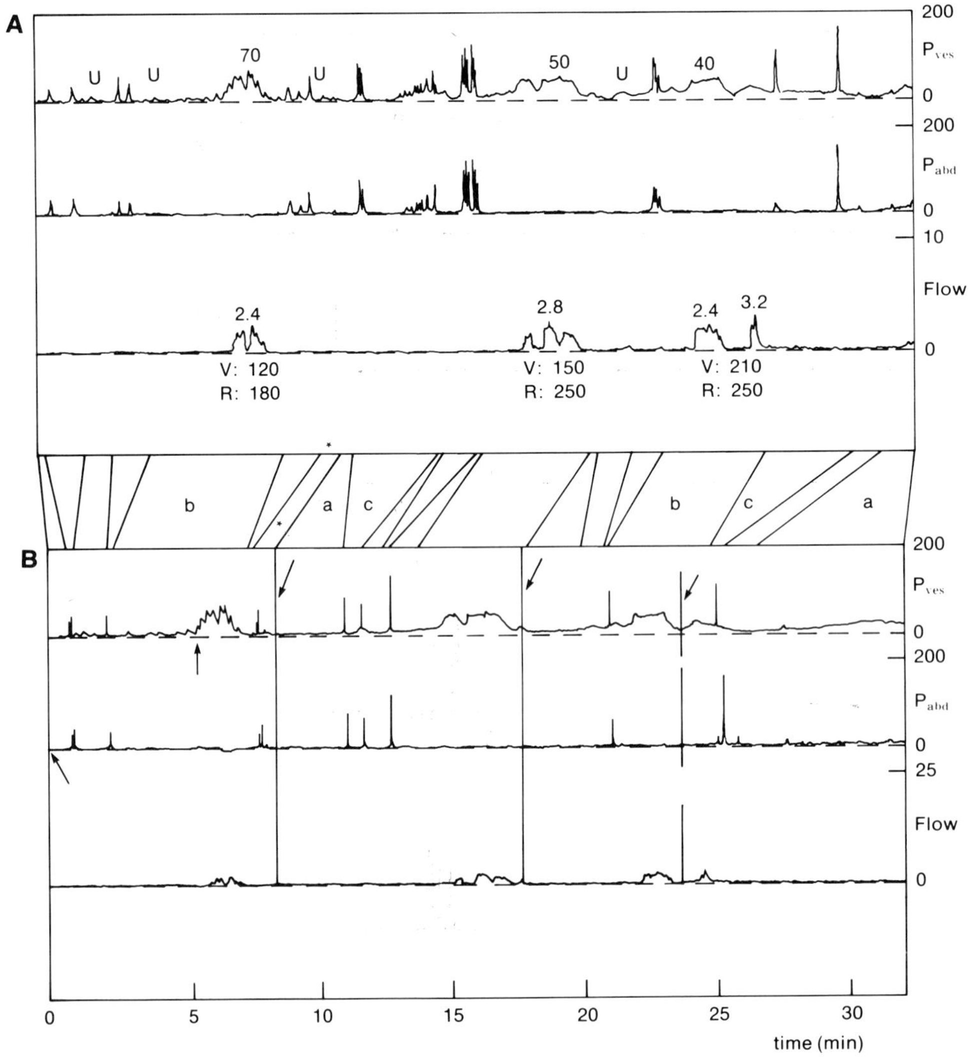

Figure Ax–5. Rescaled preview graphs of total recording (*upper part*) are ready for hard copy. Compared to the original raw data recording (*lower part;* cf. Figure Ax–3), the edited graphs feature nonlinear time scaling because of compression (a-episodes), direct reproduction (b-episodes), or extension (c-episodes) of the time scale and redefinition of resolution (flow rate scale). Artifacts have been removed (*arrows*) and various remarks inprinted on the curves. U=unstable bladder. V=voiding, voided volume. R=estimated residual volume. *:Bladder emptied by catheter. Figures: $P_{ves,\ max}$ resp. Q_{max}. Pressures are in centimeters of H_2O; flow rates are in milliliters per second; volumes are in milliliters.

evolved in urodynamics perhaps pointing to other important parameters.

Plot/Print Section. The hard copy for the patient's hospital record is an exact reproduction of the video screen display from the last section (Fig. Ax–6). Identification data and parameters are printed next to the curves. Parameters also may be printed in the curves at the appropriate times. The total record of the investigation fits on one sheet.

Advantages of Computerized Urodynamics

In addition to the advantage of a handy format for the hospital file, computerized urodynamics enables perfectly objective interpretation of the data, elimination of possible artifacts in the recorded material, the change of time resolution of recorded episodes after the recording has taken place,

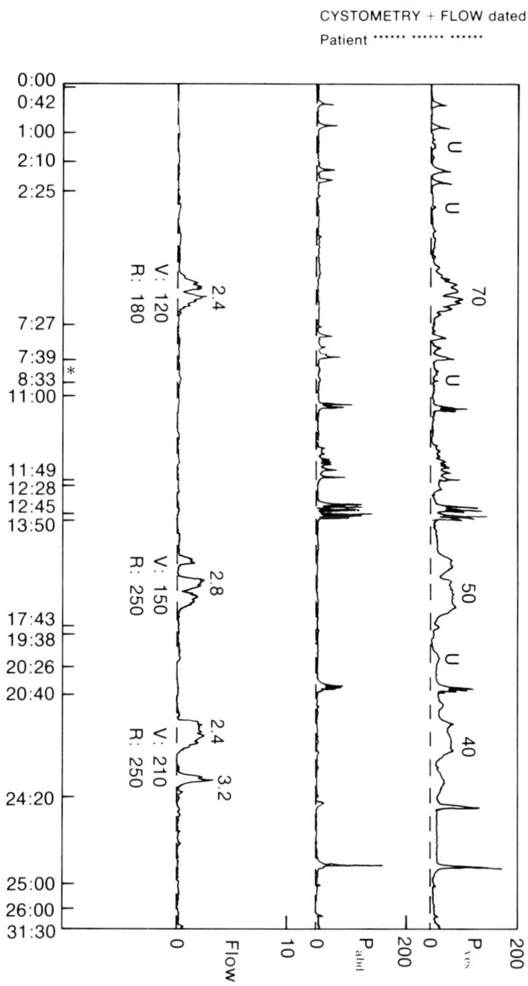

Fill rate:	50 ml/min		
Unstable bladder:	Y		
Incontinence:	N		
Voiding #:	1	2	3
$P_{ves,max}$:	70	50	40
Q_{max}:	2.4	2.8	3.2
Intermittency:	N	Y	Y
Volume voided:	120	150	210
Residual volume:	180	250	250

*: bladder emptied by catheter

Figure Ax–6. Final patient file recording of urodynamic investigation includes identification data and various parameters. Pressures are in centimeters of H_2O; flow rates are in milliliters per second; volumes are in milliliters.

easy reconnaissance by algorithm of well defined features both during and after the investigation, easy retrieval of patient data if later necessary, and easy access for retrospective (statistical) evaluation, be it for follow-up of the same patient or for group comparisons in pathology groups.

COMPUTER IN URODYNAMICS: FUTURE

Zinner (*51*) presented a "changes list" consisting of 75 items that could in future affect urologic practice. Five of these changes are directly related to computer usage but mainly in the form of fast-accessible data banks. The most challenging one on the list is number 11: *Mandatory use of computers in diagnosis and treatment.*

Indeed, if the point is reached where the computer can be the first adviser proposing (differential) diagnostics and suggesting possible therapy (*52*), benefit can probably be drawn from the collected knowledge that now is often difficult to grasp. However, much more work is necessary, by man as well as by computer, before this goal can be attained.

Rada (*53*) indicated the shallowness of the available data bases, the poor theoretical knowledge of the logic behind the diagnostic process, and the lack of theoretical knowledge of the physiology and pathology of the human system as the major stumbling stones to the development of reliable expert data bases that could be consulted for expert advice on our patients.

Progression of the current work in computer-aided urodynamics toward this goal can be foreseen for the near future. Data bases are created by protocol-controlled investigations, the results of which are fed to the computer. Off-line protocols (*19,54*) or the combination of off-line clinical data entry and the on-line recording of measurements (*42–44,46,47*) must be standardized to allow exchange of data between investigators. Statistical multivariate analyses and pattern or cluster analyses in multiple dimensions can find sensitive criteria to discriminate between normals and various patient groups (*26,49*). Trends can be followed in longitudinal studies. Complex models, incorporating theories from the various fields that foster urodynamics, can be developed and tested for their clinical significance. The results from these clinical studies can fertilize the thinking on the models again, leading to a better understanding of the physiology behind the model.

The on-line urodynamic investigation is, in our view, only the first computerized modality. We recognize that it often is just a technical progression where microprocessors are incorporated into registration units only for the sake of ease in development and flexibility. Interesting features from registrations, however, can then be edited for the user by the registration system itself (*45,55,56*). The next step might well be the coupling of such a system to a computer-interpreted radiology session, enabling the automatic evaluation of videocystometry.

In both cases the algorithms can be easily changed to select new items if new criteria must be used as the result of further investigations in model studies or of clinical developments. Moreover, the existing data base of urodynamic investigations can be used for a retrospective study on the significance of eventual new criteria.

Neurophysiologic investigations can be extended to interpret on this basis any neurologic disorders by automatic searching for deviating potentials or delay times, by averaging the signals in time or in frequency, or by untangling an intricate pattern of responses.

A computer-aided urodynamic diagnosis expert system (*46,49*) has been developed based on anamnestic data and quantitative criteria for combined parameters of urodynamic studies taken from a huge data bank. Further research can bring new parameters or longitudinal trends from the urodynamic investigations that prove to be of value for the diagnosis of lower tract pathology and thus increase the efficiency of such an automated diagnosis.

CONCLUSION

The present state of the art of computer technology makes the digital computer a well-shaped tool in urodynamics research. Although "There will never be a substitute for a careful clinical history, . . . " (*57*) and "despite sophisticated equipment, the examiner is still the key figure in diagnosing urodynamic disturbances" (*18*), it is our opinion that at this moment on-line computing in the urodynamics laboratory is feasible and rewarding. A complete history can be taken efficiently with the aid of a computer program (*50*). In the field of instrumentation, the direct advantages are the objective interpretation and the editing facilities for urodynamic curves; indirectly, the creation of urodynamic data banks will be rewarding in the future.

Advances in model theories to describe the human system and its regulatory mechanisms will bring us nearer the goal of a full understanding of any pathologic deviations of that system and the necessary measures to restore it. The ill patient who consults a computer for treatment nevertheless at this time remains a good character for science fiction.

GLOSSARY OF COMMONLY USED TERMS

Aliasing Interpretation of the signal frequency (f_0) higher than the sampling frequency (f_s) as the frequency difference ($f_s - f_0$). Caused by taking f_s too low. See: Sampling theorem.

Alphanumeric Specific: character set from letters and numbers. Most likely taken to mean all printable text characters.

Analog signal Signal to be represented by a continuous variable.

Analog-to-digital conversion (ADC) Representation of an analog signal by a finite set of discrete values.
Bit Single unit of information: "0" or "1"; "no" or "yes."
Byte Set of coherent bits, mostly eight, treated as an entity.
Central processing unit (CPU) The "heart" of the computer; that part of the electronic setup where the instructions are interpreted and executed.
Centralized system A computer system constructed in such a way that the processing and often also the memory units are physically concentrated. Input and output may be sent on terminals in other locations.
Cluster analysis Statistical technique to study groups of data.
Continuous signal A signal that can take any value inside its range.
Decentralized system System consisting of multiple interconnected CPUs.
Discrete Representation of variable values by separate elements.
Discretization error Loss of resolution of variables by discretization.
Diskette Small flexible disk-shaped magnetic storage medium.
Flexible system Computer system that can easily be reprogrammed for different tasks.
Hard copy Nonerasable output of computer results. Mostly paper or microfiche.
Image processing Processing of data that normally become available in image format (e.g., curves or imaging techniques).
Interactive Direct contact with the computer system with immediate responses to user actions.
Measure type Observation type allowing ratios and differences to be measured.
Menu Choice of available program steps.
Microcomputer, microprocessor High-density electronic circuit containing a CPU.
Multivariate analysis Statistical technique to study differences between groups of data.
Off-line Preparation of computer data by any other system than the processor itself or processor-driven peripherals.
On-line Preparation of computer data controlled by the processor itself.
Peripheral equipment Equipment connected to the computer (terminals, printers, etc.).
Permanent storage Storage of data outside the computer memory on nonerasable media. Limited meaning: Idem on computer-readable media.
Sampling theorem To get an adequate representation, the sampling frequency must be at least twice the highest frequency of interest in the signal.
Scale type Observation type allowing differences to be measured.
Score type Observation type that allows no value relations.
Storage Saving of data in the computer memory (internal) or in any other place (external); the latter mostly meant to mean in a computer-readable format.
System Total setup of computer and peripherals, including driving programs.
Video terminal Television-type peripheral with a keyboard to communicate with the computer.
Word Set of coherent bytes, 1, 2, or 4 at present, that reflect the CPU's internal architecture (8-bit, 16-bit, or 32-bit CPU).

REFERENCES

1. Scott, F. B., Quesada, E. M., and Cardus, D.: Studies on the dynamics of micturition: observations on healthy men. *J. Urol.* 92:455–463, 1964.
2. Scott, F. B., Cardus, D., Quesada, E. M., and Riles, T.: Uroflowmetry before and after prostatectomy. *South. Med. J.* 60:948–952, 1967.
3. Gleason, D. M., Bottacini, M. R., and Lattimer, J. K.: The interrelationship of some hydrodynamic parameters of voiding. *Invest. Urol.* 5:552–556, 1968.
4. Gleason, D. M., Bottacini, M. R., and Lattimer, J. K.: Some correlations between hydrodynamic and clinical findings in the urinary tract. *J. Urol.* 100:783–786, 1968.
5. Sunblad, R.: Urinary bladder dynamics in women. *Scand. J. Urol. Nephrol.* 5:(Suppl. 6), 1–51, 1971.
6. Eyrick, T. B., Many, M., and Wise, H. M., Jr.: Analysis of urethral resistance: a clinical applicable method for evaluation of urethral dynamics. *Invest. Urol.* 6:443–465, 1969.
7. Cardus, D., Scott, F. B., and Quesada, E. M.: Computer processing of data generated in micturition studies (preliminary report). *Invest. Urol.* 4:262–266, 1966.
8. Byrne, J. C., Bottacini, M. R., and Gleason, D. M.: Energy loss during micturition. *Invest. Urol.* 10:221–225, 1972.
9. Zinner, N. R., Ritter, R. C., Sterling, A. M., and Harding, D. C.: Drop spectrometer: a non-obstructive, non-interfering instrument for analyzing hy-

drodynamic properties of human urination. *J. Urol.* 101:914–918, 1969.
10. Coolsaet, B. L. R. A., van Duyl, W. A., van Mastrigt, R., and van der Zwart, A.: Stepwise cystometry of urinary bladder. *Urology* 2:255–257, 1973.
11. Coolsaet, B. L. R. A., van Duyl, W. A., van Mastrigt, R., and van der Zwart, A.: Viscoelastic properties of the bladder wall. *Urol. Int.* 30:16–26, 1975.
12. Coolsaet, B. L. R. A., van Duyl, W. A., van Mastrigt, R., and Huygen, R. E. F.: Viscoelastic properties of bladder wall strips at constant elongation. *Invest. Urol.* 13:435–440, 1976.
13. Schäfer, W.: A computing unit for the analysis of micturition. In *Digest of the 11th International Conference on Medical and Biological Engineering,* Ottawa, 1976.
14. Susset, J. G., Picker, P., Kretz, M., and Jorest, R.: Critical evaluation of uroflowmeters and analysis of normal curves. *J. Urol.* 109:414–419, 1973.
15. Shoukry, J., Susset, J. G., Elhilali, M., and Dutartre, D.: Role of uroflowmetry in the assessment of lower urinary tract obstruction in adult males. *Br. J. Urol.* 47:559–566, 1975.
16. Siroky, M. B., Olsson, C. A., and Krane, R. J.: The flow rate nomogram. I. Development. *J. Urol.* 122:665–668, 1979.
17. Siroky, M. B., Olsson, C. A., and Krane, R. J.: The flow rate nomogram. II. Clinical correlation. *J. Urol.* 123:208–210, 1980.
18. Jonas, U., Petri, E., and Banse, B.: Evaluation of urodynamic studies by computer. *Urol. Res.* 6:141–146, 1978.
19. Jonas, U., Heidler, H., and Thüroff, J.: *Urodynamik. Diagnostik der Funktionsstorungen des unteren Harntraktes.* Ferdinand Enke Verlag, Stuttgart, 1980, pp. 76–79.
20. Donkervoort, T., Sterling, A. M., van Ness, J., Zinner, N. R., Donker, P. J., and Ritter, R. C.: Megestrol acetate in treatment of benign prostatic hypertrophy. *Urology* 6:580–587, 1975.
21. Donkervoort, T., Sterling, A. M., van Ness, J., and Donker, P. J.: A clinical and urodynamic study of tadenan in the treatment of benign prostatic hypertrophy. *Eur. Urol.* 3:218–225, 1977.
22. Zinner, N. R., Ritter, R. C., Sterling, A. M., Harding, D. C., and Baker, D. W.: Detection and location of obstruction in the human male subject by analysis of the urinary stream. *J. Urol.* 106:115–121, 1971.
23. Gallandat Huet, R. C. G., Kramer, A. E. J. L., Sterling, A. M., and Donker, P. J.: The variability of normal male voiding patterns measured by drop spectrometry. *Br. J. Urol.* 52:196–203, 1980.
24. Kondo, A., Mitsuya, H., and Torii, H.: Computer analysis of micturition parameters and accuracy of uroflowmeter. *Urol. Int.* 33:337–344, 1978.
25. Rollema, H. J., Griffiths, D. J., van Duyl, W. A., van den Berg, J. w., and de Haan, R.: Flow rate versus bladder volume: an alternative way of presenting some features of the micturition of healthy males. *Urol. Int.* 32:401–412, 1977.
26. Rollema, H. J.: Uroflowmetry in males: reference values and clinical application in benign prostatic hypertrophy. M. D. thesis, Groningen, 1981.
27. Baldew, I. M.: Drop spectrometry of the urinary stream in boys with and without nocturnal enuresis. M.D. thesis, Leiden, 1980.
28. Platenkamp, G. J. J. M.: On normal values in urine drop spectrometry. M.D. thesis, Leiden, 1981 [in Dutch].
29. Bee, D., Toguri, A., and Uchida, T.: Analysis of methods to construct nomograms in uroflow studies. In Zinner, N. R., and Sterling, A. M. (eds.), *Female Incontinence.* Alan R. Liss, New York, 1981, pp. 261–268.
30. Sterling, A. M., and Donker, P. J.: A new aspect of voiding dynamics: the relationship between flow rate and the frequency of drops in the external urinary stream. *Urol. Int.* 32:184–191, 1977.
31. Abrams, P. H., Skidmore, R., Poole, A. C., and Follett, D.: The concept and measurement of bladder work. *Br. J. Urol.* 49:133–138, 1978.
32. Griffiths, D. J., and Scholtmeyer, R.: Precise urodynamic assessment of anatomic urethral obstruction in boys. *Neurourol. Urodyn.* 1:97–104, 1982.
33. Schäfer, W.: Detrusor as the energy source of micturition. In: Hinman, F., Jr. (ed.), *Benign Prostatic Hypertrophy.* Springer-Verlag, New York, 1983, pp. 450–469.
34. Schäfer, W.: The contribution of the bladder outlet to the relation between pressure and flow rate during micturition. In: Hinman, F., Jr. (ed.), *Benign Prostatic Hypertrophy.* Springer-Verlag, New York, 1983, pp. 470–496.
35. Griffiths, D. J.: *Urodynamics. The Mechanics and Hydrodynamics of the Lower Urinary Tract.* Adam Hilger, Bristol, 1980.
36. Van Mastrigt, R.: The on-line determination of the maximal contraction velocity of the urinary bladder from an isometric contraction. In Zinner, N. R., and Sterling, A. M. (eds.), *Female Incontinence.* Alan R. Liss, New York, 1981, pp. 307–310.
37. Van Mastrigt, R., and Griffiths, D. J.: The relation between female incontinence and an extremely high maximal contraction velocity of the urinary bladder. In Zinner, N. R., and Sterling, A. M., (eds.), *Female Incontinence.* Alan R. Liss, New York, 1981, pp. 67–71.
38. Schäfer, W., Hannappel, J., Gerlach, R., and Lutzeyer, W.: Computer analysis of urodynamic data in BPH. *J. Urol.* 131:166A, 1984.
39. Puers, B., Vereecken, R., Aubert, A., and de Meirsman, J.: Frequency power spectrum analysis of sphincter electromyography. In Zinner, N. R., and Sterling, A. M. (eds.), *Female Incontinence.* Alan R. Liss, New York, 1981, pp. 151–160.
40. Vodusek, D. B.: The bulbocavernosus reflex—some physiological aspects. In *Proceedings 14th Annual Meeting International Continence Society,* Innsbruck, 1984, pp. 241–243.
41. Gerstenberg, T., Hald, T., and Meyhoff, H.: Urinary cerebral evoked potentials mediated through urethral sensory nerves: a preliminary report. In Zinner, N. R., and Sterling, A. M., (eds.), *Female Incontinence.* Alan R. Liss, New York, 1981, pp. 141–143.
42. Suhel, P., Roskar, E., Kralj, B., and Dimic, D.: Urodynamic data collection system controlled by microcomputer (UDCS). In Zinner, N. R., and

Sterling, A. M. (eds.), *Female Incontinence*. Alan R. Liss, New York, 1981, pp. 295–297.

43. Kramer, A. E. J. L., and Jonas, U.: Automatic processing of urodynamic data. In *Proceedings of the XIXth Congress of the Société Internationale d'Urologie*. Abst. no. 639:184, 1982.
44. Abrams, P. H., Lewis, P., Murray, K., and MacLachlan, D.: A computerized system for the acquisition, analysis and storage of urodynamic data. *J. Urol.* 131:166A, 1984.
45. Kramer, A. E. J. L., and Jonas, U.: Computer urodynamics—evaluation of practicability of on-line computing in the urodynamics laboratory. *J. Urol.* 131:166A, 1984.
46. Deane, A. M., Gosling, P. T., Watkinson, L., Hindmarsh, J. R., and Wickham, J. E. A.: Microcomputer digital recording and expanded graphic analysis in urethrocystometry. In *Abstracts of the 6th Congress of the European Association of Urology*, Copenhagen, 1984, p. 71.
47. Gosling, P. T., Capper, V. T., and Hindmarsh, J. R.: Development of the Institute of Urology, London, urodynamic investigation system. In *Proceedings 14th Annual Meeting International Continence Society*, Innsbruck, 1984, pp. 365–366.
48. Jacobs, S. C., Sebern, M. A., Donnell, R., and Lawson, R. K.: Computer-assisted urodynamics. *J. Urol.* 132:716–717, 1984.
49. Roskar, E., Suhel, P., Kralj, B., and Dimic, D.: Microcomputer controlled urodynamic diagnostic system. In Zinner, N. R., and Sterling, A. M. (eds.), *Female Incontinence*. Alan R. Liss, New York, 1981, pp. 299–306.
50. Roskar, E., Abrams, P. H., Torrens, M. J., and Kononenko, I.: Computer assisted derivation of urodynamic diagnostic expertise for lower urinary tract disorders. In *Proceedings 14th Annual Meeting International Continence Society*, Innsbruck, 1984, pp. 173–175.

50a. Regnier, C. H.: Current and future applications of computers in urodynamics. *Neurourol. Urodyn.* 5:343–371, 1986.

51. Zinner, N. R.: The challenge from the future. In Miranda, S. I., and de Voogt, H. J. (eds.), *Current and Future Trends in Urology*. Bunge Scientific Publishers, Utrecht, 1979, pp. 1–9.
52. Glen, E. S.: Microcomputers and microprocessors in urology: present and future. *Br. J. Urol.* 55:588–590, 1983.
53. Rada, R.: Automated medical diagnosis: a summary. In Schwartz, M. D., (ed.), *Applications of Computers in Medicine*. Institute of Electrical and Electronics Engineers, New York, 1982, pp. 188–197.
54. Abrams, P. H., Feneley, R. C. G., and Torrens, M. J.: *Urodynamics*. Springer Verlag, New York, 1983, pp. 205–209.
55. Rollema, H. J.: Microprocessor controlled interpretation of urinary flow rate curves. In *Proceedings 2nd Joint Meeting ICS–UDS*, Aachen, 1983, pp. 230–231.
56. Dijkhuis, T., Klopper, P. J., and Grimbergen, C. A.: Microcomputer-based approach to the automation of flow rate measurement: a fully automatic mictiometer. *Med. Biol. Eng. Comput.* 21:768–770, 1983.
57. Ryall, R. L., and Marshall, V. R.: Measurement of urinary flow rate. *Urology* 22:556–564, 1983.

Appendix II

Practical Applications

JEFFREY R. WOODSIDE, M.D.

The application of computers in medicine has been rapidly expanding as physicians have gained familiarity with computers and the cost of hardware and software has decreased. Sophisticated computer applications to urodynamic evaluation are evolving to store and plot urodynamic data and to assist in interpretation of the data (*1*). A useful and available application for which the computer is ideally suited is the storage and retrieval of a large volume of patient urodynamic data. Many database manager programs have been written that fulfill this need, ranging in complexity from those designed for multiinstitutional use on mainframe computers (*2*) to those for minicomputers (*3*) and microcomputers (*4,5*). A recent review of computer applications in urodynamics outlines the current trends and discusses the overall impact of computers in the everyday urodynamic practice (*7*). This chapter describes the utility of a highly user-friendly computer program that was specifically written to manage a large quantity of patient urodynamic data (*6*). Additionally, it employs a popular and affordable microcomputer and printer.

HARDWARE

Although many microcomputers and database manager programs are available, this particular system consists of a Radio Shack TRS-80 model III microcomputer (Tandy Corporation, Fort Worth, TX) with 48K RAM. It is equipped with two Tandon TM 100 40 track double-sided disk drives (Tandon Magnetics Corporation, Chatsworth, CA) that use $5\frac{1}{4}$-in. floppy diskettes. Double-sided disk drives allow storage of twice the amount of data on each diskette as is possible with the more commonly used single-sided disk drives. Radio Shack does not configure the model III with double-sided disk drives, but a computer consulting firm (J & M Systems Consultants, Ltd., Albuquerque, NM) has designed the JFD-III Floppy Disk Controller to accomplish the conversion. The powerful NEWDOS/80 operating system (Apparat, Inc., Denver, CO) then controls the double-sided disk drives. The system is completed with the Epson MX 80 Printer (Epson America, Inc., Torrance, CA), a high-quality dot matrix printer. The total cost of the hardware and software is about $3000.

SOFTWARE

The program was written in BASIC language using the NEWDOS/80 operating system. For each patient record, the demographic data include name, sex, age, date of study, the hospital name, the patient's hospital number (up to 11 spaces, allowing use of the Social Security number), if the patient was referred by an outside physician, and finally if slides were made of the urodynamic study (including the capability of using up to a six-digit number to code the slides). For all other codes under the categories listed below, three-digit codes are used.

The data are recorded under four headings: general categories, specific diagnoses, urodynamic findings, and treatment. Nine general categories were chosen, under one of which any specific diagnosis may be placed

(Fig. Ax–7). This feature is useful for retrieving, for instance, all patients studied who had urinary incontinence regardless of etiology. A maximum of three specific diagnoses may be recorded for each patient (Fig. Ax–8). Similarly, a maximum of ten urodynamic findings may be recorded (Fig. Ax–9). Not all items listed are actually urodynamic findings, i.e., intermittent catheterization, myelogram, previous surgery, etc. However, they are included in this category because it is information deemed valuable to record but

001	Spinal cord injury
002	Incontinence
003	L.T. obstr.(non-NG)
004	Systemic neurol. dis.
005	Spinal crd. dis.(non-trauma)
006	Undiversion W/U
007	Drug effects
008	Loop study
999	Miscellaneous

Figure Ax–7. Code numbers and labels for general categories. (From Woodside, J. R., and Morris, F. M.: *Neurourol. Urodynam.* 1:313–318, 1982.)

001	SCI:cervical
002	SCI:T1-6
003	SCI:T7-12
004	SCI:lumbar
005	SCI:cauda equina
006	SCI:infarction
007	Myelodysplasia
008	Occult spinal dysraphism
009	Tethered cord
010	Sacral agenesis
011	SUI-I
012	SUI-II
013	SUI-III
014	Abdominal-perineal
015	Post-Wertheim
016	Post-open prost. incont.
017	Post-TURP incont.
018	Post-radical prost. incont.
019	Giggle incontinence
020	Incont.-miscellaneous
021	Dysfunctional BNO-active
022	Dysfunctional BNO-passive
023	Bladder neck contracture
024	BPH
025	Urethral stricture
026	Enuresis
027	Reflex urethral relaxation
028	V-V fistula
029	Imperforate anus
030	Spinal cord tumor
031	Spinal cord AVM
032	Pelvic plexus injury
033	Peripheral neuropathy
034	CVA
035	ALS
036	Cerebral palsy
037	Guillain-Barre
038	MS
039	Diabetes mellitus
040	Arachnoiditis
041	Herniated disk
042	Post. urethral valves
043	NNG-NGB
044	Unstable bladder
045	Distension injury
046	Infrequent voider
047	Platysbia
048	Recurrent cystitis
049	Recurrent pyelonephritis
050	Functional void. disorder
051	Seizure disorder
052	Parkinson's disease
053	Detrusor decompensation
054	Reflux
055	Post. urethral cyst
056	Extrinsic cord compression
057	Bladder diverticulum
058	Demyelinating disease-unknown
059	Transverse myelitis
060	Olivopontocerebellar degener.
061	Pain retention
062	Poor urethral milk-back
063	Irritable bladder
064	Radiation cystitis
065	Retroperitoneal fibrosis
066	Head injury
067	Prostate carcinoma
068	Urethral syndrome
069	Autonomic neuropathy
070	Megaureter
071	Zoster neuritis
072	Syringomyelia
073	Scott sphincter
074	Meningitis
075	Spinal cord lipoma
076	Diabetes insipidus
077	Uninhibited NGB
078	Muscular dystrophy
079	Urolithiasis
080	Psychogenic polydipsia
081	Prostatitis
082	Prostatodynia
083	UPJ
084	Charcot-Marie-Tooth
085	Spinocerebellar degeneration
086	Friedreich's ataxia
999	No diagnosis

Figure Ax–8. Code numbers and labels for specific diagnoses. (From Woodside, J. R., and Morris, F. M.: *Neurourol. Urodyn.* 1:313–318, 1982.)

001	Intermitt. cath.
002	Hypotonic detrusor
003	Hypertonic detrusor
004	Areflexic detrusor
005	Hyperreflexic detrusor
006	Decompensated detrusor
007	Detrusor instability
008	Elevated voiding pressure
009	Open bladder neck
010	Low urethral pressure
011	DSD
012	DSD with cord inhibition
013	Autonomic dysreflexia
014	Bladder diverticulum
015	Cystocoele
016	Normal UDS
017	Bladder only neurol. problem
018	Myelogram
019	Hydronephrosis
020	Reflux
021	Impotence
022	Spina bifida occulta
023	Drug effect
024	Diuretic renogram
025	Previous surgery
026	Poor detrusor contraction
027	Urethral catheter
028	S.P. cystostomy

Figure Ax–9. Code numbers and labels for urodynamic findings. (From Woodside, J. R., and Morris, F. M.: *Neurourol. Urodyn.* 1:313–318, 1982.)

001	Sphincterotomy	032	Y-V plasty bladder neck
002	TURBNI	033	V-V fistula repair
003	TURP	034	Cutaneous vesicostomy
004	Anterior repair	035	Bladder hydrodilation
005	MMK	036	Meatotomy
006	Stamey	037	Urethral diverticulectomy
007	Pelvic fascial sling	038	Perineal urethrostomy
008	Penile(Scott)	039	BN Foley occlusion
009	Penile(Small-Carrion)	040	Whittaker test
010	Penile(Flexi-rod)	041	Reflux-Fogarty
011	Continent vesicostomy	042	Intermitt. cath
012	Rosen sphincter	043	DMSO
013	Scott sphincter	044	Silver nitrate
014	Kaufman	045	Urecholine
015	Kaufman suspension	046	Phenoxybenzamine
016	Diverticulectomy(open)	047	Valium
017	Diverticulectomy(TUR)	048	Anticholinergic
018	Ileal conduit	049	Alpha-sympathomimetic
019	S.P. cystostomy	050	Propanalol
020	Cutaneous vesicostomy	051	Antibiotic
021	Urethral dilation	052	Laminectomy
022	Ureteroneocystostomy	053	Renacidin irrigation
023	Undiversion	054	Timed voiding
024	Partial nephrectomy	055	External catheter
025	Radical prostatectomy	056	Crede
026	Retropubic prostatectomy	057	Hysterectomy
027	Suprapubic prostatectomy	058	Biofeedback
028	Internal urethrotomy	059	Urethral catheter
029	Urethroplasty	060	Estrogens
030	Ureterolysis	997	Other medical Rx.
031	Ureteral dilation	998	Other surgical Rx.

Figure Ax–10. Code numbers and labels for treatments. (From Woodside, J. R., and Morris, F. M.: *Neurourol. Urodyn.* 1:313–318, 1982.)

that clearly does not belong in another category. Finally, a maximum of five treatments may be recorded. (Fig. Ax–10).

There is great flexibility in the manner in which data can be filtered (retrieved) from the diskette. Patient names can be filtered by last name and the date of study by year. Age may be filtered by an exact match (i.e., age 12) or a range (i.e., age 5–15). All other demographic data and all coded data are filtered by an exact match. One general category, up to three specific diagnoses, up to ten urodynamic findings, up to five treatments, and all demographic data items may be filtered simultaneously, either separately or in any combination. The computer filters data at a rate of approximately 100 patient records per minute.

All patient names listed on the printouts are automatically alphabetized. There are two choices of printout format. The short form lists the file number, patient name, sex, age, date of study, hospital name code, and patient's hospital number (Fig. Ax–11). The long form lists all demographic data and the code number and corresponding label for all other categories (Fig. Ax–12). Three patient records are printed per page in the long form.

EXAMPLE OF DATA RETRIEVAL

To demonstrate specific data retrieval, a filter is done to identify all female patients with myelodysplasia between the ages of 3 and 16 years who have areflexic, hypertonic detrusor dysfunction and who were evaluated at the University of New Mexico hospital. It requires the use of five filters: sex, age, hospital, specific diagnosis, and two codes under urodynamic findings. The six patients satisfying all these selection criteria are seen on the short-form printout (Fig. Ax–11); a long-form printout of one of the patients is shown in Figure Ax–12.

345	A, D	F	15	01/17/80	1	34-06-09
130	B, L	F	06	10/04/79	1	32-01-62
28	C, B	F	04	02/02/81	1	31-26-39
354	M, E	F	11	09/04/80	1	27-41-49
240	M, S	F	15	06/18/80	1	33-77-69
77	O, C	F	11	10/29/81	1	46-38-90

Figure Ax–11. Short form of printout. Patient names are alphabetized (initials of first and last names for publication purposes only). The sex, age, date of study, hospital name code, and patient's hospital number are shown. (From Woodside, J. R., and Morris, F. M.: *Neurourol. Urodyn.* 1:313–318, 1982.)

COMPUTER-GENERATED URODYNAMIC REPORT

In addition to data storage and retrieval, the word processing program can be used to generate a standardized urodynamic report. At the completion of a urodynamic study, the demographic, historical, physical examination, and urodynamic data are filled in on a worksheet. The Impressions, Recommendations, and Comments sections of the report are dictated. The word processing program then prompts the transcriptionist to type in all demographic, historical, physical examination, and urodynamic data (Fig. Ax–13). The dictated portions of the report

```
      NAME - M, S                             SEX - F        AGE - 15
      FILE # -    240                         STUDY DATE - 06/18/80
      HOSPITAL # - 33-77-69                          HOSPITAL - 1
      SLIDES - 64:14-20                       OUTSIDE REFERRAL - N
      GENERAL CATAGORY - 005  SPINAL CRD. DIS. (NON-TRAUM)

 * URODYNAMIC FINDINGS *                * SPECIFIC DIAGNOSES *
   001  - INTERMITTENT CATH.               007  - MYELODYSPLASIA
   003  - HYPERTONIC DETRUSOR              054  - REFLUX
   004  - AREFLEXIC DETRUSOR               000  - NONE
   020  - REFLUX
   000  - NONE                          * TREATMENT *
   000  - NONE                             039  - BN FOLEY OCCLUSION
   000  - NONE                             041  - REFLUX-FOGARTY
   000  - NONE                             022  - URETERONEOCYSTOSTOMY
   000  - NONE                             042  - INTERMITT. CATH.
   000  - NONE                             048  - ANTICHOLINERGIC
```

Figure Ax–12. Long form of printout with complete demographic data and labels for each code number. (From Woodside, J. R., and Morris, F. M.: *Neurourol. Urodyn.* 1:313–318, 1982.)

```
NAME...........................John Doe
DATE...........................11/26/82
HOSP. NO.......................515-34-7568
HOSPITAL.......................VAH
REF. DR........................Joe Jones, M.D.
AGE............................28
PARITY.........................---
HEAD INJURY....................No
SEIZURES.......................
```

Figure Ax–13. Computer screen display demonstrating prompts to which the transcriptionist responds.

URODYNAMIC REPORT

NAME: John Doe DATE: 11/26/82
HOSPITAL NUMBER: 515-34-7568 HOSPITAL: VAH
REFERRING PHYSICIAN: Joe Jones, M.D. AGE: 28 PARITY: ---

HISTORY

HEAD INJURY: No SEIZURES: No CVA: No
LOSS OF CONSCIOUSNESS: No BACK INJURY: Yes BACK SURGERY: Yes
HERNIATED DISK: No DIABETES: No BOWEL CONTROL: Suppositories
ERECTIONS: Reflex ALLERGIES: Penicillin
MEDICATIONS: Bactrim D.S., one b.i.d.
PREVIOUS SURGERY: Laminectomy, 1979
IVP: Bilateral Hydroureteronephrosis
VCUG: No reflux, trabeculated
CYSTOSCOPY: Trabeculated with cellules

PHYSICAL EXAMINATION

SPHINCTER TONE: Increased VOLUNTARY CONTRACTION: Absent
PERINEAL SENSATION: Absent BCR: Increased

URODYNAMIC DATA

FUNCTIONAL URETHRAL LENGTH: 3.0 cm. MUP: 146 cm. water
MUCP: 130 cm. water BLADDER NECK PRESSURE: 40 cm. water
BLADDER CAPACITY: 240 ml. FILLING PRESSURE: 15 cm. water
VOIDING PRESSURE: 120 cm. water REFLEX: Hyper. PVR: 110 ml.
EMG: Increased BLADDER NECK: Poor opening
REFLUX: No
TRABECULATION: Yes DIVERTICULUM: No CYSTOCOELE: ---
POSTERIOR URETHROVESICAL ANGLE: --- degrees
URETHRAL-VERTICAL ANGLE: --- degrees

IMPRESSION

1. Complete T-4 spinal cord injury.
2. Detrusor hyperreflexia with detrusor-sphincter dyssynergia.
3. Autonomic dysreflexia.
4. Bilateral hydroureteronephrosis.

RECOMMENDATIONS

1. External sphincterotomy and transurethral resection or incision of bladder neck.

COMMENTS

This man suffered a spinal cord injury in a motor vehicle accident three years ago. He initially was managed with an indwelling Foley catheter for 2 months and has been on external catheter drainage since. He has had several episodes of febrile urinary tract infections in the last year, but has had no stones. He has moderate symptoms of autonomic dysreflexia. This study shows very elevated voiding pressures and poor bladder neck opening, which have resulted in bladder and upper tract deterioration.

Jeffrey R. Woodside, M.D.
Associate Professor of Urology

Figure Ax–14. Completed computer-generated urodynamic report.

are transcribed in the usual manner. The final report is then produced by the printer (Fig. Ax–14). The secretarial time for completing a urodynamic report has been reduced from 15 to 20 minutes to only 5 minutes with this computer application.

REFERENCES

1. Lawson, R. K., Jacobs, S. C., Murphy, J. B., Halub, M. A., and Krco, M. J.: Computer assisted urodynamics. Scientific Exhibit, 78th Annual Meeting of the American Urological Association, Las Vegas, April 1983.
2. Roos, L. L., Roos, N. P., Cageorge, S. M., and Nicol, J. P.: How good are the data? Reliability of one health care data bank. *Med. Care* 20:266–274, 1982.
3. Rosen, I. I., Hall, T. C., Mettler, F., Wicks, J., Kelsey, C. A., and Gustafson, D. E.: A computerized database system for medical diagnostic studies (DIASTU). *Comput. Programs Biomed.* 12:249–261, 1980.
4. Keller, W.: Data base managers. Part II. *80 Micro* June/July: 150–157, 1982.
5. Daniel, T.: Data ace. *80 Micro* October:266–274, 1982.
6. Woodside, J. R., and Morris, F. M.: A computer program for the storage and retrieval of urodynamic data. *Neurourol. Urodyn.* 1:313–318, 1982.
7. Regnier, C.H.: Current and future applications of computers in urodynamics. *Neurourol. Urodynam.* 5:343–371, 1986.

Index

Information provided in tables is indicated by the letter *t* following page numbers; illustrations are indicated by the letter *f* following page numbers.